Apley's System of Orthopaedics and Fractures

Apley's System of Orthopaedics and Fractures

Sixth Edition

A. Graham Apley,
MB BS, FRCS
Consulting Orthopaedic Surgeon, St Thomas' Hospital, London
Emeritus Consultant Orthopaedic Surgeon, The Rowley Bristow Orthopaedic Hospital, Pyrford, and
St Peter's Hospital, Chertsey, Surrey
Formerly Honorary Director, Department of Orthopaedics, St Thomas' Hospital, London

Louis Solomon,
MB ChB, MD, FRCS
Professor of Orthopaedic Surgery, University of the Witwatersrand, Johannesburg
Chief Orthopaedic Surgeon, Johannesburg Hospital

Butterworths

London   Boston   Durban   Singapore   Sydney   Toronto   Wellington

First published	*1959*
Second Edition	*1963*
Third Edition	*1968*
Reprinted	*1970*
Reprinted	*1972*
Fourth Edition	*1973*
Reprinted	*1975*
Reprinted	*1977*
Fifth Edition	*1977*
Reprinted	*1978*
Sixth Edition	*1982*
Reprinted	*1984*
Reprinted	*1986*

British Library Cataloguing in Publication Data

Apley, A. Graham
 Apley's system of orthopaedics and fractures.
 —6th ed.
 1. Orthopedia
 I. Title   II. Solomon, Louis
 617'.3   RD731
 ISBN 0-407-40656-5

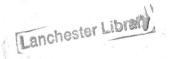
Photoset by Butterworths Litho Preparation Department
Printed in Great Britain by William Clowes Limited, Beccles and London
and bound by Anchor Brendon Ltd., Tiptree, Essex

Preface

The first outline of this book was written in 1954. The FRCS course at Pyrford was then six years old; but as it became more comprehensive the students could either pay attention or scribble notes – they couldn't do both. The obvious answer was to provide summaries of all the lectures. These were revised annually, but as the course grew longer, typed notes became unmanageable (and secretaries rebellious) so in 1959 the publishers had to take over.

For the printed version the notes were converted into more readable prose, but the systematic approach was left unchanged. Students seemed to like the idea of a standard pattern of headings and welcomed the logic of a consistent sequence for describing physical signs; learning to *look*, *feel* and *move* before turning to investigations is a habit they can profitably carry over from the lecture room (via the examination hall) to the consulting room. We like to think that in the process they will also discover that each of these deceptively simple words conveys a meaning beyond the obvious. 'Look' says more than 'inspect'; it implies contemplation of what is seen. Similarly, to 'feel' is more than to palpate, and 'move' is not merely an imperative.

Illustrations were a big problem. They are so helpful that profusion is desirable – and yet the book must not become unwieldy. The answer lay in selecting, pruning and arranging; picking only good quality illustrations, excising every scrap of surplus material, and then arranging the figures into groups so that each 'composite' tells a story. This fits in well with something every teacher knows: that, no matter how good a single illustration may be, it is more informative when combined with others in a meaningful set. Composites are the natural way of showing stages in a process, of highlighting important clinical signs, of summing up differential diagnosis and of contrasting different methods of treatment. There are some 2240 individual photographs, x-rays and drawings arranged into just over 500 composites. These can be used by themselves for quick revision; together with the text it is hoped that they provide a concise yet substantial presentation of orthopaedics and fractures in a single volume.

With the sixth edition the most important change is that there are now two authors instead of one. We have not simply divided the field; we have worked together on every chapter – differing, debating, arguing, agreeing – all the time prompting each other to further enquiry and fresh insights. In this way we have completely revised the whole *System of Orthopaedics and Fractures*. The essentially clinical character of the book has been firmly retained, but there are some changes of emphasis. The discussion of diagnostic procedures has been widened, histopathological descriptions have been enlarged and the basic sciences (notably biochemistry, biomechanics and applied anatomy) have received more attention.

Sections which have been entirely re-written include those on the rheumatic disorders, avascular necrosis of bone, the causes and pathology of osteoarthritis, metabolic bone disorders, endocrine disorders, the clinical approach to bone dysplasias, the surgery of stroke, the principles of orthopaedic operations, joint replacement and its complications, the rheumatoid hand, lumbar instability, spinal stenosis, Perthes' disease and club foot. With regard to trauma, the principles of fracture healing, cast-bracing, internal fixation, external fixation, compartment syndromes, ligamentous injuries of the knee, acetabular fractures and ankle fractures receive fresh or more detailed attention. In short, the book has been completely updated to incorporate new concepts in orthopaedics and the interdisciplinary fields into which it extends. At the same time, since two heads can be more vigilant than one, enough dead wood has been uprooted to prevent a major increase in size.

The book is designed to be used by postgraduates (and their teachers), by undergraduates (who may ignore the small print), by casualty officers (whose dangerously exposed situation in the field of trauma has been kept in mind), by general practitioners (or at any rate those who seek further understanding of their orthopaedic patients) and by our colleagues in allied professions (physiotherapists, nurses, occupational therapists, social workers, orthotists and prosthetists), who ensure that orthopaedic surgeons never lose sight of the whole patient in their concentration on the defective part.

A. Graham Apley
Louis Solomon

Acknowledgements

We have received constant help and encouragement from many friends and colleagues, especially G. Hadfield and W. Murphy, of Pyrford, F. W. Heatley and M. A. Smith, of St Thomas' Hospital, and J. J. G. Craig, S. Eisenstein, E. Erken and C. Schnitzler, of the University of the Witwatersrand, Johannesburg. To all these we owe, and gladly acknowledge, a considerable debt.

The exacting requirements of photography were carried out superbly at Pyrford by the late Ken Fensom (whose death, just as the book was nearing completion, is deeply mourned), at St Thomas' Hospital by Tom Brandon, at the Royal College of Surgeons of England by Cliff Redman, and in Johannesburg by Eric Norman.

David Seaton prepared all the new composites and drew nearly all the new diagrams; his artistic skill, unflappable good humour and untiring industry have been a tower of strength from start to finish. To Mr C. Richards and Ms B. Faiman, of Johannesburg, who did the remaining drawings, we are also extremely grateful.

The arduous secretarial work has been performed punctiliously and uncomplainingly by Ann Walker and Ruth Norman; their contributions, including keeping the notes (and the authors) in order, have been greatly appreciated. Gillian Clarke and Mary Love, who read the proofs, have been models of meticulous thoroughness. To them, and to the publishing team at Butterworths, we acknowledge our sincere thanks; the problems which dual authorship inevitably create were solved by them with commendable calmness and delightful diplomacy.

We are grateful also to colleagues elsewhere who willingly loaned illustrations to fill a few gaps. They include the following, but we apologize if, inadvertently, the name of some generous contributor has been omitted.

Mr R. C. F. Catterall, King's College Hospital, London, Fig. 24.23g

Sir John Charnley, Wrightington Centre for Hip Surgery, Figs. 12.8c, 19.44d

Mr R. A. Denham, Royal Portsmouth Hospital, Figs. 1.10d, 7.8, 8.7, 9.11a, 22.19b

Mr B. Duncan, Johannesburg, Fig. 12.13

Mr D. L. Evans, Westminster Hospital, London, Fig. 27.2c

Mr S. Eisenstein, Johannesburg, Figs. 1.16 and 18.27

Col. J. A. Feagin, West Point, New York, Fig. 22.14

Mr G. R. Fisk, Princess Alexandra Hospital, London, Fig. 27.43a, b

Mr J. Fleming, Johannesburg, Fig. 12.10

Mr B. Foster, Flinders Medical Centre, S. Australia, Fig. 19.25a

Mr G. E. Fulford, Princess Margaret Rose Hospital, Edinburgh, Fig. 8.4a

Dr N. W. T. Grieve, St Peter's Hospital, Chertsey, Fig. 22.24

Mr B. Helal, The London Hospital and Enfield Hospitals, Figs. 7.3a, 8.8c, d, 8.10c, 12.15, 16.10e, 19.8b, 21.15f, 22.21a, 25.11a, b and 27.32c

Prof. A. J. Helfet, Cape Town, Fig. 27.24

Mr R. C. Howard, Norfolk and Norwich Hospital, Fig. 12.8d

Mr G. A. Jose, Royal Adelaide Hospital, S. Australia, Fig. 8.11

Dr E. Levine, Johannesburg, Fig. 1.16

Prof. R. Lipschitz, Johannesburg, Fig. 23.5

Mr L. Nainkin, Johannesburg, Figs. 25.6b, 25.7d

Mr P. A. Ring, Redhill Group of Hospitals, Fig. 19.44b

Mr G. F. Walker, Queen Mary's Hospital for Children, Carshalton, Fig. 6.3

The following have been reproduced or re-drawn from the original articles or books in which they appeared, and we gratefully acknowledge the courtesy of the respective authors, editors and publishers for permission to do this.

Fig. 1.9: R. Wynne-Davies, *Journal of Bone and Joint Surgery*, **52B**, 704

Fig. 16.18: D. A. Bailey, *The Infected Hand*. London, H. K. Lewis

Fig. 16.19: R. J. Furlong, *Injuries of the Hand*. London, Churchill

Fig. 22.28: C. E. Holden, *Journal of Bone and Joint Surgery*, **61B**, 298

Contents

Part 3 – Fractures and Joint Injuries

Part 1 — General Orthopaedics

Diagnosis in Orthopaedics

1

'Information consists of differences that make a difference'
Gregory Bateson

Orthopaedics is concerned with bones, joints, muscles, tendons and nerves – the skeletal system and all that makes it move. An orthopaedic disorder is also part of a larger whole – a patient who has a personality, a mind and a body, a job and hobbies, a family and a home; all have a bearing upon the disorder and its treatment.

Diagnosis is not simply a process of labelling; it should also imply understanding – of the patient and how the disorder affects him and his way of life. And diagnosis begins, not with the patient on the examination couch, but from the moment we set eyes on him: we should be observing his appearance, his attitude, his gait – everything.

As the consultation and examination proceed, a cluster of symptoms and signs emerges and we begin homing-in on something we recognize. In orthopaedics this entity, the diagnosis, is likely to fall into one of seven easily remembered pairs: congenital and developmental abnormalities; infection and inflammation; injury and mechanical derangement; metabolic dysfunction and degeneration; arthritis and rheumatic disorders; sensory disturbance and muscle weakness; tumours and lesions that mimic them.

Symptoms

The word 'history' should be taken to mean 'his story' – not yours or mine. Unless the patient is allowed to tell his story in his own way, important facts can be missed and he may feel aggrieved. No matter if the story appears jumbled; it is the doctor's job to sort it out, and he should learn to think systematically. First he should consider any general symptoms; then local ones which, in orthopaedics, fall into three groups. The patient may complain that something *looks* wrong (deformity, swelling or a lump); that something *feels* wrong (pain, tingling or numbness); or that *movement* is wrong (limp, weakness, instability or stiffness). In practice, the common complaints are *pain, stiffness, swelling, deformity* and *disability*.

Moreover the history is, as the word implies, an unfolding train of events. We need to know if the onset was sudden or gradual; how long symptoms have been present; if they are constant or intermittent, static or increasing, and whether anything makes them better or worse. The patient's job and his hobbies, his previous illnesses or injuries, and any similar disorder in other members of the family also may be important.

Pain

Pain is the most common symptom in orthopaedics. Its precise location is important (ask the patient to point). So is severity; to the patient, pain is as bad as it feels. If only we could measure it! (Would the units be hells and decihells?) We can at least try to estimate severity, if only to assess therapeutic response.

Grade I	Trivial (easily ignored)
Grade II	Moderate (cannot be ignored, interferes with function and needs occasional attention)
Grade III	Severe (pain even at rest and demanding constant attention)
Grade IV	Incapacitating

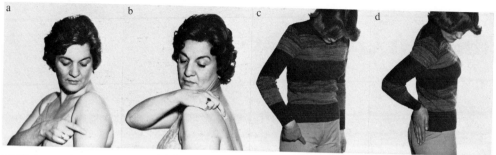

1.1 'Point to where it hurts'   In (a) and (b) the complaint would be of 'shoulder' pain; in (c) and (d) of 'hip' pain. The likely diagnoses are (a) supraspinatus tendinitis, (b) cervical spondylosis, (c) a disorder of the hip joint itself, (d) a prolapsed lumbar disc.

The term 'referred pain' is often misunderstood and incorrectly used. Pain arising in or near the skin is usually localized accurately and can be recalled with precision hours or days after it has disappeared. Pain arising in deep structures is more diffuse and is sometimes of quite unexpected distribution; thus, hip disease may manifest with pain in the knee (so might an obturator hernia!). This is not because sensory nerves connect the two sites; it is due to cortical confusion between embryologically related sites. A common example is 'sciatica' – pain at various points in the buttock, thigh and leg, supposedly following the course of the sciatic nerve. Such pain is not due to pressure on the sciatic nerve; it is 'referred' from any one of a wide variety of structures in the lumbar spine and pelvis.

Disability

Disability is not merely the sum of individual symptoms; it depends upon particular needs and is important in assessing requirements. Often symptoms are expressed in terms of disability: thus 'I can't sit for long', 'I can't hold a cup', or 'I can't put my socks on' may be offered rather than 'I have backache', 'my fingers are numb', or 'my hip is stiff'. Such disabilities suggest a more fruitful line of questioning than the mere checking of lists of symptoms.

Moreover, what to one patient is merely inconvenient may, to another, be incapacitating. Thus a doctor or a bank clerk may readily tolerate a stiff knee provided it is painless and he can walk well; but to a plumber or a parson the same disability might be economic or spiritual disaster.

Examination of a joint

General features	A brisk general appraisal of the patient is imperative
Local symptoms	Let the patient tell his story (with guidance), and point to the site of pain
Local signs	A system is the key to accurate diagnosis

Look
  Skin
  Shape
  Position
	Observe the gait
	
	At this stage *shortening* is assessed

Feel
  Skin
  Soft tissues
  Bones
	Localized tenderness may be diagnostic. Be gentle – watch the patient's face

Move
  Active
  Passive
  Power
	Examine the good limb first or both simultaneously
	At this stage *function* is assessed

X-ray	Plus other investigations

For examination, a patient must be suitably undressed; no mere rolling up of a trouser leg is sufficient. Where one limb is to be examined, the opposite one must be adequately exposed, so that the two may be compared.

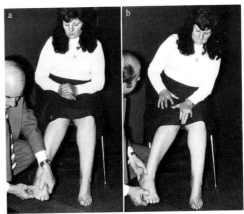

1.2 Feeling for tenderness   (a) How not to do it. It is better to watch the patient's face (b), and to stop the moment she feels pain.

● LOOK

The student, or inexperienced doctor, is inclined to rush in with his hands – a temptation which must be resisted. His motto should be 'look before you feel'. And in looking he must follow a purposeful, orderly system; otherwise he will miss vital clues.

Skin   This naturally comes first. We look systematically for colour changes, skin creases and scars. Redness usually implies inflammation; blueness, either cyanosis or bruising. Abnormal creases suggest underlying fibrosis or bony malposition (e.g. a dislocated hip); the absence of creases also may be significant. Scars reveal the past – the surgical archaeology, so to speak; they tell of natural events (e.g. an old sinus) or of operations.

Shape   Changes in shape may be generalized (e.g. dwarfism), or localized (e.g. swelling, wasting or a lump).

Position   While the position in which a joint is held may vary, if the joint is normal it 'looks natural'; any deviation from this natural appearance demands investigation. In many joint disorders and in most nerve lesions the limb adopts a characteristic attitude.

● FEEL

We must feel (as we should have looked) systematically: the good limb then the bad; the skin before the deep tissues; and the unaffected before the symptomatic area.

Skin   Is the skin warm or cold, moist or dry, rough or smooth? and – equally important – can the patient feel you touching him, or is sensation abnormal?

Soft tissues   Deep to the skin we may encounter tenderness, which is important – in two ways. First, we must avoid hurting the patient; and so we watch his face and not our hands while examining him. Secondly, tenderness is often sharply localized; if so, it may immediately locate the site of the lesion.

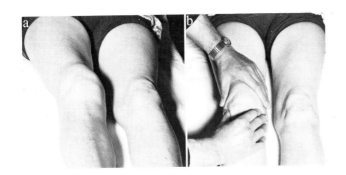

1.3 Fluid in the knee   (a) The suprapatellar pouch is bulging and the thigh wasted; (b) cross-fluctuation (see page 278).

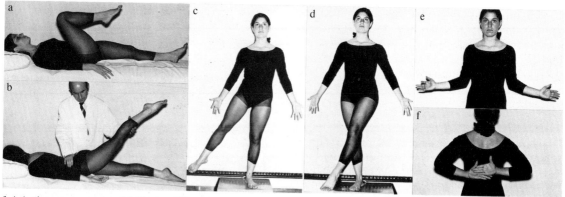

1.4 Active movements   (a) Flexion, (b) extension, (c) abduction and (d) adduction at the hip; (e) external (lateral) and (f) internal (medial) rotation at the shoulder.

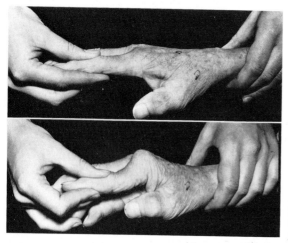

1.5 Passive movement   Stability is tested by moving the joint passively across the normal planes of action – in this case by thrusting the entire finger volarwards, thus demonstrating abnormal movement at the metacarpophalangeal joint.

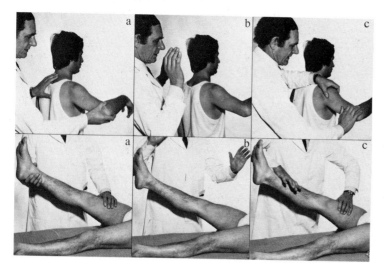

1.6 Testing muscle power   The sequence is always the same, no matter whether the deltoid, quadriceps, or any other muscle is being examined. (a)'Let me lift it.' (b) 'Hold it there.' (c) 'Keep it there.'

With superficial joints we can also feel if the synovial membrane is thickened (by rolling its edge under the fingers) and we can detect excess fluid (Fig. 1.3).

A soft tissue lump always demands careful examination to determine its size, shape, surface, consistency, edge and attachments.

Crepitus Strictly speaking this is a crackling sound which accompanies movement, but it is usually more sensitively felt than heard. Joint crepitus is fairly coarse, while tendon crepitus is fine and precisely localized to the affected tendon sheath.

● MOVE

Active The advantage of testing active movements first is that the patient is not likely to hurt himself; he stops when the point of pain is reached.

Passive We need to know if a particular movement is limited (and by how much), or painful (and at what angle); we must also be on the lookout for increased movement and for abnormal movements. To assess stability the limb is held above and below the joint and deliberately (but gently) stressed across the normal anatomical planes of movement.

Power Muscle testing is not as easy as it sounds; few patients have mastered *Gray's Anatomy*, and we must make ourselves understood. The easiest way is shown in Fig. 1.6. The sequence is important: you lift – he holds – you push – he resists while you feel. The normal limb is examined first, then the affected limb and the two are compared.

Examination of the muscle tells us something about the function of the limb. We can learn even more by watching the patient perform certain specific activities. With his upper limb he can try reaching for a high object or we can test him picking up weights and handling fine objects. To test the lower limb we can watch him stand, walk, run or hop.

The range of movement at a joint should be recorded in degrees; the eye soon acquires sufficient accuracy and a goniometer is needed only for special purposes.

Each joint moves through a characteristic range of positions in various planes, as follows.

Flexion/extension – movements in the sagittal plane towards the ventral or dorsal surface of the body.

Joints that move only – or predominantly – in flexion and extension are the knee, elbow, ankle and the joints of the fingers and toes.

Adduction/abduction – movements in the coronal plane, towards or away from the midline. The hip and shoulder have considerable ranges of adduction and abduction.

External rotation/internal rotation – torsional movements around a fixed longitudinal axis. These are seen mainly in the hip and shoulder, but some rotation takes place also at the knee.

Pronation/supination These, too, are rotatory movements, but the terms are applied only to movements of the forearm and the foot.

Circumduction – a composite movement made up of a rhythmic sequence of all the other movements. This is possible only for ball-and-socket joints (hip, shoulder). The appearance of circumduction may be given by multiple joints acting in series (e.g. the cervical spine).

Certain specialized movements, such as opposition of the thumb, lateral flexion and rotation of the spine, and inversion and eversion of the foot, will be described under the relevant regions.

Deformity

The word 'deformity' may be applied to a person, a bone or a joint. Shortness of stature is a kind of deformity; it may be due to shortness of the limbs, or of the trunk, or both (page 83). A bone also may be abnormally short; this is rarely important in the upper limbs, but it is in the lower (page 245); or a bone may be abnormally bent (page 10). A joint is said to be deformed when it is held in an unnatural position either because of faulty alignment (e.g. knock knee) or because it lacks full movement (e.g. fixed flexion). The terms describing the commoner deformities are so much a part of the everyday language of orthopaedics that a few definitions may be helpful.

Varus and valgus It may seem pedantic to replace 'bow legs' and 'knock knees' with terms such as genu varum and genu valgum. But comparable descriptive colloquialisms are not available for similar deformities of the elbow, hip or big toe. Moreover, 'varus' and 'valgus' refer not to the affected joint, but to the part distal to the joint:

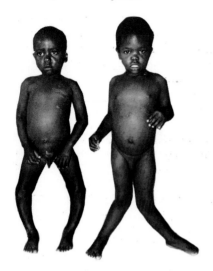

1.7 Valgus and varus These boys look like brothers; they are in fact unrelated, but came from the same village and both had a deficiency disease causing bone softening. The shorter boy has developed varus deformity, the taller one is valgus; possibly pre-existing minor deformities have become exaggerated.

varus means that the part distal to the joint is displaced towards the midline, *valgus* away from it.

Kyphosis and lordosis The spine is normally constructed as a series of rhythmic curves in the sagittal plane – concave anteriorly in the dorsal region (kyphosis), and convex anteriorly in the cervical and lumbar regions (lordosis). If any of these curves are excessive they may constitute a kyphotic or lordotic deformity.

Scoliosis Looked at in the anteroposterior plane the spine is straight. Any curvature in this (coronal) plane, whether in the dorsal or the lumbar region, whether fixed or correctible, is called a scoliosis. A combination of kyphosis and scoliosis is called kyphoscoliosis.

'Fixed' deformity This does *not* mean that the joint is fixed and unable to move. It means that movement in one plane is impossible beyond a certain point; thus a joint may flex fully but not extend fully – at the limit of its extension it is still 'fixed' in a certain amount of flexion; similarly, there may be fixed adduction, abduction or rota-

tional deformity of a joint. In the spine a fixed deformity is often called a structural deformity; it differs from a postural deformity, which the patient himself can, if properly instructed, correct by his own muscular effort.

Hysterical deformity This is usually bizarre and should not be diagnosed unless other causes of deformity have been excluded and other stigmata of hysteria are present.

Causes

Deformities affecting many joints may be due to congenital disorders (e.g. Morquio–Brailsford disease), or to acquired disease (especially rheumatoid arthritis).

In deformity of a single joint or localized group of joints, it is often possible to identify which tissue is responsible – skin, fascia, muscle, tendon, ligaments, capsule or bone. These are considered under the appropriate joints.

Gait and limp

The gait cycle (the sequence of events in each step), consists of four parts: heel strike; stance phase; toe off; and swing phase. A limp is simply an abnormal gait. Its possible causes range from a tight shoe to a 'tight' person, but the orthopaedic causes (fortunately more limited) are best analysed by noticing the point in the gait cycle at which the abnormality occurs (though if the patient is inco-ordinate or is wearing a prosthesis his limp may be obvious at more than one point in the cycle).

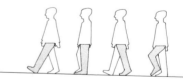

1.8 The gait cycle This oddly dressed individual's left leg shows the stages: 'heel strike' is followed by the 'stance phase'; next is 'toe off' (almost) and finally the 'swing phase'.

(1) HEEL STRIKE

The patient with heel pain steps on the toes rather than the heel. A slapping movement (and sound) immediately after heel strike is characteristic of foot drop.

(2) STANCE PHASE

Limp at this point results from pain, shortening or instability. If there is pain on weight-bearing, the patient hurries off the leg (the so-called antalgic gait). With shortening, the ipsilateral shoulder merely droops. With instability at the hip it also swings sideways over the weight-bearing leg (this, a Trendelenburg gait, is the dynamic equivalent of Trendelenburg's sign). Instability at the knee is usually self-evident, and may result from muscle weakness (e.g. polio), bony incongruity (e.g. following rheumatoid arthritis) or ligamentous injury. Fixed flexion of the knee also is easily spotted and may result from mechanical obstruction (a locked knee) or from old inflammatory disease.

(3) TOE OFF

At this point fixed flexion of the hip becomes apparent in that the heel lifts off too soon; and with a stiff straight knee the whole body is heaved up to provide clearance.

(4) SWING PHASE

Foot drop now becomes obvious and, to avoid tripping, the patient adopts a high-stepping gait. If bilateral, this must be distinguished from the gait of a tabetic: here the foot does not drop but the patient lifts it too high because he lacks position sense. Abnormality in the swing phase may also result from stiffness (usually of the hip or knee, but sometimes of the back or foot) or from spasticity. A severely painful knee is held stiff, even though passive movement may be good.

Stiffness

The term 'stiffness' is used to cover a wide variety of limitations of movement. It is convenient to consider three grades.

ALL MOVEMENTS ABSENT   Complete absence of movement may result from a suppurative arthritis in which articular cartilage has been destroyed and bony trabeculae cross the joint (bony ankylosis); or from operation (arthrodesis).

ALL MOVEMENTS LIMITED   With active inflammation of synovium, extremes of all movements are limited and the joint is said to be 'irritable'. With active arthritis there is joint rigidity, spasm preventing all but a few degrees of movement.

Tuberculous arthritis heals by fibrosis, leading to an unsound joint; that is, one in which forced movement causes spasm or pain, and deformity may increase with time. The term 'fibrous ankylosis' is used when fibrous tissue across the joint is so short that only a few degrees of movement exist. With longer fibrous tissue and more movement, the term 'ankylosis' is best avoided and 'long fibrous joint' is better.

In osteoarthritis the capsule fibroses and as the fibrous tissue matures it shrinks, limiting movement. In rheumatoid arthritis movement at several joints may be limited by pain; subsequent fibrosis may perpetuate the limitation.

After severe injury, especially compound fractures near a joint, movement in all directions may be limited as a result of oedema, infection, adhesions or loss of muscle extensibility.

SOME MOVEMENTS LIMITED   When movement in at least one direction is full and painless the cause of any limitation is usually mechanical. Thus a torn and displaced meniscus may prevent extension of the knee but not flexion.

Again, if one group of muscles acting on a joint is paralysed, the opposing group eventually loses the ability to stretch fully, and fixed deformity with stiffness in one direction results.

Bone deformity may alter the arc of movement, so that it is limited in one direction (loss of abduction in coxa vara is an example) but movement in the opposite direction is full or even increased.

Joint laxity

Increased movement at a single joint may result from muscle paralysis (especially when a joint is flail), from ligamentous injury, from ligamentous stretching (after chronic or repeated joint swelling) or from loss of cartilage or bone.

Increased movement at a few joints   also may follow paralysis, or it may be the sequel to polyarthritis. But the possibility of Charcot's disease must be borne in mind (page 57).

Generalized joint hypermobility   occurs in about 5 per cent of the general population and is inherited as a simple Mendelian dominant. The knees and elbows can be hyperextended, and the hands and feet can attain unusual positions (Fig. 1.9). A clear distinction should be made between hypermobility and instability; hypermobile joints are not necessarily unstable – as witness the controlled performances of acrobats and the legendary skill of Paganini.

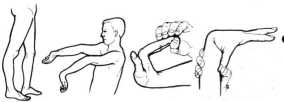

1.9 Generalized joint hypermobility   Being double-jointed is not an unmixed blessing. Recurrent dislocation and painful joints are possible sequels. (Redrawn from *Journal of Bone and Joint Surgery* vol. 25B, page 704, by courtesy of Miss R. Wynne-Davies, and the Editor.)

In people with joint hypermobility the incidence of recurrent dislocation of the patella and shoulder is higher than usual. They also have a tendency to unexplained joint pain (arthralgia). There is, however, no convincing evidence that hypermobility by itself predisposes to degenerative arthritis; only if the joint becomes unstable is this likely to develop.

Generalized hypermobility is not usually associated with any obvious disease; but severe laxity is a feature of a number of disorders, including Marfan's syndrome (page 93), osteogenesis imperfecta (page 86), Ehlers–Danlos syndrome and Larsen's disease.

In *Ehlers-Danlos syndrome* ligament laxity is combined with other connective tissue disorders: the skin is hyperextensible and splits easily to leave tissue-paper scars; and because blood-vessel walls are weak the patient bruises readily and may develop aneurysms. In *Larsen's disease* these connective tissue disorders are not present, but there is congenital dislocation of several joints.

Examination of a bone

Bones, like joints, should be examined systematically, and the pattern of headings is similar.

● LOOK
Skin   First look for scars or colour changes.

Shape   The bone may be bent or there may be a lump.

Size   The bone may be too short, too long, too wide or too narrow.

● FEEL
Skin   This may feel unduly warm or cool; sensory changes may be present.

Soft tissues   Lumps or swellings may be palpable.

The bone itself   The bone may feel too wide, surface irregularities or lumps may be palpable, and there may be localized tenderness.

● MOVE
Not only should the joints above and below the affected bone be examined, but it is wise also to examine the bone itself for movement; otherwise non-union in the forearm or leg may pass undetected.

Bent bones

The long bones are straight or have slight natural curves. If a bone is abnormally bent it must have broken, or have been relatively soft at some time, or have grown faultily.

If several bones are bent, the likely causes are multiple injury (for example, to brittle bones) or a general bone-softening disease (such as rickets or Paget's disease).

Bending of a single bone may follow injury, localized Paget's disease, a bone dysplasia or faulty growth. Fracture-separation of an epiphysis hardly ever affects growth, whereas an apparently minor fracture through the substance of the epiphysis frequently does.

1.10 Bent tibiae
Unilateral: (a) malunited fracture; (b) Paget's disease; (c) dyschondroplasia; (d) congenital pseudarthrosis; (e) syphilitic sabre tibia.

Bilateral: (f) old rickets; (g) osteogenesis imperfecta.

Bony lumps

Multiple bony lumps are uncommon. They occur in diaphyseal aclasis as squat knobs of bone around one or several joints. In syphilis and yaws there may be two or more diffuse swellings on the shaft of a bone.

A single bony lump may be due to faulty development, injury, inflammation or a tumour. Although x-ray examination is essential, a diagnosis can usually be made clinically by considering the following factors.

Size A large lump attached to bone, or a lump which is getting bigger, is nearly always a tumour.

Site A lump near a joint may be a cartilage-capped exostosis (if jutting out sharply), a benign giant-cell tumour (if ill-defined and at the very end of the bone) or a sarcoma (if ill-defined, tender and near the metaphysis). A lump in the shaft itself may be callus (which extends all round the bone), inflammatory (if tender and ill-defined) or a tumour.

Shape A benign tumour protrudes out from one aspect of the bone, malignant tumours or callus extend all round it.

Tenderness Lumps due to active inflammation, recent callus or a rapidly growing sarcoma are tender.

Edge A benign tumour has a well-defined margin; malignant tumours, inflammatory lumps and callus have a vague edge.

Consistency A benign tumour feels bony hard; malignant tumours often give the impression that they can be indented. Occasionally a small ganglion or a cyst (especially of the lateral meniscus) feels almost bony hard.

X-ray examination

'The map is not the territory'
Alfred Korzybski

X-ray examination includes not only plain radiography, but also tomography, arthrography and other specialized techniques.

How to read an x-ray

The process of reading x-ray films should be as methodical as clinical examination. It is seductively easy to be led astray by some flagrant anomaly; systematic study is the only safeguard. A convenient sequence for examination is: *patient – soft tissues – bone – joint.*

The patient

First make sure that the name on the film is that of your patient; mistaken identity is a potent source of error. Then, if the patient himself is not present, try to 'look through' the film and to visualize the living person, especially the age, build and sex.

The soft tissues

Unless examined early, these are liable to be forgotten. Look for variations in shape and variations of density.

SHAPE   Muscle planes are often visible and may reveal wasting or swelling. Bulging outlines around a hip, for example, may suggest a joint effusion; and soft-tissue swelling around interphalangeal joints may be the first radiographic sign of rheumatoid arthritis.

DENSITY   Increased density in the soft tissues follows calcification in a tendon, a blood vessel, a haematoma or an abscess; often the shape and site suggest which is involved. The radiographic density of a metallic foreign body is, of course, unmistakable; but even wood or glass may show in suitable films. The precise localization of foreign bodies necessitates multiple views.

Decreased density of soft tissues is due either to fat (the most radiolucent tissue) or to gas. The recognition of gas bubbles may be crucial in the early diagnosis of gas gangrene.

The bones

Again, variations in shape and density are sought, followed by the bone architecture. Then, if necessary, the individual components (periosteum, cortex and medulla) are examined; examples of 'visible periosteum' are shown in Fig. 1.11.

SHAPE   The bone as a whole may be bent (page 10) or may be unduly wide. Increased width is seen most often in Paget's disease; rarer causes include the deposition of subperiosteal or cortical new bone (from infection or a tumour) and some bone dysplasias.

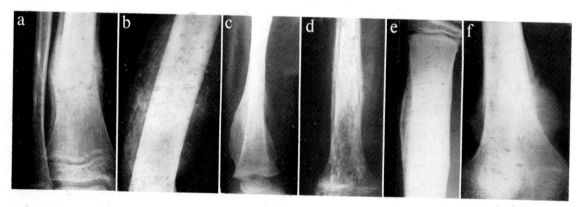

1.11 'Visible periosteum'   Ossification just outside the cortex is seen when periosteum has been lifted away from the bone. It may have been lifted by blood, as in (a) callus, (b) myositis ossificans and (c) scurvy; or by inflammatory material, as in (d) chronic osteomyelitis and (e) syphilitic periostitis; or by tumour material, as in (f) osteosarcoma.

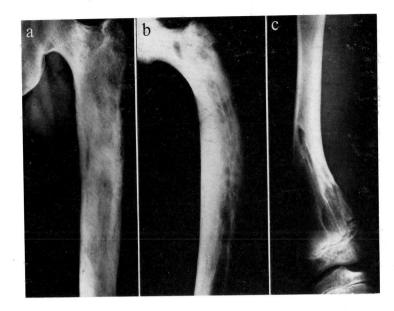

1.12 Shape and density (a) In chronic osteomyelitis the bone may show patchy increase of density and is abnormally wide – but it is straight. (b) Paget's disease looks somewhat similar except that the bone is bent. (c) In this bent femur the lower metaphysis has a streaky appearance characteristic of dyschondroplasia.

Generalized thinning of the cortex is characteristic of osteoporosis and osteomalacia. Bone loss or destruction suggests infection or a tumour. Discontinuity of the bone implies a fracture (which may be pathological). Localized swelling of a bone may be due to bulging from within (with a cyst or a tumour) or may be a bony excrescence (usually an exostosis).

DENSITY Generalized decrease of density (osteopenia) is the hallmark of advanced osteoporosis and osteomalacia; it occurs also in some bone dysplasias. Generalized increase of density occurs with marble bones (page 89) and in fluorosis. Localized increase of density occurs with metastatic deposits (especially from prostatic carcinoma), in some dysplasias and with bone necrosis. The increased density of bone necrosis has two components: (1) apparent – because the dead bone cannot share in the decalcification of the surrounding bone; and (2) real – because new bone is deposited upon the surface of the dead bone.

Localized decrease of density (rarefaction) is a common radiological feature; the following list of rare areas is by no means comprehensive.

Bone cyst – situated in the metaphysis, showing a well-defined margin.

Bone abscess – usually a small area of rarefaction with densely sclerosed surrounding bone.

Chondroma – a rarefied (though not cystic) area in the medulla, often with flecks of calcification in its centre.

Giant-cell tumour – an expanding, cyst-like lesion, usually eccentrically placed and always extending right up to the subchondral bone plate.

Fibrous dysplasia – single or multiple cysts which expand the bone.

Bone sarcoma – a malignant tumour of young people which has no well-defined edge and frequently extends into the soft tissues.

Myeloma – a globular area of rarefaction with vague margins, occurring in older people.

Lytic metastasis – ragged bone, often going on to pathological fracture.

Osteolysis – the term used when bone disappears without obvious cause, although vascular tumours must be considered. A rare area of bone is commoner and some examples of single and multiple rare areas in bone are shown in Fig. 1.13.

ARCHITECTURE Irregular alterations of density are sometimes referred to as altered architecture. Three examples are shown in Fig 1.12; rarities such as marble bones, spotted bones and striped bones are discussed under 'Dysplasias'.

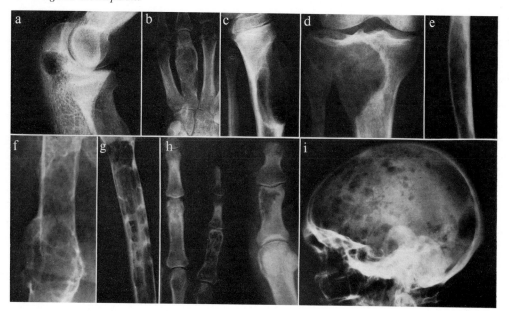

1.13 Rare areas in bone   Single: Brodie's abscess (a), tuberculous dactylitis (b), solitary cyst (c), giant-cell tumour (d), eosinophilic granuloma (e).
Multiple: Hand–Schüller–Christian disease (f), hydatid disease (g), sarcoidosis in the hand and foot (h), secondary deposits (i).

The joint

The radiological 'joint' includes both bone ends and the space between them; dislocation implies total separation of the two components; subluxation, that contact is incomplete. The joint 'space' is of course illusory; it comprises the two thicknesses of radiolucent articular cartilage. Again, it is important to look for variations in shape and in density of the joint.

SHAPE   The joint space in children is wider than in adults because more of the epiphysis is still cartilaginous and therefore radiolucent; if the bony nucleus of the epiphysis collapses, as in Perthes' disease, the space appears even wider. In adults widening of the space signifies an effusion; narrowing means cartilage loss, a characteristic of chronic arthritis. Further stages of joint destruction are revealed by interruptions in the subchondral bone plate. Erosions (periarticular bone de-

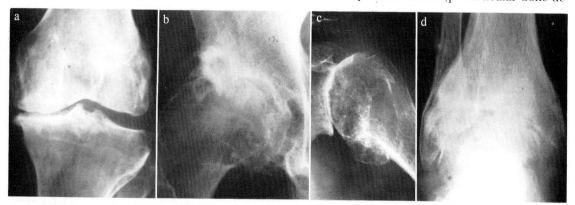

1.14 Joint x-rays   (a) The lateral compartment of this knee is normal; in the medial compartment some articular cartilage has worn away and the joint 'space' is therefore reduced. (b) In this osteoarthritic hip the superior joint space is virtually obliterated and there are juxta-articular cysts. (c) In this shoulder, degeneration has supervened on rheumatoid arthritis – the entire joint space has disappeared and there is sclerosis. (d) In this Charcot ankle the joint space is ill-defined and irregular.

fects) are characteristic of rheumatoid arthritis. Bony outgrowths from the joint margins (osteophytes) are typical of osteoarthritis.

DENSITY   Increased density in the joint 'space' occurs with calcification of articular cartilage or menisci (chondrocalcinosis).

Radiographic techniques

In addition to plain radiographs, a variety of specialized techniques is available.

Tomography

Tomography provides an image 'focused' on a selected plane. By moving the tube and the x-ray film in opposite directions on an imaginary pivot during the exposure, images on either side of the pivotal plane are deliberately blurred out. When several 'cuts' are studied, lesions obscured in conventional x-rays may be revealed. The method is particularly useful for diagnosing segmental bone necrosis, small radiolucent lesions such as osteoid osteomas, bone abscesses and difficult fractures (e.g. of the odontoid process).

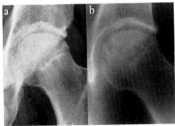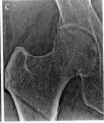

1.15 Tomography and xeroradiography   (a) The plain x-ray of this hip shows only doubtful increase in density, suggestive of avascular necrosis; but (b) the tomograph confirms the diagnosis and clearly demonstrates the triangular segment. (c) Xeroradiography, as in this patient, is often the best way to show calcification of articular cartilage (chondrocalcinosis).

Xeroradiography

Xeroradiography uses conventional x-ray exposure, but the recording plate registers the activity as an electric charge density pattern which is then transferred to plastic-coated paper as a 'positive' image. Its advantage over plain x-ray negatives is that the photoelectric process is particularly sensitive to changes in tissue density (the 'edge effect'); also, fuzzy outlines (e.g. subperiosteal erosions or faint soft-tissue calcification) are more easily displayed. Some soft-tissue shadows show well and the early stages of cartilage calcification (chondrocalcinosis) appear before they are visible in plain x-rays.

X-rays using contrast media

Substances which alter x-ray attenuation characteristics can be used to produce images which contrast with those of the normal tissues. The contrast media used in orthopaedics are mostly iodine-based liquids which can be injected into sinuses, joint cavities or the spinal theca. Air or gas also can be injected into joints to produce a 'negative image' outlining the joint cavity.

Oily iodides are not absorbed and maintain maximum concentration after injection. However, because they are non-miscible, they do not penetrate well into all the nooks and crannies. They are also tissue irritants, especially if used intrathecally. Ionic, water-soluble iodides permit much more detailed imaging and, although also somewhat irritant and neurotoxic, are rapidly absorbed and excreted. Metrizamide, a non-ionic iodide, is the least toxic and least irritant; it would be the ideal contrast medium but for its high cost.

SINOGRAPHY   is the simplest form of contrast radiography. The medium (usually one of the ionic water-soluble compounds) is injected into an open sinus; the film shows the track and whether or not it leads to the underlying bone or joint.

ARTHROGRAPHY   is a particularly useful form of contrast radiography. In the knee, torn menisci, ligament tears and capsular ruptures can be shown. In children's hips, arthrography is a useful method of defining the cartilaginous (and therefore radiolucent) femoral head; and loosening after hip replacement may be revealed by seepage of the contrast medium into the cement/bone interface. In the spine, contrast radiography can be used to diagnose disc degeneration ('discography') and abnormalities of the small facet joints ('facetography').

MYELOGRAPHY   is used extensively in the diagnosis of disc prolapse and other spinal canal lesions. Intrathecal injection of contrast media can be painful, unpleasant and dangerous; it should not be done if alternative, non-invasive methods can give the same information.

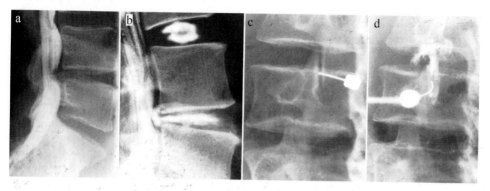

1.16 Contrast radiography   (a) Myelography outlines the spinal theca; the contrast medium has been indented by a bulging disc. (b) Contrast material can be injected into the disc itself; in this discogram the upper disc is normal, but the lower is degenerate, allowing injected material to escape. (c) Under x-ray control a needle can be inserted into the small facet joints; (d) this facetogram shows escape of contrast material from an abnormal joint (the injection reproduced the patient's pain).

The oily media are no longer used, and even with the ionic water-soluble iodides (such as iocarmic acid (Dimer X)) there is a considerable incidence of complications, such as low-pressure headache (due to the lumbar puncture), muscular spasms or convulsions (due to neurotoxicity, especially if the chemical is allowed to flow above the mid-dorsal region) and arachnoiditis (which is attributed to the hyperosmolality of these compounds in relation to cerebrospinal fluid). Precautions, such as keeping the patient sitting upright after myelography, must be strictly observed.

Metrizamide has low neurotoxicity and at working concentrations it is more or less isotonic with cerebrospinal fluid. It can, therefore, be used throughout the length of the spinal canal; the nerve roots are also well delineated ('radiculography'). A bulging disc, an intrathecal tumour or narrowing of the bony canal will produce characteristic distortions of the opaque column in the myelogram.

Computerized tomography

Like simple tomography, this is a 'cutting image' in the sense that selected planes are displayed on the final plate. However, it represents a great advance over conventional tomography in that *transverse cuts* through the body (like anatomical sections) can be represented as grey scale images. This is achieved by taking tomographic cuts from multiple directions and using a digital computer to integrate the information on x-ray absorption patterns.

The method is particularly useful for recording bone outlines and lesions that show up best in transverse section (like the shape of the spinal canal or the acetabulum) and for defining soft-tissue masses (such as a tumour, or even a bulging intervertebral disc).

The accurate measurement of x-ray attenuation also makes it possible to use this technique for assessing bone density.

Radionuclide imaging

Photon emission by radionuclides taken up in specific tissues can be recorded by either a simple rectilinear scanner or a gamma camera, to produce an image which reflects current activity in that tissue or organ.*

BONE-SEEKING COMPOUNDS
The most useful radiopharmaceutical for skeletal imaging is technetium-99m (^{99m}Tc), a single photon-emitting radionuclide with physical properties ideal for scanning, linked to a bone-seeking phosphate compound such as tripolyphosphate or methylene diphosphonate (MDP). ^{99m}Tc–MDP has a high specificity for bone and gives information of two types.

(1) *High local activity*, due to increased bone blood flow and/or new bone formation. This might occur in a fracture, infection, healing necrosis or local tumour, and nothing in the bone scan itself distinguishes between these conditions.

*Radiographs are history; scanning is news.

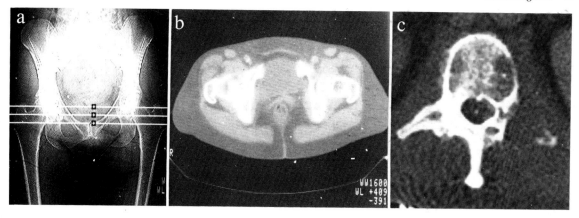

1.17 Computerized tomography The first film (a) was used to select the exact levels for subsequent tomographic 'cuts'; (b) here the hip joints have been displayed and on one side an acetabular defect is seen. The technique is particularly useful in the spine where conventional x-rays often fail to show defects; in (c) one transverse process has been almost completely destroyed by a tumour.

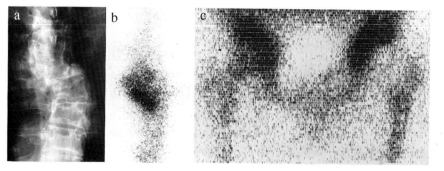

1.18 Radionuclide scanning The plain x-ray (a), though a good quality film, still looks a muddle – it shows deformity, but little else; the radionuclide scan (b) revealed that the doubtful area was 'hot', and subsequent biopsy showed a metastatic tumour. (c) This scan shows a void in the left hip where the femoral head is avascular.

However, by combining this information with the clinical picture and x-rays of the area, the diagnosis can usually be made. Even a lytic metastasis shows increased radionuclide emission, due to the reactive bone formation in the area; this has a special significance because bone scans may show areas of activity long before the lesion is big enough to be visible on the x-ray.

(2) *Low local activity*, due to an absent blood supply (e.g. in the femoral head after a fracture of the femoral neck) or to replacement of bone by pathological tissue.

The clinical applications are manifold (Hughes, 1980), and include: (1) the diagnosis of recent vertebral fractures; (2) the investigation of loosening or infection around joint prostheses; (3) the diagnosis of avascular necrosis; (4) the early detection of bone metastases; and (5) the assessment of bone vascularity in the management of Perthes' disease (Sutherland *et al.*, 1980) and of Paget's disease.

OTHER COMPOUNDS

Technetium–sulphur–colloid (^{99m}Tc–SC) is taken up by phagocytes in the reticuloendothelial system and is therefore a better indicator of marrow vascularity than the bone-seeking compounds. This may permit early diagnosis of femoral head ischaemia, but the method is not sensitive enough to justify its routine use in hip fractures or suspected femoral head necrosis.

Gallium-67 (^{67}Ga) concentrates in inflammatory cells and has been used to identify sites of hidden infection (e.g. when there is doubt about the cause of a prosthesis loosening after joint replacement).

Electrodiagnosis

Nerve and muscle function can be studied by various electrical methods. The information can supplement clinical examination – it cannot replace it. The electromyograph (EMG) is not a print-out of disease; it requires skill and experience for its interpretation.

Nerve and muscle stimulation

Electrical stimulation of a motor nerve normally produces contraction of the muscles supplied by that nerve. The stimulus is applied to the skin over the nerve and the motor unit response is measured by a concentric needle electrode inserted into the muscle; the electrical discharge is amplified and displayed on an oscilloscope.

If the nerve is divided, from the 14th day after the injury there is no response to either faradic or galvanic stimulation of the nerve, and an abnormal response from galvanic stimulation of the

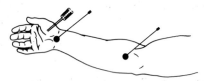

1.19 Electrodiagnosis Electrodes at different levels are used to stimulate the median nerve and one in the thenar muscle records contraction. If the distance between the electrodes is measured and the time interval (from stimulation to muscle contraction) is recorded, conduction velocity can be calculated.

muscle (the 'reaction of degeneration'). Moreover, by plotting the strength of current against the duration of stimulus necessary to produce contraction, a *strength/duration curve* can be obtained, which reflects the degree of denervation and progressive changes in nerve function over time. Other lower motor neuron disorders produce characteristic changes in the type of response and the stimulus–response interval.

Measurement of nerve conduction velocity

The time interval (*latent period*) between stimulation of a nerve and muscle contraction can be measured accurately. If the test is repeated at two points a fixed distance apart along the nerve, and the latency values obtained are subtracted from one another, the conduction velocity between those two points can be determined. Normal values are about 40–60 m per second.

Conduction velocity is slowed in peripheral nerve damage or compression, and the site of the lesion can be established by taking measurements in different segments of the nerve (e.g. in the diagnosis of nerve entrapment syndromes).

Electromyography

Electromyography does not involve electrical nerve stimulation. Instead, the concentric needle electrode in the muscle is used to record motor unit activity at rest and when attempts are made to contract the muscle.

Normally there is no electrical activity at rest, but on voluntary contraction characteristic oscilloscopic patterns appear. Spontaneous discharges at rest may occur after partial or complete denervation, with pressure on spinal nerve roots, with anterior horn cell degeneration (e.g. in progressive muscular atrophy) and in various muscle disorders. The number, shape, amplitude and duration of action potentials make up a pattern that can distinguish between neuropathic and myopathic disorders, and may permit identification of specific diseases.

Further reading

Ansell, B. M. (1972) Hypermobility of joints. In *Modern Trends in Orthopaedics—6.* Ed. by A. Graham Apley. London: Butterworths
Beighton, P. (1969) Orthopaedic aspects of Ehlers–Danlos syndrome. *Journal of Bone and Joint Surgery* **51B**, 444–453
Cheyne, C. (1971) Histiocytosis X. *Journal of Bone and Joint Surgery* **53B**, 366–382
Hoppenfeld, S. (1976) *Physical Examination of the Spine and Extremities.* New York: Appleton Century Crofts
Hughes, S. (1980) Radionuclides in orthopaedic surgery. *Journal of Bone and Joint Surgery* **62B**, 141–150
Murray, R. O. and Jacobson, H. G. (1977) *The Radiology of Skeletal Disorders*, 2nd edn. Edinburgh: Churchill Livingstone
Sutherland, A. D., Savage, J. P., Paterson, D. C. and Foster, B. K. (1980) The nuclide bone-scan in the diagnosis and management of Perthes' disease. *Journal of Bone and Joint Surgery* **62B**, 300–306

Bone Infection

2

Acute osteomyelitis

The causal organisms are usually staphylococci, though in young children streptococcal infection is not uncommon. Occasionally pneumococci, haemophilus or brucella may be responsible; and patients with sickle-cell anaemia are prone to develop salmonella bone infections.

The blood stream is invaded, usually from a minor skin abrasion, rarely from a boil. In children the organisms settle in the metaphysis at the growing end of a long bone, possibly because: (1) more blood flows to the growing end; (2) the rapidly growing cells are unduly susceptible; (3) the delicate vessels have been injured and the haematoma is a suitable medium for bacterial growth; or (4) the hairpin arrangement of capillaries has slowed down the rate of blood flow. In young infants the very end of the bone may be involved, and in adults the mid-shaft may be attacked.

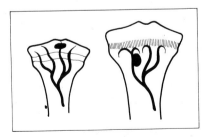

2.1 Acute osteomyelitis (1) In young infants infection may settle near the very end of the bone; joint infection and growth disturbance easily follow. In children, metaphyseal infection is usual; the growth disc acts as a barrier to spread.

Bone may be infected directly from a wound, but usually this does not present as acute osteomyelitis, because the path of infection also provides a route for drainage; a more insidious source is unsterile puncture during intravascular catheterization, haemodialysis or spinal injections.

Pathology

SUPPURATION Pus forms within the medulla and, being in a confined space under tension, forces its way along the Volkmann canals to the surface of the bone. It then spreads subperiosteally, both around the bone and along the shaft, to re-enter the bone at another level or burst out into the soft tissues. The growth disc and joint capsule are rarely penetrated except in young infants.

NECROSIS Bone dies when its blood supply is cut off by infective thrombosis, by rising tension within a rigid bony cavity or by the stripping up of the periosteum. Pieces may separate as sequestra which act as foreign-body irritants, causing persistent discharge through a sinus until they escape or are removed.

NEW BONE FORMATION New bone forms from the deep layer of the periosteum. If bone formation is extensive, it constitutes an encasing involucrum which may contain holes (cloacae); ultimately the bone often appears widened.

Clinical features

A history of a preceding skin lesion, an injury or a sore throat may be obtained. A few days later there is rapid onset of fever and malaise and of

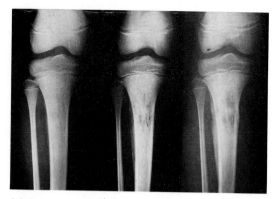

2.2 Acute osteomyelitis (2)   The first x-ray, 2 days after symptoms began, is normal – it always is; metaphyseal mottling and periosteal changes were not obvious until the second film, taken 14 days later; eventually much of the shaft was involved.

pain. The pain is localized, unrelieved by rest and often severe. The patient, usually a child, is ill and toxaemic, with a rapid pulse and high fever. There is leucocytosis and a positive blood culture.

The dramatic illness just described is by no means invariable. In children the constitutional disturbance may be misleadingly mild, and in neonates it may be absent. The local signs are as follows.

- LOOK   The limb is held still. It looks normal at first but later swelling and redness may appear.

- FEEL   If the child allows the limb to be touched, localized 'finger-tip' tenderness is felt over a metaphysis, and later warmth and oedema.

- MOVE   The child may not permit movement of the limb. Usually the neighbouring joint, though irritated, has at least a few degrees of painless movement.

- X-RAY   For the first 10 days x-rays show no abnormality. Later there is patchy rarefaction of the metaphysis, and periostitis which shows as a thin line parallel to the shaft. Later still, as healing occurs, there is sclerosis and new periosteal bone; sometimes sequestra are seen, which are very dense and separated from the surrounding bone. Hot spots on scanning are present before x-ray changes.

NOTE   Osteomyelitis in an unusual site or with an unusual organism should alert the doctor to a number of possibilities, such as: heroin addiction, sickle-cell disease or deficient host defence mechanisms (Waldvogel and Vasey, 1980).

Differential diagnosis

In acute suppurative arthritis   tenderness is diffuse, and all movement at the joint is abolished by muscle spasm.

In acute rheumatism   the pain tends to flit from one joint to another, and there may be carditis, rheumatic nodules or erythema marginatum.

In a sickle-cell crisis   the patient may present with features indistinguishable from acute osteomyelitis (page 63).

In Gaucher's disease   (page 64) a pseudo-osteitis may occur with features closely resembling infective osteomyelitis. The bone marrow is packed with macrophages containing the abnormal lipid; drilling the bone yields a milky fluid resembling thin pus. The diagnosis is made by finding other stigmata of the disease, especially enlargement of the spleen and liver.*

Treatment

ANTIBIOTICS   Blood and, if possible, aspiration material are sent immediately for culture, but the prompt administration of antibiotics is so vital that the result is not awaited. Because of the prevalence of penicillin-resistant organisms, Blockey and McAllister (1972) advise the following combination: (1) fusidic acid in aqueous suspension, 5 ml daily for children aged 1–5 years, 10 ml twice daily for older children; plus (2) erythromycin stearate 30 mg/kg body weight daily in divided doses. Other régimes are available and are used if the sensitivity tests so indicate. Antibiotic treatment should continue for a minimum of 3 weeks (6 for a severe attack or complications).

ANALGESICS   Osteomyelitis is extremely painful; adequate and repeated analgesics must be given without waiting for the patient to ask for them.

*'Osteomyelitis' + splenomegaly = Gaucher's disease (almost).

SPLINTAGE A splint is desirable but should not conceal the affected area. Often bed rest, possibly combined with traction, is sufficient. With acute osteomyelitis of the upper femur, traction or splintage is needed to prevent hip dislocation.

DRAINAGE If antibiotics are given early, drainage is often not necessary. If a subperiosteal abscess can be detected (overlying oedema is a useful sign), or if pyrexia and local tenderness persist for more than 24 hours after adequate antibiotics, the pus should be let out by aspiration or incision; it should be cultured and tested for sensitivity. Opinion is divided as to whether the medulla should be drained by drilling.

Complications

A lethal outcome from septicaemia is nowadays extremely rare; with antibiotics the child nearly always recovers and the bone may return to normal. But morbidity is common, especially if treatment is delayed, or the organism is insensitive to the chosen antibiotic. Much the most frequent sequel is chronic osteomyelitis, but the following also may occur.

METASTATIC INFECTION This may involve other bones, joints, serous cavities, the brain or lung.

SUPPURATIVE ARTHRITIS This may occur (1) in very young children, in whom the growth disc is not an impenetrable barrier; (2) where the metaphysis is intracapsular, as in the upper femur; or (3) from metastatic infection.

ALTERED LENGTH OF BONE In infants epiphyseal damage may lead to shortening, sometimes severe. In older children, however, the bone occasionally grows too long because metaphyseal hyperaemia has stimulated the growth disc.

Chronic osteomyelitis

This presents in three forms: (1) post-traumatic and postoperative; (2) the sequel to acute osteomyelitis; and (3) chronic osteomyelitis of insidious onset.

Post-traumatic and postoperative

Following an open fracture bone infection may develop. The route whereby organisms have entered serves also as an exit route, so that pressure necrosis of bone does not necessarily develop; but union of the fracture is always delayed. The essence of treatment is prophylaxis: thorough débridement, the provision of drainage by leaving the wound open, and antibiotics (see also page 349).

Postoperative osteomyelitis (the term 'osteitis' is sometime preferred) follows implanting foreign material (metal, plastic or cement) for joint replacement or for the internal fixation of fractures. The term 'iatrogenic' is salutary, even though the infection may sometimes be blood-borne from the patient himself. Again prophylaxis is the key: the cleanest possible surgical environment, a meticulous technique, careful haemostasis and suction drainage. Should infection develop soon after operation, antibiotics and early drainage are important. If these measures fail, excision of infected and necrotic material, and continuous antibiotic irrigation combined with suction drainage may enable the implant to be preserved; with an infected fracture it is important to retain the implant. Late infection is discussed on page 273.

Chronic osteomyelitis: the sequel to acute

An area of bone has been destroyed by the acute infection; cavities are therefore present and are surrounded by dense sclerosed bone. Bits of dead bone (sequestra) usually remain. They are imprisoned in fibrous tissue and sclerosed bone but may act as irritants, provoking the living tissue to produce seropus; this escapes through a sinus which tends to persist because the sequestra cannot escape. Bacteria also are imprisoned in fibrous tissue, where they often remain dormant for years, but at any time infection may flare.

The patient may present because pain, pyrexia, redness and tenderness have recurred (a 'flare'); or with a sinus which discharges seropus. X-rays show areas of bone rarefaction surrounded by dense sclerosis, and sometimes sequestra.

Treatment is usually conservative. A sinus may be painless and need a dressing simply to protect the clothing; and a flare often settles with a few days' rest, though if an abscess presents it should be incised. Most antibiotics fail to penetrate the barrier of fibrous tissue plus bone sclerosis. Fucidin is an exception and may be useful, especially

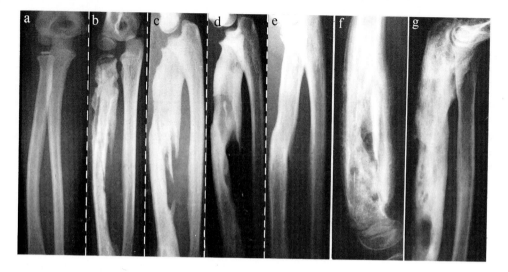

2.3 Chronic osteomyelitis (a–e) When this boy first became ill his x-ray (a) was normal. The bone was explored, but at 4 weeks it looked like this (b). A discharge persisted and the large sequestrum (c) was removed. But a tiny sequestrum (d) remained and the discharge did not clear up till this was removed. Then (e) the bone returned to normal. The remaining films show (f) early chronic osteomyelitis with a large sequestrum; and (g) the typical altered architecture of chronic osteomyelitis.

if combined with sequestrectomy, though this should be performed only if a sequestrum is radiologically visible and surgically accessible.

More radical surgery is justified only if symptoms are severe. Under antibiotic cover all infected soft tissue and all dead or devitalized bone can be excised (dead material can be identified by the preoperative injection of Disulphine Blue which stains all living tissues green, leaving dead material unstained); this is followed by the local instillation of antibiotic solution using a continuous irrigation and suction technique. An alternative is to insert a chain of cement beads which contain gentamicin, and to remove this 2 weeks later; the antibiotic leaches out into the surrounding tissues.

Chronic osteomyelitis of insidious onset

Four varieties of chronic osteomyelitis appear clinically to be chronic from the start.

BRODIE'S ABSCESS   A Brodie's abscess is usually small and situated in the metaphysis of a long bone, though it may be of any size and occur anywhere in the bone. Clinically it may remain silent for years, or present with recurrent attacks of pain. During an attack the bone is tender and there may be a little swelling.

X-rays show a translucent area with a well-defined margin and a small area of surrounding sclerosis, beyond which the bone looks normal. Confusion with osteoid osteoma may occur.

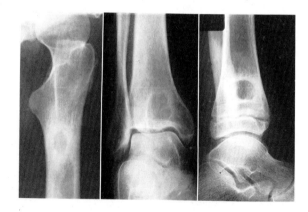

2.4 Brodie's abscess   These examples all show the characteristic features of a Brodie's abscess – a rare area with a well-defined margin and surrounding sclerosis, but no ballooning of the bone.

Treatment is operative. Under antibiotic cover the abscess is opened. Rarely it contains pus, but usually clear sterile fluid. The abscess wall is removed and the wound sutured.

TUBERCULOUS OSTEOMYELITIS (see also Chapter 3) This is a chronic infection which as a rule remains clinically silent until it presents as: (1) a joint inflammation, from irritation or eruption into a nearby joint; (2) deformity, from collapse of soft bone, as in the spine; (3) swelling, possibly of the bone itself (as in dactylitis), or a cold abscess.

X-rays show an area of bone destruction with ill-defined margins and surrounding bone atrophy, in contrast with the sclerosis around a Brodie's abscess.

SPIROCHAETAL OSTEOMYELITIS Syphilis of bone is a rare tertiary manifestation, producing localized or diffuse lesions. Localized gummata may occur in any part of the bone, but are usually subperiosteal in subcutaneous bones, and the overlying skin may break down. Diffuse periostitis may cause a sabre tibia. Diffuse osteomyelitis presents as an aching, tender bone, sometimes with sequestra and sinuses. In congenital syphilis, epiphysitis and dactylitis also occur.

In bone syphilis x-ray may show periosteal thickening and punched-out translucent areas in the midst of dense sclerosis. The lesions are often multiple. Serological tests are essential for diagnosis.

Treatment is directed to the underlying disease. Penicillin and iodides are given.

Yaws may produce bone lesions similar to those of syphilis. Several bones are usually affected. The main changes are periosteal new bone formation and areas of rarefaction in the cortex; sclerosis is less than in syphilis.

CHRONIC NON-SUPPURATIVE OSTEOMYELITIS (GARRÉ) The bone is thickened and radiologically dense (sclerosing osteitis). The clinical features, x-ray appearance and response to treatment strongly resemble those of an osteoid osteoma (page 97).

Periostitis

Following acute osteomyelitis new subperiosteal bone is laid down. The term 'periostitis' is then best avoided, for all the bony components are involved. There are two varieties of true periostitis, both chronic.

FOLLOWING INJURY A haematoma following trauma may ossify, leaving bone which is thickened on the surface (the knobbly shins of a footballer is an example). X-rays, however, show that the deep aspects of the cortex and the medulla are normal.

CHRONIC FROM THE START (SYPHILITIC PERI-OSTITIS) Spirochaetes carried by the blood stream may be deposited in bone. Cellular infiltration is succeeded by fibro-

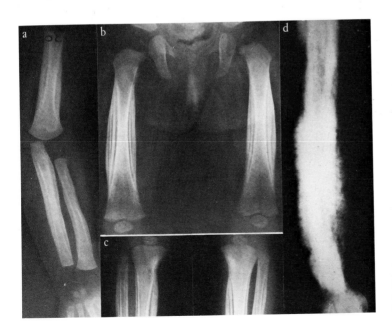

2.5 Syphilis (a, b, c) Congenital syphilis – with diffuse periostitis of many bones; (d) acquired periostitis of the femur.

sis. Subsequently, because of obliterative endarteritis, the bone locally becomes avascular, with characteristically dense sclerosis.

Diffuse periostitis This sometimes occurs in congenital syphilis; it is usually bilateral and often painless. Many bones may be involved and the appearance then is not unlike that in Caffey's disease. Occasionally only the metaphyses are involved.

Localized disease (gummatous osteoperiostitis) This occurs in congenital or acquired syphilis. Subcutaneous bones chiefly are affected and there may be more than one lump on a bone. Each lump is smooth, hard and sometimes tender; x-rays show considerable density. Later the centre may necrose and the overlying skin break down, leaving a punched-out ulcer with a yellow slough covering bare bone. When this process affects the tibia the thickening on the anterior border makes the bone appear bent (sabre tibia).

Differential diagnosis

Periostitis must be differentiated from the following conditions.

EWING'S TUMOUR (page 106) New periosteal bone is laid down in layers parallel to the shaft. The clinical and radiological features usually subside rapidly with radiotherapy, but preliminary diagnostic biopsy is essential.

OSTEOID OSTEOMA (page 97) A localized area of cortical thickening is present with a clear area (the nidus) at its centre.

HYPERTROPHIC PULMONARY OSTEOARTHRO-PATHY Ninety per cent of patients with this condition have chronic intrathoracic disease, usually bronchial carcinoma. The ends of the long bones (including the hands and feet) are symmetrically but irregularly thickened, though only the exterior of the bone is involved. Clubbing of the fingers is common and some patients complain of burning pain in the feet.

STRESS FRACTURE A teenager or young adult presents with localized pain and tenderness after activity; the tibia is a favourite site. Radiologically there is periosteal thickening overlying an area of increased density; this suggests osteosarcoma and, since the rapidly growing cells of a healing stress fracture can resemble malignant cells, biopsy may (unless the pathologist is alerted) be misleading.

SCURVY Subperiosteal bleeding occurs with minimal trauma and the haematoma calcifies. The child looks anaemic and has other stigmata of capillary fragility (see page 75).

VENOUS ULCER (STASIS) Periosteal thickening is liable to develop on the subcutaneous surface of the tibia when there is, or has been, an overlying varicose ulcer.

INFANTILE CORTICAL HYPEROSTOSIS (CAFFEY'S DISEASE) In this rare disease subperiosteal new bone is laid down over a

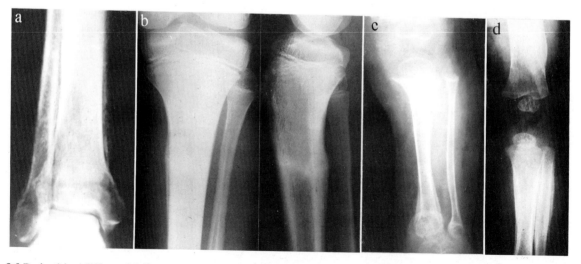

2.6 Periostitis – differential diagnosis (a) Hypertrophic pulmonary osteoarthropathy; (b) AP and lateral of a stress fracture (a tumour was suspected); (c) scurvy; (d) infantile cortical hyperostosis (Caffey's disease).

wide area of many bones. An infant under 6 months old develops swellings, which may be tender, on the mandible, long bones and sometimes the scapulae. Often there is fever. Caffey's disease recovers spontaneously and the x-ray appearance of the bones returns to normal.

Acute suppurative arthritis

Cause and pathology

The causal organisms are usually staphylococci, occasionally streptococci and, rarely, other organisms. The joint is invaded through a penetrating wound, by eruption of a bone abscess or by blood spread from a distant site. Infection spreads through the joint; the articular cartilage disintegrates and is removed by polymorphs. Pus may burst out of the joint to form abscesses and sinuses. Later, with healing, opposing surfaces may adhere (fibrous ankylosis); often, however, trabeculae grow across the joint (bony ankylosis).

Clinical features

There may have been a wound. Within a few days (sometimes only 48 hours) the patient rapidly becomes ill, with severe throbbing pain and swelling, a rapid pulse and high swinging fever. The white cell count is raised and blood culture may be positive.

Many of the local signs can be elicited only in superficial joints. The skin looks red, the joint is held flexed and it is fusiformly swollen. There is superficial warmth, diffuse tenderness and fluctuation. All movements are grossly restricted and often completely abolished by pain and spasm.

X-RAY   For the first 2–3 weeks the appearance is normal; then the bone shows widespread patchy rarefaction, and the joint space may be narrowed. With healing, the bone recalcifies; the joint space may remain narrow and irregular, or be completely obliterated and crossed by trabeculae.

Differential diagnosis

In acute osteomyelitis   tenderness is pinpointed to bone, and a little joint movement is permitted.

In rheumatic fever   the pain is less severe and is eased by large doses of salicylates; the general signs of rheumatism may be found.

In acute non-suppurative arthritis   there is less general illness and the local signs are much less severe.

With a haemarthrosis   the history (of injury or haemophilia) is important; there is little general illness.

Immediate treatment

ASPIRATION   Under anaesthesia the pus is aspirated as soon as possible and the fluid replaced by penicillin. Formal incision is advisable at the hip, or elsewhere if the pus is too thick to aspirate. The pus is cultured and the organisms are tested for sensitivity.

ANTIBIOTICS   In addition to the penicillin instilled into the joint, intramuscular injections are started immediately. With deep joints which have been opened, systemic antibiotics should be combined with continuous irrigation using an antibiotic solution.

The injections are continued for several weeks, a more effective antibiotic being substituted if tests so indicate.

SPLINTAGE   The joint must be rested either on a splint or in a widely split plaster. At the hip, traction or splintage is imperative.

Treatment of the aftermath

Once the patient's general condition is good and the joint is no longer painful or warm, further damage is unlikely.

If articular cartilage has been preserved, the aim is to regain movement. Gentle and gradually increasing active movements are encouraged. The patient is allowed up wearing a splint which is taken off for non-weight-bearing exercises. Gradually weight is taken and the splint is eventually discarded. At all stages the patient is carefully watched for signs of a flare.

If articular cartilage has been destroyed, the aim is to keep the joint immobile while ankylosis is awaited. Splintage in the optimum position is therefore continuously maintained, usually by plaster, until ankylosis is sound. The patient is allowed up; weight-bearing is resumed as the bone recalcifies.

Further reading

Blockey, N. J. and McAllister, T. A. (1972) Antibiotics in acute osteomyelitis in children. *Journal of Bone and Joint Surgery* **54B,** 299–309

Clawson, D. K. and Dunn, A. W. (1967) Management of common bacterial infections of bones and joints. *Journal of Bone and Joint Surgery* **49A,** 164–182

Mollan, R. A. B. and Piggot, J. (1977) Acute osteomyelitis in children. *Journal of Bone and Joint Surgery* **59B,** 2–7

Morrey, B. F., Bianco, A. J. and Rhodes, K. H. (1976) Suppurative arthritis of the hip in children. *Journal of Bone and Joint Surgery* **58A,** 388–392

Paterson, D. C. (1970) Acute suppurative arthritis in infancy and childhood. *Journal of Bone and Joint Surgery* **52B,** 474–482

Wahlig, H., Dingeldein, E., Bergmann, R. and Reuss, K. (1978) The release of gentamicin from polymethylmethacrylate beads. *Journal of Bone and Joint Surgery* **60B,** 270–275

Waldvogel, F. A. and Vasey, H. (1980) Osteomyelitis: the past decade. *New England Journal of Medicine* **303,** 360–370

Tuberculosis **3**

Generalized tuberculosis

Cause

The body is invaded by tubercle bacilli, human or bovine. Formerly, 85 per cent of cases were bovine in origin, but pasteurization and tuberculin-tested herds have reduced this figure to 25 per cent. The bacilli enter the body via the lung (droplet infection) or the gut (swallowing infected milk products) or, rarely, through the skin.

Pathology

PRIMARY COMPLEX   The initial lesion in lung, pharynx or gut is a small one with lymphatic spread to regional glands; this combination is the primary complex. Usually the bacilli are fixed in the glands and no clinical illness results, but occasionally the response is excessive, with enlargement of glands in the neck or abdomen.

Even though there is usually no clinical illness, the initial infection has two important sequels: (1) within glands which are apparently healed or even calcified, bacilli may survive for many years, so that a reservoir for potential reinfection exists; (2) the body has been sensitized to the toxin (a positive Heaf test being an index of sensitization), and should reinfection occur, the response is quite different, the lesion being a destructive one which spreads by contiguity.

SECONDARY SPREAD   If resistance to the original infection is low, widespread dissemination via the blood stream may occur, giving rise to miliary tuberculosis or meningitis. More often, blood spread occurs months or years later, perhaps because of lowered resistance. Bacilli escape from their lymphatic prison, and may be deposited in many tissues. Probably most of the bacilli are destroyed, but others survive giving rise to destructive lesions of which two or three often coexist.

TERTIARY LESION   The surgeon usually sees tuberculosis as a locally destructive lesion to which the term 'tertiary' may be applied. The bacilli, having gained a foothold in sensitized tissue, multiply. Giant-cell systems develop, grow and coalesce, destroying normal tissue and replacing it by caseous material. So long as this process is active, destruction and caseation continue to extend by direct contiguity, and the bone is slowly 'eaten away'. In addition the bone 'melts away'; that is, it undergoes rarefaction, a consequence of the increased blood supply occurring in chronic inflammation. Because it is being eaten away and melted away the bone tends to collapse; caseous material and tuberculous pus are squeezed out, forming a cold abscess which, if it reaches the surface, may discharge and leave a sinus. The muscles also 'melt away' and their wasting is a marked feature of joint tuberculosis.

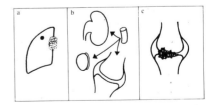

3.1 The tuberculous process   The primary infection is usually arrested in the local lymph glands (a); secondary spread is by the blood stream (b); the term 'tertiary' can be used for the local destructive lesion (c).

Clinical features

Tuberculosis of a bone or joint is merely the local manifestation of a general disease; even though the bone or joint may be the presenting feature, a second focus (for example, in the lung or urogenital tract) often coexists.

The general illness is gradual in onset, with a long history; the patient feels off-colour and may complain of lassitude, poor appetite, loss of weight and night sweats. Often he looks thin and pale, though he may have a malar flush. Slight evening pyrexia is usual, the sedimentation rate is raised and the Heaf test positive.

Frequently the illness is mild, but in those who have neither been inoculated prophylactically nor exposed to the primary disease, it is often more acute with greater systemic disturbance; thus the rural inhabitants of developing countries are at special risk when they move to an urban environment.

Treatment

Recumbency and a sanatorium life, once the cornerstones of general treatment, have been superseded by chemotherapy. Once drug treatment is stabilized and the patient reasonably fit he need not be in hospital. Until recently the standard regimen (the doses are for adults) was streptomycin (1 g by intramuscular injection daily); INAH (isonicotinic acid hydrazide – 200 mg daily by mouth); and PAS (para-aminosalicylic acid – 16 g daily by mouth). Usually streptomycin was given only every other day after 3 months and discontinued after 6 months; the other two drugs were continued for at least a year. Nowadays rifampicin (450 mg daily in divided doses) is often substituted for PAS.

Controlled trials in spinal tuberculosis have suggested that streptomycin can be omitted altogether, except in resistant cases; the cautious retain it for 3 months. Other drugs, such as ethambutol (25 mg/kg body weight daily, reducing), are also becoming available.

Complications

DISSEMINATION The secondary spread of tuberculosis is via the blood stream. Consequently, miliary tuberculosis or meningitis may occur – both used to be fatal before the introduction of chemotherapy.

AMYLOID DISEASE Associated with chronic tissue destruction there is increased production of autoantibodies which react with serum globulins and ground substance to produce an insoluble glycoprotein called amyloid. This is deposited in the ground substance of many tissues, particularly in the walls of arterioles. The main organs involved are the liver, spleen, kidneys, pancreas, adrenals and intestinal mucosa, but almost every tissue may be affected to some degree.

The disease occurs not only with tuberculosis but also with other chronic bone or joint infections, in leprosy, in malaria, and particularly in rheumatoid arthritis. The patient is pale, puffy, waxy, wasted and oedematous. The spleen, kidney and liver are enlarged. Proof of diagnosis may be obtained by the Congo red test, liver puncture or gum biopsy. The only hope is eradication of the disease, when the amyloid process may be reversed.

Joint tuberculosis

Joint tuberculosis is a local manifestation of a general disease. Nevertheless the disease as it affects any joint merits separate description. The disease is conveniently divided into three stages.

(1) ACTIVE DISEASE The disease has the upper hand and the patient may be ill in himself. There is local active inflammation as shown by warmth, muscle wasting and bone rarefaction. At first the disease is confined to the synovium or to the interior of the bone, the articular cartilage remaining normal; from this early disease restoration to normal is still possible. Later the articular cartilage may be damaged, giving a true arthritis, from which complete resolution is no longer possible.

(2) HEALING PHASE Gradually the patient gains the upper hand and masters the disease. Any general illness subsides. Locally the disease is arrested, pain and warmth disappear and the bones recalcify. If the disease was arrested before articular damage (early), healing may be by resolution to apparent normality; if articular cartilage has been damaged (late), healing is by fibrosis.

(3) AFTERMATH Once a joint has suffered a true arthritis with erosion of articular cartilage the

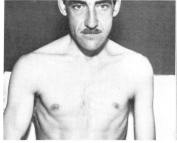
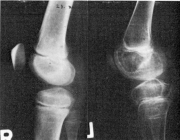

3.2 Active tuberculosis A characteristic feature is wasting of muscle (note the left deltoid) and 'wasting' of bone (note the rarefaction of the left knee).

damage is permanent and the resulting fibrous joint is unsound; i.e. increasing deformity may occur and even after many years of quiescence bacilli may be liberated from their fibrous prison, causing the infection to flare up again.

Stage 1: active disease

Bacilli carried in the blood stream are deposited in bone or synovium. A bone focus (osteomyelitis) consists of an irregular abscess cavity in the metaphysis or epiphysis; sometimes the cavity extends through the epiphyseal plate. Synovial infection (synovitis) may be directly from the blood stream or follow local extension from a bone focus. The synovial membrane becomes thick, grey and oedematous. The joint is irritated by the adjacent focus but, in this early stage, articular cartilage is undamaged.

From the bone or synovial focus the disease may extend or erupt into the interior of the joint; spread throughout the joint is now rapid. A pannus of granulation tissue spreads over the synovial membrane and across the articular cartilage. Infection also extends in the subchondral bone, so that the articular cartilage is attacked on both sides. It is extensively eroded, but not completely absorbed, for this requires phagocytes as in a septic arthritis. If unchecked, the tuberculous caseation extends into the soft tissues as an abscess; this in turn may track to the surface, forming a sinus.

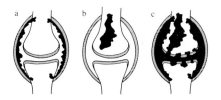

3.3 Active joint tuberculosis The disease may begin as (a) synovitis, or (b) osteomyelitis, both of which can resolve; from either it may extend to become (c) a true arthritis, which cannot.

Symptoms

With early disease (synovitis or osteomyelitis), symptoms are mild; a little ache, perhaps a limp and slight swelling – all provoked by activity and subsiding with rest. Once there is cartilaginous damage (a true arthritis) the symptoms become more severe. Pain is sometimes constant, or may take the form of 'night cries', the explanation of which is that during waking hours the joint is held immobile by muscle spasm and as this relaxes with sleep the damaged joint surfaces rub together, waking the patient. If the patient is able to walk, a pronounced limp is present. Swelling and wasting are marked, stiffness is considerable and deformity (especially shortening) usually obvious.

Signs

● LOOK The joint is held in a position of deformity and is a little swollen. Muscle wasting is marked and makes the joint swelling more apparent.

● FEEL The skin feels warm (not hot), and the joint contains some fluid (never a lot). It is sometimes possible to feel thickening of the synovial membrane, and its attachments may be tender. A bone focus may also be slightly tender. With arthritis the joint feels thick, doughy and diffusely tender. These signs can, of course, be elicited only in superficial joints.

● MOVE Movement in all directions is limited, though at first by only a few degrees; attempting to force any movement to its extreme is painful and may provoke spasm. The muscles are wasted and the patient may be unable to make them properly taut. As arthritis supervenes all movements are grossly limited and may be virtually abolished; any attempt at movement is now painful and provokes immediate spasm.

● X-RAY Rarefaction is a constant and well-marked feature; the medulla looks like ground glass and the cortex like a thin line ('pencilling'). Sometimes the epiphyses are enlarged, probably (like the rarefaction) a result of long-continued hyperaemia.

With osteomyelitis, an irregular rarefied area is seen, often extending from metaphysis into epiphysis; with synovitis, bone may be eroded at the synovial attachments.

As long as the disease is in its early stages, the joint space remains normal in width and the joint line clean and unbroken. Once arthritis has developed the joint space becomes abnormal, being narrowed if the destruction is mainly cartilaginous, or widened if much bone has been eroded; the joint line is irregular.

Management (1) The patient is put to bed for 3–6 weeks (if the hip is involved, skin traction is applied). During this time, other evidence of tuberculosis is sought by x-ray examination of the chest, the Heaf test, and so on. (2) If irritability has then disappeared, activity is gradually resumed under careful supervision. (3) If irritability has persisted or returns with activity, biopsy of synovial membrane or of regional lymph nodes is performed. The specimen is sent for section, culture and guinea-pig inoculation. Antituberculous treatment is started at once.

CHRONIC SYNOVITIS Occasionally a chronic synovitis presents with warmth, wasting, irritability and generalized rarefaction. It is clinically indistinguishable from tuberculosis but a positive Rose–Waaler test or biopsy may show it to be rheumatoid in nature; and years later other joints

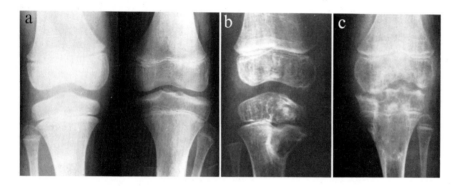

3.4 Active joint tuberculosis (a) A pair of knees, the left with synovitis – note the rarefaction. (b) A patient with osteomyelitis. (c) In this man, arthritis has supervened and complete healing by resolution cannot occur, only healing by fibrosis.

Differential diagnosis

In the early stage tuberculosis must be distinguished from the following.

TRANSIENT SYNOVITIS The cause is unknown. A joint becomes slightly painful and swollen, there is a little warmth and wasting, limitation of extremes of movement and a normal x-ray picture. In fact the joint is irritable and clinically indistinguishable from early tuberculosis.

may become involved. It is a monarticular variety of what is usually a polyarthritis.*

Once a true arthritis is present diagnosis is usually easy, but the following conditions should be considered.

ACUTE ARTHRITIS An arthritis due to pyogenic organisms is usually a dramatic condition. The onset is rapid and the patient ill with a high

*The term 'monopoly' is colloquial but appropriate.

swinging fever. There is leucocytosis and a positive blood culture.

.SUBACUTE ARTHRITIS Occasionally, diseases such as amoebic dysentery, brucellosis or smallpox are complicated by arthritis. The history, clinical features and pathological investigations usually enable a diagnosis to be made.

HAEMORRHAGIC ARTHRITIS The physical signs of blood in a joint may resemble those of tuberculous arthritis. If the bleeding has followed a single recent injury the history and absence of wasting are diagnostic. Following repeated bleeding, as in haemophilia, the clinical resemblance to tuberculosis is closer, but there is also a history of bleeding elsewhere.

Treatment

As long as a tuberculous joint remains active there are (in addition to general treatment) three principles governing local treatment.

REST By this is meant local rest as distinct from recumbency. H. O. Thomas long ago said that the rest must be prolonged, uninterrupted, rigid and enforced. For the knee, his splint is still the best. A hip is most effectively rested on a double abduction frame, though for adults this is very cumbersome and often dispensed with. The shoulder may be rested in an abduction frame and the elbow in a plaster gutter, but for both these joints a simple sling is often used.

TRACTION This overcomes spasm, prevents collapse of soft bone and keeps inflamed surfaces apart. Skin traction is used for the knee, skin or skeletal traction for the hip, and gravity plus a sling for the upper limbs.

CLEARANCE OPERATIONS Since effective antibiotics have become available, operation is seldom needed; but if, despite adequate antibiotics, the disease progresses, then surgery is advisable. A tuberculous osteomyelitis in an accessible site is best evacuated and the wound sutured; this may prevent it from bursting into the joint. With arthritis, excision of diseased synovium and gentle removal of tuberculous débris and sequestra is indicated.

Local complications

ABSCESS An abscess forms when the bone or joint is perforated. Caseous material, often in large quantities, exudes along the soft-tissue planes. The abscess walls are thick and its contents creamy. A fluctuant swelling forms which, unlike a pyogenic abscess, is not hot (hence the term 'cold abscess').

The usual treatment of an abscess is aspiration, repeated as necessary. After a while the contents become too thick to flow through a needle and it is then best, under antibiotic cover, to incise the abscess, evacuate its contents and suture the skin.

SINUS When an abscess becomes subcutaneous it is liable to perforate the skin and give rise to a sinus; often this is an index of poor resistance. The sinus track communicates with the joint and so may permit secondary infection.

Stage 2: healing phase

If the disease is arrested before articular cartilage has been damaged, healing by resolution may occur. Once there has been a true arthritis, however, although healing may occur, restoration to normal is impossible. Tuberculous granulation tissue is slowly converted to fibrous tissue in which the bacilli are imprisoned. Opposing joint surfaces stick together, giving a fibrous ankylosis which may be long (as in the hip or elbow) or short (as in the knee). Bony ankylosis almost never occurs unless there has been secondary infection.

Clinical features

The patient is fit and pain slight or absent. Wasting persists, but there is no swelling, warmth or tenderness. Movement will be slowly increasing if early disease has healed by resolution; otherwise stiffness remains.

X-RAY The bones recalcify, but some permanent alteration of bone architecture nearly always remains. Following arthritis, the joint space is irregular.

Treatment

As the disease heals, general treatment is gradually discontinued. Local treatment depends upon whether the disease was arrested early or only arrested after it had progressed to a true arthritis.

IF ARRESTED EARLY The aim is to restore movement, therefore splints are removed. The joint is, however, protected from stress, which is only gradually allowed.

Thus the patient with lower limb disease first lies in bed without splints but still on traction. The traction is then

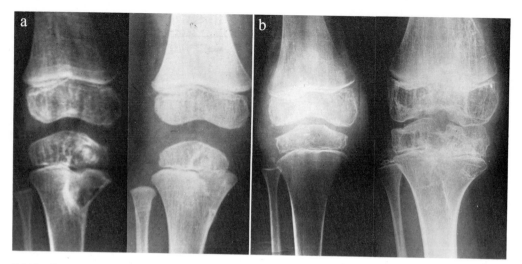

3.5 Healing tuberculosis   (a) Osteomyelitis, and the same knee after healing by resolution – the bone has recalcified without the joint becoming involved. (b) Synovitis, and the same knee after healing by fibrosis – the bone has partly recalcified but, because arthritis developed, the joint space has become irregular.

released for increasing periods and finally removed altogether. He then gets up but avoids taking weight (using a patten and crutches for the hip and a weight-relieving caliper for the knee). After a time he is allowed to take weight for gradually increasing periods until he is walking about normally.

During all this time he is continually observed. If symptoms or signs increase, he goes back a stage; if there is steady progress he goes forward (Thomas' test of recovery). At no time is movement forced; it is only permitted to return of its own accord.

In the upper limb treatment is much simpler; the splint or sling is merely dispensed with for increasing periods of time while the patient uses his arm.

IF ARRESTED LATE   The aim, once articular cartilage has been extensively destroyed, is to obtain the shortest possible fibrous ankylosis in the optimum position. Movement is therefore prevented but stress is permitted so that the joint surfaces impinge more closely together.

In the lower limb traction is taken off and a caliper or plaster applied with the joint in the optimum position. Weight-bearing is started. After some months a removable splint (of polythene, leather or metal) may be used and is taken off for bath or bed. Some form of splint may be needed permanently or until the joint is arthrodesed.

In the upper limb a somewhat longer fibrous ankylosis may be permitted and indeed is almost inevitable, because gravity exerts a constant traction force. At the shoulder, even after arthritis, splintage is gradually discarded; a sling is used for a time and gradually left off. It there is pain, the joint is arthrodesed. At the elbow, a moulded leather or polythene splint may be used permanently, but often a sling is sufficient and sometimes even this may be dispensed with.

Stage 3: aftermath

A joint which has suffered a true arthritis heals by fibrosis (unless there has been secondary infection). A fibrous joint is 'unsound' (page 9) because the fibrous tissue may: (1) shrink with time, giving increasing deformity; and (2) tear with stress, liberating bacilli and provoking a flare.

Clinical features

The limb is nearly always too thin; it may be short and the skin over it may show the scars of former sinuses. Unless there has been a recent flare, warmth and tenderness are absent. Movement is always limited: a short fibrous ankylosis with only a few degrees of movement is common at the knee, but elsewhere there may be up to half the normal range.

X-RAY   The bone is well calcified but its architecture is often faulty. The joint space may scarcely be visible and the joint line is grossly irregular. Abscesses in the vicinity of the joint may be calcified.

Differential diagnosis

The aftermath of an old tuberculous joint is usually easy to diagnose. There are, however, three other fairly common causes of a stiff, deformed or painful joint of long standing.

Old suppurative arthritis   The history is of a more acute illness and there is often bony ankylosis.

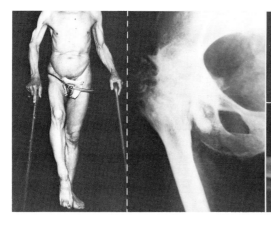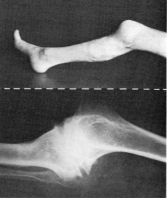

3.6 The aftermath of tuberculous arthritis Joint destruction and deformity: flexion and adduction at the hip; flexion, lateral rotation and backward subluxation (triple deformity) at the knee.

Rheumatoid arthritis   Many joints are affected, commonly small joints, particularly in the hands.

Osteoarthritis   There are no scars, little wasting and the x-ray appearance is characteristic (page 54).

Treatment

In the absence of a flare, general treatment is not required; the only local treatment needed may be a removable splint and, in the lower limb, a raised shoe.

Operations   For deformity, especially at the hip, an osteotomy is valuable.

For unsoundness at any joint arthrodesis is the best treatment. An extra-articular arthrodesis is possible at the hip or shoulder, but elsewhere it must be intra-articular. For deformity plus unsoundness at the hip it is convenient to combine extra-articular arthrodesis by means of an ischiofemoral graft with an osteotomy (Brittain's operation). After many years of quiescence, hip replacement is reasonable.

Complications

The most important complication of an old tuberculous arthritis is a flare. This is a local reactivation of the disease, though it may be accompanied by a lighting-up of the general illness. A flare may occur if the patient's resistance drops, or if trauma liberates bacilli from their fibrous prison.

If an old tuberculous joint suffers trauma it is probably wise not to await a flare, but to put the joint at rest immediately and to institute drug treatment. If a flare has actually occurred these measures are certainly necessary and it is best, once active inflammation subsides, to proceed with arthrodesis.

Extra-articular tuberculosis

Tuberculosis may involve bone without affecting a joint and may attack the synovial lining of tendon sheaths or bursae.

Tuberculous osteomyelitis

Within the bone an irregular area of destruction occurs and may be seen on x-ray. The infection, being chronic, is often not painful and may remain clinically silent until one of the following occurs.

SOFT BONE COLLAPSES   This occurs particularly in the spine where a diseased vertebral body collapses, infecting the one below and squashing caseous material into the soft tissues as an abscess (page 227).

A SWELLING APPEARS   In tuberculosis of flat bones (rib or skull) an abscess is the usual presenting feature; in tuberculous dactylitis a localized swelling or a sinus is usual.

Synovial tuberculosis

Infected synovium becomes thick, oedematous and villous. Excess fluid may be produced, giving a painless swelling and, where there is friction, particles of fibrin are moulded to resemble melon seeds. Tendon sheaths or bursae may be affected.

TENOSYNOVITIS   The commonest site for tenosynovitis is in front of the wrist (see 'Compound palmar ganglion', page 184) but the fingers or ankle region are sometimes affected. A painless swelling appears insidiously; it is fluctuant and often there is weakness and muscle wasting. Instillation of streptomycin is sometimes successful, or excision of the sheath may be necessary.

BURSITIS   The least rare sites for bursitis are the subdeltoid and gluteal bursae. A painless, cold, fluctuant swelling slowly develops, wasting is slight and the underlying joint normal. Treatment is by excision under drug cover.

Further reading

Hodgson, A. R., Wong, W. and Yau, A. (1969) *X-ray Appearances of Tuberculosis of the Spine*. Springfield, Illinois: Charles C Thomas

Nicholson, R. A. (1974) Twenty years of bone and joint tuberculosis in Bradford. *Journal of Bone and Joint Surgery* **56B,** 760–765

Robins, R. H. C. (1967) Tuberculosis of the wrist and hand. *British Journal of Surgery* **54,** 211–218

Seddon, H. J. (1976) The choice of treatment in Pott's disease (Editorial). *Journal of Bone and Joint Surgery* **58B,** 395–397

Somerville, E. W. and Wilkinson, M. C. (1965) *Girdlestone's Tuberculosis of Bone and Joint*, 3rd edn. London: Oxford University Press

Rheumatic Disorders

4

'Rheumatic disorder' is a descriptive term linking a number of conditions which cause chronic pain and swelling of joints and tendon sheaths. This does not imply a causal connection, but they do share certain pathological features: (1) a faulty immune mechanism; (2) an inflammatory response which persists almost indefinitely; and (3) progressive damage to joints and tendons.

Rheumatoid arthritis

Rheumatoid arthritis is a systemic, inflammatory disease in which the changes are most marked in the synovial tissue of tendons and joints. It is characterized by a chronic, symmetrical polysynovitis, morning stiffness, elevation of the ESR and the appearance of anti-IgG globulins (rheumatoid factors) in the serum. It affects about 3 per cent of the population, usually starting in the fourth decade, and is three times as common in women as in men. Both the prevalence and the clinical expression vary in different populations: it is most common (and generally more severe) in the urban communities of Europe and America, but is seldom seen in the tribal populations of Africa (Solomon *et al.*, 1975).

Cause

Some antigen – possibly a virus – sets off a chain of events suggesting a seriously disturbed immune response. This type of reaction may be genetically predetermined, for patients show increased frequencies of certain histocompatibility anti-

gens (HLA-CW3 and HLA-DW4). An important sequence is the appearance of antigen–antibody complexes in the joint which, after complement activation, stimulate a local phagocytic reaction, release of lysosomal enzymes and inflammation. These immune complexes probably also stimulate the production of autoantibodies which appear in the synovial fluid and blood as the antiglobulin rheumatoid factor.

Pathology

The condition is widespread, affecting tissues throughout the body, and should be called rheumatoid *disease*. However, the brunt of the attack falls on synovium. The constant and characteristic feature is a chronic inflammation; an inconstant but pathognomonic lesion is the rheumatoid nodule.

JOINTS AND TENDONS
The pathological changes, if unchecked, proceed in three stages.

Stage 1: synovitis   Early changes are proliferation of synoviocytes and infiltration of the subsynovial

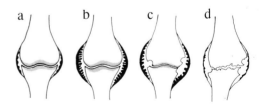

4.1 Pathology of rheumatoid arthritis   (a) The normal joint. (b) Stage 1 – synovitis and joint swelling. (c) Stage 2 – early joint destruction with periarticular erosions. (d) Stage 3 – advanced joint destruction and deformity.

layers by polymorphs, lymphocytes and plasma cells. There is thickening of the capsular structures, villous formation of the synovium and a cell-rich effusion into the joints and tendon sheaths. Though painful, swollen and tender, these structures are still intact and mobile, and the disorder is potentially reversible.

Stage 2: destruction Persistent inflammation causes joint and tendon destruction. Articular cartilage is eroded, partly by proteolytic enzymes, partly by vascular tissue in the folds of the synovial reflection, and partly due to direct invasion of the cartilage by a pannus of granulation tissue creeping over the articular surface. There is also erosion of the periarticular bone caused by osteoclastic activity at the margins of the joint.

Similar destructive changes and granuloma formation between the collagen bundles may cause partial or complete rupture of tendons.

Stage 3: deformity The combination of articular destruction, capsular stretching and tendon rupture leads to progressive instability and deformity of the joints. By this time the inflammatory process may have long since subsided; the emphasis is now on the mechanical and functional effects of joint and tendon disruption.*

EXTRA-ARTICULAR TISSUES

The rheumatoid nodule is a small granulomatous lesion consisting of a central necrotic zone surrounded by a radially disposed palisade of local histiocytes, and beyond that by inflammatory granulation tissue. Nodules occur under the skin (especially over bony prominences), in the synovium, on tendons, in the sclera and in many of the viscera.

Lymphadenopathy can affect not only the glands draining inflamed joints, but those at a distance such as the mediastinal nodes. *Vasculitis*, more usually associated with disseminated lupus, may be fairly widespread. *Muscle weakness* may be due to a rheumatoid myopathy or neuropathy, but it can also result from spinal cord involvement or cervical spine displacement. *Sensory changes* may be part of a neuropathy, but isolated symptoms can result from nerve compression by thickened synovium. *Visceral disease* can occur in the lungs, heart, kidneys, brain and gastrointestinal tract.

Clinical features

The usual pattern is an insidious emergence of malaise, tiredness, loss of weight, muscle pain and stiffness, followed by pain and swelling of peripheral joints and tendon sheaths; gradually more and more joints are involved as the disease spreads relentlessly, resulting in widespread deformities and loss of function. Sometimes the joint symptoms are less severe and there are alternating spells of acute exacerbation and relative quiescence. Occasionally, in older individuals, the onset is explosive, with severe joint pain and systemic illness; paradoxically these patients have a relatively good prognosis.

During stage 1 (synovitis) the predominant – sometimes the only – feature is a symmetrical polysynovitis, most commonly affecting the proximal joints of the hands and feet, the wrists, ankles, knees and shoulders, the flexor tendons of the fingers and the extensors of the wrists. There is local tenderness, and thickened synovium can often be felt at the margins of joints and along superficial tendons. Tenosynovitis of the finger flexors is easily diagnosed by feeling the coarse crepitation over the flexor sheaths in the palm as the patient's fingers are alternately flexed and extended. Movement is usually limited but the joints are still stable and deformity is unusual.

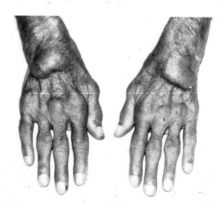

4.2 Rheumatoid arthritis – early features This patient, with a 3-month history of joint pains, has swelling of the proximal interphalangeal joints ('spindling'), of some metacarpophalangeal joints and extensor tendon sheaths, and of both wrists. The changes are remarkably symmetrical.

*RA does not burn itself out; it burns itself in.

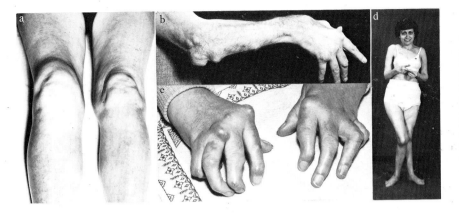

4.3 Manifestations of rheumatoid arthritis (a) Monarticular disease – but years later it became polyarticular; the term 'monopoly' seems appropriate. (b) Rheumatoid nodules. (c) The combination of nodules and deformities is pathognomonic. (d) Despite multiple deformities this patient looks happy – such euphoria is fortunately not uncommon.

In stage 2 (destruction) deformities appear: e.g. a dropped finger due to rupture of an extensor tendon; radial deviation of the wrist due to weakness of extensor carpi ulnaris; inability to straighten the elbow because of capsular thickening.

It is usually at about this time that subcutaneous nodules can be felt over the olecranon process, though they occur in only 25 per cent of patients. Other extra-articular features such as muscle weakness and wasting, lymph node enlargement and skin atrophy may also be present.

In stage 3 (deformity) the diagnosis is obvious at a glance. Fingers are deviated ulnarwards, often with subluxation or dislocation of the metacarpophalangeal joints; wrists show radial and volar deflection; elbows cannot be straightened and shoulders have lost abduction and external rotation; knees may be swollen and unable to extend fully; ankles are usually in valgus; the toes are clawed; there is dislocation of the metatarsophalangeal joints and painful callosities under the prominent metatarsal heads. About a third of all patients develop pain and stiffness in the cervical spine.

In long-standing cases muscle wasting may be extreme. Vasculitis and peripheral neuropathy are uncommon features of severe disease. Marked visceral disease also is rare.

X-rays

In stage 1, x-rays show only the features of synovitis: soft-tissue swelling and periarticular osteoporosis.

Stage 2 is marked by the appearance of marginal bony erosions and narrowing of the 'joint space', especially in the proximal joints of the hands and feet, the wrists and the acromioclavicular joints.

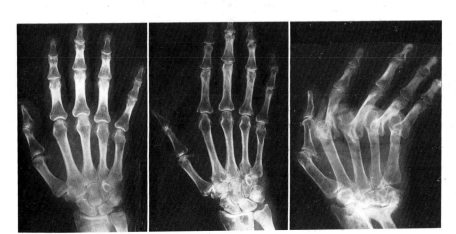

4.4 Rheumatoid arthritis – sequence of changes The progress of disease is well shown in this patient's x-rays. First there was only soft-tissue swelling and periarticular osteoporosis; later juxta-articular erosions appeared; ultimately the joints became unstable and deformed, with four of the metacarpophalangeal joints dislocated.

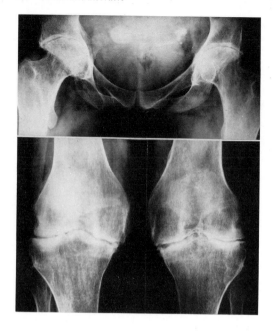

4.5 Joint damage   With destruction of articular cartilage the joint space becomes irregular, and narrowed or obliterated. Many joints may be wrecked.

In stage 3 articular destruction and joint deformity are usually obvious. Flexion and extension views of the cervical spine often show subluxation at the atlantoaxial or mid-cervical levels; surprisingly, this causes few symptoms in the majority of cases.

Blood investigations

Some degree of normocytic, hypochromic anaemia is common. In active phases the ESR is raised, C-reactive protein may be present and mucoprotein levels are high. Serological tests for rheumatoid factor are positive in about 80 per cent of patients with full-blown rheumatoid arthritis.

Diagnosis

The minimal criteria for considering a diagnosis of rheumatoid disease are: (1) bilateral, symmetrical polyarthritis involving (2) the proximal joints of the hands or feet, present for (3) at least 6 weeks. If, in addition, there are subcutaneous nodules or x-ray signs of periarticular erosions, the diagnosis is certain. *A positive test for rheumatoid factor in the absence of the above features is not sufficient evidence of rheumatoid arthritis, nor does a negative test exclude the diagnosis if the other features are all present.* The chief value of the rheumatoid factor tests is in the assessment of prognosis: persistently high titres herald more serious disease.

In the differential diagnosis of polyarthritis several disorders must be considered.

HEBERDEN'S ARTHROPATHY   affects the *distal* interphalangeal joints, and causes a nodular arthritis with radiologically obvious osteophytes – all of which are absent in the erosive arthritis of rheumatoid disease.

REITER'S DISEASE   usually affects the larger joints and the lumbosacral spine. There is a history of urethritis or colitis and often also conjunctivitis.

ANKYLOSING SPONDYLITIS   may involve the peripheral joints, but it is primarily a disease of the sacroiliac and intervertebral joints, causing back pain and progressive stiffness.

POLYARTICULAR GOUT   affects large and small joints, and tophi on fingers and toes may be mistaken for joint effusions. On x-ray the erosions are quite different from those of rheumatoid arthritis; the diagnosis can be clinched by finding birefringent crystals in the joint fluid.

SERONEGATIVE POLYARTHRITIS   is a feature of a number of conditions vaguely related to rheumatoid arthritis: psoriatic arthritis, juvenile chronic arthritis (Still's disease), systemic lupus erythematosus and other connective-tissue diseases. These are considered in later sections.

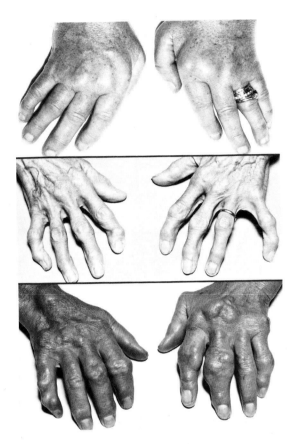

4.6 Rheumatoid arthritis – differential diagnosis These three patients all presented with painful swollen finger joints. In the upper figure it is the proximal joints which are enlarged and deformed (rheumatoid arthritis); in the middle figure the distal joints are the worst (Heberden's osteoarthritis); while in the lower the asymmetrical nodules are actually large tophi (gout).

SARCOIDOSIS may present with a symmetrical small joint polyarthritis and no bone involvement. Erythema nodosum and hilar lymphadenopathy are clues to the diagnosis. Another form of the disease, with granulomatous infiltration of bone, synovium and other organs, is more common in Negroes. In addition to arthritis and tenosynovitis, x-rays show punched-out 'cysts' and cortical destruction of the bones of the hand and foot. The ESR is raised and the Kveim test may be positive.

POLYMYALGIA RHEUMATICA occurs mostly in middle-aged or elderly women, causing marked post-inactivity stiffness and weakness. Pain is most severe around the pectoral and pelvic girdles; tenderness is in muscles rather than joints. The ESR is almost always high. This is a form of giant-cell arteritis and carries the risk of temporal arteritis resulting in blindness. Corticosteroids provide rapid and dramatic relief of all symptoms.

Treatment

The management of rheumatoid arthritis is guided by four simple injunctions: (1) *stop the synovitis;* (2) *prevent deformity;* (3) *reconstruct*; and (4) *rehabilitate.* A multidisciplinary approach is needed from the beginning; the physician, surgeon, physiotherapist, occupational therapist, orthotist and social worker must co-operate as a team.

(1) STOP THE SYNOVITIS

Anti-inflammatory drugs Mild to moderate synovitis can be controlled with appropriate non-steroidal anti-inflammatory drugs (NSAID). Such drugs are not curative, do not influence the progress of erosions and do not lower the ESR, but they do control pain and stiffness and therefore improve function. Side-effects are common (rashes, gastrointestinal symptoms, peptic ulceration) but reversible.

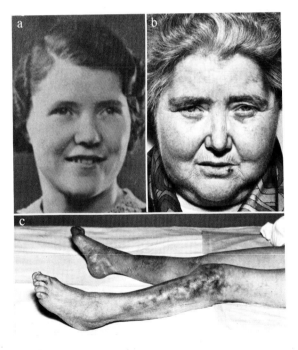

4.7 Treatment of rheumatoid arthritis – (1) control the synovitis Anti-inflammatory drugs are necessary – but can be harmful. (a) This young woman on corticosteroids became (b) severely Cushingoid. (c) This patient had multiple ecchymoses which, combined with tissue-paper skin, increase the risk of limb surgery.

Specific anti-rheumatic drugs Gold, penicillamine and immunosuppressive drugs have a direct action on the immunopathological process and can control disease progress. However, they all have unpredictable – and potentially lethal – side-effects on the kidney, liver and haemopoietic system. They are, therefore, usually introduced only when other measures have failed; but in severe cases with florid synovitis, high ESR and strongly positive rheumatoid factor tests (when simpler measures are likely to fail) they may be used much earlier. Their effects must always be monitored by regular blood tests and by liver and renal function tests. Dosage should be adjusted with great caution; the rule is: 'Start low, go slow'. It may take 6–12 weeks before the patient improves.

Corticosteroids So effectively do these relieve joint pain and stiffness that their use is a constant temptation; a temptation to be resisted, however, because of their adverse effects on metabolism, adrenal function, bone structure and soft-tissue integrity. With experience and discipline they can be used (a) during severe, incapacitating exacerbations, to help weather the storm while waiting for gold or penicillamine to start acting; (b) when no other treatment helps; and (c) in the rare instances of fulminating disease.

Rest and splintage No drug will reduce joint inflammation more effectively than rest and immobilization. This is ideally indicated for acute exacerbations but night splints can be used intermittently at any stage of the disease.

Intra-articular injections Corticosteroids and cytotoxic drugs, like nitrogen mustard, are highly effective when injected into inflamed joints or tendon sheaths. However, they should be used sparingly, for repeated injections can cause cartilage or tendon damage. Radiocolloids have been used to produce synovial irradiation. Yttrium-90 (5 mCi) can be injected on an outpatient basis, provided the limb is firmly splinted to reduce absorption of the isotope.

Synovectomy Even at an early stage of the disease, if all other measures fail, operative synovectomy is justified. With the appearance of increasingly potent drugs, this is seldom called for.

(2) PREVENT DEFORMITY

Physiotherapy Inflamed joints must be rested, but should also be put through a full passive range of

movement each day. As disease activity subsides, active exercises are encouraged.

Splintage Established deformities are seldom correctable by splints, but, if anticipated, can often be prevented by judicious splinting.

Tendon surgery Tendon rupture leads to fixed deformity. It should be diagnosed early and treated by tendon suture or replacement, particularly in the wrist and hand.

Joint surgery Soft-tissue stabilization of the wrist or finger joints can prevent increasing destruction and deformity. Excision of the radial head or the distal end of the ulna are simple methods of relieving local pain and stiffness.

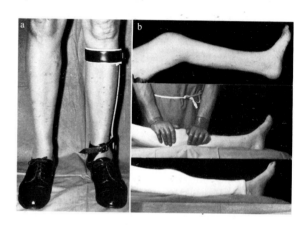

4.8 Treatment of rheumatoid arthritis – (2) prevent deformity (a) Splintage to rest inflamed joints may, if started early, halt the progress of deformity. (b) An early fixed deformity of the knee can be corrected by gentle manipulation and temporary plaster splintage.

(3) RECONSTRUCT

Advanced joint destruction, instability and deformity are clear indications for reconstructive surgery, often combined with synovectomy of the joint or tendons. Arthrodesis, osteotomy and replacement all have their place and are considered in the appropriate chapters.

(4) REHABILITATE

Rehabilitation should not be seen as a rearguard action; it accompanies all stages of treatment

ARTHRODESIS

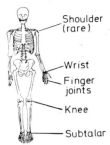

EXCISION

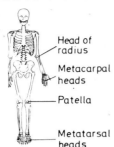

JOINT REPLACEMENT

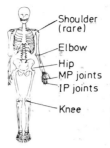

4.9 Treatment of rheumatoid arthritis – (3) reconstruct Sites where each operation may be useful.

from the start, and includes functional assessment, special training, social integration and psychological adjustment.

A full understanding of the patient's specific needs must influence treatment. Some patients are well motivated and crave to return to work and domestic independence; others are passive and dependent. For the one group mechanical aids, special utensils, adjustment of home and work space are essential adjuncts to medical and surgical treatment; for the other the support of family and friends may be all that is wanted.

Ankylosing spondylitis

This chronic inflammatory disorder of the spine and sacroiliac joints is characterized by pain and stiffness of the back, with variable involvement of peripheral joints. Its prevalence is about 0.1 per cent in western Europe, but is much lower in American blacks and African Negroes. Males are affected more frequently than females (ratios vary from 4:1 to 10:1) and the usual age of onset is between 15 and 25 years.

Cause

Genetic predisposition is important. The disease is much commoner in family members than in the general population, and HLA-B27 is present in both patients and half of their first-degree relatives. But, as only a fraction of people with HLA-B27 develop ankylosing spondylitis, there must be some additional 'trigger'. Since classic ankylosing spondylitis is sometimes associated with genitourinary or bowel infection, and disorders such as Reiter's disease and ulcerative colitis cause vertebral and sacroiliac changes indistinguishable from those of ankylosing spondylitis, it is thought that lymphatic drainage to the spine may be important.

Pathology

There are two basic lesions; synovitis of diarthrodial joints; and inflammation at the fibro-osseous junctions of syndesmotic joints and tendons.

Synovitis of the sacroiliac and vertebral facet joints causes destruction of articular cartilage and periarticular bone. The costovertebral joints also are frequently involved, leading to diminished respiratory excursion. When peripheral joints are affected the same changes occur.

Inflammation of the fibro-osseous junctions affects the intervertebral discs, sacroiliac ligaments, symphysis pubis, manubrium sterni and the bony insertions of large tendons. Pathological changes proceed in three stages: (1) an inflammatory reaction with round-cell infiltration, granulation tissue formation and erosion of adjacent bone; (2) replacement of the granulation tissue by fibrous tissue; and (3) ossification of the fibrous tissue, leading to ankylosis of the joint.

Ossification across the surface of the disc gives rise to small bony bridges or *syndesmophytes* linking adjacent vertebral bodies. If many vertebrae are involved the spine may become absolutely rigid.

Symptoms

The disease starts insidiously, with intermittent backache and stiffness recurring at intervals over a number of years.* Symptoms are worse in the early morning and after inactivity. Referred pain may appear as sciatica and some patients are mistakenly treated for intervertebral disc prolapse. Gradually pain and stiffness become continuous and other symptoms, such as pain and swelling of joints or tenderness at the insertion of the tendo Achillis, may appear. In 10 per cent of patients the disease starts with an asymmetrical polyarthritis.

Signs

Early on there is little to see apart from some loss of spinal mobility. In established cases the posture is typical: flattening of the lumbar lordosis, a forward thrust of the neck and slight flexion of the hips and knees. There may be tenderness over the dorsolumbar spine and sacroiliac joints.

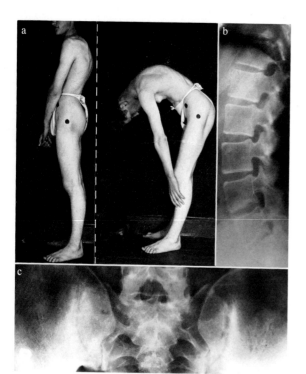

4.10 Ankylosing spondylitis – early The early features are (a) a stiff spine, (b) 'squaring' of the lumbar vertebrae, and (c) bilateral sacroiliac erosion.

Spinal movements are diminished in all directions, but loss of extension is both the earliest and the most severe disability. It is revealed dramatically by the 'wall test': the patient is asked to stand with his back to the wall; heels, buttocks, scapulae and occiput should all be able to touch the wall simultaneously. If extension is seriously diminished the patient will find this impossible. In the most advanced stage the spine may be completely ankylosed from occiput to sacrum – sometimes in positions of grotesque deformity.

Chest expansion, which should be at least 5 cm in young men, is often markedly decreased. In old people, who may have pulmonary disease, this test is unreliable.

If peripheral joints are involved (usually shoulders, hips and knees) they show the features of inflammatory arthritis: swelling, tenderness, effusion and loss of mobility.

EXTRASKELETAL MANIFESTATIONS include ocular inflammation (in about one-third of patients), aortic valve disease, carditis and, occasionally, pulmonary fibrosis.

X-rays

The cardinal sign – and often the earliest – is erosion and fuzziness of the *sacroiliac joints*. Later there may be periarticular sclerosis, especially on the iliac side of the joint, and finally bony ankylosis.

The earliest *vertebral* change is flattening of the normal anterior concavity of the vertebral body ('squaring'). Later, ossification across the intervertebral discs produces delicate syndesmophytes spanning the gaps between adjacent vertebrae. Bridging at several levels gives the appearance of a 'bamboo spine'.

Peripheral joints may show erosive arthritis, or progressive bony ankylosis.

Special investigations

Serological tests for rheumatoid factor are negative. The ESR is elevated during active phases of the disease. HLA-B27 is present in 90 per cent of cases.

---

*Persistent backache in a youth is due to ankylosing spondylitis, infection or a tumour.

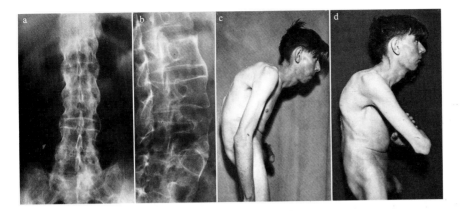

4.11 Ankylosing spondylitis – late   (a, b) Bony bridges (syndesmophytes) between the vertebral bodies convert the spine into a rigid column ('bamboo spine'); note that the sacroiliac joints have fused. Spinal osteotomy may be necessary at this stage: (c) before operation this man could see only a few paces ahead; (d) after osteotomy his back is still rigid, but his posture, function and outlook are vastly improved.

Differential diagnosis

THE SERONEGATIVE SPONDARTHRITIDES A number of disorders are associated with vertebral and sacroiliac lesions indistinguishable from those of ankylosing spondylitis. They are Reiter's disease, psoriatic arthritis, ulcerative colitis, Crohn's disease, Whipple's disease and Behçet's syndrome (Moll *et al.*, 1974). In each there are certain characteristic features: the rash or nail changes of psoriasis, intestinal ulceration in enterocolitis, genitourinary and ocular inflammation in Reiter's disease, buccal and genital ulceration in Behçet's syndrome. Yet there is considerable overlap between them; all show some familial aggregation and all share the antigen, HLA-B27.

ANKYLOSING HYPEROSTOSIS (FORESTIER'S DISEASE) This is a fairly common disorder, predominantly of elderly men, characterized by widespread ossification of ligaments and tendon insertions. X-rays show pronounced but asymmetrical intervertebral spur formation and bridging throughout the dorsolumbar spine; the anterior and right lateral aspects are the most severely affected (Forestier and Rotes-Querol, 1950). Although it bears a superficial resemblance to ankylosing spondylitis, it is not an inflammatory disease, spinal pain and stiffness are seldom severe, the sacroiliac joints are not eroded and the ESR is normal. The cause of this condition is unknown, but it is said to be associated with diabetes and obesity.

Treatment

In the absence of a specific agent, treatment consists of anti-inflammatory and analgesic drugs, the preservation of movement and the prevention of deformity. Active movement and exercises are encouraged, under cover of a potent analgesic/anti-inflammatory drug such as indomethacin or phenylbutazone. Postural training is aimed at preventing deformity; if ankylosis is inevitable, let it at least be in a good position. Prolonged rest and immobilization, effective in most inflammatory joint diseases, are *contraindicated* because they tend to increase osteoporosis and ankylosis.

Stiffness of the hips can be treated by joint replacement, though this seldom provides more than moderate mobility. Deformity of the spine may be severe enough to warrant lumbar or cervical osteotomy; these are difficult and potentially hazardous procedures.

Psoriatic arthritis

About 4 per cent of patients with chronic polyarthritis have psoriasis; not all, however, have psoriatic arthritis, which is a distinct entity and not simply 'RA plus psoriasis'. Unlike rheumatoid arthritis, it is common in men and runs in families. Individual joints and tendons show the features of a chronic synovitis, with cartilage and bone destruction which may be unusually severe ('arthritis mutilans'). However, rheumatoid nodules are not seen.

Symptoms and signs

Psoriasis of the skin or nails usually precedes the arthritis. Occasionally the condition starts with recurrent tenosynovitis. The distinctive feature is involvement of the *distal* joints of the hands and feet. This may go on to such severe destruction that the finger-tips are either completely flail or are severely

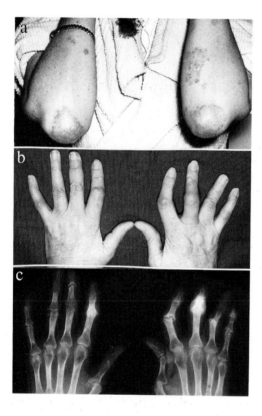

4.12 Psoriatic arthritis (1) (a) Psoriasis of the elbows and forearms; (b) typical finger deformities, and (c) x-rays show *distal* joint involvement – so clearly the disease is not simply rheumatoid arthritis in a patient with psoriasis.

deformed. Large joints also may be involved and tenosynovitis may cause fixed deformities of the fingers. About a quarter of the patients develop sacroiliitis and/or ankylosing spondylitis. Ocular inflammation occurs in about 30 per cent.

X-RAYS show destruction of the distal and/or proximal inter-phalangeal joints; changes in the large joints are similar to the erosive arthritis of rheumatoid disease. Sacroiliac erosion is fairly common; if the spine is involved the appearances are identical to those of ankylosing spondylitis.

SPECIAL INVESTIGATIONS   Tests for rheumatoid factor are almost always negative; HLA-B27 occurs in 50–60 per cent, especially in those with overt sacroiliitis.

Treatment

GENERAL TREATMENT   aims at controlling the skin disorder with topical preparations, and alleviating joint symptoms with non-steroidal anti-inflammatory drugs. In resistant forms of arthritis immunosuppressive agents (azathioprine and methotrexate) have proved effective.

LOCAL TREATMENT   consists of judicious splintage to avoid undue deformity, and surgery for unstable joints. Arthrodesis of the distal interphalangeal joints may greatly improve function.

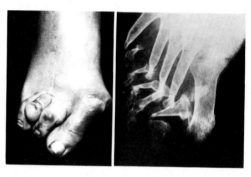

4.13 Psoriatic arthritis (2)   The feet also may be affected, and this patient first presented at an ortho-paedic clinic.

Reiter's disease and reactive arthritis

'Classic' Reiter's disease is a clinical triad: poly-arthritis, conjunctivitis and non-specific urethritis. However, the term is now used more loosely for a *reactive arthritis* associated with non-specific urogenital or bowel infection. It is probably the commonest type of large-joint polyarthritis in young men. Familial aggregation, overlap with other forms of seronegative spondyloarthritis in first-degree relatives, and an increased frequency of HLA-B27 in all these disorders point to a genetic predisposition. *Lymphogranuloma venereum* and *Chlamydia trachomatis* have been implicated as urogenital infective agents, but arthritis also occurs with bowel infection due to *Shigella, Salmonella* or *Yersinia enterocolitica*.

The joints themselves are not infected; the synovitis is the end stage of an abnormal immune response to infection elsewhere or to the products of that infection.

Symptoms and signs

Reiter's disease affects mainly the large joints and especially the knee and ankle. Often it starts as an acute arthritis with marked effusion (usually of the knee), suggesting gout or mechanical derangement, until other joints become involved. Tenosynovitis and plantar fasciitis are common. Backache and stiffness, due to sacroiliitis and spondylitis, occur in the majority of patients at some stage. Although this is said to be a self-limiting disease, 80 per cent of patients continue to have symptoms for many years.

Urogenital and bowel infections can take the form of urethritis, cystitis, prostatitis, cervicitis and dysentery. The urethritis is not necessarily sexually acquired and the condition may occur in children.

Ocular lesions include conjunctivitis, episcleritis and uveitis. *Buccal ulceration* and *skin lesions*, including balanitis, also occur.

X-RAYS are at first normal, but after many months may show an erosive arthritis. Sacroiliac and vertebral changes are similar to those of ankylosing spondylitis.

SPECIAL INVESTIGATIONS Tests for HLA-B27 are positive in 75 per cent of patients with sacroiliitis. The ESR may be high in the active phase of the disease. The causative organism can sometimes be isolated from urethral fluids or faeces, and tests for antibodies may be positive.

Differential diagnosis

GOUT OR INFECTIVE ARTHRITIS may be mistaken for Reiter's disease. Examination of synovial fluid for organisms and crystals excludes these disorders.

ENTEROPATHIC ARTHRITIS Ulcerative colitis and Crohn's disease may be associated with subacute synovitis, causing pain and swelling of one or more of the peripheral joints. This subsides when the intestinal disease is controlled.

GONOCOCCAL ARTHRITIS takes two forms: (1) bacterial infection of the joint; and (2) a reactive arthritis with sterile joint fluid. A history of venereal infection further complicates the distinction from Reiter's disease, and diagnosis may depend on identifying the organism or gonococcal antibodies.

Treatment

GENERAL TREATMENT is indicated for active urogenital or bowel infection; a short course of antibiotics is usually sufficient, but for *Chlamydia* tetracycline daily for 6 months is recommended.

LOCAL TREATMENT is non-specific and palliative: rest and splintage if arthritis is severe, and then prolonged administration of anti-inflammatory agents while waiting for spontaneous remission.

Juvenile chronic polyarthritis

Juvenile chronic polyarthritis is the preferred term for non-infective inflammatory joint disease in children under 16 years. It embraces a cluster of disorders which includes rheumatoid arthritis, ankylosing spondylitis, psoriatic arthritis and systemic lupus erythematosus that may happen to start before the age of 16; it includes also an inflammatory polyarthritis that *characteristically* affects young children and which was first described by George Frederick Still in 1897.

Symptoms and signs

Still's disease occurs in three overlapping forms.

A pauciarticular arthritis (L. *paucus* = few) causing pain and swelling, usually of medium-sized joints (knees, ankles, elbows and wrists) as well as the cervical spine. In about 10 per cent there is chronic iridocyclitis. Systemic features are not marked.

A monarticular arthritis – at least at the onset – usually affecting the knee. In about half of these patients the disease remains confined to one or two joints; in the remainder it becomes polyarticular.

Systemic Still's disease which starts with intermittent fever, rashes and malaise, the joints being affected only after several months. In severe,

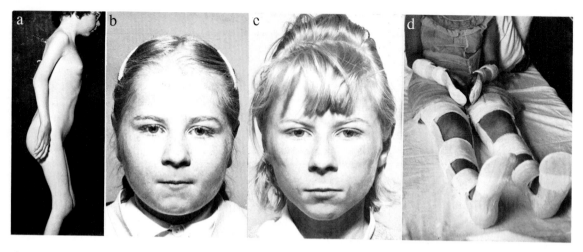

4.14 Juvenile chronic polyarthritis (a) Polyarthritis results in flexion deformities of the elbows, wrists, hips and knees. Steroids are rarely necessary, and in this young girl (b) they produced stunting of growth and Cushing's syndrome, which fortunately recovered (c) after steroids were discontinued. In the acute stage, splints (d) are useful.

active disease there may also be lymphadeno-pathy, splenomegaly and hepatomegaly. In long-standing cases there is a serious risk of amyloid-osis, which (according to Ansell and Bywaters, 1978) is nearly always fatal.

Complications

Ankylosis While most patients recover good function, some loss of movement is common. Hips, knees and elbows may be unable to extend fully, and in the ankylosing spondylitic form of juvenile chronic polyarthritis the spine, hips and knees may be almost rigid. Temporomandibular ankylosis and stiffness of the cervical spine can make general anaesthesia difficult and dangerous.

Growth defects There is a general retardation of growth, aggravated by prolonged corticosteroid therapy. In addition, epiphyseal disturbances lead to characteristic deformities (external torsion of the tibia, dysplasia of the distal ulna, underdevelopment of the mandible, shortness of the neck and scoliosis).

Fractures Children aged under 5 years with chronic joint disease may suffer osteoporosis and they are prone to fractures.

Treatment

GENERAL TREATMENT is similar to that of rheumatoid arthritis. Corticosteroids should be used only for severe systemic disease and chronic iridocyclitis unresponsive to topical therapy.

LOCAL TREATMENT aims to prevent stiffness and deformity. Night splints are useful for the wrists, hands, knees and ankles; prone lying for some period each day may prevent flexion contracture of the hips. If cervical ankylosis threatens, a collar should be used to prevent stiffening in flexion. Between periods of splinting, active exercises are encouraged.

Fixed deformities may need correction by serial plasters; when progress is no longer being made, joint capsulotomy may help.

For painful, eroded joints operation is indicated. Useful procedures include: custom-designed arthroplasties of the hip and knee (even in children), and arthrodesis of wrists, ankles and talar joints.

Systemic lupus erythematosus

Systemic lupus erythematosus occurs mainly in young females (F:M ratio = 9:1). As with rheumatoid arthritis, there is probably a viral infection in a genetically predisposed individual, resulting in disturbance of the immunoregulatory system.

The characteristic pathological lesion is fibrinoid necrosis of the small vessels. A wide variety of inflammatory lesions occurs in the kidney, spleen, lung and other organs. Fibrinoid deposits in the synovium are associated with mild inflammation, and cartilage destruction is seldom severe.

Symptoms and signs

Although joint pain is usual, it is not a salient feature; systemic changes (malaise, anorexia, weight loss and fever) are more conspicuous. The arthritis of systemic lupus is described as non-destructive and non-deforming. In fact, pain may be due to tenosynovitis rather than joint involvement, and sometimes this goes on to tendon rupture. Occasionally polyarthritis is more severe and may even resemble rheumatoid arthritis. Aseptic necrosis of the hip and other joints is not uncommon, but it is uncertain whether this occurs except in patients on corticosteroid therapy.

The diagnosis of systemic lupus erythematosus rests on the pattern of systemic involvement, which includes skin rashes and ulceration, Raynaud's phenomenon, splenomegaly, hepatomegaly, and disorders of the kidney, heart, lung, eyes and central nervous system. Anaemia, leucopenia and elevation of the ESR are common. Tests for antinuclear factor are always positive. Rheumatoid factor tests also are positive in 25 per cent of cases.

Treatment

Corticosteroids are indicated for severe systemic disease. Joint symptoms can usually be controlled with anti-inflammatory drugs; physiotherapy and night splints may be needed.

Further reading

Ansell, B. M. and Bywaters, E. G. L. (1978) Juvenile chronic polyarthritis. In *Copeman's Textbook of the Rheumatic Diseases*, 5th edn. Ed. by J. T. Scott. Edinburgh: Churchill Livingstone

Forestier, J. and Rotes-Querol, J. (1950) Senile ankylosing hyperostosis of the spine. *Annals of the Rheumatic Diseases* **9**, 321–330

Kammer, G. M., Soter, N. A., Gibson, D. J. and Scher, P. H. (1979) Psoriatic arthritis: a clinical, immunologic and HLA study of 100 patients. *Seminars in Arthritis and Rheumatism* **9**, 75–97

Moll, J. M. H., Haslock, I., Macrae, I. F. and Wright, V. (1974) Associations between ankylosing spondylitis, psoriatic arthritis, Reiter's disease, the intestinal arthropathies and Behçet's syndrome. *Medicine* **53**, 343

Solomon, L. (1979) Surgery of the major joints in arthritis. *Medicine* **12**, 600

Solomon, L. and Berman, L. (1979) Rheumatic disorders of the lumbar spine. In *Disorders of the Lumbar Spine*. Ed. by A. J. Helfet and D. M. G. Lee. Philadelphia: Lippincott

Solomon, L., Beighton, P., Valkenburg, H. A., Robin, G. and Soskolne, C. L. (1975) Rheumatic disorders in the South African Negro. *South African Medical Journal* **49**, 1292–1296

Ziff, M. (1973) Pathophysiology of rheumatoid arthritis. *Federation Proceedings* **32**, 131–133

Degenerative Arthritis

5

In contrast to the rheumatic disorders, there is a group of conditions in which some physical or chemical agent causes a local reaction resulting, eventually, in degeneration of articular cartilage. At one end of the spectrum is the acute synovitis associated with abnormal crystal deposition; at the other extreme is the slow cartilage disintegration of osteoarthritis.

Gout

This is a disorder of purine metabolism characterized by hyperuricaemia and recurrent attacks of acute synovitis due to urate crystal deposition. Late changes include cartilage degeneration. It is much commoner in males (20:1) and is rarely seen before the menopause in females. Two forms are recognized: (1) *primary* (95 per cent), an inherited disorder with overproduction or underexcretion of uric acid; and (2) *secondary* (5 per cent), resulting from acquired conditions that cause uric acid overproduction (e.g. myeloproliferative disorders) or underexcretion (e.g. renal failure).

Pathology

Uric acid crystals are deposited in synovium, tendons and articular cartilage and appear in synovial fluid. They excite attacks of acute inflammation. In chronic gouty arthritis there is cartilage degeneration and periarticular 'cyst' formation due to accumulation of monosodium urate. Large urate deposits cause cartilage and soft-tissue tophi (L. *tophus* = porous stone); juxta-articular bone may show extensive destruction and replacement by pultaceous material.

Symptoms and signs

THE ACUTE ATTACK   The sudden onset of severe joint pain which lasts for a few days is typical of acute gout. This is usually spontaneous but may be precipitated by minor trauma, operation, un-accustomed exercise or alcohol. The commonest sites are the metatarsophalangeal joint of the big toe, the ankle and finger joints, and the olecranon bursa. The skin looks red and shiny and there is considerable swelling. The joint feels hot and extremely tender, suggesting a cellulitis or septic arthritis. Sometimes the only feature is acute pain and tenderness in the heel or the sole of the foot.

Hyperuricaemia is present at some stage, though not necessarily during an acute attack. The diagnosis can be established beyond doubt by finding the characteristic negatively birefringent urate crystals in the synovial fluid (a drop is examined by polarized light).

CHRONIC GOUT   Recurrent acute attacks may eventually merge into polyarticular gout. Joint erosion causes chronic pain, stiffness and deformity; if the finger joints are affected this may be mistaken for rheumatoid arthritis. Tophi may appear around joints, over the olecranon, in the pinna of the ear and – less frequently – in almost any other tissue. A large tophus can ulcerate through the skin and discharge its chalky material. Renal lesions include calculi, due to uric acid precipitation in the urine, and parenchymal disease due to deposition of monosodium urate from the blood.

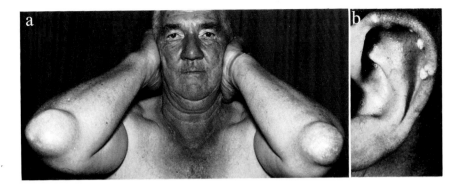

5.1 Gout This man with chronic gout declares his diagnosis at a glance, with his rubicund face, bulging olecranon bursae, and tophi.

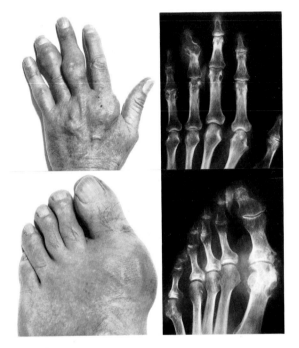

5.2 Gout In both the hand and the foot, joints are asymmetrically swollen; x-rays show large periarticular excavations, which are filled with uric acid deposits. The joints felt curiously 'pulpy'.

X-rays

During the acute attack x-rays show only soft-tissue swelling. Chronic gout may show: (1) symmetrical, punched-out 'cysts' in the periarticular bone; (2) joint space narrowing and secondary osteoarthritis; or (3) ill-defined bone destruction, which may be so marked as to resemble malignant disease.

Differential diagnosis

INFECTION   Cellulitis, septic bursitis, an infected bunion or septic arthritis must all be excluded, if necessary by immediate joint aspiration.

REITER'S DISEASE   This may present with acute pain and swelling of a knee or ankle, but the history is more protracted and the response to anti-inflammatory drugs less dramatic.

PSEUDOGOUT   Pyrophosphate crystal deposition may cause an acute arthritis indistinguishable from gout – except that it tends to affect large rather than small joints and is equally common in women and men. Articular calcification may show on x-ray. Demonstrating the crystals in synovial fluid establishes the diagnosis.

RHEUMATOID ARTHRITIS   Polyarticular gout affecting the fingers may be mistaken for rheumatoid arthritis, and elbow tophi for rheumatoid nodules. In difficult cases biopsy will establish the diagnosis.

Treatment

The acute attack should be treated by resting the joint and giving indomethacin 50 mg or phenylbutazone 200 mg 6-hourly. Colchicine is less effective and may cause diarrhoea, nausea and vomiting. A tense joint effusion may require aspiration and local injection of hydrocortisone.

Interval therapy is indicated only if the serum urate (uric acid) is above 0.48 mmol/l (8 mg/100 ml), if acute attacks are frequent, for chronic tophaceous gout or for renal complications. If renal function is normal, uricosuric drugs (probenecid or ethebenecid) can be used. Allopurinol, a xanthine oxidase inhibitor, is usually preferred, and is specifically indicated for severe tophaceous gout and for cases associated with marked uric acid overproduction and renal involvement.

These drugs should never be started except under cover of an anti-inflammatory preparation, otherwise they may actually precipitate an acute attack.

Chondrocalcinosis

Deposition of calcium pyrophosphate dihydrate (CPPD) crystals in joint tissues is common, especially in the elderly. Usually it is asymptomatic; sometimes, however, the effects resemble those of gout. Chondrocalcinosis is sometimes familial. Though usually idiopathic, it may be associated with hyperparathyroidism, idiopathic haemochromatosis, gout and diabetes.

Pathology

CPPD crystals are probably formed around chondrocytes in articular cartilage and then extruded into the joint, giving rise to an inflammatory reaction similar to gout. This is more likely in ageing and abnormal cartilage and is, therefore, often associated with other arthritides. The immediate cause of crystal shedding is believed to be a sudden change in ionic calcium and pyrophosphate equilibrium in cartilage (e.g. after acute illness or operation), or physical disruption of cartilage (e.g. due to trauma), or enzymatic degradation of the matrix (e.g. in inflammatory arthritis). Chronic chondrocalcinosis often precedes, and is assumed to predispose to, the development of osteoarthritis. In about one-third of cases there is intervertebral calcification.

Symptoms and signs

The patient may present with an *acute non-septic arthritis* ('pseudogout'); this is even more puzzling if the serum uric acid is raised; CPPD and urate gout often go together. The knee is the usual site but other large joints can be involved. Unlike urate gout, it seldom affects the big toe. Diagnosis may be confirmed by finding positively birefringent crystals in the synovial fluid.

Chronic chondrocalcinosis is usually asymptomatic, but some patients develop polyarticular osteoarthritis. Spine changes may be similar to those of ankylosing hyperostosis (page 43).

X-rays

The characteristic feature is calcification of articular cartilage and of fibrocartilaginous structures such as the menisci of the knee, the triangular plate of the wrist, the symphysis pubis and intervertebral discs. Long-standing cases may show the chronic degenerative changes of osteoarthritis and pronounced, widespread vertebral spur formation.

Differential diagnosis

GOUT   The differentiation from gout is discussed on page 49.

HYPERPARATHYROIDISM   Intra-articular calcification is a feature of primary hyperparathyroidism. Investigations should include x-rays of the fingers for subperiosteal erosions and blood tests for hypercalcaemia and raised parathyroid hormone levels.

HAEMOCHROMATOSIS   Although uncommon, the arthropathy of haemochromatosis is so characteristic that the diagnosis should not be missed. There is progressive degenerative arthritis of the finger joints, and x-rays show calcification in multiple joints and in the intervertebral discs. The serum iron and iron-binding capacity are raised.

OCHRONOSIS   This inborn error of metabolism is due to the absence of homogentisic acid oxidase in the liver and kidney. Homogentisic acid is deposited as a dark brown pigment in connective tissues, including hyaline and fibrocartilage. Clinically the disease presents at around the fourth decade with pain and stiffness of the spine and the larger joints. X-rays show calcification of the intervertebral discs progressing to obliteration of the disc spaces and ankylosis.* The peripheral joints may show chondrocalcinosis and severe osteoarthritis. Excretion of homogentisic acid causes the urine to turn black on standing.

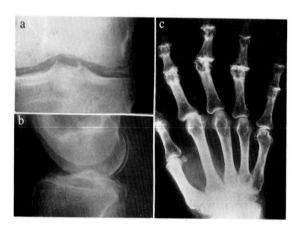

5.3 Chondrocalcinosis Calcium pyrophosphate crystals may be deposited in cartilage, causing (a) calcification of menisci and (b) a thin, dense line on the surface of the articular cartilage. Usually no specific cause is found, but chondrocalcinosis may be associated with a variety of disorders. (c) This patient has haemochromatosis; degenerative arthritis of the proximal finger joints is typical – the spine also was affected.

*Gout strikes the small joints, pseudogout the large joints, and ochronosis the spine.

OTHER CRYSTAL DEPOSITION DISORDERS   Mixed deposits of pyrophosphate and hydroxyapatite are fairly common in joint disorders (Dieppe *et al.*, 1979). However, it is unclear under what conditions they may cause symptoms.

Treatment

The treatment of pseudogout is the same as that of acute gout: rest and appropriate anti-inflammatory therapy.

Chronic chondrocalcinosis appears to be irreversible. Fortunately it usually causes few symptoms and little disability. When it is associated with progressive joint degeneration the treatment is essentially that for secondary osteoarthritis.

manifest as clinical osteoarthritis (Byers *et al.*, 1970).

We distinguish, therefore, between two types of cartilage degeneration: (1) *limited cartilage loss*, seen mainly away from load-bearing areas and probably due to 'wear and tear'; and (2) *progressive cartilage destruction*, which is always maximal in the major load-bearing area and is associated with symptomatic osteoarthritis.

There is no single cause of osteoarthritis; it results from a disparity between the stress applied to articular cartilage and the ability of the cartilage to withstand that stress. This may be due to increased stress, weak cartilage or poor subchondral bone.

Osteoarthritis

Osteoarthritis is a degenerative joint disorder in which there is progressive loss of articular cartilage accompanied by new bone formation and capsular fibrosis. It is defined as *primary* when no cause is obvious, and as *secondary* when it follows a demonstrable abnormality.

It is much more common in some joints (the hip, knee and spine) than in others (the elbow and ankle). Moreover, individual joints are affected with differing frequency in men and women (terminal interphalangeal osteoarthritis chiefly affects postmenopausal women), and in different ethnic groups (the hip is seldom involved in Africans).

Cause

The most obvious thing about osteoarthritis is that it increases in frequency with age. This does not mean that it is an expression of senescence; it simply shows that osteoarthritis takes many years to develop. To be sure, cartilage ageing does occur, resulting in splitting and flaking of the surface, diminished cellularity, reduction of the proteoglycan ground substance, and loss of elasticity with a concomitant decrease in breaking strength. But, although these changes are qualitatively similar to those of osteoarthritis, they differ from it in two important respects: they are not progressive, and they occur in areas that seldom

5.4 Osteoarthritis – causal factors (1)   In the normal joint (a) the forces are evenly distributed. The remaining diagrams show the three ways in which cartilage may be damaged: (b) deformity increases the stress in a localized area by concentrating the load at this point; (c) cartilage which has been weakened by some preceding disorder is unable to bear even normal loads; (d) if the subarticular bone is abnormal it may be unable to support the cartilage adequately.

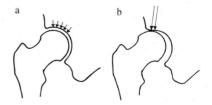

5.5 Osteoarthritis – causal factors (2)   (a) Normally, loading forces are widely distributed over the articular surfaces and stress is minimal. (b) Instability, subluxation or deformity may decrease the area of contact; the same force is now concentrated over a smaller area, stress is greatly increased, and the surface may break down.

INCREASED STRESS

Stress is load per unit area. It may increase because of *increased load* (e.g. in deformities which affect the lever system around a joint) or because of *decreased contact area* (e.g. due to joint incongruity or instability). Both factors operate in varus deformity of the knee – a common precursor of osteoarthritis.

WEAK CARTILAGE

There is normally a loss of cartilage tensile strength with age; add to this any disorder which stiffens the cartilage, making it less resilient (e.g. ochronosis), or softens the cartilage (e.g. chronic inflammation), and progressive destruction may ensue. Crystal deposition has been implicated as a cause of osteoarthritis (Ali, 1980), but the evidence is still incomplete. Polyarticular osteoarthritis and Heberden's arthritis are more likely due to a generalized cartilage defect than to mechanical dysfunction. Generalized bone dysplasias also tend to give osteoarthritis in more than one joint.

POOR ARTICULAR SUPPORT

The subchondral bone may be abnormally fragile (e.g. in osteonecrosis) providing inadequate support for the articular cartilage, or abnormally dense (e.g. following fracture healing), and so a poor shock absorber.

Pathology

ARTICULAR CARTILAGE AND BONE   The earliest abnormality is an increase in water content of the cartilage; this is followed by disruption of the large chondromucoprotein molecules and loss of proteoglycans (McDevitt and Muir, 1976). These findings have been ascribed to fatigue failure of the collagen network (Freeman, 1975). As the cartilage becomes oedematous and soft, secondary damage to chondrocytes may cause further matrix breakdown due to release of cell enzymes. Progressive cartilage deformation adds further stress to the collagen network. The first visible signs are softening and splitting of the cartilage surface. Gradually the clefts become more pronounced until there is obvious fraying, or *fibrillation*, of the normally smooth and glistening cartilage.

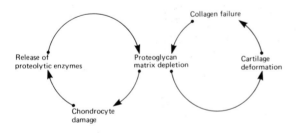

The early changes are sometimes described as *chondromalacia* and, if they are not actually reversible, neither do they necessarily advance to complete articular destruction. There

is even evidence of attempts at repair in the appearance of chondrocyte clusters ('cloning') in the matrix-depleted cartilage, and some workers claim that proteoglycan synthesis is increased up to the time of cartilage failure (Mankin and Lippiello, 1970). The subarticular bone reacts to the increased stress by thickening, which appears on x-ray as sclerosis in the overloaded segment. Cracks in the subchondral bone plate permit pressure transmission to the cancellous bone, resulting in cyst formation. Progressive cartilage disintegration may eventually lead to surface abrasion and complete exposure of bone in areas of peak overload.

As instability increases, the intact cartilage in peripheral unstressed areas proliferates and ossifies, producing bony outgrowths (osteophytes). This 'remodelling' process restores a measure of congruity to the increasingly malopposed joint surfaces. The final appearance is, therefore, determined by the interplay between cartilage loss, bone fragmentation, trabecular sclerosis and osteophytic remodelling; i.e. the balance between destruction and repair.

SYNOVIAL MEMBRANE AND CAPSULE   Some degree of inflammation is usually present in osteoarthritis; occasionally inflammation precedes cartilage damage, but usually it results from the deposition of cartilage and bone detritus onto the synovium. The particles then penetrate to the subsynovial layers and the resultant fibrosis may extend to the capsule which becomes thickened and inelastic; as the fibrous tissue matures it shrinks, thus limiting movement.

Symptoms

There may be a history of some previous disorder or injury of the joint. A typical feature of osteoarthritis is its intermittent course, with periods of symptomatic remission lasting for months or even years. Sometimes, as the joint becomes stiffer (and more stable) it becomes less painful.

PAIN   is the usual presenting symptom. Often it is worse on rising from bed, and again at the end of a day's activity. It is aggravated by extremes of movement or by unaccustomed exertion. Early on it is relieved by rest, but with time, relief comes more slowly and is less complete. The worst is pain in bed at night, when the patient has difficulty finding any position of comfort. Helal (1965) has attributed the pain to three distinct sources: capsular (on forcing extremes), muscular (after exertion) and venous (rest pain). It may also be referred to a distant site – e.g. pain in the knee from osteoarthritis of the hip.

STIFFNESS   is common; at first it occurs after periods of inactivity, later it is constant and progressive.

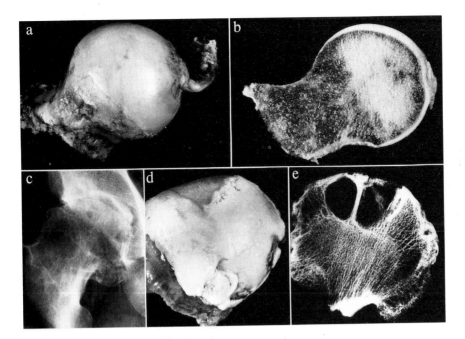

5.6 Osteoarthritis – pathology (a) Normal ageing causes slight degeneration of the articular surface, but the coronal section (b) shows that the cartilage thickness is well preserved even in old age. By contrast, in progressive osteoarthritis (lower row) the weight-bearing area is severely damaged: the x-ray (c) shows cartilage loss at the superior pole and cysts in the underlying bone; the specimen (d) shows that the top of the head was completely denuded of cartilage; and a fine-detail x-ray of the specimen (e) shows that the subchondral bone plate has been perforated.

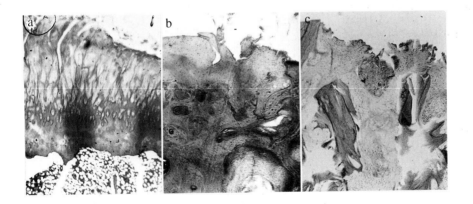

5.7 Osteoarthritis – histology In progressive osteoarthritis (a) deep clefts appear in the cartilage; this is known as fibrillation. Later (b) the cartilage structure is disorganized. Finally, when cartilage gives way (c) the underlying bone also crumbles (note the small trabecular fragments and the complete absence of cartilage).

SWELLING   in peripheral joints may be due to an effusion, to synovial and capsular thickening, or to osteophytes.

DEFORMITY   often precedes the onset of osteo-arthritis (e.g. genu varum), but it may also result from muscle imbalance, capsular contracture or joint instability.

Signs

The pattern of joint involvement varies consider-ably. Usually the patient complains of only one or two joints, but examination may show that others also are affected in varying degrees.

Swelling and deformity may be obvious in peripheral joints; at the hip, deformity is usually masked by postural adjustments of the pelvis and spine. In long-standing cases there is muscle wasting. Tell-tale scars denote previous abnor-malities. Local tenderness is common, and in superficial joints fluid, synovial thickening or osteophytes may be felt.

Movement is always restricted, but is often painless within the permitted range; it may be accompanied by crepitus. Some movements are more curtailed than others; thus, at the hip extension, abduction and internal rotation are the most severely limited.

In the late stages joint instability may occur for any of three reasons: loss of cartilage and bone; asymmetrical capsular contracture; and muscle weakness.

X-rays

The cardinal features are: (1) narrowing of the joint space; (2) subarticular sclerosis; (3) bone cysts; (4) osteophytes. Initially the first three features are usually restricted to the major load-bearing part of the joint, but in late cases and in osteoarthritis following inflammatory disease, the entire joint is affected. Bone density is either normal or increased. Evidence of previous dis-orders (congenital defects, old fractures, rheuma-toid arthritis, chondrocalcinosis) may be present.

Occasionally serial x-rays show a rapid and startling amount of bone destruction. This occurs especially in patients taking large amounts of analgesic and anti-inflammatory drugs and con-tinuing with strenuous activity.

Differential diagnosis

MONARTICULAR SYNOVITIS   Pain, stiffness and swelling of a single large joint may herald the onset of Reiter's disease or rheumatoid arthritis, but eventually other joints become involved.

CRYSTAL DEPOSITION DISEASE   Chronic gout or chondrocalci-nosis may coexist with osteoarthritis or precede it.

ASEPTIC NECROSIS   Idiopathic necrosis causes pain and local effusion. The diagnosis is made on the typical x-ray appear-ances; unlike osteoarthritis, the joint 'space' is preserved because the articular cartilage remains viable.

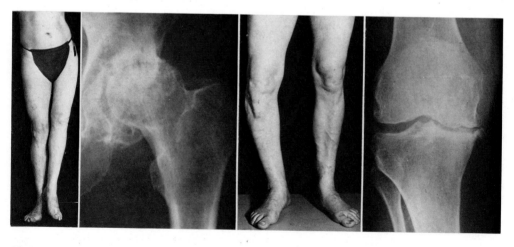

5.8 Osteoarthritis – clinical   Deformity and diminished joint space at the hip and the knee.

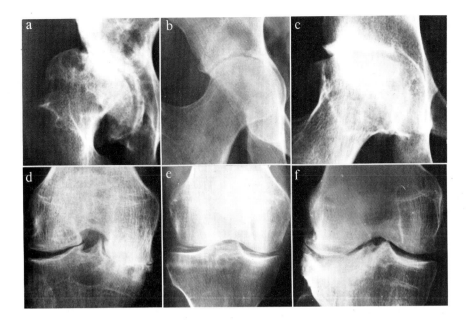

5.9 Osteoarthritis – x-rays   The three types of osteoarthritis are shown in the hip (a, b, c) and the knee (d, e, f). In type I mechanical overload has damaged a localized area of cartilage – the upper pole in this hip (a) and the medial compartment in this knee (d). In type II the articular cartilage was already abnormal – following an inflammatory arthritis of the hip (b) and chondrocalcinosis of the knee (e), so that even normal loads damaged the surfaces. In type III the underlying bone was defective – either too weak as in osteonecrosis of the hip (c) or too sclerotic, as in this old tibial plateau fracture (f) – causing breakdown of the covering cartilage.

Treatment

EARLY
There are three principles in the treatment of early osteoarthritis: (1) relieve pain; (2) increase movement; (3) reduce load.

Pain relief   Analgesics and anti-inflammatory agents can control pain for many years. But overmedication must be avoided; it may lead to rapid 'analgesic degeneration'. Measures to provide local warmth usually give only short-lived relief. Rest periods and modification of activities may be necessary.

Mobilization   A strict programme of exercises is important. Early on, pain is felt mainly at the extremes of movement, so that increasing the range (by exercise or gentle manipulation) reduces capsular strain.

Load reduction   Commonsense measures to reduce joint load include weight loss, the use of a walking

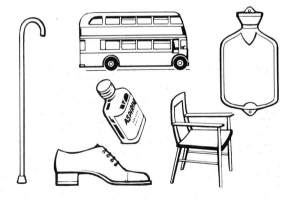

5.10 Osteoarthritis – conservative treatment   Simple measures to relieve pain in osteoarthritis of the hip: analgesics, warmth, a raised heel and a stick; 'don't stand when you can sit, don't walk when you can ride'.

stick, avoidance of unnecessary stress (such as jogging or climbing stairs) and even intermittent periods of complete rest.

INTERMEDIATE

If symptoms and signs increase, then at some joints (chiefly the hip and knee) realignment osteotomy is indicated. It should be done while the joint is still stable and mobile and x-rays show that a major part of the joint 'space' is preserved. Pain relief is often dramatic and is ascribed to (1) vascular decompression of the subchondral bone, and (2) redistribution of loading forces towards less damaged parts of the joint. After femoral osteotomy fibrocartilage may grow to cover exposed bone.

LATE

Progressive joint destruction, with increasing pain, disability and deformity, usually requires reconstructive surgery. Arthrodesis is indicated if the stiffness is acceptable and neighbouring joints are not likely to be prejudiced. With arthroplasty timing is essential. Too early, and the odds against a durable result lengthen in proportion to the demands of strenuous activity and time; too late, and bone destruction, deformity, stiffness and muscle atrophy make the operation more difficult and the results more unpredictable.

Primary generalized osteoarthritis

A common form of osteoarthritis presents as a polyarthritis, affecting finger joints (chiefly distal), thumb joints (basal), big toe joints (metatarsophalangeal), and often also the knees and the facet joints of the spine. It mainly affects postmenopausal women and has a marked familial incidence. Sometimes only the distal interphalangeal joints of the fingers are affected ('Heberden's arthropathy'); sometimes – especially in men – the fingers escape but other joints are symmetrically involved and the spinal changes are pronounced. In all forms there is a greater than usual incidence of carpal tunnel compression and isolated tenosynovitis. The pathology of individual joints is the same as that in monarticular osteoarthritis.

Symptoms and signs

Many joints may eventually become involved but typically pain starts in the hands and slowly spreads from finger to finger. In the late stages stiffness, swelling and deformity may be marked but pain is usually minimal. The knobbly appearance and bony hard feel of the distal finger joints have engendered the term 'nodal arthritis' as a synonym for Heberden's arthropathy.

X-rays show the characteristic features of osteoarthritis affecting multiple joints. In the fingers, young osteophytes may look like periarticular ossicles; this appearance is due to

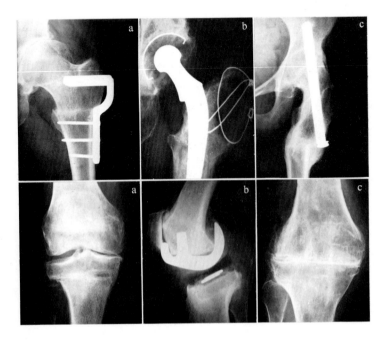

5.11 Operative treatment The three basic operations: (a) osteotomy, (b) arthroplasty, (c) arthrodesis:

at the hip

at the knee

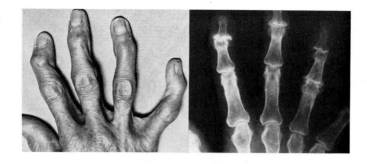

5.12 Heberden's nodes Osteoarthritis of the terminal interphalangeal joints is common. The pain always improves, but the knobbly deformities remain.

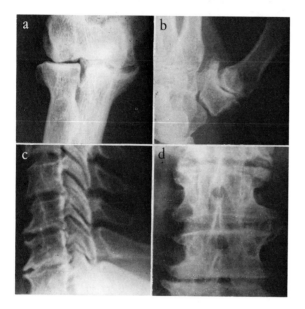

5.13 Primary generalized osteoarthritis The most obvious feature may be deformity of the fingers; but x-rays often show that other joints also are affected – in this case (a) the elbow (where symptoms are rare) and (b) the carpometacarpal thumb joint (where they are common). Often the spine shows marked disc degeneration and large bony spurs (c, d)

people, characterized by bone proliferation at the ligament and tendon insertions around peripheral joints and the intervertebral discs (Resnick *et al.*, 1975). These are, in fact, the generalized manifestations of ankylosing hyperostosis (Forestier's disease), and x-rays of the spine show the characteristic 'flowing' intervertebral ossification.

GOUT Chronic polyarticular gout produces knobbly finger joints, but the lumps are due to tophi and x-rays show periarticular bone destruction.

Treatment

The patient with Heberden's nodes should be reassured that the joints will become painless. At other sites operation may be needed, but the possible multiplicity of joint involvement must be borne in mind.

ossification within cartilaginous outgrowths at the joint margin, the early stage of osteophyte formation.

Differential diagnosis

RHEUMATOID ARTHRITIS This does not affect the terminal finger joints, so confusion should not arise.

PSORIATIC ARTHRITIS This does involve the terminal joints but is an erosive arthritis, causing marked destruction and no osteophytes.

DIFFUSE IDIOPATHIC SKELETAL HYPEROSTOSIS (DISH) This is a fairly common (though long overlooked) disorder of elderly

Neuropathic joints (Charcot's disease)

Cause and pathology

A neuropathic joint is one in which the appreciation of pain and position sense is lost. Consequently there is no reflex safeguard against injuries and a rapidly progressive degeneration occurs. In some cases the changes appear to begin suddenly and to be initiated by a fracture into the joint.

The underlying neurological conditions include tabes, syringomyelia, myelomeningocele and peripheral neuritis, usually diabetic. Leprosy and congenital indifference to pain are other possibilities. A Charcot-like neuropathy has also been reported following frequently repeated hydrocortisone injections into rheumatoid joints.

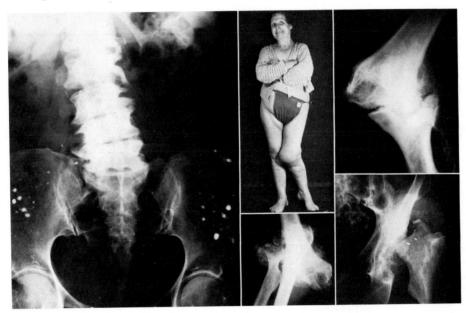

5.14 Charcot's disease   The vertebrae are distorted and dense, the buttocks show the radio-opaque remains of former injections; the knee, elbow and hip joints look grotesque. Moral: 'If it's bizarre, do a WR'. Note also the happy smile (though not all Charcot joints are tabetic, nor are they always painless).

General features

In tabes, adults over 45 are usually affected. They often complain of lightning pains. The pupils may be Argyll Robertson in type; knee and ankle jerks are often lost, and there is no pain on squeezing the tendo Achillis.

In syringomyelia the condition often dates from early adult life. Characteristically there is dissociated sensation (loss of pain and temperature sense, but not of touch). Scoliosis is common.

Symptoms and signs

The patient complains of weakness, instability, swelling and deformity of the affected joint; the symptoms may progress surprisingly rapidly. The appearance of an established Charcot's joint suggests that movement would be agonizing and yet it is painless. The paradox is diagnostic.

Swelling and deformity are marked. The joint may be subluxed or even dislocated. There is no warmth or tenderness. Fluid is greatly increased and bits of bone can be felt everywhere. Often the joint is flail, normal movements being increased and painless abnormal movements present.

X-RAY   The joint is subluxed or dislocated, gross bone erosion is obvious and there are irregular calcified masses in the capsule.

Treatment

The underlying condition may need treatment, but the affected joints cannot recover. They should, if possible, be stabilized by external splintage (e.g. a caliper). Operation is not advised.

Haemophilic arthropathy

Of the various bleeding disorders, only two are associated with recurrent haemarthroses and progressive joint destruction: classic haemophilia, in which there is a deficiency of clotting factor VIII; and Christmas disease, due to deficiency of factor IX. Both are X-linked recessive disorders manifesting in males but carried by females. Their incidence is about 1 per 10 000 male births.

Plasma-clotting factor levels above 40 per cent of the normal are compatible with normal control of haemorrhage; levels of 20–40 per cent may cause prolonged bleeding after injury or operation; only with levels below 5 per cent does spontaneous bleeding occur.

ACUTE BLEEDING INTO A JOINT OR MUSCLE With trivial injury a joint (usually the knee, elbow or ankle) may rapidly fill with blood. Pain, warmth, boggy swelling, tenderness and limited movement are the outstanding features. The resemblance to a low-grade inflammatory joint is striking, but the history is diagnostic.

The appropriate factor in the form of a cryoprecipitate must be given without delay; early factor replacement is the only method of controlling a bleed – external pressure is useless and has caused loss of a limb. If the factor is not available, fresh-frozen plasma is given. Aspiration is avoided unless distension is severe. A removable splint is wise, but once the acute episode has passed movement is encouraged.

Acute bleeding into muscles (especially the forearm, calf or thigh) is less common. A painful swelling appears with deformity of the related joint. Occasional complications are acute Volkmann's ischaemia and pressure on a peripheral nerve, but decompression is unwise and ineffective. The treatment is early factor replacement and splintage. Later, operation may be needed to correct fixed deformity.

Home treatment with freeze-dried factor concentrate is being developed; it is effective as emergency treatment, avoids delay and may be all that is needed for minor bleeds.

JOINT DEGENERATION This, the sequel to repeated bleeding, usually begins before the age of

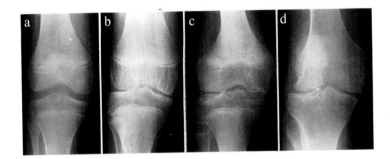

5.15 Haemophilic arthritis (a) At first there is blood in the joint but the surfaces are intact; (b) later the cartilage is attacked and the joint 'space' narrows; (c) bony erosions appear and eventually the joint becomes deformed and unstable; in (d) early subluxation is obvious.

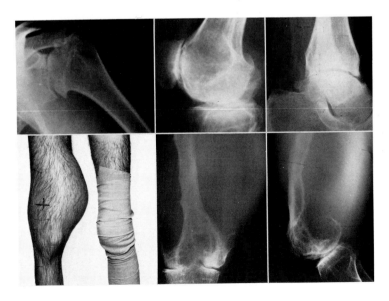

5.16 Haemophilia Top row: degeneration in several joints after repeated bleeding.

Bottom row: since it threatened the integrity of the femur, this large pseudotumour was extirpated; at the same time massive bone grafts were inserted – no light undertaking in a haemophilic.

15. Chronic synovitis is followed by cartilage degeneration, probably from the action of local hydrolytic enzymes. An affected joint shows wasting and fixed deformity not unlike a tuberculous or rheumatoid joint.

On x-ray several stages can be identified (Arnold and Hilgartner, 1977); I, soft-tissue swelling only; II, osteoporosis and epiphyseal overgrowth; III, slight narrowing of the joint space and squaring of the patella and femoral condyles; IV, marked narrowing of the joint space and joint disorganization; and V, joint disintegration.

Up to stage III progressive degeneration is preventable by controlling bleeds, encouraging movement and counteracting joint deformity. Operative treatment (including osteotomy and joint replacement) is feasible but must be covered by factor replacement, which should continue throughout the period of healing and subsequent mobilization.

PSEUDOTUMOURS AND CYSTS   These follow repeated local bleeding. The size of the bleed is critical; if absorption of the blood is not accomplished, there is increased fluid absorption by osmosis with pressure on the surrounding tissues, in which fragile capillaries allow further bleeding. A swelling appears which may slowly increase in size. Bone is eroded, giving rise either to a cystic appearance resembling a giant-cell tumour, or to extensive osteolysis. In addition to factor replacement, the tumour may need to be excised, and weakened bone may need reinforcement by grafting.

FRACTURES   The bleeding which accompanies any fracture must first be controlled. The fracture is then treated on its merits; internal fixation (under factor replacement) is often used for unstable fractures. Union is not delayed.

Further reading

Ali, S. Y. (1980) Mineral-containing matrix vesicles in human osteoarthrotic cartilage. In *The Aetiopathogenesis of Osteoarthrosis*. Ed. by G. Nuki. Tunbridge Wells: Pitman Medical

Arnold, W. D. and Hilgartner, M. W. (1977) Hemophilic arthropathy. *Journal of Bone and Joint Surgery* **59A**, 287–305

Byers, P. D., Contepomi, C. A. and Farkas, T. A. (1970) A post mortem study of the hip joint including the prevalence of features on the right side. *Annals of the Rheumatic Diseases* **29**, 15–31

Dieppe, P. A., Crocker, P. R., Corke, C. F., Doyle, D. V., Huskisson, E. C. and Willoughby, D. A. (1979) Synovial fluid crystals. *Quarterly Journal of Medicine* **48**, 533–553

Freeman, M. A. R. (1975) The fatigue of cartilage in the pathogenesis of osteoarthrosis. *Acta Orthopaedica Scandinavica* **46**, 323–328

Helal, B. (1965) The pain in primary osteoarthritis of the knee. *Postgraduate Medical Journal* **41**, 172–181

McCarty, D. J. (1976) Calcium pyrophosphate dihydrate crystal deposition disease. *Arthritis and Rheumatism* **19**, Suppl. 3, 275–285

McDevitt, C. A. and Muir, H. (1976) Biochemical changes in the cartilage of the knee in experimental and natural osteoarthritis in the dog. *Journal of Bone and Joint Surgery* **58B**, 94–101

Mankin, H. J. and Lippiello, L. (1971) The glycosaminoglycans of normal and arthritic cartilage. *Journal of Clinical Investigation* **50**, 1712–1719

Resnick, D., Shaul, S. R. and Robins, J. M. (1975) Diffuse idiopathic skeletal hyperostosis (DISH): Forestier's disease with extraspinal manifestations. *Radiology* **115**, 513–524

Solomon, L. (1976). Patterns of osteoarthritis of the hip. *Journal of Bone and Joint Surgery* **58B**, 176–183

Bone Necrosis

6

Bone may die as the result of infection (page 19), or if its blood supply is cut off by injury (page 357); bone death is also the major feature of Perthes' disease (page 258). Because they are discussed elsewhere, these are omitted from the present chapter, which deals with: (1) the general principles of bone necrosis; (2) those specific disorders not considered elsewhere (sickle-cell disease, caisson disease, Gaucher's disease and drug-induced necrosis); (3) osteochondritis, which is included for convenience and because in some varieties bone necrosis is important.

Bone necrosis – general principles

Pathology

Dead bone is structurally and radiologically indistinguishable from live bone. However, lacking a blood supply it does not undergo turnover or renewal, and after a limited period of repetitive stress it suffers fatigue failure. The pathological changes develop in four overlapping stages.

Stage 1: bone death without structural change After interruption of the blood supply there is, within a few days, evidence of marrow necrosis and cell death. However, for weeks or even months the bone and articular cartilage may show no alteration in macroscopic appearance.

Stage 2: repair and early structural failure At a variable interval after infarction the surrounding bone shows a vascular reaction. Small capillaries infiltrate the necrotic area and osteoblasts lay down new bone upon the dead trabeculae; the increase in bone mass shows on the x-ray as exaggerated density. Despite this active repair, small fractures appear in the dead bone and there may be some compression of the necrotic segment.

Stage 3: major structural failure As new bone infiltrates the infarct, trabecular collapse continues, so that healing may actually be accompanied by increased distortion.

Stage 4: articular destruction Cartilage, being nourished mainly by synovial fluid, is preserved even in advanced osteonecrosis. However, severe distortion of the surface eventually leads to cartilage breakdown.

Symptoms and signs

The earliest stage of bone death is asymptomatic; by the time the patient presents, the lesion is well advanced. Pain is the usual complaint; it is felt near a joint and is accompanied by stiffness. Local tenderness may be present and, if a superficial bone (such as the carpal lunate or a metatarsal head) is affected, there may be some swelling. Movements are usually restricted.

X-rays

The distinctive feature of avascular necrosis is increased bone density. This may be due, in part, to trabecular compression in a collapsed segment, but the main reason is the reactive new bone

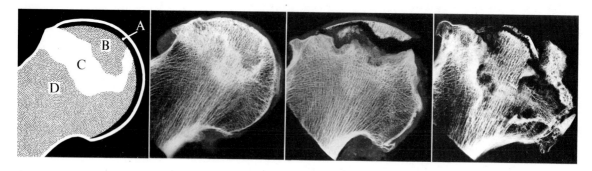

6.1 Avascular necrosis of bone – pathology These fine-detail x-rays of necrotic femoral heads show the progress of osteonecrosis. The articular cartilage (A) remains intact for a long time. The necrotic segment (B) has a texture similar to that of normal bone, but it may develop fine cracks. New bone surrounds the dead trabeculae and causes marked sclerosis (C). Beyond this the bone remains unchanged (D). In the later stages the necrotic bone breaks up and finally the joint surface is destroyed.

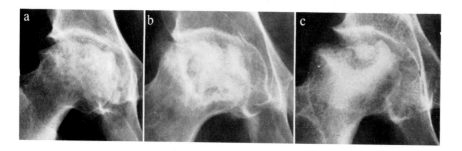

6.2 Avascular necrosis – x-rays (a, b) Though details may differ, the major features are constant: increased bone density and distortion of bone architecture, but an intact joint space. Sometimes the necrotic segment separates ('dissects') as a discrete fragment (c).

formation in the surrounding tissue. It appears months or even years after the infarction. Other changes are subarticular fracturing and bone deformation. Occasionally the necrotic segment separates from the parent bone.

Radionuclide scanning with ^{99m}Tc-sulphur-colloid, which is taken up in myeloid tissue, may reveal an avascular segment. This is most likely in sickle-cell disease where a 'cold' area contrasts significantly with the generally high nuclide uptake due to increased erythroblastic activity.

Treatment

If possible, the cause should be eliminated. In stages 1 and 2, bone collapse can sometimes be prevented by a combination of weight-relief and splintage. Once bone collapse has occurred (stage 3), an osteotomy, by transferring stress to an

undamaged area, may be useful. In stage 4 the treatment is the same as for osteoarthritis.

Specific types of avascular necrosis (AVN)

Sickle-cell disease

Red cells containing the abnormal haemoglobin S (Hb S) may become sickle-shaped, leading to bone infarction. This is particularly likely in homozygous sickle-cell disease (where two Hb S genes have been inherited), but may also occur in the heterozygous disorders, Hb S/C haemoglobinopathy and Hb S/thalassaemia. Inheritance of one Hb S gene and one normal β-globin gene results in the *sickle-cell trait*, in which

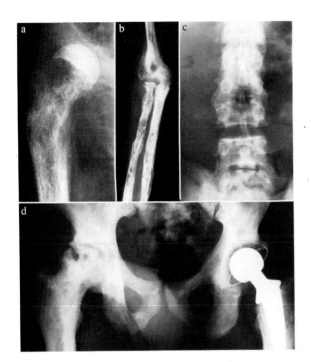

6.3 Sickle-cell disease (a) Typical changes in the femur due to marrow hyperplasia, with bone infarction and necrosis of the femoral head. (b) In severe cases infarctions of tubular bones may resemble osteomyelitis, with sequestra and a marked periosteal reaction (sometimes a true salmonella infection supervenes). (c) The spine also may be involved. (d) In adults osteoporosis is followed by endosteal sclerosis, seen clearly in the right femur; the left hip has already been replaced following femoral head necrosis.

crises') or, if more severe, ischaemic necrosis. Almost any bone may be involved and there is a tendency for the infarcts to become infected, sometimes with unusual organisms such as *Salmonella*.

On x-ray the tubular bones (including the phalanges) may show irregular endosteal destruction and medullary sclerosis, together with periosteal new bone formation. Not only does this resemble osteitis, but true infection is often superimposed on the infarct. Medullary calcification is common and may be very extensive. In children, femoral head necrosis could be mistaken for Perthes' disease were it not that the latter is known to be uncommon in Africans.* Involvement of the spine may lead to vertebral collapse. Bone scanning with ^{99m}Tc-sulphur-colloid may show localized areas of diminished uptake, many of which are asymptomatic. The definitive diagnosis of the underlying haemoglobinopathy is made by special haematological tests.

Treatment Bone crises are treated by rest and analgesics, followed by physiotherapy to minimize stiffness. Established necrosis is treated according to the principles on page 62, but with the emphasis on conservatism. Anaesthesia carries serious risks and may even precipitate vascular occlusion in the central nervous system, lungs or kidneys; moreover, the chances of postoperative infection are high.

sickling occurs only under conditions of hypoxia (e.g. under anaesthesia, in extreme cold or at high altitudes).

The abnormal Hb S gene is limited to people of Central and West African Negro descent; it is fairly common in Nigeria, around the Mediterranean, in the West Indies and in the USA (about 10 per cent of American Negroes have the sickle-cell trait). Below the equator it is virtually unknown.

In the established disorder there is increased aggregation of the haemoglobin molecules and subsequent distortion of red cell shape; this is most marked in deoxygenated blood. Clumping of the sickle-shaped cells causes diminished capillary flow and repeated episodes of pain ('bone

Caisson disease

Decompression sickness (caisson disease) and osteonecrosis are important causes of disability in deep-sea divers and compressed-air workers building tunnels or underwater structures. Under increased air pressure the blood and other tissues (especially fat) become supersaturated with nitrogen; if decompression is too rapid the gas is released as bubbles, which cause local tissue damage and generalized embolic phenomena. The symptoms of decompression sickness, which may develop within minutes, are pain near the

*'Perthes' disease' in a black child – look for sickling.

joints ('the bends'), breathing difficulty and vertigo ('the staggers'). In the most acute cases there can be circulatory and respiratory collapse, severe neurological changes, coma and death. Only 10 per cent of patients with bone necrosis give a history of decompression sickness.

Radiological bone lesions have been found in 17 per cent of compressed-air workers in Britain; almost half the lesions are juxta-articular – mainly in the humeral head and femoral head – but microscopic bone death is much more widespread than x-rays suggest.

The bone infarction may be due to one or more of the following: (1) intravascular capillary obstruction by nitrogen bubbles; (2) extravascular capillary compression by gas released from the supersaturated marrow fat in the non-expandable bone; (3) intravascular fat embolism or thromboembolism resulting from tissue disruption when gas bubbles are released (Cryssanthou, 1978).

Clinical and x-ray features   The necrosis may cause pain and loss of joint movement, but many lesions remain 'silent' and are found only on routine x-ray examination. Medullary infarcts cause mottled calcification or areas of dense sclerosis. Juxta-articular changes are similar to those in other forms of osteonecrosis.

Management   The aim is prevention; the incidence of osteonecrosis is proportional to the working pressure, the length of exposure, the rate of decompression and the number of exposures. Strict enforcement of suitable working schedules has reduced the risks considerably. The treatment of established lesions follows the principles already outlined.

Gaucher's disease

This familial disease occurs predominantly in Ashkenazi Jews. Deficiency of the specific enzyme causes an abnormal accumulation of glucocerebroside in the macrophages of the reticuloendothelial system. The effects are seen chiefly in the liver, spleen and bone marrow, where the large, polyhedral 'Gaucher cells' accumulate; their pressure on the bone sinusoids may be the cause of the bone necrosis.

Necrosis of the femoral head is not uncommon. It may occur at any age and presents with pain and limp; movement becomes gradually more restricted. Other areas may be similarly affected. There is a tendency for the Gaucher deposits to become infected and the patient may present

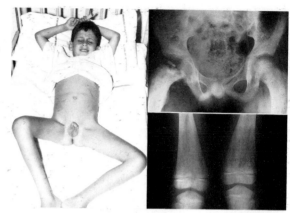

6.4 Gaucher's disease   This young boy, whose sister also had Gaucher's disease, developed pain in the right hip; abduction was limited and painful. X-rays show necrosis of the right femoral head and widening of the femoral shafts (the Erlenmeyer flask appearance).

with septicaemia. Blood tests show anaemia, leucopenia and thrombocytopenia. A diagnostic, though inconstant, finding is a raised serum acid phosphatase level.

X-ray   The appearances resemble those in other types of osteonecrosis, and 'silent' lesions may be found in a number of bones. A special feature (due to replacement of myeloid tissue by Gaucher cells) is expansion of the tubular bones, especially the distal femur, producing the Erlenmeyer flask appearance. Cortical thinning may lead to pathological fracture.

Treatment   of the osteonecrosis follows the general principles outlined on page 62. Femoral head replacement is often advisable.

Drug-induced necrosis

Corticosteroids, given in high dosage, may give rise to 'spontaneous' osteonecrosis; thus, in renal transplant patients on immunosuppressive corticosteroids, the incidence is about 16 per cent. Excessive alcohol (an average daily consumption of more than 175 g) is another potent cause. Both conditions cause fatty infiltration of the liver and bone marrow, often associated with hyperlipidaemia. But why they cause bone ischaemia is unknown. Repeated fat embolism may occlude the intraosseous end arteries; or fat-cell distension in the marrow may compress the venous sinusoids.

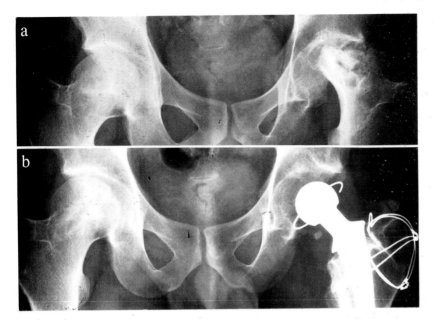

6.5 Drug-induced necrosis (a) Alcohol abuse has led to bilateral femoral head necrosis, advanced on the left but early on the right. (b) Drilling of the femoral neck to decompress the bone was in time to save the right hip; the left had to be replaced.

Necrosis occurs at the ends of the tubular bones and is most common in the femoral head. The pathological changes are those described on page 61, but new bone formation is tardy, probably because both drugs adversely affect osteogenesis.

Pain may be present for many months before x-rays show any abnormality; the earliest signs are a small subarticular fracture and a vague blush of increased bone density. Even before this, the intraosseous pressure is raised and local venography shows circulatory congestion. In the late stage there is bone collapse or sequestration of the necrotic fragment.

Treatment is controversial. In the earliest stage the condition is potentially reversible if the cortisone or alcohol is stopped. Symptomatic treatment for pain, weight relief and physiotherapy are often all that is required, even when the x-rays show bone collapse. Decompression of the affected bone by drilling is justified if one accepts that the raised intraosseous pressure causes the ischaemia. If pain is severe and joint disruption is advanced, reconstructive surgery – usually joint replacement – is required.

Table 6.1 Summary of causes of osteonecrosis

Trauma	Fracture	Femoral neck
		Scaphoid
		Talus
	Dislocation	Hip
		Talus
		Lunate
	Forcible reduction of CDH	
Infection	Osteomyelitis	Any bone
	Septic arthritis	Hip
	Tuberculosis	Hip
Sickle-cell disease		Any bone
Gaucher's disease		Hip
		Knee
Caisson disease		Shoulder
		Hip
		Knee
Irradiation		Any bone
'Idiopathic'	Perthes' disease	Hip
	Corticosteroids	Hip
		Knee
		Shoulder
	Alcohol	Hip

Osteochondritis
(osteochondrosis)

Osteochondritis is a collection of entities falling into three unrelated groups: (1) 'crushing' osteochondritis (or osteochondrosis); (2) 'splitting' osteochondritis (dissecans); and (3) 'pulling' osteochondritis (traction apophysitis). The first two are associated with bone necrosis.

Table 6.2 The types of osteochondritis

Type	Bone	Eponym
Crushing	Metatarsal	Freiberg
	Navicular	Köhler
	Lunate	Kienböck
	Capitulum	Panner
Splitting	Femoral condyle	
	Elbow	
	Talus	
	Metatarsal	
Pulling	Tibial tuberosity	Osgood–Schlatter
	Calcaneum	Sever

Crushing osteochondritis

This mainly occurs during phases of rapid growth or increased physical activity. It is characterized by apparently spontaneous necrosis of the ossific nucleus in a long-bone epiphysis or one of the cuboidal bones of the wrist or foot. A local anatomical or mechanical feature, which could markedly raise the compressive or shearing stress on the bone, can sometimes be identified, and it is thought that this may interrupt the blood supply. The pathological changes are the same as those in other forms of osteonecrosis: bone death, fragmentation or distortion of the necrotic segment, and new bone formation on the ischaemic trabeculae.

Pain and limitation of joint movement are the usual complaints. Tenderness is sharply localized to the affected bone. X-rays show the characteristic increased density, accompanied in the later stages by distortion and collapse of the necrotic segment.

The common examples of osteochondritis have, by long tradition, acquired eponymous labels: Freiberg's disease of the metatarsal (page 327); Köhler's disease of the navicular (page 326); Kienböck's disease of the carpal lunate (page 181); and Panner's disease of the capitulum.

Scheuermann's disease (page 225)   Compression and fragmentation of the vertebral epiphyseal plates during adolescence lead to wedging and dorsal kyphosis. Although x-rays show sclerosis and irregularity of the vertebral end plates, this is not necrosis. Similar changes in the lumbar spine predispose to later disc degeneration.

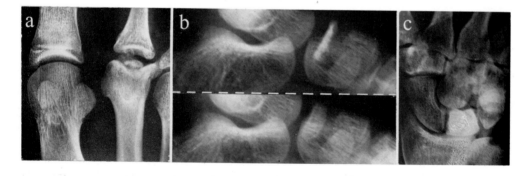

6.6 Crushing osteochondritis   (a) Freiberg's disease of the second metatarsal; (b) Köhler's disease of the navicular, compared with the normal side below; (c) Kienböck's disease of the lunate.

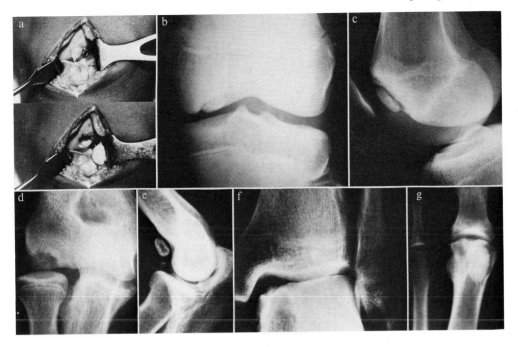

6.7 Splitting osteochondritis   (a) The fragment becomes separated and may break away. The knee (b, c) and elbow (d, e) are the commonest sites; but the process may affect any convex articular surface such as the talus (f) or the first metatarsal head (g).

Splitting osteochondritis (dissecans)

A small segment of articular cartilage and the subjacent bone may separate (dissect) as an avascular fragment. It occurs typically in young adults, usually men, and affects certain particular sites: the lateral surface of the medial femoral condyle in the knee, the anteromedial corner of the talus in the ankle, the superomedial part of the femoral head, the humeral capitulum and the first metatarsal head.

The cause is almost certainly repeated minor trauma causing osteochondral fracture of a convex surface; the fragment loses its blood supply. However, there must be other predisposing factors, for the condition is sometimes multifocal and sometimes runs in families. Necrosis of articular surfaces may follow treatment with large doses of corticosteroids but these lesions are more extensive and affect the weight-bearing part of the joint.

The knee is much the commonest joint to be affected. The patient presents with intermittent pain, swelling and joint effusion. If the necrotic fragment becomes completely detached, it may cause locking of the joint or unexpected episodes of giving way. Similar but less frequent episodes occur in the hip or ankle.

X-rays must be taken with the joint in the appropriate position to show the affected part of the articular surface in tangential projection. The dissecting fragment is defined by a radiolucent line of demarcation. When it separates, the resulting 'crater' may be obvious.

If the fragment is in position, treatment consists of weight relief and restriction of activity. In children complete healing may occur, though it takes up to 2 years; in adults it is doubtful whether the future course of events can be significantly influenced. If the fragment becomes detached and causes symptoms it should be pinned back in position or else completely removed.

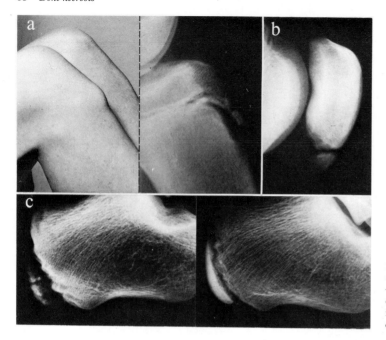

6.8 Pulling osteochondritis These are merely traction lesions, but dignified by eponyms: (a) Osgood–Schlatter's disease involves the apophysis into which the extensor mechanism is inserted; (b) in Johannson –Larsen's disease the calcification is a sequel to the patellar ligament partially pulling away from the bone; (c) Sever's disease, compared with the normal side.

Pulling osteochondritis (traction apophysitis)

Excessive pull by a large tendon may damage the unfused apophysis to which it is attached; this occurs typically at two sites – the tibial tuberosity (Osgood–Schlatter's disease, page 293) and the calcaneal apophysis (Sever's disease, page 325). These lesions do not produce bone necrosis. The traumatized apophysis becomes painful and there may be an associated tenosynovitis of the attached tendon.

Further reading

Amstutz, H. C. (1973) The hip in Gaucher's disease. *Clinical Orthopaedics* **90,** 83–89

Chung, S. M. K., Alavi, A. and Russell, M. O. (1978) Management of osteonecrosis in sickle-cell anemia and its genetic variants. *Clinical Orthopaedics 130,* 158–174

Cryssanthou, C. P. (1978) Dysbaric osteonecrosis. Etiological and pathogenetic concepts. *Clinical Orthopaedics* **130,** 94–106

Jaffe, H. L. (1972) *Metabolic, Degenerative and Inflammatory Disease of Bones and Joints.* Philadelphia: Lee and Febiger

Solomon, L. and Spivey, J. (1978) Avascular necrosis of the femoral head in adults. *Clinics in Rheumatic Disease* **4,** 347–374

Metabolic and Endocrine Disorders   7

Calcium and bone control

Bone is not merely for support; equally important is its role in maintaining a steady calcium ion concentration in the extracellular fluid. For all its solidity it is in a continuous state of flux, and the control of osteoblastic formation and osteoclastic resorption is linked inescapably to that of calcium exchange.

In children, epiphyseal growth is followed by ossification and remodelling, while the tubular shaft enlarges by subperiosteal apposition and endosteal resorption. Up to the fourth decade bone formation continues to exceed bone loss, so that the tubular cortices become thicker and cancellous bone more dense. This optimal state persists for some years, but after the climacteric (around 50 years in women, 65 in men) there is a dramatic and progressive loss of cortical thickness and bone mass; cavities enlarge and trabeculae become thinner, making the skeleton increasingly frail.

These long-term changes in the mineral pool are complemented by rapid alterations that occur from moment to moment throughout life.

Calcium and phosphate exchange

Most of the body's calcium and phosphate is in bone, chiefly in the form of hydroxyapatite crystals and capable of only very slow exchange. The rapidly exchangeable mineral is in the extracellular fluid and in partially formed bone crystals.

Both calcium and phosphate concentration depend largely on intestinal absorption and renal excretion; transient alterations in serum levels can be accommodated rapidly by changes in renal tubular reabsorption. The control of calcium levels is, however, far more rigid than that of phosphate; in persistent calcium deficiency the extracellular calcium ion concentration is maintained, even at the expense of bone, whereas phosphate deficiency simply leads to lowered serum phosphate concentration. Hence the pre-eminence of calcium in bone metabolism.

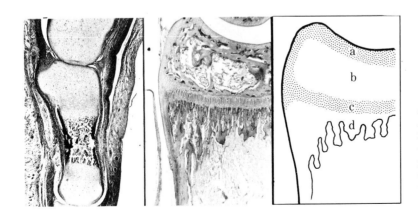

7.1 Bone growth On the left a fetal phalanx, with bone forming in its cartilage model. By the time the child is born, the bone (on the right) shows the familiar separation into (a) articular cartilage, (b) epiphysis, (c) cartilaginous growth plate (or physis), and (d) newly formed juxta-epiphyseal bone.

The organs mainly concerned in calcium balance are the gut, kidney and bone; consequently these are the targets for the hormones regulating its metabolism, and the battlegrounds for metabolic bone disease.

Vitamin D

Naturally occurring vitamin D_3 (cholecalciferol) is derived from two sources: directly from the diet and indirectly by the action of ultraviolet light on precursors in the skin. Vitamin D itself is inactive. Conversion to active metabolites (which function as hormones) takes place first in the liver by 25-hydroxylation to form 25-hydroxycholecalciferol (25-HCC), and then in the kidney by a further 1α-hydroxylation to give 1,25-dihydroxycholecalciferol (1,25-DHCC).

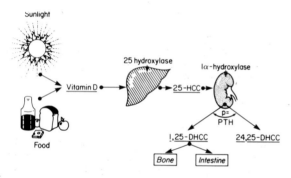

7.2 Vitamin D metabolism   Cholecalciferol is derived either from the diet or by conversion of precursors when the skin is exposed to sunlight. This inactive 'vitamin' is hydroxylated, first in the liver and then in the kidney, to form the active metabolite 1,25-dihydroxycholecalciferol.

The terminal metabolite, 1,25-DHCC, is the most active form; it stimulates the uptake of calcium by the small intestine and promotes increased bone resorption. The liver metabolite, 25-HCC, has similar though weaker effects. Other, less active, vitamin D metabolites are formed by the kidney. Indeed, 24,25-DHCC is normally present in far greater quantity than 1,25-DHCC, and it is only under conditions of need that the production of 1,25-HCC increases. This switch is controlled by parathyroid hormone (PTH) and by the serum phosphate concentration; a rise in PTH or a fall in phosphate increases 1,25-DHCC synthesis and decreases 24,25-DHCC production proportionately. A fall in serum calcium does the same indirectly, by stimulating PTH production; the increased 1,25-DHCC then promotes intestinal absorption of calcium and the serum level is restored.

Parathyroid hormone

While vitamin D is concerned with the mass movement of calcium into and out of bone, parathyroid hormone (PTH) is the fine regulator of calcium exchange. Its production is stimulated by a fall and suppressed by a rise in serum calcium ion concentration. PTH has two independent actions: it increases phosphate excretion by restricting tubular reabsorption, and it conserves calcium by increasing its tubular reabsorption. These rapid responses give the kidney its important role in calcium homoeostasis.

In the skeleton PTH causes bone resorption, resulting in a rise in serum calcium. There is both a rapid effect (osteocytic bone lysis) and a prolonged effect (osteoclastic resorption). In the intestine PTH indirectly stimulates calcium absorption via its effect on 1,25-DHCC production in the kidney.

Calcitonin

Calcitonin, which is secreted by the C cells of the thyroid, exerts a rapid hypocalcaemic effect by inhibiting bone resorption. This occurs especially when bone turnover is high, as in Paget's disease. Its secretion is stimulated by a rise in serum calcium.

Other hormones

A number of hormones which influence epiphyseal growth, bone formation and bone resorption play a secondary role in calcium balance. Oestrogen is thought to stimulate calcium absorption and to protect bone from the unrestrained action of PTH. Its withdrawal leads to osteoporosis. Adrenal corticosteroids in excess cause osteoporosis due to a combination of increased bone resorption, diminished formation and defective collagen synthesis. Thyroxine increases both formation and resorption, but more so the latter; hyperthyroidism is associated with high bone turnover and osteoporosis.

Non-hormonal factors

Mechanical stress markedly affects bone formation and remodelling. Under physiological conditions the important mechanical forces are gravity, load-bearing and muscle action. Weightlessness, prolonged bed rest, lack of exercise and muscular weakness are all associated with osteoporosis.

Prostaglandin E stimulates bone resorption and may account, at least in part, for the bone destruction and hypercalcaemia in metastatic bone disease (Tashjian, 1975). Acid–base balance affects bone resorption, which is increased in acidosis and decreased in alkalosis. Increased phosphate or pyrophosphate concentration can inhibit bone resorption: the same effect is achieved by giving diphosphonates (pyrophosphate analogues).

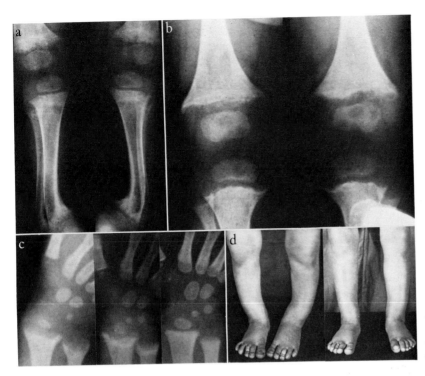

7.3 Rickets   (a, b) Florid disease; (c) series showing the response to treatment; (d) before and after osteotomy for the neglected case.

Rickets and osteomalacia

Rickets and osteomalacia are different expressions of the same disease: inadequate mineralization of bone. In children (rickets) this chiefly affects areas of active endochondral growth; in adults new bone throughout the skeleton is incompletely calcified, and therefore 'softened' (osteomalacia). The inadequacy may be due to calcium deficiency, marked hypophosphataemia, or defects anywhere along the metabolic pathway for vitamin D: nutritional lack, underexposure to sunlight, intestinal malabsorption, decreased 25-hydroxylation (liver disease, anticonvulsants) and reduced 1α-hydroxylation (renal disease, nephrectomy, 1α-hydroxylase deficiency).

Symptoms and signs

The infant with *rickets* may present with tetany or convulsions. There is failure to thrive, listlessness and muscular flaccidity. Early bone changes are deformity of the skull (craniotabes), and thicken-ing of the knees, ankles and wrists from epiphyseal overgrowth. Enlargement of the costo-chondral junctions ('rickety rosary') and lateral

Table 7.1 Characteristics of different types of rickets

	Vitamin D deficiency	Renal tubular	Renal glomerular
Family history	−	+	−
Myopathy	+	−	+
Growth defect	±	+ +	+ +
Serum			
Ca	↓	N	↓
P	↓	↓	↑
Alk. phos.	↑	↑	↑
Urine			
Ca	↓	↓	↓
P	↓	↑	↓
Osteitis fibrosa	±	+	+ +
Other	Dietary deficiency or malabsorption	Amino-aciduria	Renal failure Anaemia

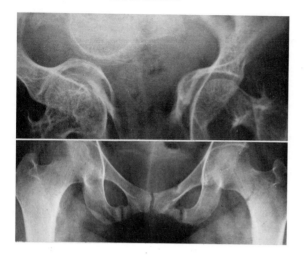

7.4 Osteomalacia   Two characteristic features of osteomalacia: above, indentation of the pelvic walls producing the 'trefoil pelvis'; and (below) Looser's zones in the pubic rami and left femoral neck.

indentation of the chest (Harrison's sulcus) may also appear. Distal tibial bowing has been attributed to sitting or lying cross-legged. Once the child stands, lower limb deformities increase, and stunting of growth may be obvious. In severe rickets there may be spinal curvature, coxa vara and bending or fractures of the long bones.

Osteomalacia has a much more insidious course and patients may complain of bone pain, backache and muscle weakness for many years before the diagnosis is made. Vertebral collapse causes loss of height, and existing deformities such as mild kyphosis or knock knees – themselves perhaps due to adolescent rickets – may increase in later life. Unexplained pain in the hip or one of the long bones may presage a stress fracture.

X-rays

In active rickets there is thickening and widening of the growth plate, cupping of the metaphysis and, sometimes, bowing of the diaphysis. The metaphysis may remain abnormally wide even after healing has occurred.

The stamp of osteomalacia is the Looser zone, a thin transverse band of rarefaction in an otherwise normal-looking bone. These zones, seen especially in the shafts of long bones and the axillary edge of the scapula, are due to incomplete stress fractures

which heal with callus lacking in calcium. More often, however, there is simply a slow fading of skeletal structure, resulting in biconcave vertebrae (from disc pressure), lateral indentation of the acetabula ('trefoil' pelvis) and spontaneous fractures of the ribs, pubic rami, femoral neck or the metaphyses above and below the knee.

Secondary hyperparathyroidism occurs if the serum calcium is low. In children the resulting subperiosteal erosions are at the sites of maximal remodelling (medial borders of the proximal humerus, femoral neck, distal femur and proximal tibia, lateral borders of the distal radius and ulna). In adults the middle phalanges of the fingers are more often affected, and in severe cases brown tumours ('cysts') are seen in the long bones.

Biochemistry

Changes common to almost all types of rickets and osteomalacia are diminished serum calcium and phosphate levels, increased alkaline phosphatase and diminished urinary excretion of calcium. In vitamin D deficiency the 25-HCC levels also are low. The 'calcium phosphate product' (derived by multiplying calcium and phosphorus levels expressed in mmol/l), normally about 3, is diminished in rickets and osteomalacia, and values of less than 2.4 are diagnostic.

Varieties of rickets and osteomalacia

Vitamin D deficiency

Vitamin D deficiency may be due to dietary lack, underexposure to sunlight, malabsorption or a combination of these. Classic rickets responds rapidly to small doses of calciferol (2000 i.u. a day for 3–6 weeks) and residual deformity is slight.

Osteomalacia is fairly common in the elderly; diagnosis is difficult because they are also osteoporotic (Solomon, 1974). It is possible that they have a metabolic disorder together with vitamin D deficiency, because very large doses of calciferol and calcium are required to produce improvement.

Renal tubular rickets

Impaired renal tubular reabsorption of phosphate results in hypophosphataemia with normal calcium levels but defective bone mineralization.

Familial hypophosphataemia, probably the commonest cause of rickets today, is an X-linked genetic disorder with dominant inheritance, starting in infancy or soon after and causing severe bony deformity. The children are dwarfed, boys more so than girls. There is no myopathy. X-rays show marked epiphyseal changes but, because the serum calcium is normal, there is no secondary hyperparathyroidism. Treatment is by large doses of vitamin D (50000i.u. or more) and up to 4g of inorganic phosphate per day (with careful monitoring to prevent overdosage), continued until growth ceases. Bony deformities may require bracing or osteotomy. If the child needs to be immobilized, vitamin D must be stopped temporarily to prevent hypercalcaemia from the combined effects of treatment and disuse bone resorption.

Adult-onset hypophosphataemia, though rare, must be remembered as a cause of unexplained bone loss and myopathy.

Renal glomerular osteodystrophy

The patient has chronic renal disease involving both glomeruli and tubules. Uraemia and phosphate retention are accompanied by a fall in serum calcium which is due partly to the hyperphosphataemia and partly to 1,25-DHCC deficiency. Skeletal consequences are (1) rickets or osteomalacia; (2) widespread osteitis fibrosa, the hallmark of secondary hyperparathyroidism; and (3) osteosclerosis (and soft-tissue calcification), which is related in some way to the hyperphosphataemia.

Renal abnormalities precede the bone changes by several years. Children are clinically more severely affected than adults: they are stunted, pasty-faced and have marked rachitic deformities. Myopathy is common. X-rays show widened and irregular epiphyseal plates. In older children with long-standing disease there may be displacement of the epiphyses (epiphyseolysis). Osteosclerosis is seen mainly in the axial skeleton and is more common in young patients: it may produce a 'rugger jersey' appearance in lateral x-rays of the spine, due to alternating bands of increased and decreased bone density. Signs of secondary hyperparathyroidism may be widespread and severe.

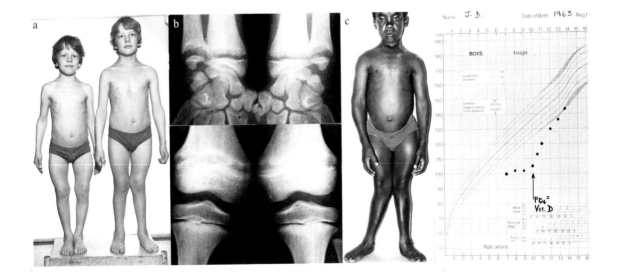

7.5 Renal tubular rickets – familial hypophosphataemia (a) These brothers presented with knee deformities: their x-rays (b) show defective juxta-epiphyseal calcification. (c) Another example of hypophosphataemic rickets; his growth chart shows that he was well below the normal range in height, but improved dramatically on treatment with vitamin D and inorganic phosphate.

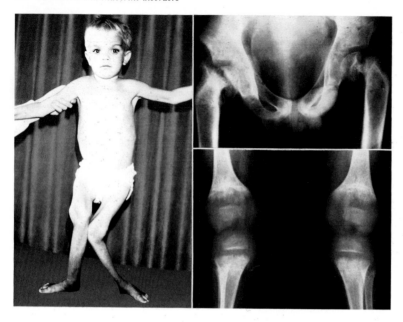

7.6 Renal glomerular osteodystrophy   This young boy with chronic renal failure has severe abnormality of epiphyseal growth; the upper femoral epiphyses are grossly displaced.

Biochemical features are low serum calcium, high serum phosphate and elevated alkaline phosphatase levels. Urinary excretion of calcium and phosphate is diminished. Plasma PTH levels may be raised.

The renal failure, if irreversible, may require haemodialysis or renal transplantation. The osteodystrophy should be treated, in the first instance, with large doses of vitamin D (up to 500 000 i.u. daily); in resistant cases, small doses of 1,25-DHCC may be effective. Epiphysiolysis may need internal fixation and residual deformities can be corrected once the disease is under control.

Hyperparathyroidism

Excessive secretion of parathyroid hormone may be primary (usually due to an adenoma or hyperplasia), secondary (due to persistent hypolcalcaemia) or tertiary (when secondary hyperplasia leads to autonomous overactivity).

Pathology

Overproduction of PTH enhances calcium conservation by stimulating renal tubular absorption, intestinal absorption and bone resorption. The resulting hypercalcaemia so increases glomerular filtration of calcium that there is hypercalciuria despite the augmented tubular reabsorption. Urinary phosphate also is increased, due to suppressed tubular reabsorption. The main effects of these changes are seen in the kidney: calcinosis, stone formation, recurrent infection and impaired function. There may also be calcification of soft tissues.

There is a general loss of bone substance. In more severe cases, osteoclastic hyperactivity produces subperiosteal erosions, endosteal cavitation and replacement of the marrow spaces by vascular granulations and fibrous tissue ('osteitis fibrosa cystica'). Haemorrhage and giant-cell reaction within the fibrous stroma may give rise to brownish, tumour-like masses, whose liquefaction leads to fluid-filled cysts.

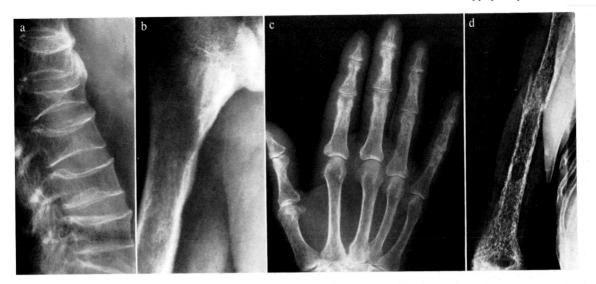

7.7 Hyperparathyroidism (a) This hyperparathyroid patient with spinal osteoporosis later developed pain in the right arm; an x-ray (b) showed cortical erosion of the humerus; he also showed (c) typical erosions of the phalanges. (d) Another case, showing 'brown tumours' of the humerus and a pathological fracture.

Symptoms*

The commonest features are due to the hypercalcaemia: anorexia, nausea and depression, abdominal pain, polyuria and recurrent kidney stones. Bone rarefaction may cause pain, pathological fracture and deformity. Curiously, patients with marked bone disease seldom have renal stones, and *vice versa*.

Biochemical tests show hypercalcaemia, hypophosphataemia and, sometimes, hyperuricaemia. Alkaline phosphatase is raised with osteitis fibrosa. Serum PTH levels may be high.

X-rays

The diagnostic sign is subperiosteal bone resorption, best seen on the radial borders of the middle phalanges of the second and third fingers. Generalized loss of bone density is common and cysts may be seen. Chondrocalcinosis sometimes occurs in the knees, wrists and shoulders.

Treatment

Removal of the adenoma or hyperplastic parathyroid tissue is usually indicated. Postoperatively there is a danger of severe hypocalcaemia due to brisk new bone formation (the 'hungry bone syndrome'). This must be treated promptly, with one of the vitamin D metabolites.

Scurvy

Vitamin C (ascorbic acid) deficiency causes failure of collagen synthesis and osteoid formation. The result is osteoporosis, which in infants is most marked in the juxtaepiphyseal bone. Spontaneous bleeding is common.

The infant is irritable and anaemic. The gums may be spongy and bleeding. Subperiosteal haemorrhage causes excruciating pain and tenderness near the large joints. Fractures or epiphyseal separations may occur.

*Bones, stones, moans and groans.

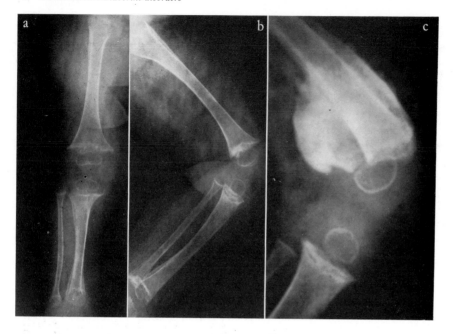

7.8 Scurvy   (a, b) The ring sign, the corner sign, and small subperiosteal haemorrhages;
(c) the femoral epiphysis has displaced, and the subperiosteal haemorrhage has calcified.

X-rays show generalized bone rarefaction, most marked in the long bone metaphyses. The normal calcification in growing cartilage produces dense transverse bands at the juxta-epiphyseal zones, and around the ossific centres of the epiphyses (the 'ring sign'). The metaphyses may be deformed or fractured. Subperiosteal haematomas show as soft-tissue swellings or periosseous calcification.

Treatment with large doses of vitamin C results in prompt recovery.

Hypervitaminosis

Hypervitaminosis A occurs in children following excessive dosage: in adults it occurs only in explorers who eat Polar bear livers. There may be bone pain, and headache and vomiting due to raised intracranial pressure. X-ray shows increased density in the metaphyseal region and subperiosteal calcification.

Hypervitaminosis D occurs if too much vitamin D is given. It exerts a PTH-like effect so that, as in the underlying rickets, calcium is withdrawn from bones; but metastatic calcification occurs. In treatment the dose of vitamin D must be properly regulated and the infant given a low calcium diet but plentiful fluids.

Osteoporosis

In osteoporosis the composition of bone is normal, but the amount of bone per unit volume is less than normal. By this definition everyone from 40 years onwards gradually becomes more osteoporotic. After the climacteric (about 50 years in women and 65 years in men) this process is markedly accelerated. Clearly gonadal involution is the most important factor and the same changes occur in younger women after oöphorectomy.

In addition to age-related bone loss, there are many diseases in which generalized osteoporosis is a feature. A clinical classification is presented (page 78), though to keep a sense of perspective certain practical truths must be recognized:

(1) Most cases of osteoporosis remain unexplained even after extensive investigation.
(2) Osteoporosis is so common in old people that it is impractical to investigate them for all possible causes (though malignant disease, dietary insufficiency and iatrogenic factors must always be excluded).

(3) Patients under 45 need full investigation; an important cause in the fifth decade is multiple myeloma.
(4) In any particular case, several factors may be involved.
(5) Radiological loss of bone density may be due to osteomalacia or osteoporosis, or to a combination of both.

Symptoms and signs

Bone loss is not in itself disabling: it only becomes so when it results in structural failure. Fractures occur with minimal force, especially in the spine, lower radius and femoral neck. Vertebral fractures lead to backache, kyphosis and loss of height. Unsuspected rib fractures may cause chest pain. Unless there is some associated metabolic bone disorder, biochemical tests are normal.

X-rays

General loss of bone density may be obvious, but does not differentiate osteoporosis from osteomalacia. Wedging or biconcave indentation of the vertebrae is common (but isolated fractures in the upper thoracic spine suggest malignant disease). In long bones the cortex is unduly thin.

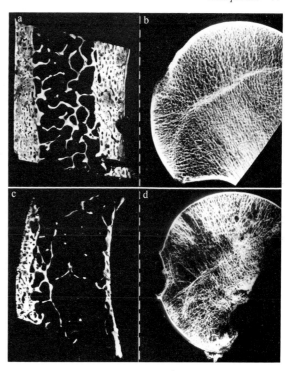

7.9 Osteoporosis Fine-detail x-rays of iliac crest biopsies and femoral head slices, showing the contrast between trabecular density at the age of 40 (a, b) and aged 70 (c, d). No wonder old bones break easily.

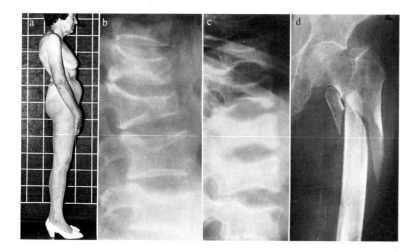

7.10 Osteoporosis (a) This woman noticed that she was becoming more and more 'round-shouldered'; she also had chronic backache and her x-rays (b) show compression of vertebral bodies. (c) Shows the spine of a similar patient who, 6 years after this film was taken, fell in her kitchen and sustained the fracture shown·in (d).

Measurement   Subjective x-ray evaluation of density is inaccurate because half the bone mass must be lost before rarefaction is detectable. Measuring cortical thickness (Nordin, 1971) and assessing the proximal femoral trabecular pattern (Singh *et al.*, 1972) are better. Other methods (photon absorptiometry, *in vivo* neutron activation analysis of bone mineral and computer-assisted axial tomography) require special equipment.

NOTE   Many elderly patients with 'osteoporotic' fractures also have osteomalacia. Unless tell-tale clinical or x-ray signs are present, the diagnosis can only be made on biopsy.

Table 7.2   Some causes of osteoporosis

Nutritional	*Malignant disease*
Scurvy	Carcinomatosis
Malnutrition	Multiple myeloma
Malabsorption	Leukaemia
Endocrine disorders	*Non-malignant disease*
Hyperparathyroidism	Rheumatoid arthritis
Gonadal insufficiency	Ankylosing spondylitis
Cushing's disease	Tuberculosis
Thyrotoxicosis	Chronic renal disease
Drug-induced	*Idiopathic*
Corticosteroids	Juvenile osteoporosis
Alcohol	Postclimacteric osteoporosis
Heparin	

Treatment

If there is a specific underlying disorder it may be correctable. Complications, such as femoral neck fracture or vertebral collapse, must be treated; and it is important to keep the patient active and to correct dietary deficiencies.*

Bone mass, once lost, is extremely difficult to restore. Bone formation can be stimulated by giving fluoride but, because the new bone is poorly calcified, this has to be combined with large doses of calcium and vitamin D (Jowsey, 1976). This 'triple therapy' has been used not only in postclimacteric osteoporosis, but in other forms also; careful monitoring is essential.

Prevention   There is now good evidence that oestrogens, given from the onset of the menopause, can prevent progressive bone loss (Lindsay *et al.*, 1976). However, there is still a fear of possible harmful side-effects of long-term oestrogen therapy.

Table 7.3

Osteomalacia	*Osteoporosis*
	Common in ageing women
	Prone to pathological fracture
	Decreased bone density
Ill	Not ill
Generalized chronic ache	Pain only after fracture
Muscles weak	Muscles normal
Looser's zones	No Looser's zones
Alkaline phosphatase increased	Normal
Serum phosphorus decreased	Normal
Ca × P < 2.4 mmol/l	Ca × P > 2.4 mmol/l

Endocrine disorders

Hypopituitarism

Growth hormone deficiency produces two distinct disorders: (1) proportionate dwarfism ('Lorain type') due to epiphyseal growth retardation; and (2) delayed skeletal maturation associated with adiposity and hypogonadism (Fröhlich's 'adiposogenital syndrome'). In both, the epiphyses remain unfused and, especially in those with the adiposogenital syndrome, there is danger of epiphyseal slipping at the hip or knee.

In the acquired types, the disorder may be reversible; e.g. by removing a craniopharyngioma. In others, growth hormone has been used.

*Dietary fads – a cause of starvation in the midst of plenty.

Hyperpituitarism

Acidophil cell hypersecretion results in skeletal overgrowth, the effects of which vary according to the age of onset.

Gigantism An acidophil adenoma in childhood stimulates epiphyseal growth. Patients are excessively tall, often with sexual immaturity and mental retardation. Slipping of the upper femoral epiphysis may occur.

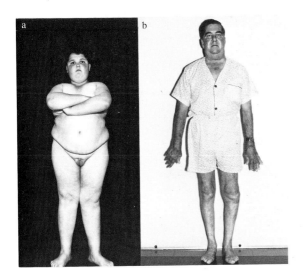

7.11 Endocrine disorders Two endocrine disorders which affect bone: (a) Fröhlich's adiposogenital syndrome; and (b) Cushing's syndrome, due in this instance to prolonged corticosteroid treatment for rheumatoid disease.

Acromegaly Hyperpituitarism starting in adulthood stimulates appositional bone growth and hypertrophy of articular cartilage. The jaw enlarges; together with thickening of the skull this produces a characteristic facies. The hands and feet are big and the long bone ends are markedly thickened; osteoarthritis is common.

Cushing's syndrome

Cushing's syndrome may be due to hypersecretion by the adrenal cortex, but is more often due to corticosteroid therapy. There is a characteristic obesity of the face and trunk, and generalized osteoporosis. With very large doses of steroids there is danger of bone necrosis.

Cretinism

With congenital thyroid deficiency the child is severely dwarfed and mentally retarded. Irregular epiphyseal ossification may be mistaken for avascular necrosis. These changes can be prevented by early treatment with thyroid hormone.

Paget's disease (osteitis deformans)

Paget's disease has a curious ethnic and geographic distribution, being relatively common in Britain, Germany and Australia (more than 3 per cent of people aged over 40), but rare in Asia, Africa and the Middle East. The cause is unknown, although recent work suggests a viral infection. The condition is characterized by high rates of bone resorption and formation;* plasma alkaline phosphatase and hydroxyproline are high and there is increased excretion of hydroxyproline in the urine.

In the osteolytic (or 'vascular') stage there is avid resorption of existing bone by large osteoclasts, the excavations being filled with vascular fibrous tissue. In adjacent areas osteoblastic activity produces new woven and lamellar bone, which in turn is attacked by osteoclasts. This alternating activity extends on both endosteal and periosteal surfaces, so that the bone increases in thickness but is structurally weak and easily deformed. Gradually osteoclastic activity abates and the eroded areas fill with new lamellar bone, leaving an irregular pattern of cement lines that mark the limits of the old resorption cavities; these 'tidemarks' produce a marbled or mosaic appearance on microscopy. In the late, osteoblastic, stage the thickened bone becomes increasingly sclerotic and brittle.

Clinical features

Paget's disease affects men and women equally. Only occasionally does it present in patients

---

*Paget bone is busy bone; busy but disorganized.

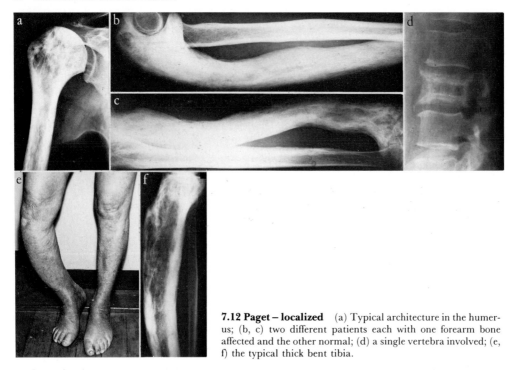

7.12 Paget – localized (a) Typical architecture in the humerus; (b, c) two different patients each with one forearm bone affected and the other normal; (d) a single vertebra involved; (e, f) the typical thick bent tibia.

under 50, but from that age onwards it becomes increasingly common. The disease may for many years remain localized to part or the whole of one bone – the pelvis and tibia being the commonest sites, the femur, skull, spine and clavicle the next commonest.

When a single bone is affected it may remain asymptomatic, or it may become painful and bent. The pain is a dull constant ache, worse at night, but rarely severe unless fracture occurs or sarcoma supervenes. Diagnosis is easy: the bone looks bent, feels thick and the skin over it is unduly warm; hence the term 'osteitis deformans'.

The patient with generalized Paget's disease may have few complaints, but a wide variety can occur: headache, deafness, deformities, stiffness, limb pain and sometimes fractures and heart failure. The skull enlarges so that bigger hats are required. Otosclerosis may produce deafness, and occasionally pressure on the optic nerve produces blindness. There is considerable kyphosis so that the patient becomes shorter and ape-like, with bent legs and arms hanging in front of him. Backache and root pain are common, and thickening of a single vertebra can produce all the symptoms of spinal stenosis. There is slight coxa vara, and considerable anterolateral bowing of the legs. When the disease extends up to a joint surface it may result in a painful, erosive arthritis.

X-rays show that the bone as a whole is thick and bent; its density in the vascular stage is decreased and in the sclerotic stage increased.* The trabeculae are coarse and widely separated, giving a streaky or honeycomb appearance. In the vascular stage, areas of porosis shaped like a candle flame are seen in the cortex. Later the thick cortex often shows, on its convex aspect, fine subperiosteal cracks probably resulting from stress; the junction of cortex and medulla is indistinct.

Disease activity is gauged by the increase in serum alkaline phosphatase and urinary hydroxyproline levels.

---

* Regular enlargement of bone suggests Paget's disease.

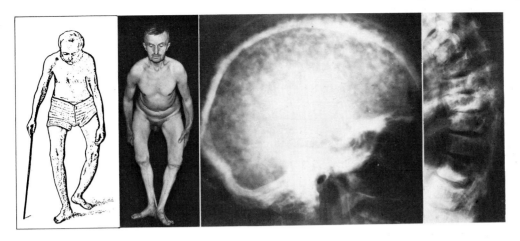

7.13 Paget – generalized   Paget's original case compared with a modern photograph. The skull and spine are characteristic.

Complications

FRACTURES are common, especially in the weight-bearing long bones. In the femoral neck they are often vertical; elsewhere the fracture line is usually partly transverse and partly oblique, like the line of section of a felled tree. In the femur there is a high rate of non-union; for femoral neck fractures prosthetic replacement, and for shaft fractures early internal fixation are recommended. Small stress fractures may be very painful; they resemble Looser zones on x-ray, except that they occur on convex surfaces.

BONE SARCOMA in the elderly is almost always due to Paget's disease. The frequency of malignant change is reported as between 1 and 11 per cent. It should always be suspected if a previously diseased bone becomes more painful, swollen and tender. Occasionally it presents as the first evidence of Paget's disease. The prognosis is extremely grave.

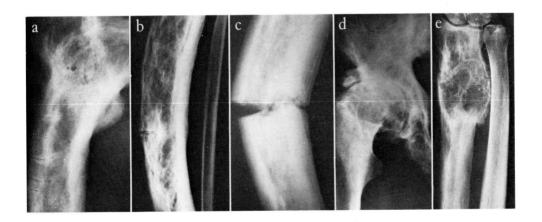

7.14 Paget – complications   (a) Fine cracks (microfractures) on the convex aspect, often associated with pain; (b) incomplete fracture; (c) the characteristic line of a complete fracture; (d) secondary osteoarthritis; (e) sarcoma.

NERVE COMPRESSION may cause peripheral pain or deafness.

NARROWING OF THE SPINAL CANAL can produce 'spinal claudication' and weakness in the lower limbs.

ARTHRITIS of the hip or knee occurs only if the subarticular bone is involved.

HIGH-OUTPUT CARDIAC FAILURE, though uncommon, is an important general complication. It is due to prolonged, increased bone blood flow.

HYPERCALCAEMIA may occur if the patient is immobilized for long.

In spite of all these complications most patients with Paget's disease come to terms with the condition and live to a ripe old age.

Treatment

Most patients with Paget's disease never have any symptoms and require no treatment. Drugs which suppress bone turnover, notably calcitonin and diphosphonates, are available as specific therapy; they are most effective when the disease is active and bone turnover is high. Indications for treatment are: (1) persistent bone pain; (2) repeated fractures; (3) neurological complications; (4) high output cardiac failure; (5) hypercalcaemia due to immobilization; and (6) for some months before and after major bone surgery where there is a risk of excessive haemorrhage. Drugs have also been used in the hope of slowing the process in the relatively young.

Calcitonin is the most widely used. It reduces bone resorption by decreasing both the activity and the number of osteoclasts; serum alkaline phosphatase and urinary hydroxyproline levels are lowered. Salmon calcitonin is more effective than the porcine variety; subcutaneous injections of 50–100 MRC units are given daily until pain is relieved and the alkaline phosphatase levels are reduced and stabilized. Maintenance injections once or twice weekly may have to be continued indefinitely, but some authorities advocate stopping the drug and resuming treatment if symptoms recur. Drug resistance due to antibody formation may occur, but this will be avoided when human calcitonin is more generally available.

Diphosphonates can be given orally (5 mg/kg per day for 6 months). If relapse occurs the treatment can be repeated. Higher doses carry the risk of a mineralization defect and increased fracture rate (Siris *et al.*, 1980).

Fractures occurring in the sclerotic stage unite slowly and usually require internal fixation. When the fracture is treated, the opportunity should be taken to straighten the bone.

Further reading

Chalmers, J., Conacher, W. D. H., Gardner, D. L. and Scott, P. J. (1967) Osteomalacia – a common disease in elderly women. *Journal of Bone and Joint Surgery* **49B**, 403–423

DeLuca, H. F. (1978) Vitamin D metabolism and function. *Archives of Internal Medicine* **138**, 836–847

Editorial (1978) Ten years' treatment for Paget's disease. *Lancet* **i**, 914–915

Jowsey, J. (1976) Advances in osteoporosis. *Lancet* **ii**, 524–525

Krane, S. M. (1977) Paget's disease of bone. *Clinical Orthopedics* **127**, 24–36

Lindsay, R., Hart, D. M., Aitken, J. M., MacDonald, E. B., Anderson, J. B. and Clarke, A. C. (1976) Long-term prevention of postmenopausal osteoporosis by oestrogen. *Lancet* **i**, 1038–1040

Nordin, B. E. C. (1971) Clinical significance and pathogenesis of osteoporosis. *British Medical Journal* **1**, 571–576

Parfitt, A. M. (1976) The actions of parathyroid hormone on bone: relation to bone remodelling to turnover, calcium homeostasis and metabolic bone disease. *Metabolism* **25**, 809–844, 909–955, 1033–1069 and 1157–1188 (in 4 parts)

Singh, M., Riggs, B. L., Reabout, J. W. and Jowsey, J. (1972) Femoral trabecular pattern index for evaluation of spinal osteoporosis. *Annals of Internal Medicine* **77**, 63–67

Siris, E. S., Caufield, R. E., Jacobs, T. P. and Baquiran, D. C. (1980) Long-term therapy of Paget's disease of bone with EHDP. *Arthritis and Rheumatism* **23**, 1177–1184

Solomon, L. (1974) Fracture of the femoral neck: bone ageing or disease? *South African Journal of Surgery* **2**, 269–279

Tashjian, A. (1975) Prostaglandins, hypercalcemia and cancer. *New England Journal of Medicine* **293**, 1317–1318

Dysplasias

8

Bone dysplasia is taken to mean a generalized disorder of bone and cartilage. Malformations may involve bone, though not necessarily; but there are structural defects in more than one system.

Genetic considerations

DOMINANT INHERITANCE   Only one gene of a pair is abnormal. The resulting disorder typically affects both sexes and all generations; up to 50 per cent of first-degree relatives are affected, though with varying severity.

RECESSIVE INHERITANCE   Both genes of a pair are abnormal. The resulting disorder appears in the child of apparently normal parents, each of whom has one abnormal gene. Up to one in four siblings may be affected. If the same dysplasia has two forms of inheritance, the recessive is the more severe.

X-LINKED INHERITANCE   The gene concerned is on the X chromosome (of which males have one, but females two). An X-linked disorder can never pass from father to son. The father inevitably passes his X chromosome only to his daughters, who may be unaffected carriers. X-linked recessive disorders affect only males; X-linked dominant disorders are commoner in females.

MULTIFACTORIAL INHERITANCE   Multiple genes and environmental factors combine to produce the disorder, so that inheritance is complex. Many common orthopaedic disorders such as club foot and congenital hip dislocation are in this group.

A clinical approach

From the moment the patient appears it may be obvious that he has a generalized dysplasia of some kind. But these disorders are . rare and precise diagnosis is difficult. The following section is intended as an introductory guide to identification, which is important for prognosis, treatment and genetic counselling.

HISTORY

Family history   Most dysplasias are familial, but any individual patient may be the first in his family to be affected. Such sporadic cases arise either from new mutations (this is common with achondroplasia) or from environmental damage (e.g. thalidomide deformities).

Fractures   A history of many fractures suggests the possibility of osteogenesis imperfecta or of osteopetrosis.

CLINICAL EXAMINATION

Stature   Many dysplastic patients are short enough to be classified as dwarfs (less than 1.25 m in height). If so, it is helpful to know which kind:

(1) Proportionate dwarfs (with trunk and limbs equally affected). Possible diagnoses include Hurler's disease, hypophosphatasia, hypophosphataemia, and the severe (congenita) varieties of osteogenesis imperfecta and osteopetrosis.
(2) Short-limbed dwarfs with a normal (or nearly normal) spine. Possible diagnoses include achondroplasia, hypochondroplasia, diastrophic dwarfism and chondroectodermal dysplasia.

(3) Short-limbed dwarfs with considerable spine involvement. Possible diagnoses include spondyloepiphyseal dysplasia, metatropic dwarfism and Morquio's disease.

Joints Excessive joint laxity is a feature of a number of connective-tissue disorders, including Ehlers–Danlos syndrome, Marfan's syndrome, Morquio's disease and osteogenesis imperfecta.

Distribution Some dysplasias (e.g. dyschondroplasia, dysplasia epiphysealis hemimelica and melorheostosis) are not generalized; they affect only one side of the body or only one limb. Such disorders are not familial.

X-RAYS
Anatomical site Even if clinical examination does not reveal which portion of the long bones is affected, radiographs do; they may enable one to label the disorder as epiphyseal, metaphyseal or diaphyseal; and they demonstrate whether or not the spine is involved. Three films often suffice: an AP of the wrists and hands, an AP of the pelvis and hips, and a lateral of the spine.

Bone density There is generalized decrease of bone density in osteoporosis, homocystinuria, osteogenesis imperfecta and Albright's disease. Increased bone density is seen in osteopetrosis, Engelmann's disease, melorheostosis and osteopoikilosis.

Achondroplasia

This disease is of autosomal dominant inheritance, but since most individuals do not marry and have children, cases are usually sporadic. Cartilage cells produced by the epiphyses fail to line up properly and undergo degeneration.

Clinical features

If the child survives the first year he becomes a short-limbed dwarf with normal intelligence and often with excellent muscles. The skull is large

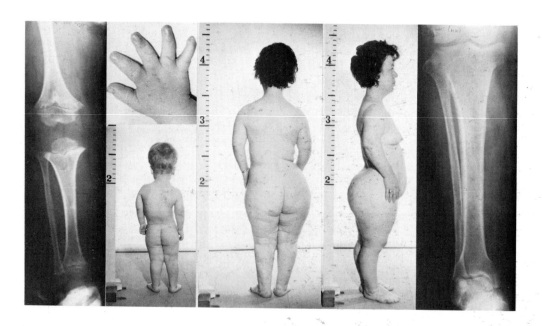

8.1 Achondroplasia This boy and his mother show the typical features of the classic disease, although their slight scoliosis is uncommon. The child's epiphyses have V-shaped notches. If his mother had them also, her present x-rays clearly show that they did not distort growth.

and brachycephalic, with bulging vault and forehead, and a flat nose. The limbs are grossly short, notably the proximal segments, so that the hands do not reach the buttocks and the patient may be able to kiss his toes while keeping his knees straight. The fingers are short, stubby and unusually equal in length. The trunk, though not very short, may have a kyphosis (which occasionally persists and becomes severe) and a lumbar lordosis, producing the prominent buttocks which, together with the other features described, account for the popularity of achondroplastics as circus dwarfs.

The vertebral pedicles are short and, in the lumbar spine, too close together; consequently the spinal canal is narrow (spinal stenosis), and disc prolapse (which is common) has exceptionally severe effects (a feature noted also in dachshunds, who are of course achondroplastic).

X-rays

The tubular bones are short and relatively thick. The metaphyses at the knee are splayed out peripherally and may contain a central notch into which the central part of the epiphysis dips. The skull as a whole is large but its base is too short. The pelvis is too small for normal delivery.

Diagnosis

The 'classic' disorder described above must be differentiated from its variants, and from other causes of short-limbed dwarfism.

In *hypochondroplasia* dwarfism is less marked and the skull is normal.

In *diastrophic dwarfism* other deformities are associated, notably severe club foot, scoliosis, cauliflower ear, joint contractures and a widely abducted 'hitch-hiker's' thumb.

In *chondroectodermal dysplasia* (Ellis–van Creveld syndrome) dwarfism is associated with cardiac disorders, polydactyly and hypoplastic nails and teeth. The limb shortness, unlike that in achondroplasia, affects distal segments more than proximal.

In *spondyloepiphyseal dysplasia* dwarfism is associated with grossly distorted large proximal joints, a normal skull and irregular platyspondyly. The term covers a group of disorders, including one which is X-linked and affects only males. In most, the trunk (unlike that in achondroplasia) is disproportionately short; but one variety is short-limbed and is called pseudoachondroplasia, although the distorted joints preclude the supple agility of classic achondroplasia.

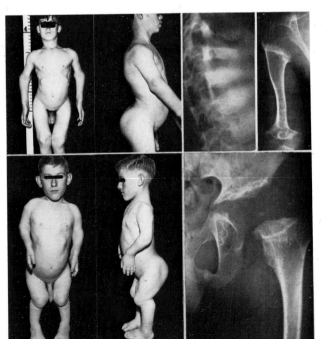

8.2 Spondyloepiphyseal dysplasia

Usual variety

Pseudoachondroplastic type

Osteogenesis imperfecta (brittle bones)

The process of bone manufacture is faulty and stops short at the 'woven bone' stage. Consequently the bones bend too easily and break too easily. There are two distinct varieties: (1) congenita (recessive) – multiple fractures occur before, during or soon after birth; and (2) tarda (dominant) – this is less severe, and the patient is likely to survive into adult life. The tendency to fracture diminishes after puberty.

Clinical features

As well as short stature and limb deformities, the clinical features may include: a broad skull (with Wormian bones visible on x-ray), blue sclera, otosclerosis (although deafness does not come on until adult life), scoliosis, ligament laxity and a tendency to bruise easily. The limb deformities result from the bending of soft bone combined with malunion of fractures. Coxa vara, bowing of the femur and tibia, knock knees, valgus feet and dislocation of the radial head are all fairly common.

The appearance depends upon the variety. In the *congenita* type dwarfism and deformities are severe; the limbs are bent and the spine scoliotic, but deafness and blue sclerae are not marked features. In the *tarda* variety deformity is much less; the spine and limbs are often straight, but the sclerae are blue and deafness is common in middle life. Shortly before a fracture, blue sclerae may look darker, the sweat may smell different and the child become more clinging.

The shafts of the long bones are bent and slender; the ends, however, appear large and are sometimes cystic. A triradiate pelvis and biconcave vertebral bodies are other sequels of the bone softening; osteoporosis is marked.

Complications and treatment

The fractures are frequently greenstick in type and unite rapidly with routine treatment. Very occasionally a tremendous periosteal reaction develops; the appearance of this 'hyperplastic callus' mimics that of a bone sarcoma.

No general treatment is known. To prevent malunion of fractures intramedullary nailing is useful; and where severe deformity has already occurred, the shaft can be divided into segments and held straight with an intramedullary nail (the 'kebab' treatment). To allow for growth, telescopic rods may be used.

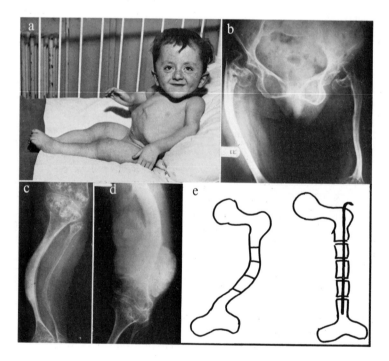

8.3 Brittle bones (a) The patient may look like Humpty Dumpty (who probably had brittle bones); (b, c) the bones develop characteristic deformities; (d) hyperplastic callus – a rare complication; (e) the 'kebab' procedure for straightening a bent bone.

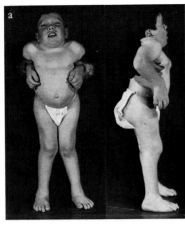
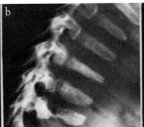
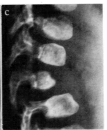

8.4 Mucopolysaccharide disorders (a) Morquio–Brailsford disease—note the manubriosternal angle; (b) irregular platyspondyly in a similar patient, contrasted with (c) the sabot appearance in Hurler's disease.

Mucopolysaccharide disorders

This group is characterized by inborn errors of mucopolysaccharide (MPS) metabolism. They differ from each other in mode of inheritance, type of MPS found in the urine, and in their clinical features – which may include dwarfism. Among the least rare are the following.

MORQUIO–BRAILSFORD DISEASE   Development is apparently normal for the first year or two; thereafter dwarfism becomes progressively obvious. The spine is kyphotic and the manubriosternal angle is 90 degrees (a pathognomonic feature). The vertebrae are too flat (platyspondyly) with a narrow tongue of bone projecting forwards. The hips are grossly distorted and genu valgum or varum often severe. Ligamentous laxity is marked, but the skull and mentality are both normal. Keratan sulphate is found in the urine

HURLER'S DISEASE   The synonym 'gargoylism' is justified by coarse skin, bloated lips and eyelids, wide-set eyes and corneal opacities. Mental retardation is noted early. The limb deformities may resemble those in Morquio–Brailsford disease. There is, however, no platyspondyly or 'tonguing', although the lower part of a vertebra may protrude forwards. There is no ligament laxity; indeed these children are stiff-jointed. Dermatan sulphate and heparan sulphate are found in the urine. Cardiopulmonary complications are common, so that, in contrast to Morquio–Brailsford disease, these patients rarely survive into adult life.

HUNTER'S DISEASE   differs slightly from Hurler's and is less severe. It is of X-linked recessive inheritance and all patients are male.

Hereditary multiple exostoses (diaphyseal aclasis)

In this disorder of autosomal dominant inheritance there is failure of bone remodelling: as tubular bones grow in length, the excess metaphyseal bone is not resorbed but forms irregular cartilage-capped exostoses. It has been suggested that the affected bones 'squander their growth potential'; the cartilage columns of the epiphyseal plate grow less rapidly in length, while appositional growth of cartilage continues and leads to wide, poorly modelled metaphyses.

Clinical features

The skull and spine are normal, although often the patient is slightly short. Multiple lumps are found on the upper humerus, the lower end of the radius and ulna, around the knee, above the ankle and occasionally on flat bones. No lumps grow on the epiphyses, and only rarely does an exostosis migrate with growth as far as the middle third of the shaft. In contrast with dyschondroplasia the fingers have only tiny knobs, or none at all. Bowing of the radius and valgus deformity at the knees and ankles are not uncommon; some deformities may be produced by an exostosis from one bone pressing on its neighbour. X-rays show irregular metaphyses, with sessile or pedunculated exostoses projecting from the surface.

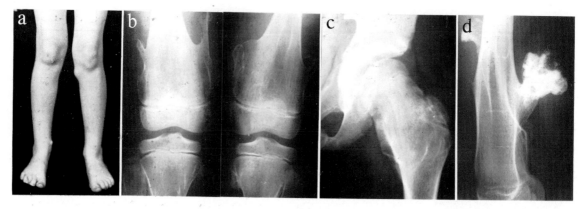

8.5 Diaphyseal aclasis (a) This boy's brother and father had similar lumps. (b) Another patient with typical exostoses near the bone ends. (c) Sometimes the metaphyses are broad and their architecture is irregular. (d) Wide metaphysis and a large cartilage-capped exostosis.

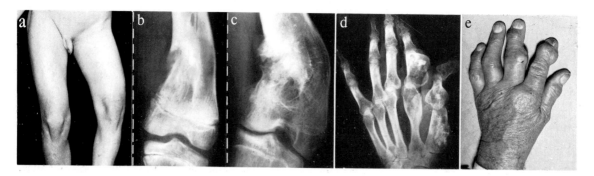

8.6 Dyschondroplasia (a) This boy with a bent femur had, when first seen, the x-ray shown in (b); deformity progressed to (c) before an osteotomy was performed. (d) and (e) show two patients with multiple chondromas.

Treatment and complications

A lump may interfere with tendon action and need removal. The exostoses stop growing when the parent bone does; any subsequent increase in size is suggestive of malignancy (chondrosarcoma), which is said to occur in 5 per cent of patients.

Dyschondroplasia (Ollier's disease)

This rare disease is not familial. Ossification of cartilage at the growth discs is faulty, islands of cartilage remaining unossified within the shaft.

Clinical features

Typically the disorder is unilateral; indeed only one limb or even one bone may be involved. An affected limb is short and, if the growth plate is asymmetrically involved, the bone grows bent. Common deformities are valgus or varus at the knee and ankle, and relative shortening of the ulna so that the radius is curved and sometimes dislocated. The fingers or toes frequently contain multiple enchondromata, which are characteristic of the disease and may be so numerous that the hand is crippled. Malignant change in 1 per cent of the chondromata has been reported. A rare variety of dyschondroplasia is associated with multiple haemangiomata (Maffucci's disease).

X-rays show large translucent islands or columns of cartilage in the metaphysis. As the child grows, these islands develop irregular dense spots. The shaft, although often curved, is usually of normal structure. The metaphysis may be mottled or streaky. The fingers nearly always show multiple chondromata with stippled calcification. Even when the disease is clinically unilateral, the other side may show radiographic abnormalities.

Treatment includes the correction of deformity, but osteotomy should, if possible, be deferred until growth is complete – otherwise it is likely to recur.

Osteopetrosis (marble bones, Albers–Schönberg disease)

The bones are excessively dense and structureless on x-ray; they look like marble and break easily. There are two forms. (1) *Tarda* (dominant): this, the common form, may be asymptomatic and only discovered during radiography for other conditions. The general appearance and life span are normal, and complications (other than pathological fracture) are uncommon. (2) *Congenita* (recessive): this form is rare. Progressive anaemia, infection (dental caries may lead to osteomyelitis of the jaw) and pancytopenia may lead to death in the first or second decade. Cranial nerve palsies and encroachment on the pituitary fossa may occur.

Candle bones, spotted bones and striped bones

Candle bones (melorheostosis, Leri's disease) is not familial. The patient presents with pain and stiffness, usually confined to one limb. X-rays show irregular patches of sclerosis, usually distributed in linear fashion through the limb; the appearance is reminiscent of the wax which congeals on the side of a burning candle. Scleroderma and joint contractures may be associated.

In *spotted bones* (osteopoikilosis) numerous white spots are seen in the x-rays of many bones; there may also be whitish spots in the skin (disseminated lenticular dermatofibrosis).

In *striped bones* (osteopathia striata) x-rays show lines of increased density parallel to the shafts of long bones, but radiating like a fan in the pelvis. The condition is symptomless.

Cleidocranial dysplasia

In this condition of autosomal dominant inheritance there is faulty development of membrane bones, chiefly the clavicles and skull. The patient is somewhat short, with a large head, flat-looking face and drooping shoulders. The skull is brachycephalic, the teeth appear late and develop poorly. Because the clavicles are partly absent, the patient can bring his shoulders together in front of the chest. Spinal curvature

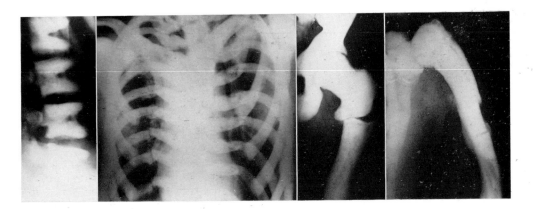

8.7 Marble bones Despite the remarkable density, the bones break easily; but, as in this humerus, union occurs without special difficulty.

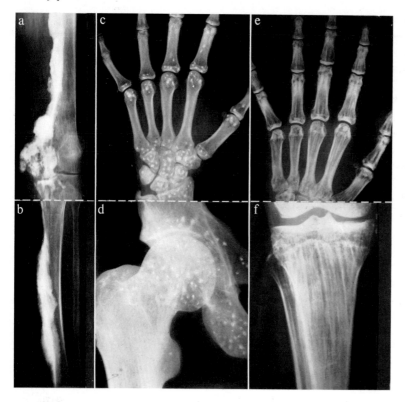

8.8 Radiological curiosities

(a) (b)
Candle
bones

(c) (d)
Spotted
bones

(e) (f)
Striped
bones

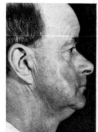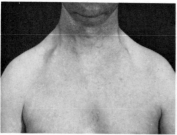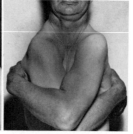

8.9 Cleidocranial dysplasia
The squashed face, sloping shoulders and trick movement are unmistakable.

and widening of the symphysis pubis are not uncommon. The radius may be short and the elbows valgus. The hands are curious in that the index finger is often too long, while the terminal phalanx of the thumb (or other fingers) is too short. The mentality is normal.

X-rays show that a part of each clavicle is absent; usually the outer half, sometimes the middle third and, rarely, the inner quarter. Wormian bones occur in the skull, the pubis usually shows deficient ossification and sometimes there is coxa vara.

Epiphyseal dysplasias

Dysplasia epiphysealis multiplex is the least rare of this group, some of which are familial. The face, skull and spine are normal. Many major epiphyses are affected. On x-ray they appear late and close early; they are ill-formed, irregular and mottled. In time their architecture becomes normal but not their shape, so that deformity and stiffness result. Secondary osteoarthritis is common.

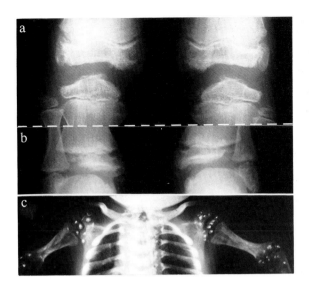

8.10 Epiphyseal dysplasias (a, b) This girl with multiple epiphyseal dysplasia had many epiphyses as irregular as these; her sister was similarly affected. (c) This infant probably has Conradi's disease – the spots usually disappear with growth.

Dysplasia epiphysealis punctata may be a variation of multiplex, but a severe one, with epiphyseal mottling obvious at birth. Conradi's disease (chondrodysplasia calcificans congenita), in which mental retardation, dwarfism, congenital heart disease and cataracts occur, also has epiphyseal mottling visible from birth, but the mottling disappears with growth.

Dysplasia epiphysealis hemimelica affects epiphyses, usually of the ankle but sometimes also of the knee. One limb only is involved and usually only half the epiphysis (medial or lateral); in the affected area a bony lump develops. The child presents because of the lump or because of stiffness. Treatment consists of removing the excess epiphyseal material.

Craniometaphyseal dysplasia (of autosomal dominant inheritance) is sometimes confused with Pyle's disease. It is less rare and, in addition to the metaphyseal widening, there is progressive thickening of the skull and mandible, resulting in a curiously prominent forehead, a large jaw and a squashed-looking nose.

Metaphyseal chondrodysplasia is of autosomal dominant inheritance. The metaphyses are an odd shape and may look irregularly cystic. Varus hips and knees are common. Schmid's disease is the mildest variety. In Jansen's disease dwarfing is severe and deafness may occur. In McKusick's disease there is dwarfing, sparse hair and sometimes also Hirschsprung's disease; the condition is often mistaken for rickets.

Diaphyseal dysplasias

Progressive diaphyseal dysplasia (Camurati's or Engelmann's disease) is characterized by fusiform widening and sclerosis of the shafts of the long bones and sometimes also of the skull. Often the femur, tibia and forearm bones are symmetrically

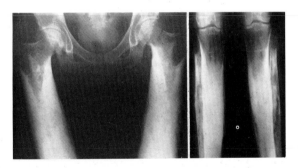

8.11 Engelmann's disease This patient had considerable discomfort from her long bones – all of which were wide and looked dense on x-ray.

Metaphyseal dysplasias

Metaphyseal dysplasia (Pyle's disease) is of autosomal recessive inheritance. There is failure of modelling in the long bone metaphyses, resulting in 'Erlenmeyer flask' deformities of the distal femora and proximal tibiae; this may be associated with genu valgum.

affected. Cortical thickening is both superficial (causing widening) and deep (sometimes causing medullary obliteration); the bone ends are normal. The patient presents with painful limbs, weakness or a waddling gait. Steroids are said to relieve pain.

Craniodiaphyseal dysplasia is characterized by expansion of the long bone shafts coupled with gross bony thickening of the skull and face, so that the term leontiasis ossea is sometimes used.

Fibrous dysplasia (fibrocystic disease)

Fibrous dysplasia is probably a developmental defect. The process may affect one bone (monostotic), one limb (monomelic) or many bones (polyostotic). In all varieties the cellular fibrous tissue in the medullary spaces of the bone proliferates, destroying trabeculae; the resulting cavities contain fluid or fibro-osseous tissue and the walls contain giant cells.

The patients present in childhood or adolescence with ache, limp, bony enlargement, deformity or, occasionally, a pathological fracture. Radiologically, translucent 'cystic' areas are found in the affected metaphyses and shafts, but not in the epiphyses; the abnormal areas are crisscrossed by dense lamellae, or have a uniform ground-glass appearance. In contrast to hyperparathyroidism the bones are not markedly osteoporotic. Girls are affected more often than boys, and the polyostotic variety is more common than the monostotic.

Yellowish-brown pigmentation of the skin may be associated, especially with the polyostotic variety. In girls this may be associated with sexual precocity (Albright's disease).

The possibilities of treatment are: excision and bone-grafting if the area is not too extensive; osteotomy if the bone is bent.

Fibrodysplasia ossificans progressiva

Fibrodysplasia ossificans progressiva is very rare; its cause is unknown. In the first years of life episodes of fever occur and tender swellings appear, chiefly in the head, neck or trunk. Subsequently ectopic ossification develops in the connective tissue of muscle, mainly in the trunk. An associated anomaly is undue shortness of the big toes and sometimes also the thumbs. The ossification gradually extends, limiting movement more and more; the outcome used to be fatal but it is hoped that treatment with diphosphonates will be effective.

The condition was formerly called *myositis ossificans progressiva*, but it has no connection with *myositis ossificans traumatica*, which follows injury or operation (page 362); nor with *myositis ossificans circumscripta*, which particularly affects patients with brain or cord damage and which may involve several joints (especially the hips, knees and shoulders), sometimes totally stiffening these joints.

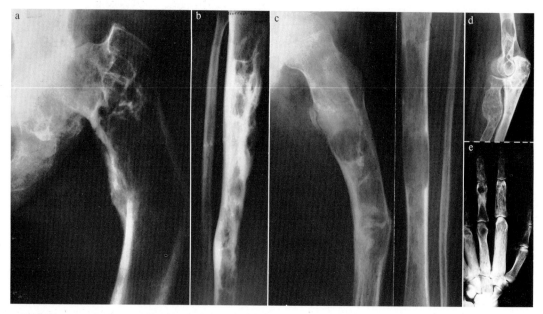

8.12 Fibrous dysplasia   (a) Monostotic fibrous dysplasia of the upper femur, with the so-called 'shepherd's crook' appearance; (b) monostotic fibrous dysplasia of the tibia. (c, d, e) are from three patients with polyostotic fibrous dysplasia.

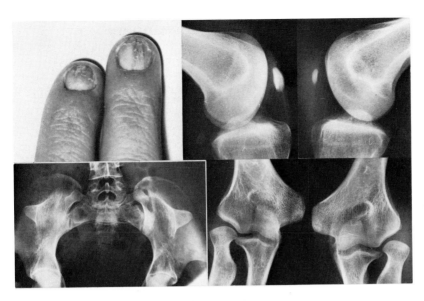

8.13 The nail–patella syndrome   The dystrophic nails, minute patellae, pelvic 'horns' and subluxed radii combine to make an unmistakable picture.

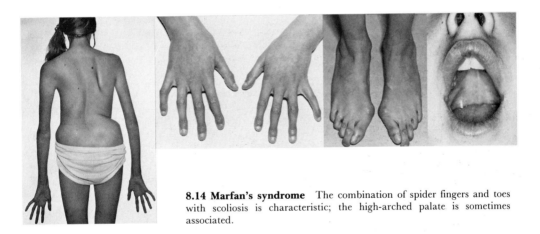

8.14 Marfan's syndrome   The combination of spider fingers and toes with scoliosis is characteristic; the high-arched palate is sometimes associated.

Nail–patella syndrome (osteo-onychodysplasia)

A dominant autosomal gene is responsible for this curious familial disorder. The nails are hypoplastic and the patellae unduly small or absent. The radial head may be subluxed laterally and bony excrescences ('horns') develop on the lateral aspect of the ilium. Congenital nephropathy may be associated.

Marfan's syndrome

In this disorder of autosomal dominant inheritance there is a defect in elastin or collagen, or both. Ocular lens dislocation and aortic aneurysms are often the presenting features. The patients are tall, with disproportionately long legs, and often with chest deformities. Despite the absence of vertebral anomalies scoliosis is common. The digits are unusually long, giving rise to the term 'arachnodactyly' (spider fingers).

Generalized joint laxity is usual, but often the finger and toe joints have contractures. Other features include a high arched palate and hernias.

HOMOCYSTINURIA   This metabolic disorder of autosomal recessive inheritance resembles Marfan's disease in general build and proneness to lens dislocation. But osteoporosis and widening of epiphyses and metaphyses occur only in homocystinuria (the osteoporotic vertebrae may be flat or biconcave); scoliosis and arachnodactyly, however, are less frequent. Moreover, mental defect is much commoner in homocystinuria and stickiness of platelets increases the risk of postoperative thrombosis. The diagnostic feature is of course the presence of homocystine in the urine.

Acrocephalosyndactyly (Apert's syndrome)

In this disease of dominant inheritance the head is peculiar in shape, with a high broad forehead ('tower-shaped'), a flattened occiput, bulging eyes and a prominent jaw. Unless premature fusion of the cranial sutures can be prevented, eye changes and mental retardation occur. The associated syndactyly of fingers and toes is of an unusual type; the three 'inboard' digits are joined together.

The combination of Apert's syndrome with polydactyly of the toes is called *Carpenter's syndrome*.

Chromosome anomalies

These include numerical anomalies (e.g. too few chromosomes, as in Turner's syndrome; or too many, as in Down's syndrome), and structural anomalies such as translocation of a group of genes. Chromosome anomalies are always associated with multiple defects and usually with mental retardation.

Localized malformations

CONGENITAL VERTEBRAL ANOMALIES
These are of three main kinds: (1) agenesis, with total absence of vertebrae; (2) dysgenesis, with hemivertebrae, or with vertebrae fused together (sometimes called errors of segmentation); and (3) dysraphism, with deficiencies of the neural arch. These are considered under scoliosis (page 219), kyphosis (page 224) and spina bifida (page 119). Corresponding sacral anomalies also occur: agenesis has a low incidence of visceral anomalies; dysgenesis a high incidence; and dysraphism may have urogenital problems but is otherwise usually normal.

CONGENITAL LIMB ANOMALIES
These include extra bones, absent bones and fusions. Complete absence of a limb is called amelia, almost complete absence (a mere stub remaining) phocomelia and partial

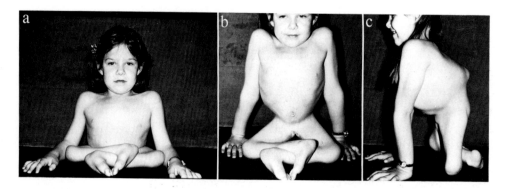

8.15 Sacral agenesis   This girl with sacral agenesis shows (a) the characteristic sitting posture, (b) the underdeveloped pelvic girdle, and (c) the spinal 'hump'.

absence ectromelia; defects may be transverse or axial. In the hands and feet brachydactyly, syndactyly, polydactyly and symphalangism are among the many possibilities. When genetic factors are present at all, the inheritance is dominant. Detailed elaboration of terminology interests the philologist more than the surgeon.

ABSENT RADIUS Although sometimes an isolated phenomenon (page 177) absence (or dysplasia) of the radius may be associated with pancytopenia; this condition (Fanconi's anaemia) leads to early death. In another syndrome with radial absence the blood cells are normal but there is a deficiency of platelets.

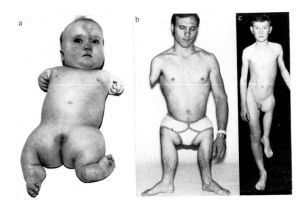

8.16 Congenital limb anomalies (a) A thalidomide baby, with all four limbs severely affected. (b) This man, with three limbs affected, had almost complete absence of his femora. (c) Severe dysplasia of one femur – leg length inequality was the major problem here.

DYSPLASIA OF THE UPPER FEMUR In its most benign form shortening is less than 7 cm and treatment no different from that for leg inequality in poliomyelitis (page 142). But if the dysplasia is combined with coxa vara, shortening may be too severe for practicable leg lengthening; an artifical extension may be feasible but amputation often permits greater prosthetic elegance. If the entire upper third of the femur is missing the situation is still worse; but the 'absent' part may in fact be cartilaginous, in which case bone grafting can provide hip stability and therefore more satisfactory limb-fitting. Good prognostic features are: a good acetabulum; a large gap between the acetabulum and the radiologically visible part of the upper femur; and a bulbous end to the upper femur. If the upper third (or even more) is truly absent the only prospect for even mediocre prosthetic fitting is to perform one of several heroic operations described by van Nes: e.g. femoral osteotomies to make the foot point backwards so that its muscles activate the 'knee' of a prosthesis.

CONGENITAL PSEUDARTHROSIS OF THE TIBIA As usual, the term 'congenital' is ambiguous for the fracture is not necessarily present at birth; the unbroken tibia may contain an area of neurofibromatosis, or of fibrous dysplasia, or may simply be bowed forwards. Fracture below the mid-shaft occurs within the first 2 years of life; if treated by conservative methods non-union is inevitable.

Treatment McFarland's technique is reasonably successful; a graft is inserted from healthy bone above to healthy bone below, bypassing the angulated abnormal area. Alternatives are onlay grafting with rigid internal fixation, or electrical stimulation (page 361). If these measures fail, amputation is kinder than repeated operations. It should be noted that, whereas anterior bowing (tibial kyphosis) is dangerous, posterior bowing is said to be innocuous, and to correct itself without fracture.

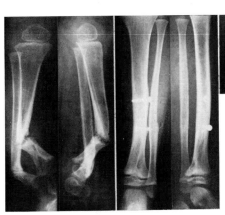

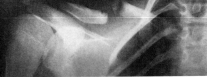

8.17 Congenital pseudarthrosis The tibia is the commonest site; in this case bone-grafting was successful. This clavicular pseudarthrosis (from a different patient) is of course on the right.

OTHER ANOMALIES OF THE LEG   Absence of the tibia usually demands amputation. Absence of the whole or part of the fibula may be associated with tibial bowing, with leg shortening or with absence of the fourth or fifth rays of the foot. Leg lengthening is exceedingly difficult, and if osteotomy seems inappropriate, amputation (preferably Syme's) is needed.

CONGENITAL PSEUDARTHROSIS OF THE CLAVICLE   is probably due to pressure by the subclavian artery on the developing clavicle. In every reported unilateral case the right side has been affected—except in one patient with dextrocardia. The child is brought up with a painless lump. Treatment, if required, is by excision or grafting.

Further reading

Aegerter, F. and Kirkpatrick, J. A. (1975) *Orthopaedic Diseases*, 4th edn. Philadelphia: Saunders

Bailey, J. A. (1970) Orthopaedic aspects of achondroplasia. *Journal of Bone and Joint Surgery* **52A**, 1285–1301

Fixsen, J. A. and Lloyd-Roberts, G. C. (1974) The natural history and early treatment of proximal femoral dysplasia. *Journal of Bone and Joint Surgery* **56B**, 86–95

King, J. D. and Bobechko, W. P. (1971). Osteogenesis imperfecta. *Journal of Bone and Joint Surgery* **53B**, 72–89

Lloyd-Roberts, G. C. (1971) *Orthopaedics in Infancy and Childhood*. London: Butterworths

Lloyd-Roberts, G. C., Apley, A. G. and Owen, R. (1975) Reflections upon the aetiology of congenital pseudarthrosis of the clavicle. *Journal of Bone and Joint Surgery* **57B**, 24–29

Marafioti, R. L. and Westin, G. W. (1977) Elongating intramedullary rods in the treatment of osteogenesis imperfecta. *Journal of Bone and Joint Surgery* **59A**, 467–472

Shapiro, F., Simon, S. and Glimcher, M. J. (1979) Hereditary multiple exostoses. *Journal of Bone and Joint Surgery* **61A**, 815–824

Shapiro, F., Glimcher, M. J., Holtrop, M. E., Tashjian, A. H., Brickley-Parsons, D. and Kenzora, J. E. (1980) Human osteopetrosis. *Journal of Bone and Joint Surgery* **62A**, 384–399

Wynne-Davies, R. (1973) *Heritable Disorders in Orthopaedic Practice*. Oxford: Blackwell Scientific

Wynne-Davies, R. and Fairbank, T. J. (1976) *Fairbank's Atlas of General Affections of the Skeleton*. Edinburgh: Churchill Livingstone

Tumours

9

Classification

In 1972 the World Health Organization proposed a classification of bone tumours, of which the following is an abstract:

Bone-forming tumours – including osteoma, osteoblastoma and osteosarcoma.

Cartilage-forming tumours – including chondroma, chondroblastoma and chondrosarcoma.

Giant-cell tumours – which form a group on their own.

Marrow tumours – including Ewing's tumour and myeloma.

Vascular tumours – including haemangioma, glomus tumours and angiosarcoma.

Other connective-tissue tumours – including lipoma, liposarcoma and fibrosarcoma.

Other tumours – including adamantinoma, neurilemmoma and neurofibroma.

For completeness they add a further group of 'tumour-like lesions', such as bone cysts, fibrous dysplasia and eosinophilic granuloma. In the present chapter benign tumours of bone are described first, doubtful ones next, then malignant bone tumours; the final section deals with soft-tissue tumours and lumps.

Benign or malignant?

A benign tumour remains local, and on x-ray usually has a well-defined edge. A malignant tumour has the potential to metastasize and its edges often look ill-defined.

Nearly all benign tumours occur in adolescents or young adults and stop growing when bone growth is complete; they may be large, but size alone is not evidence of malignancy, though progressive increase of size may well be. Other features suggesting malignancy are pain, warmth, tenderness, cortical destruction (as distinct from thinning), calcification extending into the soft tissues and 'hot spots' on bone scanning.

It should be clearly understood that all primary bone tumours, whether benign or malignant, are rare; this is in contrast with secondary deposits in bone which, especially in those over the age of 50, are relatively common.

Osteoma

The word 'osteoma' is often used loosely and applied to any bony overgrowth, whether or not this is a tumour. Even with the two varieties described below (the least equivocal), the terminology is doubtful; thus a compact osteoma is regarded by some pathologists as a variety of fibro-osseous dysplasia; and osteoid osteoma, though generally thought to be a true tumour, often behaves like a granuloma.

COMPACT OSTEOMA (ivory exostosis)
This rarity consists of a squat sessile knob of ivory-hard bone which microscopically shows only normal bone cells. It does not metastasize.

An adolescent or young adult presents with a painless lump, usually on the outer surface of the skull. It can occur on the inner surface (focal epilepsy is then a possibility), or it may grow into the paranasal sinuses. On x-ray a sessile plaque of exceedingly dense bone with a well-circumscribed edge is seen.

The tumour is best excised. It is so hard that a small area of surrounding normal bone must be excised with the tumour.

OSTEOID OSTEOMA
Microscopically the tumour consists of osteoid tissue with trabeculae of newly formed bone, in a vascular connective-tissue groundwork. It is

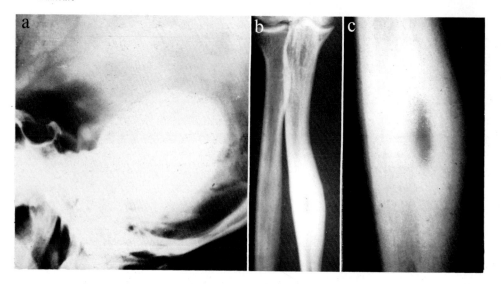

9.1 Osteoma (a) Compact osteoma – as hard as ivory, but painless. (b) Osteoid osteoma – a source of considerable pain; (c) enlarged view of the same case to show the translucent nidus.

small (usually less than 1 cm in size), round or oval in shape and is encased in dense bone.

Osteoid osteoma is most commonly seen in patients aged under 30; males predominate. Any bone except the skull may be affected, but over half the cases occur in the femur or tibia. The leading symptom is pain, which is sometimes severe and is not relieved by rest; limp and wasting may occur. Salicylates often relieve the pain.

The important x-ray feature is a small radio-lucent area, the so-called 'nidus'. In medullary lesions there may be slight surrounding sclerosis, but in the cortex thickening and sclerosis are often so dense that the nidus (which may itself contain a radio-opaque centre) can be seen only in tomograms.

It is sometimes difficult to distinguish an osteoid osteoma from a small Brodie's abscess without biopsy. Ewing's tumour and chronic periostitis must also be excluded (see page 24). Rarely, regional osteoporosis occurs with an osteoid osteoma and the x-ray appearance then resembles joint tuberculosis. Diagnostic doubt, especially in children, is often dispelled by a bone scan using ^{99m}Tc.

Excision of the affected area cures the pain and the tumour does not recur.

BENIGN OSTEOBLASTOMA
This rare vascular tumour, sometimes called a giant osteoid osteoma, usually affects adults. Histologically it is indistinguishable from an osteoid osteoma. It occurs in the spine (often with scoliosis) or the major limb bones. Pain and tenderness are features. X-ray shows a well-demarcated osteolytic lesion which sometimes contains flecks of calcification. Treatment consists of excision and bone grafting. Malignant change has been reported.

Cartilaginous tumours

SHORT-BONE CHONDROMA
This, the commonest variety, consists only of mature cartilage cells. The tumour is well encapsulated, often lobulated, and rarely becomes malignant. It occurs in one of the short pipe bones – a metacarpal, metatarsal or proximal phalanx.

The patient presents with a swelling or, more commonly, with a fracture after trivial injury. X-ray shows a well-defined rare area, often with characteristic specks of calcification.

The differential diagnosis is from a solitary cyst (which has no calcification) and from dyschondroplasia (in which the chondromas are multiple). The tumour with its lining capsule should be excised and a bone graft or chips inserted.

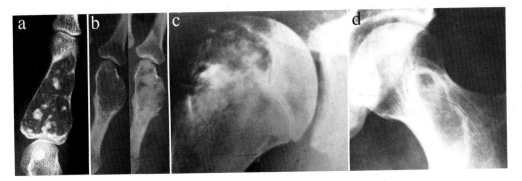

9.2 Cartilaginous tumours (a) Chondroma of a finger. (b) Another digital chondroma, before and after curettage and grafting. (c) Chondroblastoma. (d) Chondromyxoid fibroma.

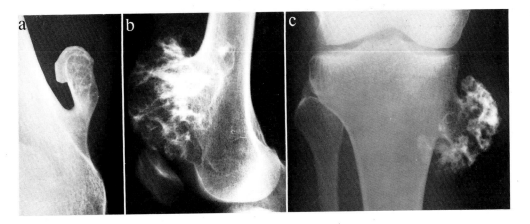

9.3 Cartilage-capped exostosis (osteochondroma) The two main varieties: (a) is conical and the cartilage does not show on x-ray; (b) and (c) are cauliflower-shaped and the cartilage cap has partly calcified.

LONG-BONE CHONDROMA

A true chondroma may involve a long bone. The patient is usually aged over 30. X-ray shows a rare area, usually well defined and with a mottled appearance due to irregular calcification. Malignancy may supervene and the tumour is therefore best excised.

BENIGN CHONDROBLASTOMA

The cells of this rarity are chondroblasts. The tumour starts in the epiphysis, usually of the proximal humerus or femur, though the pelvis or other bones can be affected. Males are more commonly affected, especially in their teens or twenties, and the presenting symptom is a constant ache gradually increasing in severity. X-ray shows a well-defined area of rarefaction eccentrically placed in the epiphysis or across the epiphyseal plate, with no reaction in the surrounding bone.

Malignant change does not occur, and simple curettage is the best treatment.

CHONDROMYXOID FIBROMA

This presents as a chronic ache, chiefly in patients aged 10–40; the lower limb is usually involved. X-rays show a round or oval rare area, often eccentrically placed in the metaphysis but occasionally crossing the growth disc. It is distinguishable by its sclerosed endosteal margin. Malignant change has been recorded and though curettage may prove adequate, where feasible the tumour should be resected.

CARTILAGE-CAPPED EXOSTOSIS
(osteochondroma)

This, the commonest benign 'tumour' of bone, is really a hamartoma. It consists of normal bone covered by a cap of normal cartilage. Any bone which develops by endochondral ossification may be involved; the commonest site is the metaphysis

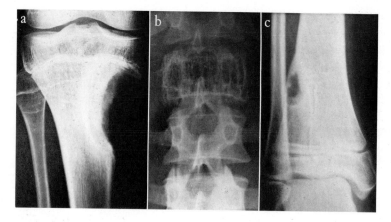

9.4 Other benign tumours   (a) Aneurysmal bone cyst. (b) Haemangioma of vertebra. (c) Fibrous cortical defect – if these defects are large, the term 'non-ossifying fibroma' is sometimes used.

of a long bone, especially around the knee. The tumour may be broad and cauliflower-shaped, or an elegant cone. In either case the lump should stop growing when bone growth ceases.

The patient is usually aged between 10 and 40. Any symptoms (other than the presence of a lump) such as pain or interference with tendon action, depend upon the anatomical site. The lump is bony hard, though sometimes covered by a bursa which may be tender. It is attached to the parent bone, but not to skin or muscle. On x-ray it is well defined; often it looks smaller than it feels, because the cartilage cap is invisible. The diagnosis is from diaphyseal aclasis, a familial disorder in which the lumps are multiple (page 87).

If the tumour causes symptoms it should be excised; if, in an adult, it has recently become bigger or painful then operation is urgent, for these features (together with a fluffy outline on x-ray) suggest malignancy. In about 1 per cent of cases the cartilage cap continues to grow in adult life and gives rise to a chondrosarcoma. This is seen most often with pelvic exostoses – not because they are inherently different, but because considerable enlargement may, for long periods, pass unnoticed.

Other benign tumours

ANEURYSMAL BONE CYST

This tumour-like lesion contains cavities filled with blood. It chiefly occurs in the spine and the metaphysis of long bones. It is an expanding lesion, thinning and destroying the cortex. X-rays show a well-defined rare area, often trabeculated and eccentrically placed. Radiologically it may resemble a giant-cell tumour, but that tumour extends to the articular surface whereas aneurysmal bone cysts are confined to the metaphyseal side of the growth plate. Curettage and packing with bone chips gives good results.

HAEMANGIOMA

When this rare tumour occurs in the spine it is a source of persistent backache. X-rays show vertical striations which can be distinguished from Paget's disease by the lack of bone expansion. In the skull and pelvis the so-called 'sun-burst' or 'soap-bubble' appearance with radiating spicules is typical and may suggest malignancy, but there is no associated cortical or medullary destruction. In the pipe bones a haemangioma may cause elongation of the bone; usually it presents as a pathological fracture. X-ray shows a shaggy trabeculated tumour expanding the bone. At operation these tumours bleed profusely, and radiotherapy is a wiser method of treatment.

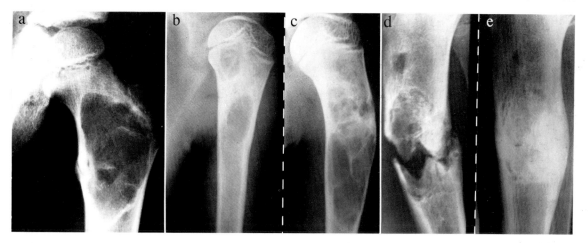

9.5 Solitary cyst   (a) A typical solitary (or unicameral) cyst – on the shaft side of the growth disc and expanding the cortex. (b, c) Cyst extending as the patient grows. (d, e) Fracture through a cyst, leading to healing.

FIBROUS CORTICAL DEFECT (non-ossifying fibroma)

This is a benign 'tumour' of children. It is discovered accidentally on x-ray, which shows a lucent area in the cortex of a long bone metaphysis; the margin is well defined, sometimes scalloped and often sclerosed. Most of these defects heal spontaneously, but it seems likely that some may grow, so that pathological fracture is a possibility.

SOLITARY CYST

This is not strictly a tumour. It usually occurs in the upper humerus, femur or tibia, but other bones may be affected. Solitary cysts are seen in children up to the age of puberty and after that become increasingly rare. Clinically a cyst presents with local ache, or as a pathological fracture.

X-rays show a translucent area on the shaft side of the growth disc. The cortex may be thinned and the bone expanded. The cyst is rounded and has a clear-cut edge but no surrounding sclerosis (for differential diagnosis, see page 13).

Because cysts are hardly ever seen in adults, it is presumed that many disappear spontaneously. A fracture through a cyst often results in the cyst becoming obliterated. Injecting steroids into the cyst, after penetrating its wall with a trocar, may lead to its obliteration (Scaglietti *et al.*, 1979). If not it can be evacuated, the wall scraped and the cavity filled with bone chips.

Giant-cell tumour

Pathology

The adjective 'benign' was formerly used but is misleading: only about one-third remain truly benign, one-third become locally invasive and one-third metastasize.

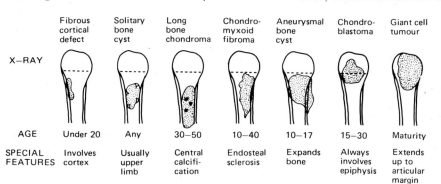

	Fibrous cortical defect	Solitary bone cyst	Long bone chondroma	Chondro-myxoid fibroma	Aneurysmal bone cyst	Chondro-blastoma	Giant cell tumour
X–RAY							
AGE	Under 20	Any	30–50	10–40	10–17	15–30	Maturity
SPECIAL FEATURES	Involves cortex	Usually upper limb	Central calcification	Endosteal sclerosis	Expands bone	Always involves epiphysis	Extends up to articular margin

9.6 Cyst-like lesions of bone

The tumour derives its name from multinucleated giant cells which are seen in large numbers; but these are less significant than mononuclear stromal cells, from whose proliferation they probably arise (Dahlin, 1978). Typically there is no definite intercellular substance, but blood-filled spaces are not uncommon and sometimes there are fibrogenic zones. Macroscopically the tumour is usually large, soft and friable; it may look grey or reddish-brown, and sometimes oozes blood. Grading on a cellular basis is used but is not prognostically reliable.

Clinical features

The tumour usually occurs between the ages of 20 and 40. It is nearly always situated at the very end of a long bone. Possibly, however, it originates in the metaphysis but grows so rapidly that, by the time it is seen clinically, it abuts against the joint. The usual presenting symptom is vague discomfort, sometimes with slight swelling. A history of trauma is not uncommon and pathological fracture occurs in 10–15 per cent of cases.

On examination, there is a vague swelling of the end of a long bone. (Egg-shell crackling is rare nowadays because of early diagnosis.) The neighbouring joint is often irritated.

X-rays show a rarefied area situated asymmetrically at the end of a long bone abutting against the articular surface. Often there are trabeculae and a 'soap-bubble' appearance. The junction with normal bone is often ill-defined; but even a well-defined junction must not be taken to ensure

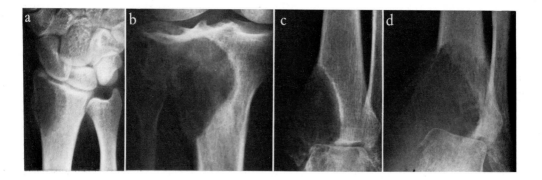

9.7 Giant-cell tumours (a, b, c) In each of these the tumour abuts against the joint margin, and is asymmetrically placed – these are characteristic features; in (d) malignant change has supervened and the junction of the tumour with the rest of the bone is no longer well-defined.

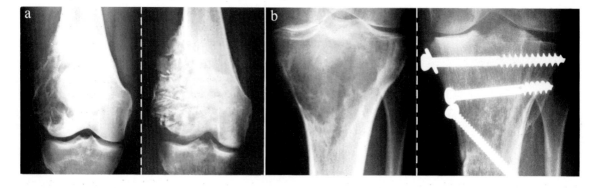

9.8 Giant-cell tumour – treatment (a) Excision and bone grafts. (b) Block resection and replacement with a large osteocartilaginous graft from another individual (who had died after a road accident).

a good prognosis. The cortex is very thin and sometimes ballooned, but is intact unless a fracture has occurred or the tumour is frankly malignant.

Treatment

The simplest treatment is curettage (followed by cauterization of the wall and instillation of bone chips), but recurrence is common. Total excision is therefore the treatment of choice, with replacement by specially designed prostheses or by osteocartilaginous grafts. Amputation is indicated for tumours which recur with increasing evidence of malignancy. Radiotherapy is reserved for surgically inaccessible tumours.

Chordoma

This rare tumour arises from notochordal remnants. The usual site is the sacrococcygeal spine but the cervical spine can be affected. The tumour has been called 'benign' because metastasis is rare; but it is locally malignant, growing to a large size and invading surrounding structures. It may present as a lump, or with pain from nerve involvement, or with pelvic obstruction and oedema of one or both lower limbs. The usual x-ray appearance is a large osteolytic area in the midline, occasionally containing flecks of calcification. If excision is not feasible, radiotherapy should be tried.

Osteosarcoma

Pathology

Osteosarcoma (formerly called osteogenic sarcoma) implies a primary tumour arising from bone and producing bone.

Primitive spindle cells with numerous mitoses are characteristic. Their products may be predominantly fibroblasts (when the tumour looks like a 'fibrosarcoma'), chondroblasts (when it looks like a 'chondrosarcoma') or mucoid cells (when it looks like a 'myxosarcoma'). But these are all variants of one

tumour. In addition, there are bone cells of two main varieties: osteoblasts which lay down osteoid, and giant osteoclasts which destroy bone.

The macroscopic appearance is enormously variable, but the tumour is a big one situated in the metaphysis. If bone destruction predominates, the tumour is very soft and vascular (osteolytic); if there is a fair amount of bone formation, it is more grey and gritty (osteoblastic).

The tumour at first extends within the medulla but soon perforates the cortex. The periosteum is pushed away from the shaft and new bone is laid down at the angles of periosteal elevation (Codman's triangle). As the bone invades the soft tissues, new bone forms along the vascular channels at right angles to the shaft (sun-ray spicules). The tumour metastasizes via the blood stream, chiefly to the lungs but also to other bones, commonly the skull and femur.

Clinical features

The incidence is highest between the ages of 10 and 20 years, but a second peak occurs in the sixth and seventh decades due to malignant change in Paget's disease. The commonest site is at the metaphysis of a long bone, especially around the knee.

A history of trauma is present in more than half the cases but is thought to have no aetiological significance; it merely draws attention to the underlying disorder. Pain is usually the first symptom; it is constant, worse at night and gradually becomes severe. Sometimes the patient presents with a lump. A pathological fracture is rare.

On examination, a lump (usually large) can nearly always be seen or felt. The overlying skin may be shiny with prominent veins. The lump feels tender and lacks a definite edge. It is attached to bone and often to muscles. If growing rapidly, it feels warm and it may pulsate. The erythrocyte sedimentation rate is raised.

X-ray appearances are very variable but show a combination of bone destruction and bone formation. The medulla contains an area of rarefaction, sometimes with ill-defined clouds of increased density; the tumour has an ill-defined junction with the rest of the shaft. The cortex is somewhere perforated. The periosteum may show sun-ray spicules and Codman's triangle; these are not common but when they do occur are characteristic. An adjacent soft tissue mass, containing spicules of new bone, may be seen.

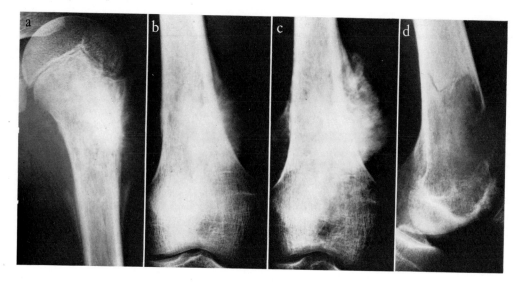

9.9 Osteosarcoma   (a, b) Characteristic appearance with sun-ray spicules and Codman's triangle; (c) the same patient as (b), after radiotherapy; (d) a predominantly osteolytic tumour.

Scanning techniques may help in determining the extent of the tumour and investigating the possibility of metastases.

Differential diagnosis

A painful lump near the end of a long bone in a young person must be presumed to be a sarcoma until the contrary is proved, if necessary with the aid of biopsy. Other conditions which must be considered are as follows.

Post-traumatic swellings   such as callus and myositis ossificans.

A stress fracture   may show a small area of cortical interruption with overlying subperiosteal new bone; this, together with the histological appearance of disorganized callus, easily gives rise to a tragically mistaken diagnosis of osteosarcoma.

Infective conditions   such as osteomyelitis or syphilis of bone; in every case a white cell count and tests for syphilis are essential.

Benign tumours   usually have a well-defined edge, but not always. If there is any doubt, a biopsy is needed.

Treatment

The former appalling prognosis has markedly improved with combined therapy, though precise figures are not yet available. The fundamentals are simple: amputation for the primary, chemotherapy for mini-secondaries, radiotherapy in reserve. But an x-ray of the chest and a biopsy of the tumour are essential preliminaries.

Amputation   is the mainstay of treatment. Formerly very high amputations were needed (e.g. above-knee for even a low tibial tumour); effective chemotherapy protects against stump recurrence, and amputation through the affected bone (provided it ensures complete removal of the primary tumour) is now sufficient.

Chemotherapy   aims to destroy undetectably minute metastases. It must begin soon after amputation, certainly within 10 days. The drugs are highly toxic, so must be given in centres equipped to deal with bone marrow, renal, cardiac and other complications. Various protocols are under trial. In Britain the drugs used are doxorubicin, vincristine and methotrexate (a folic acid antagonist). Huge doses of methotrexate are used; a few hours later the patient's normal cellular activity is 'rescued' by citrovorum factor. Vincristine, methotrexate and citrovorum factor are administered at 21-day intervals, or alternating with doxorubicin. This regimen may have debilitating side-effects and requires hospital admission for a day or two every 3 weeks, for at least a year. Unsuspected secondaries may be revealed by bone scanning.

Radiotherapy is used to control tumours at surgically inaccessible sites, such as the pelvis and jaw, or for patients who refuse amputation.

Other methods include: (1) resection of solitary (or even multiple) pulmonary metastases when rendered 'static' by chemotherapy; (2) excision of stump recurrences, also combined with chemotherapy; (3) immunotherapeutic techniques are being tried (a portion of the excised tumour is implanted into a sarcoma survivor, removed after 14 days, and 'sensitized' lymphocytes from it infused into the patient); (4) interferon also is being tried.

Parosteal sarcoma

This rare tumour is on the outer surface of the bone. The cells are well differentiated, often with fibroblasts; macroscopically the tumour is firm, grey and encapsulated. It is prone to be mistakenly diagnosed as a benign fibrous lesion.

The patient is aged over 30. He presents with constant ache, or a lump which is growing and which feels like hard rubber. X-ray shows an irregular amorphous mass of ossified tissue on the surface of the bone and tending to encircle it; the cortex is not eroded and usually a fine linear gap remains between cortex and tumour. Amputation gives a high cure rate but, if the site is unsuitable, local excision followed by radiotherapy carries a reasonably good prognosis.

Chondrosarcoma

Chondrosarcoma can occur either as a primary tumour or as secondary change in a pre-existing cartilaginous tumour. It affects people aged 35–55. They complain of a constant ache or of recent increase in size of a previously stationary lump. The x-ray appearances are variable: a primary (central) chondrosarcoma gives a large cystic lesion with cortical destruction and central calcification; malignant change in a cartilage-capped exostosis gives increase in size and a fuzzy outline.

These tumours tend to metastasize late, and at least one attempt at wide local excision is justified. Where neither excision nor amputation is practicable, radiotherapy may be tried.

Fibrosarcoma of bone

Fibrosarcoma of bone may arise in previously abnormal bone. (Paget's disease and irradiated giant-cell tumours are examples.) The patients are aged over 30 (often over 50) and present

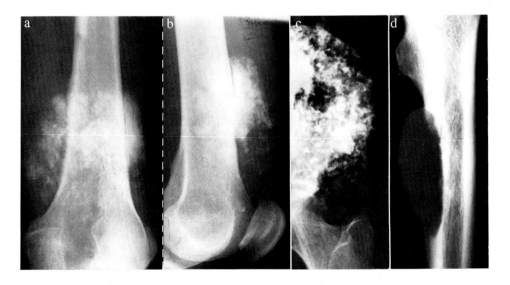

9.10 Some other bone sarcomas   (a, b) Parosteal sarcoma – note the linear gap between cortex and tumour; (c) this chondrosarcoma developed in a cartilage-capped exostosis; (d) fibrosarcoma.

with pain or a pathological fracture. X-rays show an osteolytic lesion which may be completely surrounded by reactive subperiosteal new bone. Treatment is by amputation or radiotherapy; the survival rate is better than that for osteo-sarcoma.

Ewing's tumour

Pathology

Microscopically, sheets of small dark polyhedral cells with no regular arrangement and no ground substance are seen. Macroscopically, the tumour is lobulated and often fairly large. It may look grey (like brain), or red (like red-currant jelly) if haemorrhage has occurred into it.

Local spread is similar to that of osteogenic sarcoma. The periosteum appears to resist the tumour and may lay down layers like an onion. Distal spread is (1) via the blood to the lungs and also often to other bones; (2) via the lymphatics.

Clinical features

The tumour occurs most commonly between the ages of 10 and 20 years (rarely, 5–30). A long bone is usually affected, especially the tibia. The tumour is situated anywhere in the bone.

Pain and a limp are the chief presenting symptoms; the pain is throbbing, worse at night and often severe; a history of trauma is common. The patient is sometimes ill and may be pyrexial. The lump is warm, tender, has an ill-defined edge and is attached to bone and to soft tissues. The pain, swelling and pyrexia may all fluctuate from time to time.

The x-ray appearances vary widely. Sometimes a rarefied area can be seen in the medulla and often the cortex is perforated. 'Onion-layers' of periosteal new bone are said to be characteristic.

Differential diagnosis

Blood examination is important to exclude staphylococcal osteomyelitis (which Ewing's tumour may closely resemble) and to exclude syphilis.

Biopsy is essential to exclude other tumours affecting bone, notably adrenal neuroblastoma and reticulum-cell sarcoma; both these conditions, as well as Ewing's tumour, are sometimes called 'round-cell sarcomas of bone' but there are important differences.

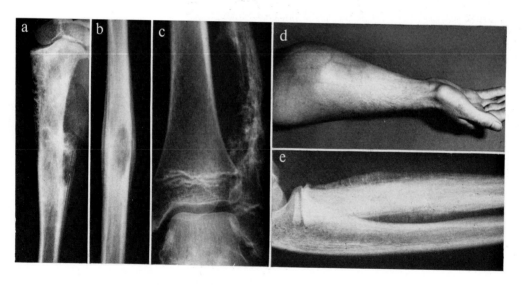

9.11 Ewing's tumour   (a) Of the humerus; (b) of the mid-shaft of the fibula; (c) of the lower fibula; (d, e) secondary adrenal neuroblastoma mimicking Ewing's tumour.

Adrenal neuroblastoma metastasizes to bone and the deposits strongly resemble Ewing's tumour. Histologically, however, the round cells of neuroblastoma are arranged in characteristic rosettes. In 60 per cent of neuroblastomas the urine contains the catecholamine derivative vanilmandelic acid.

Reticulum-cell sarcoma in bone is sometimes a solitary lesion; in which case (after biopsy has established the diagnosis) radiotherapy may effect a cure. If, however, there is generalized involvement of the reticuloendothelial system (malignant lymphoma) the prognosis is poor and treatment is by chemotherapy.

Eosinophilic granuloma of the mid-shaft may give onion-layering and be indistinguishable from Ewing's tumour without biopsy.

Treatment

The outlook is poor, but the best results so far reported were from a combination of wide excision, radiotherapy and triple chemotherapy.

Multiple myeloma

Pathology

The tumours are said to arise from plasma cells of the bone marrow. The typical microscopic picture is of plasmacytes with a large eccentric nucleus containing a spoke-like arrangement of chromatin. The tumours are found wherever red marrow occurs; that is, in the trunk bones, skull and root bones. They are usually multiple from the start; they are small, and grey or purple in colour. They look like multiple secondaries, but no primary tumour is ever found.

Clinical features

The patient, aged 45–65, presents with weakness, bone pain or a pathological fracture. The bone pain is constant and backache in particular is common, sometimes with root pain and occasionally paraplegia. Anaemia, cachexia and chronic nephritis all contribute to the general ill-

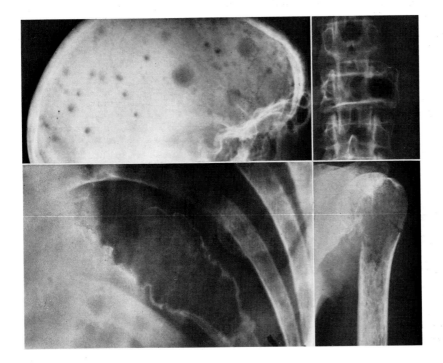

9.12 Myelomatosis   In the skull and spine the appearance resembles that of secondary carcinoma; the rib and humerus are more characteristic of myelomatosis.

health. There is almost invariably a high sedimentation rate. The usual cause of death is renal failure.

X-rays may show nothing more than overall reduction in density; more often there are multiple punched-out defects with no marginal new bone around them. These make it difficult to exclude those cases of multiple secondary deposits in which no primary can be found.

Investigations of importance in establishing a diagnosis are: urinalysis, which in over half the cases shows Bence Jones protein; electrophoretic analysis of plasma and urine proteins, which shows a characteristic pattern; and sternal marrow puncture, which reveals the typical myeloma cells. Often an unusually high sedimentation rate (over 100) alerts suspicion and prompts the surgeon to undertake these investigations.*

Treatment

Radiotherapy and chemotherapy relieve pain and pressure effects for a time, and may prolong survival. Pathological fractures in the limbs are best treated by internal fixation. Spinal fractures are treated with a brace; unrelieved cord pressure may need decompression.

Plasmacytoma

This is the name often applied to a solitary myeloma. The patient presents with pain, a lump or a pathological fracture. X-ray shows a multilocular expanding osteolytic lesion in a red marrow area. Years may elapse before multiplicity becomes apparent. Treatment is by radiotherapy.

Secondary carcinoma of bone

Pathology

In two-thirds of cases, secondary bone deposits arise from carcinoma of the breast or prostate, because these are the most common primary tumours. In a further one-sixth of cases, the deposits arise from other carcinomas (of thyroid gland, kidney, bronchus, genitalia, bladder, gastrointestinal tract). In the remaining one-sixth, no primary tumour is found. The macroscopic and microscopic appearances correspond to those of the primary tumour.

There are three possible routes whereby the deposit may travel from the primary tumour to the bone.

(1) Most bone secondaries arise from tissue whose veins do not drain via the portal system into the liver. The cells travel via the vena cava and heart to the lung (where carcinoma cells can always be found microscopically in cases of bone deposits). In the lung, clumps of cells multiply, then probably penetrate capillaries to enter the systemic circulation and so reach bone.
(2) There is also a direct connection between the pelvic plexus of veins and the vertebral veins, which explains why pelvic primaries are especially liable to give deposits in the pelvic bones and spine.
(3) Tumours of the rectum and of some other epithelial tissues may invade bone directly.

The above theories fail to explain why the muscles, heart and spleen enjoy immunity from secondary deposits.

Clinical features

The patient is usually aged 50–70 years and secondary deposits are found chiefly where red bone marrow is plentiful; namely, in the trunk bones (vertebrae, skull, pelvis, ribs) and 'root' bones (upper ends of the humerus and femur).

The primary tumour may be obvious but sometimes even a meticulous search fails to reveal it. The neck, breasts, axillae, lungs, abdomen and genitalia should be examined, and rectal or vaginal examination is usually necessary. Investigations which may be required include x-rays of the chest and urogenital tract, blood count, sedimentation rate, protein electrophoresis and estimation of the serum phosphatases.

The secondary deposit usually presents either with local ache or as a pathological fracture. Some deposits, however, are clinically silent, being revealed only by x-ray. Many fail to show even on x-ray but can be revealed by bone scanning using radioactive isotopes.

---

*Osteoporosis, aged 45–60 + a high ESR = myelomatosis until proved otherwise.

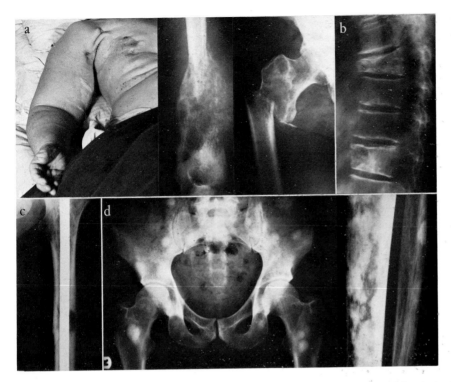

9.13 Secondary deposits (a) This patient presents an all-too familiar picture; (b) spinal secondaries; (c) osteolytic deposits are liable to fracture and invite internal fixation; (d) osteoblastic deposits in the pelvis and tibia, from prostatic carcinoma.

X-ray appearances

OSTEOLYTIC DEPOSITS These are much the commoner variety and 90 per cent of breast secondaries are of this type. One or more rare areas are seen in the medulla. Later the cortex appears mottled and may be destroyed so that the bone collapses. There is little or no periosteal reaction.

OSTEOBLASTIC DEPOSITS Deposits from carcinoma of breast or bowel are occasionally osteoblastic, but much the commonest are prostatic secondaries, probably because the cells contain much phosphatase (serum acid phosphatase is increased). A single vertebral body may look too dense. More often the pelvis shows mottled increase of density; and this latter must be distinguished from Paget's disease, in which the alkaline phosphatase (not the acid) is increased. Lymphoma deposits also may resemble prostatic metastases.

Treatment

By the time a patient has developed secondary deposits the prognosis, as far as life is concerned, is almost hopeless. Occasionally, radical treatment (by combined surgery and radiotherapy) of a solitary secondary deposit and of its parent primary may be rewarding and even apparently curative. This applies particularly to hypernephroma and thyroid tumours; but in the great majority of cases, and certainly in those with multiple secondaries, treatment is entirely symptomatic. For that reason elaborate witch-hunts to discover the source of an occult primary tumour are to be deprecated; the search may be diagnostically satisfying, but is therapeutically valueless and psychologically harmful.

Most patients with secondary deposits can, however, be made comfortable for a time by one or more of the following measures: drug therapy, irradiation or operative treatment.

DRUGS Ordinary analgesics should be tried first; later, larger doses or more powerful drugs become necessary. Although a fatal outcome is inevitable it may be long delayed, so caution must be exercised in using habit-forming drugs until the condition is advanced.

The pain of secondary deposits from the breast or prostate can often be relieved by drugs which control the hormone environment; moreover, these drugs sometimes delay the advance of the condition and relief may last for several years. For prostatic secondaries, stilboestrol is the most effective drug. With secondary deposits from the breast, androgenic drugs are usually best in premenopausal patients, and oestrogens in those past the menopause.

Cytotoxic drugs, which damage cells in proportion to their mitotic activity, are often valuable. They include alkylating agents such as the nitrogen mustards, and antimetabolites such as various folic acid antagonists; actinomycin D possibly comes into this second category.

IRRADIATION Deep x-ray therapy and other forms of irradiation are exceedingly valuable. A primary tumour may shrink in size and become painless, the pain from secondary deposits also is usually relieved at least for a time, and paraplegia due to spinal deposits sometimes recovers. Moreover, irradiation can usefully be combined with other forms of treatment.

OPERATIVE TREATMENT A fungating tumour is usually best excised, although occasionally it can be controlled by radiotherapy. Intractable pain from secondary deposits may occasionally require surgical methods for its relief; these include division of sensory nerves, nerve roots, nerve tracts in the spinal cord and the intrathecal injection of alcohol. In addition, the hormone environment of secondary breast deposits can sometimes be controlled by oöphorectomy combined with adrenalectomy, or by hypophyseal ablation.

THE TREATMENT OF FRACTURES A patient with secondary deposits often does not present until pathological fracture occurs. In treating these fractures it is important not to be too timid. An overcautious conservative approach often means a painful, lingering death. It is better to accept the small risk of operative methods with internal fixation; if the bone is too weak for effective plating it may first be plugged with acrylic cement. The pain of the fracture is immediately relieved and the patient usually able to get up and about. If operation is followed by radiotherapy, the fracture often unites satisfactorily; moreover, the use of internal fixation enables the patient to be taken to the radiotherapy department without discomfort. Vertebral fractures through secondary deposits are treated by radiotherapy and a spinal support.

Prophylactic internal fixation is a neglected but valuable technique; if x-rays suggest the possibility of subsequent fracture, fixation by plating or an intramedullary nail is well worth considering.

Soft-tissue tumours and lumps

The vital question (as with bone tumours) is whether the tumour is benign or malignant. The features of a lump which arouse suspicion are: pain, especially in a previously painless lump; recent or rapid increase of size; an indefinite edge; and attachment to surrounding structures. When doubt exists, a biopsy is essential. The regional lymph nodes should be palpated and, since malignant soft-tissue tumours almost invariably metastasize to the lungs, the chest should be x-rayed. The account which follows is intended only as a summary of those soft-tissue tumours likely to be encountered in orthopaedics.

FATTY TUMOURS
A *lipoma,* one of the commonest of all tumours, may occur almost anywhere, the subcutaneous layer being a favourite site. It consists of lobules of fat with a surrounding capsule which may become tethered to surrounding structures. The patient, usually aged over 50, complains of a painless swelling. The lump is soft and almost fluctuant; the well-defined edge and lobulated surface distinguish it from a chronic abscess. Fat is notably radiotranslucent, a feature which betrays the occasional subperiosteal lipoma. Lipoma may be multiple.

Liposarcoma is exceedingly rare but should be suspected if a previously existing lipoma (especially in the buttock or thigh) grows rapidly or becomes painful.

FIBROUS TUMOURS
Fibromas are widely distributed and not uncommon. They consist of masses of fibrous tissue often arranged in whorls. A hard fibroma is usually round and has a well-defined edge. A soft fibroma contains many blood vessels, is often diffuse and its edges may be ill-defined; differentiation from a fibrosarcoma is difficult and indeed the risk of a soft fibroma becoming malignant is sufficient to justify early excision-biopsy. Recurrence of any fibroma after excision (Paget's recurring fibroid) is suspicious.

Fibrosarcoma, the commonest malignant soft-tissue tumour, is composed of spindle cells with elongated nuclei. The tumour appears to be encapsulated but the capsule is not effective in preventing penetration of surrounding tissues. The lack of a definite edge and attachment to surrounding structures are the main clinical features. Treatment is wide excision or amputation, combined with radiotherapy.

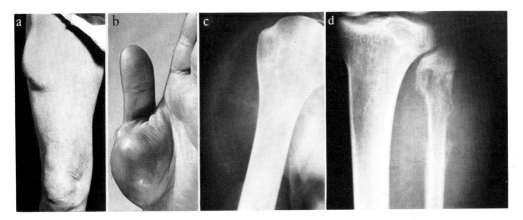

9.14 Fatty tumours (a) Subcutaneous lipoma – like so many lipomas, this one felt almost fluctuant; (b) intramuscular lipoma; (c) subperiosteal lipoma; (d) liposarcoma – the cortex of the fibula has been eroded.

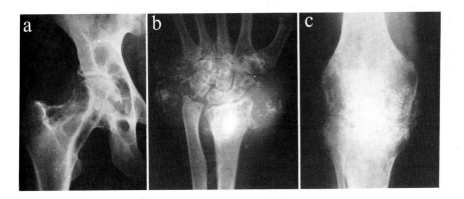

9.15 Synovial tumours (a) Pigmented villonodular synovitis – note the cystic excavations on both sides of the joint; (b) and (c) malignant synoviomas, with the typical snowstorm appearance.

Fibromatosis includes a wide spectrum of disorders in which fibroblasts behave anarchically. At one end are disorders such as Dupuytren's contracture, in which the deformity progresses slowly unless the abnormal tissue is excised. At the other end, and much rarer, is a tumour-like mass which behaves aggressively; neighbouring structures are compressed or destroyed, and only if excision includes a wide margin of normal tissues (which may even need to include nerves and vessels) can recurrence be prevented. Between these extremes are such conditions as desmoid tumour.

Microscopically these lesions vary from those with clearly benign cells, to some whose appearance suggests malignancy (multinucleated cells with many mitoses). The differentiation from fibrosarcoma is difficult and demands considerable histological expertise; but it is important, because fibromatosis does not metastasize and can be eradicated if surgery is sufficiently thorough.

SYNOVIAL TUMOURS

Pigmented villonodular synovitis (giant-cell tumour of synovium) may occur wherever synovial membrane is found – in joints, tendon sheaths or bursae; apart from giant cells, foam cells are a prominent feature and the term 'xanthoma' is often applied. There is diffuse hyperplasia of the synovium, which develops yellowish-brown pigmentation and grows progressively. In tendon sheaths a fairly common site is the back or front of the hand; the patient complains of a lump or of interference with tendon action. In a joint a large boggy swelling develops and, on x-ray, both bones have a cystic appearance. The treatment is synovectomy; though it does not become malignant, if the tumour recurs (which it often does) radiotherapy is worth trying.

Malignant synovioma is totally different. The patient presents with a rapidly growing swelling. The lack of a well-defined edge may be apparent if a tendon sheath is involved; but in a joint (the knee is the commonest site) the swelling may become very large before its malignant character is obvious. On x-ray the combination of bone defects and a soft-tissue 'snowstorm' is characteristic. With a combination of radiotherapy, chemotherapy and excision (or amputation) about half the patients survive.

BLOOD VESSEL TUMOURS

A haemangioma may be capillary or cavernous. The capillary variety is commoner and the congenital skin naevus ('birthmark') its most familiar example. A cavernous haemangioma may be deep or superficial; because it consists of a sponge-like collection of blood spaces, it feels soft and can be emptied by pressure. Haemangiomata may calcify, and sometimes there is associated hypertrophy of an affected limb.

Aneurysms may be (1) congenital (e.g. cerebral); (2) the sequel to disease (nowadays arteriosclerosis is a much commoner cause than syphilis); or (3) traumatic (in half of these the accompanying vein also is damaged, causing an arteriovenous fistula). The cardinal sign is a pulsating lump. The lump is in the course of an artery and can be reduced by proximal pressure. The pulsation is expansile not transmitted; it is visible, palpable and audible. Distally the pulse may be diminished in volume and the tissues poorly nourished. An aneurysm which has been present since childhood may cause overgrowth of a limb.

The diagnosis of an aneurysm is easy – provided the possibility is borne in mind; the consequence of failure may be alarming or disastrous. The nurse who ostentatiously sprinkles sawdust on the floor when a house surgeon is about to incise an 'abscess' has observed pulsation which he has missed.

NERVE TUMOURS

A *neuroma* is not a true tumour but an overgrowth of connective tissue following trauma. In an amputation stump the lump is round and may be tender. On a plantar digital nerve it may be too small to feel, but causes pain and localized tenderness (Morton's metatarsalgia, page 327). A *schwannoma* is a tumour arising from Schwann cells occurring within a nerve and forming a round well-defined lump which causes little numbness or weakness. Its removal without damaging the nerve is difficult. A *neurilemmoma* is clinically similar but grows from the nerve sheath and is easier to remove.

A neurofibroma contains whorls of cellular fibrous tissue and arises from the interstitial tissue of a peripheral nerve. The lump is in the line of a nerve and can be moved only from side to side across the nerve; it may be soft or firm and is sometimes tender. Paraesthesia is not uncommon. Sometimes a nerve root is involved and compression of the spinal cord or cauda equina may occur.

Multiple neurofibromatosis (von Recklinghausen's disease) is said to occur in 1 in 3000 of the population; half the cases are genetic (of autosomal dominant inheritance) and half are new mutations. The neurofibromas are associated with café-au-lait spots and sometimes with skin nodules (molluscum fibrosum). Scoliosis develops

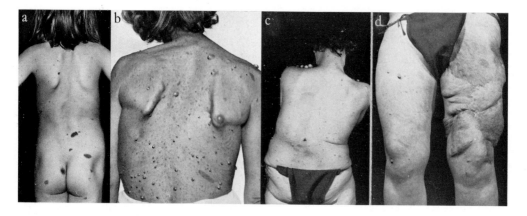

9.16 Neurofibromatosis　(a) Café-au-lait spots, (b) molluscum fibrosum with slight scoliosis; (c) and (d) a patient with scoliosis and elephantiasis.

in 30 per cent of patients, and occasionally hypertrophy of one limb. The nerve tumours themselves may be palpable or may cause symptoms when situated in a confined space such as the spinal canal. Occasionally x-ray reveals pressure erosion of bone; rarely, one of the tumours undergoes malignant change. Neurofibromatosis has other curious skeletal associations including disturbance of bone growth, anomalies of bone architecture and pseudarthrosis of the tibia (page 95).

OTHER TUMOURS

A *ganglion* (page 183) is probably not a true tumour. Ganglia occur chiefly in the hand or foot, occasionally round the knee. The lump may be soft and fluctuant, or so tensely cystic as to feel almost bony. It is well defined and, except in the fingers, not usually tender. Occasionally a ganglion presses on a nerve or penetrates between its fibres, causing paraesthesia and weakness. 'Ganglion cyst of bone' is the term applied to a well-defined rare area in bone (near a joint) which histologically resembles a ganglion.

A *rhabdomyoma* (tumour of a striped muscle) is rare and should not be confused with the lump which follows muscle rupture. Both are in the line of a muscle, can be moved across but not along it, and harden with muscle action; the muscle rupture, however, has a depression distal to the lump and the lump is not getting bigger. If a tumour is suspected, early exploration is advisable because malignant change is not uncommon; not infrequently the swelling proves to be normal muscle fibres in an anomalous situation. A *rhabdomyosarcoma* is very rare. It occurs mainly in the buttock, thigh or leg. The patient presents with ache and a rapidly growing ill-defined mass attached to and moving with the affected muscle.

A *glomus tumour* is rare but very painful. It consists of mixed neural, vascular and muscle elements. The overlying skin is often bluish, but the tumour, which is subcutaneous, is often minute in size and never bigger than a pea. The characteristic features are pain, sensitivity to cold and exquisite tenderness. Any part of the body may be affected, especially the fingers and toes; sometimes it occurs beneath the nail and it may erode the bone. The treatment is excision.

Further reading

Bacci, G., Campanacci, M. and Pagani, P. A. (1978) Adjuvant chemotherapy in the treatment of clinically localized Ewing's sarcoma. *Journal of Bone and Joint Surgery* **60B**, 567–574

Campbell, C. J., Cohen, J. and Enneking, W. F. (1975) New therapies for osteogenic sarcoma (Editorial). *Journal of Bone and Joint Surgery* **57A**, 143–144

Carroll, R. E. and Berman, A. T. (1972) Glomus tumors of the hand. *Journal of Bone and Joint Surgery* **54A**, 691–703

Dahlin, D. C. (1978) *Bone Tumors*, 3rd edn. Springfield, Illinois: Charles C Thomas

Eyre-Brook, A. L. and Price, C. H. G. (1969) Fibrosarcoma of bone. *Journal of Bone and Joint Surgery* **51B**, 20–37

Friedman, B. and Hanaoka, H. (1971) Round-cell sarcomas of bone. *Journal of Bone and Joint Surgery* **53A** 1118–1136

Larsson, S.-E., Lorentzon, R. and Boquist, L. (1975) Giant-cell tumour of bone. *Journal of Bone and Joint Surgery* **57A** 167–173

McGrath, P. J. (1972) Giant-cell tumour of bone. *Journal of Bone and Joint Surgery* **54B**, 216–229

Mankin, H. J., Cantley, K. P., Lippiello, L., Schiller, A. L. and Campbell, C. J. (1980) The biology of human chondrosarcoma. *Journal of Bone and Joint Surgery* **62A**, 160–194

Price, C. H. G. and Goldie, W. (1969) Paget's sarcoma of bone. *Journal of Bone and Joint Surgery* **51B**, 205–224

Scaglietti, O., Marchetti, P. G. and Bartolozzi, P. (1979) The effects of methylprednisolone acetate in the treatment of bone cysts. *Journal of Bone and Joint Surgery* **61B**, 200–208

Schajowicz, F. (1981) *Tumors and Tumorlike Lesions of Bone and Joint*. Berlin, Heidelberg, New York: Springer-Verlag

Sweetnam, R. (1976) Surgical treatment of osteogenic sarcoma. *Proceedings of the Royal College of Medicine* **69**, 547–549

Neuromuscular Disorders

10

Weak or paralysed muscles

Assessment

Muscle weakness may be due to upper motor neuron lesions (spastic paresis), lower motor neuron disorders (flaccid paresis) or muscular dystrophy. If diagnosis is inconclusive, special investigations may help: serum creatinine phosphokinase is raised in muscular dystrophies; electromyography may distinguish neurological from muscle disease; and muscle biopsy is essential if dystrophy is suspected.

In assessment it is important to examine not only individual muscles but also functional groups. Grading muscle power is most valuable in the floppy type of paralysis associated with spina bifida and poliomyelitis; in cerebral palsy it is useful but more difficult because spasticity obscures the undoubted weakness. Muscle charting pinpoints the site and severity of paralysis; repetition enables progress to be recorded. The following grades are standard:

0   total paralysis
1   barely detectable contracture
2   not enough power to act against gravity
3   strong enough to act against gravity
4   still stronger but less than normal
5   full power

Effects

Instability   This occurs when the muscles which control opposing movements at a joint are both equally weak (the term 'balanced paralysis' is convenient). The joint is then floppy or flail.

Deformity   This occurs when one group of muscles overpowers its antagonist – unbalanced

paralysis. At first it can be overcome passively, but later the deformity becomes fixed. It must be appreciated that the action of some muscles is aided by gravity (e.g. ankle plantarflexors); consequently, in assessment, gravity must not be overlooked as it is often worth at least 1 point.

Shortening   A paralysed limb fails to grow normally. Consequently paralysis which is predominantly unilateral and which arises in childhood causes limb inequality.

Principles of treatment

Assessment of the whole patient   This is an essential prerequisite of definitive treatment, especially if operation is contemplated. Has the patient the mental capacity to co-operate or to utilize any local improvement? Will a 'better' position lead to improved function? And is the situation complicated by skin anaesthesia, making splintage hazardous?

Instability   Floppy joints often need to be stabilized. In the leg, stability is essential for walking; but even in the arm it may be important to stabilize proximal joints in order to allow use of a normal hand. Stability can be achieved by splintage or by arthrodesis. Some examples of splintage for instability are shown in Fig. 10.2.

Deformity   Sometimes the establishment of deformity can be postponed (though rarely prevented) by passive stretching combined with intermittent splintage. It is often better to divide shortened tendons. Of necessity they belong to acting muscles, and the possibility of rerouting them more usefully must always be considered.

Tendon rerouting (transfer) is used, not only to correct deformity, but also to restore a valuable

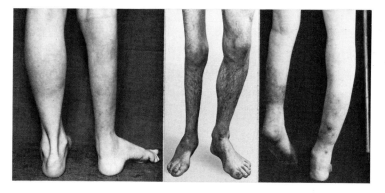

10.1 Some effects of neurological lesions These patients, all of whom had polio, illustrate some of the effects of paralysis – deformity, wasting and shortening; the trophic changes in the patient on the right suggest that, in her, the anterolateral horn cells also may have been damaged.

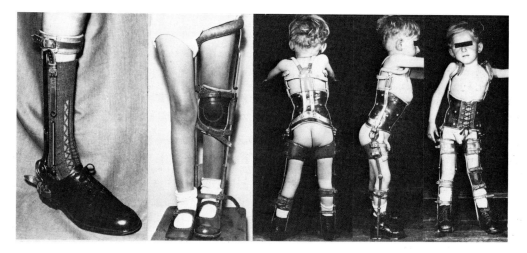

10.2 Equipment for stabilization The paralysed patient may need equipment, sometimes very extensive.

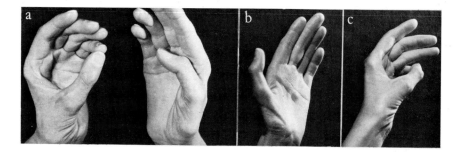

10.3 Tendon transfer (a) In both hands the opponens pollicis was paralysed; in the left hand a sublimis transfer has restored opposition: (b) and (c) show the transferred tendon in action.

action at the expense of one less important (see Fig. 10.3). Any fixed deformity must first be corrected.*

Once deformity has become fixed, tendon surgery alone is not enough: bone carpentry is needed. Thus, fixed varus deformity of the foot may be treated by subtalar fusion (which provides stability) combined with excising a laterally based wedge of bone to make the foot plantigrade. Even then, deformity is likely to recur unless muscle imbalance is eliminated by dividing or reattaching the deforming tendons.

Shortening   This is of importance only in the legs, where inequality of more than 2.5 cm needs treatment (see page 142).

Cerebral palsy

The term 'cerebral palsy' includes a group of disorders which result from non-progressive cerebral dysfunction, originating before the central nervous system has matured. It is not due to a single or specific type of brain damage although perinatal anoxia is almost certainly the commonest causal factor; others include trauma (to the brain or its vessels), kernicterus (with or without Rhesus incompatibility) and infection (perinatal or in early infancy).

General features

The incidence is from 0.5 to 2 per 1000 live births, so that, as with spina bifida, the social and medical problems are immense. A history of difficult labour or early kernicterus may suggest the diagnosis, but at birth the disease is rarely recognized. Early symptoms include difficulty in sucking and swallowing, with dribbling at the mouth; the mother may notice that the baby feels stiff or wriggles awkwardly. Gradually it becomes apparent that the milestones are delayed (the normal child usually holds up its head at 3 months, sits up at 6 months and begins walking at about 1 year).

Intelligence is often impaired, but not as often as formerly supposed. Accurate assessment is important, for severe mental defect precludes useful treatment. The IQ is often assessed too low because spasticity has hampered learning, and because of speech and hearing difficulties. The children are often emotionally unstable and may suffer from fits; skin sensation is usually normal.

Limb signs

The characteristic deformities take months or years to develop. They result from muscle incoordination and muscle imbalance, both the product of the upper motor neuron damage.

There are four main varieties of cerebral palsy: spastic, athetotic, ataxic and rigid. However, mixed syndromes are not uncommon.

SPASTIC PALSY   This is the commonest variety (50 per cent of cases) and the only one with which the orthopaedic surgeon is likely to be concerned. The muscles feel rigid and resist stretching, and there is inability to relax; but stiffness takes time to develop and the severely spastic child may have been a floppy infant. Tendon reflexes are increased and the plantar responses extensor. Some muscles, however, may feel flaccid and it must be realized that paresis is always an important feature. Imbalance gives rise to the characteristic deformities: adduction and internal rotation of the shoulder, flexion of the elbow, pronation of the forearm, flexion of the wrist, adduction of the thumb, flexion and adduction of the hips, flexion of the knee and equinus of the foot. Equinus may not be obvious while the child is lying down but appears immediately when the feet touch the ground and the child attempts to walk.

In nearly one-third of cases the arm and leg on one side are affected (hemiplegia); in nearly one-third both legs are much more severely affected than the arms (diplegia); and in nearly one-third all four limbs are involved (quadriplegia).

ATHETOSIS   This type, due to kernicterus, is seldom seen nowadays. Typically the limbs wave about with continual, irregular, worm-like movements which are purposeless. Usually the movements are uncontrollable, but sometimes the

---

*A tendon transfer will never correct a fixed deformity; at best it will hold position after correction of the deformity.

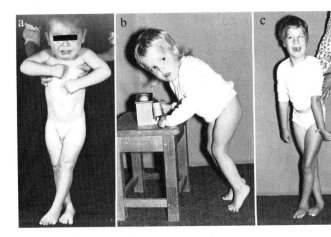

10.4 Cerebral palsy (1) (a) Scissors stance; (b) flexion deformity of hips and knees with equinus of the feet; (c) characteristic facial expression and limb deformities.

patient tries to keep the limb still by voluntarily contracting all the muscles of a particular joint. The condition may then be confused with the spastic type of cerebral palsy.

Often the face, tongue and speech muscles share in the athetoid movements and it is hard to resist incorrectly calling the children mental defectives.

ATAXIA   This type is relatively rare. There is an irregular intention tremor and incoordination, but no spasticity, flaccidity or athetosis.

RIGIDITY   This was formerly confused with the spastic type, but the muscles are in a constant state of increased tone and, on examination, do not 'give' like spastic muscles.

Conservative treatment

MENTAL TRAINING   It is important to decide early whether the child is educable, for, if not, treatment is useless. But it is easy to underestimate mental ability; the child should be given the benefit of the doubt. A calm atmosphere in the home, but with adequate and affectionate stimulation, helps to make the most of the child's abilities. Education should start young, and special schools can provide suitable equipment as well as competition with similarly afflicted children. Speech therapy is important.

PHYSICAL TRAINING   The aim is to teach new patterns of posture and movement. This is obviously easier if faulty habits, say, of walking, have not first to be unlearnt. Enthusiasm, gentleness and patience are the keynotes of success;

when instructed, an intelligent mother with plenty of time is often the best physiotherapist.

Temporary splints are often necessary to prevent deformity or to maintain a correction obtained by manipulation. Splints should be taken off daily and the joints put through their full range of movement.

Operative treatment

Operations have a definite, if limited, place in treatment. Hemiplegics respond best, partly because their mentality is usually normal. With diplegia or quadriplegia the results are often disappointing and surgery should certainly be avoided in patients with low intelligence and in those with athetosis or rigidity. Careful selection of patients is imperative, for the child who has struggled to learn to get about may, despite theoretically attractive operations, be unable to do so if he is off his feet for a few weeks.

The main task is to prevent or correct deformity, thereby improving posture and reducing the weight of splintage which the weak muscles have to carry around. The principles described on page 114 apply, but timing is difficult because spasticity hampers accurate muscle charting. If it can be established that deformity is progressing in spite of adequate conservative treatment, tendon surgery is worth while even in young children. Thereafter it usually needs to be combined with bone surgery and joint stabilization. Postoperative physiotherapy is essential.

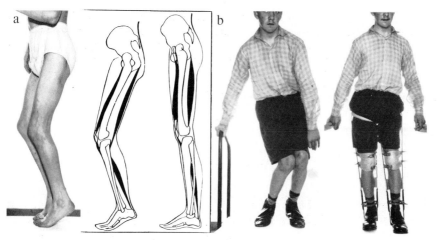

10.5 Cerebral palsy (2) – treatment   (a) Showing how deformities in the lower limb can be improved by moving the insertion of the hamstrings from tibia to femur; (b) sometimes, however, splintage alone is appropriate.

Regional survey

UPPER LIMB   Operative treatment is delayed longer than in the lower limb and is rarely indicated before the age of 12. Even then it is almost exclusively confined to the forearm, wrist and thumb.

For the pronated forearm, release of pronator teres is a possibility, or the tendon can be rerouted round the back of the forearm in the hope that it may act as a supinator. The combination of forearm pronation with wrist palmarflexion can sometimes be improved by transferring flexor carpi ulnaris into one of the wrist extensors. If the fingers work better when held extended, the best operation is wrist arthrodesis in slight dorsiflexion; when flexion deformity is severe the lower radius can usefully be tapered and embedded into the carpal bones.

The chief hand deformities are clenched fingers and thumb-in-palm. Finger function can be improved by elongating the flexor tendons, but it is important first to ensure that deformity can be overcome by steady pressure, for if there is joint contracture operation is useless. The thumb-in-palm deformity (flexion–adduction contracture) is very disabling and best treated by Matev's procedure: first the flexor pollicis longus is elongated; then, through a palmar incision, all the thenar muscles are released; and finally abduction and extension are reinforced by shortening the appropriate tendons or by tendon transfers.

SPINE   Significant scoliosis develops in 12 per cent of cerebral palsy patients, but correction and stabilization are rarely needed.

LOWER LIMB   Although it is customary to consider each deformity individually, Burke Evans (1971) has emphasized the inter-relationship between the various posture problems, especially lumbar lordosis, hip flexion, knee flexion and ankle equinus; this must be constantly borne in mind when surgery is being planned.

At the hip   adductor overaction or contracture may be treated by tenotomy; this can be combined with obturator neurectomy, or the adductor origin can be moved to the ischial tuberosity. Flexion deformity can be helped by dividing the psoas tendon, and medial rotation by dividing the front half of gluteus medius. These operations may prevent the hip from dislocating – a constant danger. If dislocation has already occurred they may be combined with varus osteotomy of the upper femur. A long-standing dislocation may be irreducible; if discomfort makes operation imperative the femoral head can be excised.

At the knee   flexion contracture can be treated by a modification of Eggers' operation: the medial hamstrings are reinserted into the femoral condyle, the biceps tendon is elongated and, if necessary, the patellar retinacula are divided. Probably this combined procedure should be reserved for severe cases.

In the foot   equinus deformity is common; it may indeed be useful in a limb with flexed hip and knee. But if correction is needed, elongation of the tendo Achillis is probably best combined with a gastrocnemius slide operation. Tendo Achillis elongation is combined with lengthening of the peronei if there is also valgus deformity, or with lengthening of tibialis posterior for varus deformity. (Alternatively the tibialis posterior may be rerouted through the interosseus membrane to the front of the foot.) But when these combined deformities are fixed, bone surgery is needed: either calcaneal osteotomy or, more often, subtalar fusion. Flexion deformity of the hallux or other toes is best treated by arthrodesis.

Stroke

Cerebral damage following a stroke may cause persistent spastic paresis in the adult; disturbance of proprioception and stereognosis may coexist. In the early recuperative stage, physiotherapy and splintage are important in preventing fixed contractures; all affected joints should be put through a full range of movement every day, and deformities should be corrected and splinted until controlled muscle power returns. Proprioception and co-ordination can be improved by occupational therapy. Once maximal motor recovery has been achieved – usually by 9 months – residual deformity or joint instability may need surgical correction or permanent splinting.

In the lower limbs the principal deformities requiring correction are equinus or equinovarus of the foot, flexion of the knee and adduction of the hip causing a 'scissors gait'. In the upper limb (where the chances of regaining controlled movement are less) the common residual deformities are adduction and internal rotation of the shoulder (often accompanied by shoulder pain), and flexion of the elbow, wrist and metacarpophalangeal joints. The appropriate treatment is summarized in Table 10.1

Friedreich's ataxia

In this condition, of autosomal recessive inheritance, there is degeneration of the spinocerebellar tracts, the corticospinal tracts, the posterior columns of the cord and part of the cerebellum. It usually presents at the age of 5 or 6 with an awkward, unsteady gait, a tendency to fall and clumsiness. Typical deformities are pes cavovarus with claw toes, and scoliosis, sometimes very mild. Neurological examination shows ataxia and loss of vibration sense and two-point discrimination.

In severe cases there is progressive disability and cardiac involvement; patients eventually take to a wheelchair and may die before they are 20. In milder cases operative correction of the foot and spine deformities is well worth while (Makin, 1953).

Arthrogryposis multiplex congenita

This disorder, always rare, has now become even rarer. It is characterized by stiffness of many joints, contractures, shapelessly cylindrical limbs and absent skin creases. The deformities are due to muscle imbalance and do not progress after birth. The condition is thought to be an intrauterine neuropathy, perhaps in association with oligohydramnios. Deformities such as club foot are common and may be the only obvious expression of what is usually a more widespread disorder.

Spina bifida

The incidence of spina bifida in Great Britain is approximately 3 per 1000 live births. Formerly

Table 10.1 Treatment of the principal deformities of the limbs

	Deformity	Splintage	Surgery
Foot	Equinus	Spring-loaded dorsiflexion	Lengthen tendo Achillis
	Equinovarus	Bracing in eversion and dorsiflexion	Lengthen tendo Achillis and transfer lateral half of tibialis anterior to cuboid
Knee	Flexion	Long caliper	Hamstring release
Hip	Adduction	—	Obturator neurectomy Adductor muscle release
Shoulder	Adduction	—	Subscapularis release
Elbow	Flexion	—	Release elbow flexors
Wrist	Flexion	Wrist splint	Lengthen or release wrist flexors

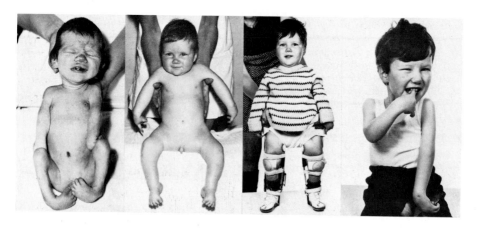

10.6 Arthrogryposis multiplex congenita Severe deformities are present at birth but surgery is possible and, as this bright lad shows, worth while. The lower limbs are tackled first (aiming at straight legs with plantigrade feet), then the upper limbs (where the minimum aim is getting a hand to the mouth).

many of these babies soon died because of infection or hydrocephalus; early operation has increased the survival rate and highlighted the enormous surgical and social problems.

The cause is unknown, but there is a great geographic variation in frequency, even between different localities in Great Britain. The incidence is higher in certain races, in firstborn children and in poor families. The familial incidence has made prophylaxis feasible. If one parent, or a previous child, has a neural tube defect, there is a 5 per cent risk to the next child. Estimation of alpha-fetoprotein in the amniotic fluid (obtained by amniocentesis) shows if the fetus is affected and whether termination of pregnancy should be considered.

The term 'spina bifida' simply means that the two halves of the neural arch have failed to fuse. Through the defect the membranes or cord may protrude; the cord itself may be undeveloped (dysplastic). The simplest classification is into closed lesions in which the skin is intact, and open lesions (aperta) in which it is not.

Closed spina bifida

Closed spina bifida may be associated with any of the following: dermal cysts; lipoma of the cauda equina; diastematomyelia (in which the cord is bifurcated by bone projecting backwards from the vertebral body); partial or complete absence of the sacrum; and, finally, meningocele. Meningocele is very rare and is merely a thecal hernia containing no neural elements, so that neurological lesions are said not to occur.

Clinical features

Although the skin is intact it is almost never normal. Some midline anomaly suggests the diagnosis, so that the term 'occulta' (meaning 'secret') seems inappropriate. The possible lesions range from a tiny dimple or excess of 'down', to a large pigmented naevus or a veritable 'faun's tail'. A bulge deep to the skin is suggestive of an associated lesion.

X-rays show the gap in the neural arch; widening of the spinal canal is common and the bony spur of diastematomyelia should be sought.

Treatment

The most important indications for treatment are neurological deficit, disturbance of bladder function, and weakness, numbness or trophic changes in one or both legs. These features may develop during growth, either because the cord is tethered at the defect or because its distal portion is bulky and too immobile to escape damage when the patient moves his back. The state of affairs is best revealed by a cisternal air myelogram.

Should operation be needed it is best done by a neurosurgeon. Tethering bands or adhesions are divided and the cord is mobilized; lipomas, dermoid cysts or bony spurs are excised.

Open spina bifida

In 60 per cent of open spina bifidas the lesion is a myelomeningocele of the lumbar or lumbosacral region. Through the bony defect protrudes a meningeal sac containing nerve roots and cord remnants which may be adherent to it. The sac is exposed with no skin cover. Hydrocephalus may be present at birth; with a communicating hydrocephalus the intracranial pressure may not be elevated until leakage from the spinal lesion is arrested by surgical closure.

Clinical features

The newborn baby has a translucent cystic lump in the midline of the back. The baby's posture may suggest paralysis and sometimes indicates its neurological level. Associated deformities are common, especially hip dislocation, genu recurvatum, talipes and claw toes. Such deformities may be due to intrauterine paralysis or they may develop later because of unbalanced paralysis; sometimes they are primary, i.e. independent of the paralysis.

Muscle charting (page 114) should be performed within 24 hours of birth. Sharrard has shown convincingly that this is perfectly practicable; he suggests that the untreated child may, within a few days, become increasingly paralysed as enlargement of the meningeal sac exerts traction on adherent nerve roots.

Treatment

Selection of patients for operation is ethically controversial. Most centres avoid urgent operation if the neurological lesion is high, the skull is enlarged or spinal deformities are severe. In the remainder (about half) the skin lesion is closed early.

For subsequent management teamwork is essential. The ideal is a combined clinic at which neurosurgery, orthopaedics, urology and paediatrics are all represented; but the key figure is the physiotherapist. As the child grows, help is likely to be needed from the splint maker, the social worker and possibly the psychotherapist. But above all, the child will need parental understanding and ceaseless devotion.

EARLY MANAGEMENT

(1) *Skin closure* should, in those patients with good prognostic signs, be performed within 48 hours.

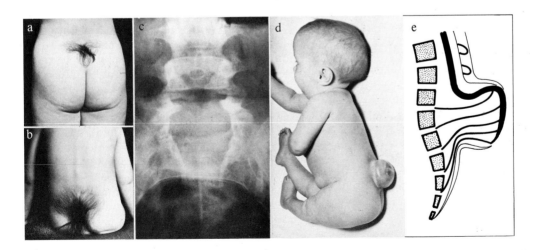

10.7 Spina bifida (1) (a, b) Examples of the hairy patches which suggest a bony defect such as that in (c). (d, e) Myelomeningocele: the diagram shows the neural plaque on the surface, and also why traction lesions of the nerve roots develop with growth.

LEVELS		EARLY MANAGEMENT – TIMING	
HIP	KNEE	AGE	PROCEDURE
		1 DAY	Close skin defect
Flexion — L1, L2		1 WEEK	Ventriculo-caval shunt
Adduction — L3 — Extension		1 MONTH	Stretch and strap
Abduction — L4, L5 — Flexion		6 MONTHS TO 3 YEARS	Orthopaedic operations
Extension — S1, S2		WHENEVER NEEDED	Urogenital operations

10.8 Spina bifida (2)   The diagram shows the root levels concerned with hip and knee movements. The table is a simple guide to the timing of operations.

The neural plaque is carefully preserved and the skin widely undercut to facilitate closure. Only in this way can drying and ulceration be prevented.

(2) *Hydrocephalus* is the next priority. Usually it develops within a few days; treatment must not be delayed or brain damage follows. A ventriculocaval shunt containing a valve (e.g. Spitz–Holter) is inserted. As the baby grows, the shunt may need to be replaced.

(3) *Deformities* must be kept under control. The orthopaedic surgeon is usually not called upon for 3 weeks, and then only if the child is thriving, the back healed and a shunt (if needed) working. At this stage muscle charting is repeated and a programme of stretching and strapping begun: stretching to keep deformity at a minimum; elastic strapping (or simple splints) to hold correction.

Two features dominate orthopaedic management: the bones are somewhat fragile (spontaneous fractures are common and frequently unite with excessive callus); and the skin is anaesthetic. Consequently manipulations must not be too forcible, and splintage should be intermittent. The skin must be protected from localized pressure and watched with extravagant vigilance.*

(4) *Urinary problems* develop in 90 per cent of cases. Intravenous pyelography is used to detect any upper urinary tract dilatation, and is repeated at intervals. Males can usually be fitted with a penile appliance but in females urinary diversion is needed.

SUBSEQUENT MANAGEMENT OF PARALYSIS AND DEFORMITY

The guiding principles are:

(1) For the first 6–12 months deformities are treated by stretching and strapping (see above). Forcible overcorrection followed by plaster is forbidden: this combination, useful in other varieties of paralysis, is disastrous with spina bifida; the bones may break and the skin will ulcerate.
(2) Open methods of correcting deformity are best, but should be delayed until the child is several months old. Then short tendons are the main problem: they should be divided and, where appropriate, transferred. Only when balance has been restored should any residual deformity be corrected by osteotomy.
(3) Splints alone are never used to obtain correction; they may be used to maintain it but even then only intermittently; their action is reinforced by frequently repeated stretching.

*A sore which takes a day to form may take a month to heal.

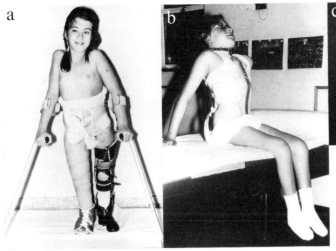
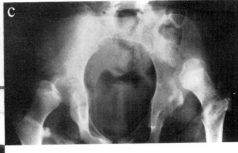

10.9 Spina bifida (3)   (a) Paralysis may require permanent splintage in a caliper, and crutch-walking for life. (b) Scoliosis is common and is treated in a brace until the child is old enough for fusion. (c) Muscle imbalance may lead to bilateral hip dislocation.

Regional survey

SPINE   Apart from the posterior defect which constitutes spina bifida, many other vertebral anomalies can occur, such as unsegmented bars, hemivertebrae and fused ribs, resulting in scoliosis, lordosis or kyphosis. Neonatal kyphosis may be so severe that spinal osteotomy is needed if the skin defect is to be closed.

Even moderate kyphosis or kyphos may later cause persistent skin ulceration; treatment consists in excising the kyphotic vertebrae and fixing the two halves of the spine together – a procedure less alarming than it sounds because the cord is already non-functioning. Many patients with high neurological lesions develop progressive lordoscoliosis aged 5 or 6. Bracing at best slows deterioration. When the child is old enough (aged about 10) operative correction and stabilization is often needed using a combination of Dwyer and Harrington instrumentation.

HIP   The aim is to secure hips straight enough to enable the child to stand in calipers, and flexible enough for him to sit. If the neurological level of the lesion is above L1, all muscle groups are equally paralysed (balanced); the hips are flail and no treatment other than splintage is needed. With a lesion from S1 downwards there may be pure flexion deformity; this can be corrected by elongation of the psoas tendon combined with detachment of the flexors from the ilium (Soutter).

Usually the lesion is between these levels and the commonest hip problem is dislocation: 50 per cent of spina bifida children have subluxed or dislocated hips by the age of 2. Some may be coincidental congenital dislocations, but most result from unbalanced paralysis; if the flexors and adductors can over-power the extensors and abductors, dislocation is almost inevitable. In infancy reduction (closed or open) is usually possible, perhaps aided by adductor tenotomy; but, because postoperative splintage must be minimized, it is important to improve muscle balance. This is achieved by transferring the psoas tendon from the lesser to the greater trochanter; flexor power is reduced and extensor–abductor power may be increased. Sharrard advocates threading the detached psoas through a large hole in the ilium, while Mustard prefers moving the tendon across the front of the bone.

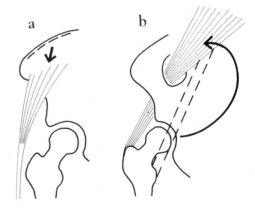

10.10 Spina bifida (4)   Two procedures for hip deformity. (a) Soutter's muscle slide, (b) Sharrard's iliopsoas transfer.

In older children it may be difficult or impossible to reduce a dislocation. The possibilities then are varus osteotomy of the upper femur or innominate osteotomy; often it is best not to intervene.

KNEE   Unlike the hip, the knee usually presents no problem, because the aim is simple – a straight knee suitable for straight calipers. Occasionally recurvatum develops and cautious elongation of the quadriceps may be called for. In older children fixed flexion may follow prolonged sitting. If stretching and splintage fail, one or more of the hamstrings may be lengthened, divided or reinserted into the femur or patella. Not uncommonly the knees are straight and will not bend, making sitting difficult; extensive soft-tissue release may be needed if subcutaneous tenotomy proves inadequate.

FOOT   The aim is a plantigrade foot with plantar skin strong enough not to break down easily. The floppy foot of balanced paralysis needs no surgery; accurately fitting footwear with strong external bracing is adequate. The same is true of any deformity which can be corrected passively, though in every case the patient and parents must be taught an elaborate ritual of skin care; pressure sores must, at all costs, be prevented.

Fixed deformities are common and varied. Tendon operations are often helpful and are best performed at or before the age of 6 months: preoperative electrical testing may help in deciding if the short tendon is paralysed but contracted (in which case simple division is satisfactory), or is active but unopposed (in which case transfer is better). The common equinovarus deformity often requires extensive posteromedial release, also at the age of 6 months.

Vertical talus is not uncommon, with a rigid boat-shaped foot and possibly skin ulceration. Operative reduction is important and preferable to astragalectomy; it is performed at the age of 3 years or over. Still older children may need bone operations to restore a plantigrade foot. Should claw toes prove troublesome, flexor-to-extensor transfer is suitable for the outer four toes, and tenodesis of the long flexor (anchoring it to the proximal phalanx) for the hallux.

Anterior poliomyelitis

In developed countries immunization has been so successful that poliomyelitis has become a rare disease, though the victims of earlier epidemics continue to pose challenging problems. In developing countries the acute disease is not uncommon. Following a trivial and often unrecognized minor illness (a sore throat or diarrhoea) the patient develops meningitis; soon afterwards paralysis may follow, reaching its maximum in a day or two. If he does not succumb from respiratory paralysis, pain and pyrexia subside – the convalescent stage has been reached; this is when the surgeon may be called in.

Some anterior horn cells will have been destroyed by the virus; others, merely damaged by oedema, survive, and the muscles they supply can regain their lost power. Vigorous physiotherapy is needed to hasten recovery; consequently splintage must be kept to a minimum. Because of the associated trophic changes hydrotherapy also is useful. Operative treatment should await the definitive stage – at least a year from onset

Clinical features (in the definitive stage)

The patient, except for residual paralysis, is fit; although, if the trunk muscles were involved, he may have respiratory difficulty and he may have scoliosis. An affected limb often looks bluish, wasted and deformed; if the disease occurred in childhood there may also be shortening. There are frequently extensive chilblains and the skin feels cold. When a badly paralysed limb is picked up it has a floppy feel which, in the presence of normal sensation, is characteristic.

Treatment

Further recovery is, by definition, impossible; further physiotherapy is useless. Severe trophic changes may need sympathectomy; and leg shortening is treated as described on page 142. The two remaining problems are deformity due to unbalanced paralysis, and instability from balanced paralysis (page 114); their management is described in the section which follows, but the importance of muscle charting is self-evident.

Regional survey

UPPER LIMB
Provided the scapular muscles are strong, abduction at the shoulder can be restored (Fig. 10.12) by arthrodesing the glenohumeral joint (50 degrees abducted and 25 degrees flexed). Contracted adductors may need division, but a strong pectoralis major can, if needed, be used to provide elbow flexion; it is detached from its insertion and sutured to the biceps tendon. Proximal advancement of the forearm flexors is a less effective way of restoring elbow flexion.

Arthrodesis of the wrist is sometimes useful; deformity can be corrected and any active wrist muscle rerouted more usefully.

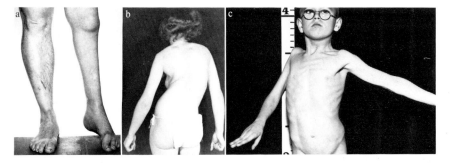

10.11 Polio (a) Shortening and wasting of the left leg, with equinus of the ankle. (b) This long curve is typical of a paralytic scoliosis. (c) This boy is trying to abduct both arms, but the right deltoid and supraspinatus are paralysed.

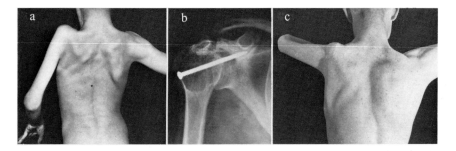

10.12 Polio treatment (a) This patient had paralysis of the left deltoid; after arthrodesis (b) he could lift his arm (c) by using his scapular muscles.

In the thumb, weakness of opposition can be overcome by a sublimis transfer (Fig. 10.3); the tendon (usually of the ring finger) is wound round that of flexor carpi ulnaris (which acts as a pulley), threaded across the palm and fixed to the distal end of the first metacarpal.

TRUNK

Unbalanced paralysis causes scoliosis, frequently a long thoracolumbar curve which may involve the lumbosacral junction, causing pelvic obliquity. Operative treatment is often needed, the most effective being a combination of Dwyer's anterior fusion with posterior Harrington rod instrumentation.

LOWER LIMB

At the hip balanced paralysis causes instability; the resulting Trendelenburg gait cannot be avoided except by arthrodesis, which is rarely advisable. Unbalanced paralysis causes deformities similar to those in spina bifida and cerebral palsy. Fixed flexion can be treated by Soutter's muscle slide operation or by transferring psoas to the greater trochanter. For fixed adduction with pelvic obliquity, the fascia lata and iliotibial band may need division.

At the knee instability is dangerous. Unaided walking may still be possible provided the hip has good extensor power and the foot good plantarflexion power (or fixed equinus); with this combination the knee is stabilized by being thrust into hyperextension as body weight comes onto the leg. In the absence of such passive stabilization a full-length caliper is needed. Fixed flexion with flexors stronger than extensors is commoner and must be corrected; the possibilities are hamstring division or hamstring to quadriceps transfer; but if fixed flexion remains, supracondylar osteotomy is needed.

In the foot instability can be controlled by a below-knee caliper, and foot drop by a toe-raising spring. Often there is imbalance causing varus, valgus or calcaneocavus deformity: fusion alone is unsatisfactory and should be combined with tendon rerouting to restore balance.

For varus or valgus the simplest procedure (Grice) is to slot bone grafts into vertical grooves on each side of the sinus tarsi; alternatively a triple arthrodesis (Dunn) of subtalar and mid-tarsal joints is performed, relying on bone carpentry to correct deformity. With associated foot drop Lambrinudi's modification is valuable: triple arthrodesis is performed but the fully plantarflexed talus is slotted into the navicular with the forefoot in only slight equinus; foot drop is corrected because the talus cannot plantarflex further, and slight equinus helps to stabilize the knee. With calcaneocavus deformity Elmslie's operation is useful: triple arthrodesis is performed in the calcaneus position, but corrected at a second stage by posterior wedge excision combined with tenodesis using half of the tendo Achillis. Claw toes, if the deformity is mobile, are corrected by transferring the toe flexors to the extensors; if the deformity is fixed, the interphalangeal joints should be arthrodesed in the straight position and the long extensor tendons reinserted into the metatarsal necks.

most peripheral muscles are the most affected. Deformities include pes cavus, peroneal wasting and claw hand (from intrinsic muscle weakness). Sensation is less affected. Electrical stimulation shows marked slowing of peripheral nerve conduction.

The worst cases (those of recessive inheritance) begin in early childhood and are soon completely disabled. Mild cases (of dominant inheritance) present in adolescence, usually with pes cavus which may need operation: soft-tissue release, transfer of tibialis posterior to the lateral side and flexor-to-extensor transfers. Uncorrected cavus may later require triple arthrodesis.

Other lower motor neuron disorders

SPINAL MUSCULAR ATROPHY

In this rare disorder anterior horn cells and cranial nerve motor nuclei degenerate. Severe cases (Werdnig–Hoffmann's disease) die soon after birth. Less severely affected children (Kugelberg–Welander's disease) present with weakness, chiefly of the proximal limb muscles. These patients may live to 20 or 30 years, but are usually confined to a wheelchair. Scoliosis may need bracing or fusion.

PERONEAL MUSCULAR ATROPHY (CHARCOT–MARIE–TOOTH)

In this familial disorder peripheral nerves (motor and sensory), motor nerve roots and the spinal cord degenerate. The

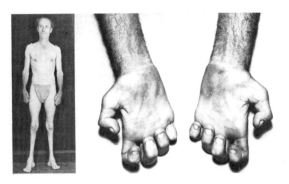

10.13 Peroneal muscular atrophy   The most peripheral muscles are the most severely affected, producing cavus feet, claw toes and claw hands. This man could ride a bicycle, but scarcely walk – until his feet were straightened surgically. His hands were left untreated – it seems incredible, but he made beautiful model ships as a hobby.

Muscular dystrophies

DUCHENNE DYSTROPHY

This progressive disease, of sex-linked recessive inheritance, is usually unsuspected until the child starts to walk. He has difficulty standing and falls frequently. The muscle bulk

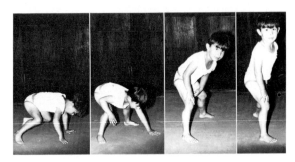

10.14 Muscle dystrophy   This boy, with a Duchenne type of dystrophy, has to climb up his legs in order to achieve the upright position.

(pseudohypertrophy) is due to fat and belies the weakness, which is progressive and generalized. By 10 the child is unable to walk and he rarely survives into adult life. Manipulation, splintage or even tendon operations may help to prevent and correct joint deformities and to keep the child mobile.

LIMB GIRDLE DYSTROPHY

This disorder, of autosomal recessive inheritance, is even rarer than the Duchenne type and much less disabling. Symptoms usually start in late adolescence. Pelvic girdle weakness causes a waddling gait and difficulty in rising from a low chair;

pectoral girdle weakness makes it difficult to raise the arms above the head. The disease is slowly progressive and by the fifth decade disability is usually marked. Treatment consists of physiotherapy and splintage to prevent contractures, and operative correction when necessary. Because the deltoid muscles are spared, shoulder movements can be improved by fixing the scapula to the ribs posteriorly, so improving deltoid leverage.

FACIOSCAPULOHUMERAL DYSTROPHY

This condition, of autosomal dominant inheritance, presents in early adult life with facial muscle weakness, winging of the scapula and slight pelvic girdle weakness. Deterioration is slow and the life span normal. Treatment is the same as for limb girdle dystrophy.

Further reading

Burke Evans, E. (1971) Hip flexion deformity in spastic cerebral palsy (Editorial). *Journal of Bone and Joint Surgery* **53A,** 1465–1467

Lloyd-Roberts, G. C. (1971) *Orthopaedics in Infancy and Childhood.* London: Butterworths

Makin, M. (1953) The surgical management of Friedreich's ataxia. *Journal of Bone and Joint Surgery* **35A,** 425–436

Menelaus, M. B. (1980) *The Orthopaedic Management of Spina Bifida Cystica,* 2nd edn. Edinburgh: Churchill Livingstone

Merle d'Aubigné, R. and Dubousset, J. (1971) Surgical correction of large length discrepancies in the lower extremities of children and adults. *Journal of Bone and Joint Surgery* **53A,** 411–430

Sharrard, W. J. W. (1979) *Paediatric Orthopaedics and Fractures,* 2nd edn. Oxford: Blackwell Scientific

Peripheral Nerve Lesions

11

Classification

NEUROTMESIS (complete division) Although 'neurotmesis' means 'nerve cutting', the term is applied not only to a nerve which has been cut across but also to one which is so severely scarred that it cannot regenerate spontaneously. Neurotmesis may be caused therefore by open wounds, traction injuries, compression or intraneural injections.

AXONOTMESIS (incomplete division) Axonotmesis is incomplete in the sense that only the axons are divided; the endoneural tubes are undamaged. It occurs with closed fractures, dislocations and pressure injuries. Clinically it is at first indistinguishable from neurotmesis, but spontaneous recovery is likely.

NEURAPRAXIA (physiological interruption) The axons are intact; the only lesion is degeneration of the myelin sheaths. The larger motor fibres are mainly affected, the smaller sensory fibres less so; hence motor loss may at first be total but sensory loss is rare (though subjective tingling is common). Spontaneous recovery is the rule.

Pathology

THE NERVE The space between the cut ends fills with blood clot, the clot organizes and Schwann cells from each stump grow into it. Distally, the axons degenerate and are removed by phagocytes. The Schwann cells of the endoneural tubes multiply and, if the tube is not soon occupied by a growing axon, this multiplication narrows it.

Proximally, degeneration also occurs, but only for about 1 cm. Within a few days the cut axons proliferate and streams of axoplasm grow towards the gap. If obstructed by clot they form a bulky nerve bulb, often loosely called a neuroma. Otherwise they enter the Schwann tubes (not necessarily the

correct ones) and grow along them. The advancing axon is followed by advancing myelinization. Eventually, the axon joins an end organ which enlarges unless it has in the

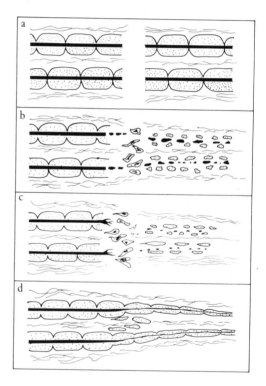

11.1 Regeneration after nerve division (a) Two axons with their myelin sheaths immediately after the nerve has been cut. (b) Axons and myelin sheaths degenerate distal to the cut (on the right) and for a short distance proximal to it; Schwann cells grow into the gap. (c) Proximal to the cut the axons sprout branches which grow into the gap. Eventually (d) they find their way into distal endoneural tubes (Schwann tubes) and acquire a new myelin sheath.

meantime become too degenerate. The nerve fibre has 'matured' when the myelinated axon is connected to an end organ.

Experimentally the axons grow at a speed of 4mm a day, but there is delay in starting, in crossing the gap and in connecting with the end organ. In practice, the speed of recovery is 1–1.5mm a day.

OTHER STRUCTURES Denervated muscles waste, and the joints they control are liable to become deformed and stiff. The skin and nails may undergo trophic changes. The brain may 'forget' the pattern of muscle behaviour.

Clinical features

Numbness and weakness are the chief symptoms. With some partial lesions there may be pain and increased sweating (see page 137)

● LOOK There may be a scar of the causal wound. Anaesthetic skin looks smooth and shiny, the affected fingers are thin and tapering and their nails abnormal. Trophic ulcers may be present, especially in the foot. Muscle wasting is apparent and the attitude of a paralysed limb is characteristic.

● FEEL The anaesthetic skin feels smooth, cool and dry. A nerve bulb may be palpable and may be tender. Where sensory nerve damage exists, the patient himself will point to the anaesthetic areas; however, it is useful for the surgeon to map out the area of loss and to chart the quality of sensation in four grades, from total sensory loss up to two-point discrimination.

● MOVE The patient cannot perform certain movements, though passive range may be full. Muscle tone and power are lost, and bulk is diminished. In testing individual muscles errors may occur, especially in the hand, because of anomalous innervation, trick movements or supplementary movements. To assess recovery, power may usefully be charted in five grades (page 114).

● X-RAY The bones may decalcify.

Diagnosis

With a suspected nerve injury, the following questions arise.

Is a nerve lesion present? A quick test for each nerve, in which a distal area of skin or a distally supplied muscle is examined, is useful.

At what level is the lesion? Usually this is obvious from the injury; if it is not, individual muscles whose branches arise at successive levels must be tested. Special investigations are occasionally useful (see below).

What type of lesion is present? Clinical examination may suggest a neurotmesis; a palpable nerve bulb confirms it. Partial division is liable to produce hyperaesthesia or excess sweating. With neurapraxia, paralysis is not total and recovery begins early.

Is the lesion recovering? The earliest evidence is Tinel's sign: the nerve is tapped lightly, starting peripherally; the point at which the patient feels pain or tingling in the distribution of the nerve indicates how far (if at all) recovery has progressed.

Special investigations

Nerve blocking A small quantity of local anaesthetic may be injected into the injured nerve. If this is followed by greater sensory or motor loss the lesion is partial. Similarly, by injecting undamaged nerves, overlap can be recognized.

Electrical tests Precise information of the nature, level and extent of recovery in nerve lesions can be obtained by: (1) the assessment of strength/duration curves; (2) electromyographic study of voluntary action potentials; and (3) the measurement of motor and sensory conduction velocities at varying levels.

Treatment

NERVE REPAIR A divided nerve needs to be repaired. Difficulties arise in deciding whether the division is complete (neurotmesis) and in knowing when to operate. Nerve exploration with a view to repair is indicated when (1) the nerve is known to be divided because the lesion was seen at the wound toilet operation; (2) the nerve is likely to have been divided because of the nature of the injury – e.g. a knife wound; (3) the nerve is presumed to be divided because recovery of the highest supplied muscle has not occurred in the calculated time, or because a palpable nerve bulb has developed; and (4) occasionally for diagnostic purposes.

CARE OF PARALYSED PARTS While recovery is awaited, the skin should be guarded against burns and the circulation assisted by massage. The joints should be moved through their full range twice daily to prevent stiffness. Splints may be necessary and 'lively splints' are the best; they hold the paralysed muscle in its shortened position by means of a spring which is weak enough to allow the unparalysed muscles to work against it.

SECONDARY OPERATION   Even if recovery of the nerve cannot occur, the function of the limb may be improved by splints or operations. For example, tendon transfers are useful for an irrecoverable radial nerve injury; in the foot, stabilization may be helpful; occasionally a high sciatic nerve lesion may necessitate below-knee amputation.

TIMING OF NERVE EXPLORATION

A divided nerve is best repaired as soon as this can be done safely. Primary suture at the time of wound toilet, though not easy (because the sheath is very thin) has considerable advantages: the nerve ends have not retracted much; their relative rotation is usually undisturbed; and there is no fibrosis. But if repair would involve groping about in the depths of a dirty wound it should be postponed, at least until the wound has healed. It may also be wise to postpone repair if the nature of the lesion is uncertain; thus with closed fractures four out of five nerve lesions recover spontaneously and it is worth waiting until the most proximally supplied muscle should have recovered.

With the passage of time the prospects of recovery diminish, for several reasons: (1) the activity of the sprouting axons and of the Schwann cells (which bridge the gap and guide the axons) declines after 7–12 days; (2) the Schwann tubes become narrow, the motor end plates degenerate and the muscles atrophy; and (3) the brain 'forgets' how to use the limb. Consequently it is better to explore too soon (even if the nerve is found to be intact) than too late.

TECHNIQUE OF OPERATION

Tourniquet   If a tourniquet is necessary it should be a pneumatic one; it should be released and bleeding stopped before the wound is closed.

Exposure   A long incision is essential, and the nerve must be widely exposed well above and below the lesion, before the lesion itself is cleared. The nerve must be handled gently with rubber loops or with non-toothed forceps holding only the sheath. To obtain adequate mobilization branches may be stripped up.

Magnification   A loupe or a simple watchmaker's headpiece is of considerable value; but if fascicular repair or grafting is to be attempted an operating microscope is essential.

Resection   With complete division, the fibrous tissue of the proximal end is pared away with a razor blade until axons pout from the stump; similarly at the distal end until the empty tubes are seen. When the lesion is in continuity it is sometimes difficult to know whether resection is necessary or not; if the nerve looks and feels normal or only slightly thick, resection is not advised; if there is a soft fusiform lump resection is again inadvisable; if the lump is hard, it should be resected. A lateral nerve bulb usually needs resection; the cut ends are best joined by a graft, but can be sutured directly leaving the undamaged part of the nerve as a loop.

Suture   The sheath only is sutured, using atraumatic needles with fine silk ('virgin silk' is best) or wire. There must be no tension at the suture line, so gaps must be bridged by mobilization of the nerve and, if necessary, transposition. Flexion of the appropriate joint also helps but it should not be too acute, nor should the process of straightening begin until at least 3 weeks after operation.

After-care   After closure of the wound, the limb is splinted for 3–6 weeks to relieve the suture line from tension. Physiotherapy is then started and is designed to keep the skin, muscles and joints in good condition.

NERVE GRAFTS

In nerve repair there is a critical resection length above which it is useless to try to bridge a gap. The length varies from 7 to 10 cm according to the individual nerve.

With greater gaps autogenous grafts are worth considering. Cutaneous nerves which can be spared for use as grafts include the lateral cutaneous nerve of the thigh, the saphenous, the sural, and the medial cutaneous nerve of the forearm. Because their diameter is small, several strips may be used (cable graft). Nerve grafts should aim at being 15 per cent too long.

If the ulnar and median nerves are both irreparable, a pedicle graft from the ulnar nerve may be used to bridge the gap in the median.

BONE SHORTENING

This is a theoretical possibility to bridge a large gap; it is permissible only when there is established non-union of a fracture, and then but rarely.

Prognosis

Type of lesion   Neurapraxia always recovers fully; axonotmesis usually recovers well; neurotmesis carries the worst prognosis.

Level of lesion   The higher the lesion, the worse the prognosis.

Type of nerve   Purely motor or purely sensory nerves recover better than mixed nerves, because there is less likelihood of axonal confusion.

Size of gap   Above the critical resection length, suture is not successful.

Age   In children the prognosis is better than in adults.

Delay in suture This is a most important adverse factor. After a few months, recovery following suture becomes progressively less likely.

Associated lesions Damage to vessels, tendons and other structures makes it more difficult to obtain recovery of a useful limb even if the nerve itself recovers.

Brachial plexus: birth injuries

Upper arm type (Erb's palsy)

A traction injury during difficult labour damages the plexus just proximal to Erb's point. The nerves involved are C5 and C6; sometimes C7 is slightly affected.

The mother notices that one arm is not being used. The abductors and external rotators of the shoulder and the forearm supinators are paralysed. The arm is therefore held to the side, internally rotated and pronated. If recovery does not occur, contractures develop and x-rays show that the acromion and coracoid processes are elongated and droop downwards.

Most cases (75 per cent) recover without treatment, but it is traditional to hold the arm abducted, externally rotated and supinated either on a splint or by tying the wrist behind the neck to the opposite axilla. If contracture threatens, splintage and daily stretching are important.

If fixed deformities have been allowed to develop, they may require operative correction; for example, by osteotomy of the neck of the humerus for fixed internal rotation, or division of soft tissues for fixed adduction and pronation.

Lower arm type (Klumpke)

This rare lesion follows breech delivery with the arm above the head. The nerves damaged are C8 and T1, especially T1.

The intrinsic muscles of the hand and the finger flexors are paralysed. There may be some sensory loss in the ulnar forearm and hand, and sometimes a Horner's syndrome.

The fingers should be kept supple in the hope of recovery, which is a slender one. Splints and operations are useless.

Brachial plexus: later lesions

The commonest cause is a motorcycle accident; the resulting traction may avulse the roots. Shoulder dislocation may give a partial paralysis, but it

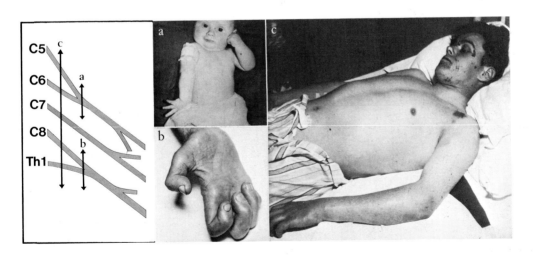

11.2 Brachial plexus Site of the lesions and clinical appearance of brachial plexus injuries: (a) Erb's palsy; (b) Klumpke type; (c) tell-tale abrasions on the face and shoulder show how this motorcyclist pulled his entire plexus apart.

usually recovers. Fractures of the clavicle rarely damage the plexus, and only do so if caused by a direct blow. A cervical rib may compress the lower trunk.

Clinical features

In the whole-arm type, all the arm, forearm and hand muscles and some scapular muscles are paralysed. Most of the limb is numb. With injury at the level of the roots there is often a Horner's syndrome and sometimes associated cord damage; at the level of the trunks, the rhomboid muscles and serratus anterior muscle escape; and at the level of the cords the supraspinatus muscle escapes. The closer the lesion to the cord, the worse is the outlook; bad prognostic signs include considerable pain, a tilted cervical spine in the anteroposterior view and a fracture of the appropriate transverse process. Prognostic aids include myelography, electromyography and skin testing with histamine injections.

In the upper-arm type, the nerves involved are C5 and C6. As in Erb's palsy, the shoulder abductors and external rotators and the forearm supinators are paralysed. Sensory loss involves the outer aspect of the arm and forearm.

The lower-arm type is rare. Wrist and finger flexors are weak, and the intrinsic hand muscles are paralysed so that a claw hand develops. Sensation is lost in the ulnar forearm and hand. There may be an associated Horner's syndrome.

Treatment

Suture, using grafts and microsurgical techniques, is sometimes possible; it is painstaking and difficult, but worth while.

The limb should be maintained in good condition because, with incomplete lesions, a useful amount of recovery sometimes occurs after 2–3 years.

When the lower trunk is not involved, the hand remains useful. It is then sometimes worthwhile arthrodesing the shoulder so that the arm can be abducted by the scapular muscles. The latissimus dorsi can be used to restore elbow flexion. Wrist and finger extension can, in suitable patients, be restored by means of tendon transfers. If there has been a preganglionic avulsion of all the nerve roots, leaving a flail insensitive limb, the best treatment is probably amputation through the mid-humerus combined with arthrodesis of the shoulder.

Median nerve

Gunshot wounds or fractures may give high lesions. Cuts in front of the wrist may divide the nerve. Dislocations of the carpal lunate often cause temporary nerve compression. Compression within the carpal tunnel is common.

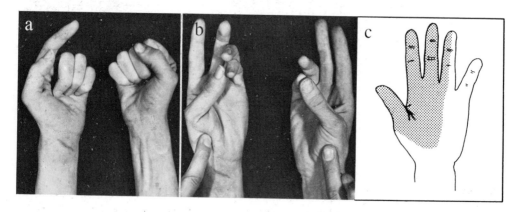

11.3 Cut median nerve (a) The pointing index when trying to clench the hand; (b) opponens wasting; (c) sensory loss.

Clinical features

In low lesions the thenar eminence is wasted and the opponens pollicis muscle paralysed (this should be tested by feeling the muscle as contraction is attempted, because opposition can be faked by a trick movement). Sensation is lost over the radial three and a half digits, and this causes clumsiness, so that the patient cannot pick up a pin.

In high lesions the front of the forearm also is wasted; the thumb, index and middle finger flexors, the radial wrist flexor and the forearm pronator muscles are all paralysed. Often the hand is held with the ulnar fingers flexed and the index straight (pointing index). The middle finger may be flexed because its deep flexor, though paralysed, is joined to the unparalysed ulnar half of flexor profundus. Trophic changes are common.

Treatment

Suture should always be attempted in median nerve lesions. Extensive mobilization may be necessary; thus for lesions just above the wrist it may be necessary to extend the incision to above the elbow and to divide the bicipital fascia. Incomplete, but useful, recovery is common.

While recovery is awaited wrist dorsiflexion should be prevented.

If no recovery occurs, the disability is severe because of sensory loss and loss of pincer action. If sensation recovers, but not opposition, a sublimis–opponens tendon transfer may help.

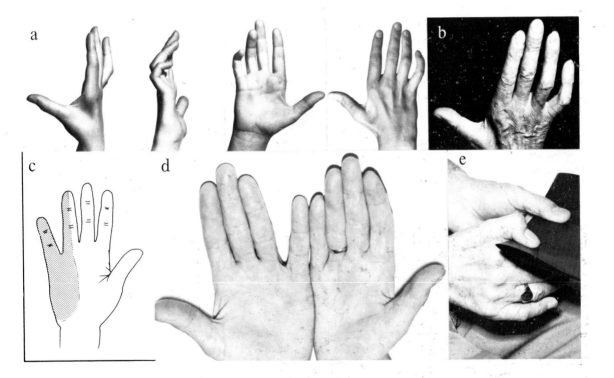

11.4 Ulnar nerve lesions (a) Low ulnar palsy: intrinsic muscle wasting; in the ring and little fingers the knuckle joints are hyperextended (paralysed lumbricals) and the interphalangeal joints are flexed (paralysed interossei). (b) High ulnar palsy: profundus action is lost, so the terminal interphalangeal joints are not flexed (ulnar paradox). (c) Sensory loss. (d) When the patient tries to push his little fingers apart, weakness of one abductor digiti minimi is displayed. (e) Froment's sign – because adductor pollicis is weak, the flexor pollicis longus is being used.

Ulnar nerve

An open wound may injure the nerve at any level. At the elbow, fracture of the medial epicondyle often causes damage, usually temporary. Fracture of the lateral condyle, if ununited, leads to a cubitus valgus with delayed ulnar palsy. Osteoarthritis of the elbow may cause ulnar palsy from friction neuritis. At the wrist, cuts with glass are common and a deep carpal ganglion may compress the nerve, especially at the exit of the pisohamate tunnel. Bilateral ulnar nerve lesion occurs in leprosy.

Clinical features

In low lesions (wrist) the hand is clawed, the ring and little fingers being hyperextended at the metacarpophalangeal joints and flexed at the interphalangeal joints. Wasting of the intrinsic muscles is especially obvious in the first cleft which, on being pinched, feels much too thin. Neither the index nor the little finger can be abducted actively against resistance, nor the middle finger waggled sideways. Sensation is lost over the ulnar one and a half fingers.

In high lesions (elbow) the visible deformity is actually less marked, in that the terminal joints of the ring and little fingers are not flexed; this is because the ulnar half of flexor digitorum profundus is paralysed (loss of active flexion of the terminal joint of the fifth finger is a useful test). Otherwise sensory and motor loss are the same as in low lesions. In lesions well above the elbow, the flexor carpi ulnaris muscle also is paralysed.

Treatment

Exploration and suture of a divided ulnar nerve is well worth while and anterior transposition permits a gap to be bridged. Transposition is also advised when a deformed or degenerate elbow has caused the lesion; not only is the palsy prevented from advancing further, but some degree of recovery usually occurs. Some lesions at the elbow are due to compression of the nerve by a fibrous band at the proximal end of the flexor carpi ulnaris muscle. Division of this band is not always sufficient and transposition is preferable.

While recovery is awaited, the skin should be guarded against burns. 'Lively' splints keep the hand supple and useful.

If recovery does not occur, the hand still has reasonable function. Bunnell's operation (sublimis-to-extensor tendon transfer) is sometimes used but Zancolli's operation is probably better; through four longitudinal palmar incisions the volar capsule of each metacarpophalangeal joint is shortened by proximal advancement of a distally based flap.

Radial nerve

Open wounds may injure the nerve at any level. At the elbow, fractures may cause damage which is usually temporary. In the axilla a crutch palsy may occur; this always recovers.

Clinical features

In low lesions (posterior interosseus nerve) the posterior forearm looks flat and the patient can extend neither the interphalangeal joint of the thumb nor the metacarpophalangeal joints of the fingers and thumb. There is no detectable sensory loss.

In high lesions (around the elbow) the radial wrist extensors and the supinator muscle also are paralysed (the patient can still supinate the flexed elbow with his biceps muscle).

In very high lesions (axilla) the triceps muscle also may be paralysed. There is a small area of sensory loss on the dorsum of the first cleft.

Treatment

Suture below the elbow is rarely possible, because the nerve cannot be sufficiently mobilized. At or above the elbow, suture may be worth while.

While recovery is awaited, a Brian Thomas splint is worn; this is a 'lively' splint holding the metacarpophalangeal joints straight and the thumb straight and abducted, while still permitting active use of the hand.

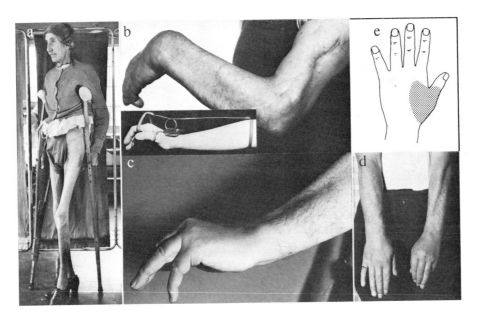

11.5 Radial nerve lesions   (a) Crutches should not be thrust high into the axilla, or palsy may follow; (b) complete division with drop wrist (*inset* – Brian Thomas' splint); (c) this patient demonstrates the inability to extend the fingers at the knuckle joints, but he can straighten the interphalangeal joints with his intrinsic muscles; (d) wasting; (e) sensory loss.

If recovery does not occur, the disability can be almost completely overcome by tendon transfers; the commonest is described on page 145.

NOTE   Tourniquet palsy is more common in the upper than in the lower limb. It usually affects only or predominantly the motor fibres. Spontaneous recovery is usual.

Lumbosacral plexus

INDIVIDUAL ROOTS   may be compressed by a tumour or by a prolapsed intervertebral disc.

Pressure on L3 and 4 roots may cause quadriceps wasting, depression of the knee reflex and loss of sensation over the anterior thigh and medial side of the leg. Pressure on L4 alone causes weakness of the hamstrings; this produces a hyperactive knee jerk (because of the unopposed extensor action).

Pressure on L5 root may cause weak gluteal muscles, weak foot and big toe dorsiflexors and altered sensation over the front of the leg and dorsum of the foot.

Pressure on S1 root may cause weak gluteal muscles, weak foot plantarflexors, a depressed ankle jerk and altered sensation along the sole of the foot.

INDIVIDUAL NERVES   (other than the sciatic) may be affected.

The lateral cutaneous nerve (L2 and 3)   may be compressed within fibres of the inguinal ligament, causing local tenderness and hyperaesthesia or numbness over the outer thigh. This is known as meralgia paraesthetica and is an example of a tunnel syndrome. If severe, the condition may be relieved by freeing the nerve or, if necessary, dividing it.

The femoral nerve (L2, 3, 4)   may be injured by a gunshot wound (rarely seen, because associated femoral artery damage often proves fatal) or by traction during an operation. There is quadriceps paralysis and numbness of the anterior thigh and medial aspects of the leg.

Sciatic nerve

Division of the main sciatic nerve is rare except in gunshot wounds. Traction lesions may occur with traumatic hip dislocations and with pelvic fractures.

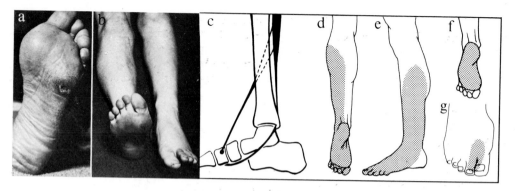

11.6 Sciatic nerve   Two problems in sciatic lesions are: (a) sensory loss, which may lead to trophic ulcer; and (b) foot drop, which can be treated with a toe-raising spring, or by rerouting tibialis posterior to the front (c). The remaining diagrams show the areas of sensory loss following division of (d) complete sciatic nerve, (e) lateral popliteal nerve, (f) posterior tibial nerve, and (g) anterior tibial nerve.

Clinical features

The calf and leg are thin and the patient walks with a drop foot; all muscles below the knee are paralysed. Because the quadriceps muscle is supplied by the anterior crural nerve it functions normally, but knee flexion is weak because the hamstring supply has been damaged. Sensation is absent below the knee (except on the medial side of the leg) and trophic ulcers often develop on the sole.

Treatment

Suture should be performed if possible.

While recovery is awaited, below-knee irons and a toe-raising spring are worn. Great care is taken with socks, shoes and foot toilet to try to prevent trophic ulcers.

If recovery fails and sores develop, a below-knee amputation may be necessary.

'SCIATICA'
Pain along the distribution of the sciatic nerve may be due to root compression by a prolapsed intervertebral disc (see page 232); or it may be referred from the facet joints or from neighbouring structures.

Lateral popliteal nerve

The main nerve may be damaged at the level of the neck of the fibula by traction when the knee is forced into gross varus (or if gross valgus deformity is corrected overenthusiastically), by pressure from a splint, from lying with the leg externally rotated, by skin traction, by an intraneural ganglion or by wounds. The branches are rarely injured except by gunshot wounds.

Clinical features

With a high lesion (the main lateral popliteal nerve), the outer side of the leg is wasted and the patient cannot dorsiflex or evert the foot and toes. He has a foot drop and therefore walks with a high-stepping gait. Sensation is lost over the front and outer half of the leg and the dorsum of the foot and toes.

A low lesion involving only the musculocutaneous branch causes paralysis of the peroneal muscles with wasting; on dorsiflexion the foot is pulled into varus. Sensation is lost over the outer side of the leg, foot and toes.

A lesion involving only the anterior tibial branch causes paralysis of the tibialis anterior muscle and the long toe extensors. The front of the leg is wasted and the patient cannot dorsiflex his foot without everting it. Sensation is lost only in the first cleft.

Treatment

Where possible, the nerve is sutured.

While recovery is awaited a splint may be worn; the skin must be guarded against ulceration.

If recovery does not occur, any disability can be minimized by tendon transfers (e.g. detaching tibialis posterior, threading it through the interosseous membrane and attaching it in front), or foot stabilization.

Medial popliteal nerve

The nerve is rarely injured except in open wounds.

Clinical features

With a complete lesion of the main medial popliteal nerve, the calf is thin and the heel valgus. The patient cannot plantarflex his ankle. The intrinsic muscles of the foot are paralysed so that the toes are clawed. Sensation is absent over the sole (where there may be a trophic ulcer) and part of the calf.

A lesion of the posterior tibial branch alone causes much less wasting of the calf and weakness of plantarflexion. The toes are clawed from intrinsic muscle paralysis. Sensation is lost over the sole of the foot, but the sural supply remains.

Unlike the lateral popliteal nerve, the medial popliteal or the posterior tibial nerve may suffer from the irritation syndrome, especially when incomplete division is associated with sepsis.

Treatment

A complete lesion should be sutured if possible.

While recovery of a high lesion is awaited, a side-iron is worn which fits into a square socket in the heel of the shoe; this prevents the foot dorsiflexing too far. A lesion confined to the posterior tibial branch needs no splintage. Care is taken to prevent ulcers on the sole.

Occasionally an irritation syndrome is so severe as to warrant below-knee amputation.

Tunnel syndromes (nerve entrapment)

Wherever peripheral nerves traverse fibro-osseous tunnels they are at risk of compression, especially if the soft tissues increase in bulk, as they may in pregnancy, myxoedema or with rheumatoid synovitis. The underlying pathology is probably not simple nerve compression, but an ischaemic neuropathy due to venous stasis and impedance of arterial flow. Common sites are the carpal tunnel (median nerve) and the epicondylar tunnel at the elbow (ulnar nerve); less common sites are the tarsal tunnel (posterior tibial nerve), Guyon's canal at the wrist (ulnar nerve) and the inguinal ligament (lateral cutaneous nerve of the thigh causing meralgia paraesthetica).

The patient complains of tingling or numbness distal to the point of entrapment; except in the carpal tunnel, pain is seldom severe. Typically symptoms occur at night, when the related joint may be held still for several hours; relief is obtained by moving the hand or foot 'to get the circulation going'. Symptoms can sometimes be reproduced by proximal compression; e.g. with a sphygmomanometer cuff. Nerve conduction is slowed.

Tunnel syndromes can be cured by operative decompression.

Reflex sympathetic dystrophy (irritation syndrome)

A number of clinical syndromes are now collected under this heading, including causalgia, the shoulder–hand syndrome and Sudeck's atrophy. What they have in common is pain, trophic skin changes, vasomotor instability and osteoporosis. Precipitating causes may be trauma (often trivial), a peripheral nerve lesion, myocardial infarction or stroke. The cause is unknown (despite a plethora of theories) but autonomic nerve dysfunction is suspected.

Clinical features

The patient complains – bitterly – of burning or penetrating pain: usually in the hand or foot, sometimes the shoulder and occasionally progressing up the limb. The limb is held immobile and may be swollen. The skin looks sweaty, blotchy and sometimes patchily cyanosed. It feels warm, but the slightest touch may provoke a spasm of withdrawal. Later, joint stiffness and fixed deformities may develop. X-rays show patchy osteoporosis, and on radionuclide scanning there is increased activity.

The acute symptoms sometimes subside after 6–18 months, but established deformities remain and some degree of pain may persist indefinitely.

Treatment

Treatment should be started as soon as the diagnosis is suspected; the earlier the better. Analgesics, ice-packs and active exercises may help. Specific measures include: (1) 'chemical sympathectomy' – an arterial tourniquet is applied proximal to the affected area, 20 mg of guanethidine diluted with saline is injected intravenously, and after 20 minutes the tourniquet is removed (Hannington-Kiff, 1979); (2) sympathetic interruption by injection or operation; and (3) a short course of steroids in fairly high dosage.

Further reading

Aids to the Examination of the Peripheral Nervous System (1976) *MRC Memorandum No. 45.* London: HMSO
Editorial (1972) Causalgia. *Lancet* **i,** 1170–1171
Editorial (1980) Brachial plexus injuries in motorcyclists. *British Medical Journal* **280,** 1242
Hannington-Kiff, J. G. (1979) Relief of causalgia in limbs by regional intravenous guanethidine. *British Medical Journal* **2,** 367–368
Omer, G. E. (1968) Evaluation and reconstruction of the forearm and hand after traumatic peripheral nerve injuries. *Journal of Bone and Joint Surgery* **50A,** 1454–1478
Seddon, Sir H. J. (1975) *Surgical Disorders of the Peripheral Nerves,* 2nd edn. Edinburgh and London: Churchill Livingstone

Fundamentals of Orthopaedic Operations

12

To operate on bone requires the tools of a carpenter, yet orthopaedic surgery is not carpentry; biological imperatives ensure that this can never be. *The art and skill of orthopaedic surgery is directed not to constructing a particular arrangement of parts, but to restoring function to the whole.*

Preparation

PLANNING   Operations upon bone must be carefully planned in advance, when accurate measurements can be made and bones can be compared for symmetry with those of the opposite limb.

STERILITY   The need for sterility is even greater in bone surgery than in soft-tissue surgery; any wound infection represents a setback, but bone infection can be a disaster.

X-RAY CONTROL   Procedures involving realignment of bones and joints or accurate placement of pins and nails should always be checked by intraoperative x-rays – preferably fluoroscopy and image intensification.

EQUIPMENT   Bone operations need special instruments, the minimum requirements being drills (for boring holes), osteotomes (for cutting cancellous bone), saws (for cutting cortical bone), chisels (for shaping bone), gouges (for removing bone) and plates, screws and screwdrivers (for fixing bone).

THE 'BLOODLESS FIELD'   Many operations on limbs can be done more rapidly and accurately if bleeding is prevented by a tourniquet. This should always be a pneumatic cuff, applied over bulky soft tissues to avoid nerve pressure, inflated to not more than 100 mmHg above the systolic pressure and removed within 2 hours; whenever practicable it should be removed before the wound is closed, so that bleeding can be controlled and a 'silent' postoperative haematoma avoided. Excessive or prolonged pressure can cause permanent nerve or muscle damage (Klenerman, 1980).

Basic procedures

DRILLING   Drilling may be necessary simply to evacuate a bone abscess, or a series of holes may facilitate cutting through cortex with an osteotome. Most commonly, however, the drill is used to prepare seat-holes for screws.

CUTTING   Cancellous bone can be cut with an osteotome; the tapered edge cleaves soft bone, but may shatter cortical bone. The tubular shaft, therefore, has to be weakened by drilling a series of holes before applying the osteotome. Less hazardous, and more accurate, is a motorized saw.

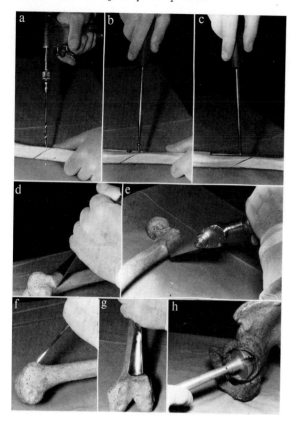

12.1 Basic operative procedures   (a) Drilling. (b) Inserting a screw. (c) Plating. (d) Cutting with an osteotome and (e) with a motorized saw. (f) Shaping bone with a chisel, and (g) with a gouge. (h) Reaming.

MODELLING   The bone surface can be shaped with a chisel; concave surfaces are more easily worked with a gouge.

REAMING   To ream means (literally) to widen. A joint socket, or the medullary cavity of a tubular bone, may need reaming before it will accept a prosthesis or a nail of suitable size.

FIXING   Bone fragments can be firmly joined by simple *screwing* (especially if a small piece has to be fixed back in position), by *attaching a bridging plate* to the bone with a row of screws, by passing a *long nail* down the medullary canal, by transfixing the fragments with *pins or wires*, by *stapling* the pieces together (only in soft bone), by securing the pieces with *malleable wire*, or by a *combination* of these methods. All these will eventually loosen or break unless natural union occurs.

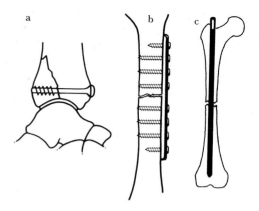

12.2 Three ways of fixing bone   (a) With a single screw – this is a lag screw (threaded only distally) and therefore interfragmentary compression is achieved; (b) plate and screws – the commonest way of fixing a shaft fracture; (c) intramedullary nail.

Operations on bones

Osteotomy

Osteotomy may be used to correct deformity, or to relieve pain in arthritis. Preoperative planning is essential, with precise measurements of the patient and the x-rays. The following must be determined.

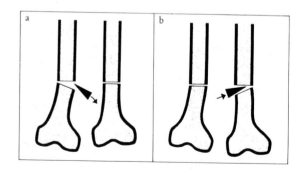

12.3 Osteotomy   A bent bone can be straightened (a) by removing a wedge of bone, or (b) by inserting one: (a) is sometimes called a 'closing wedge osteotomy' – it is easier, but leaves the bone shorter; (b) is an 'opening wedge' – it maintains length but may be more difficult to do.

The exact site of bone division For corrective osteotomy this should be as near as possible to the site of deformity. For joint realignment, local geometry dictates the level.

The amount of correction required The intended angular or rotational shift must be measured in degrees.

The method of correction To change an angular deformity a wedge of bone may have to be removed ('closing wedge') or inserted ('opening wedge'). The size of the wedge should be calculated accurately and reproduced on a template for use during the operation.

The method of fixation Sometimes plaster splintage alone will suffice. Usually internal fixation is preferred. The bone must be splinted or protected from weight-bearing until union is complete.

Complications

(1) The commonest is over- or undercorrection of the deformity: hence the importance of preoperative planning. (2) Non-union may occur if fixation is inadequate; raw bone surfaces must be firmly apposed and rigidly splinted. (3) Joint stiffness may occur if the limb is not exercised. (4) As with all bone operations, infection is a calculated risk.

Bone grafts*

Bone grafts serve three purposes: (1) to provide stability (e.g. for fractures, arthrodesis or to buttress unstable joints) – for this purpose cortical bone is best; (2) to provide linkage (e.g. to replace missing bone or to fill cavities); (3) to stimulate osteogenesis—for this purpose cancellous bone is best. Pedicle grafts (swung on a pedicle of muscle direct to the new site) retain their blood supply, but are seldom feasible.

Autografts Bone taken from the patient himself has the best chance of survival and incorporation.

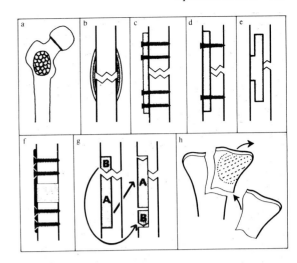

12.4 Bone grafts (a) Chip grafts to fill a cavity; (b) onlay strips of cancellous bone (Phemister technique); (c) onlay cortical graft; (d) inlay cortical graft; (e) latch graft; (f) cancellous block graft plus plating (Nicoll technique); (g) sliding graft – the portion marked A is slid up to bridge the fracture; (h) large cadaveric osteocartilaginous graft obtained fresh and sterile from an organ donor.

Even then, only the surface cells survive and, nourished by tissue fluids, are capable of a little osteogenesis. Most of the transplanted bone dies, but it acts as a scaffold which is invaded by vessels and bone cells of the host bed and is slowly replaced by new bone. Cancellous bone is more readily incorporated than compact bone.

Allografts (homografts) Bone transferred from one individual (living or dead) to another of the same species is immunologically unacceptable; resorption and replacement are therefore delayed and may even cease. Its antigenicity can, however, be modified by freezing or by nuclear irradiation. Irradiation sterilizes bone, but it also alters collagen structure and depresses graft incorporation. Freezing is not harmful, but the donor bone must then be harvested under sterile conditions. Allografts are plentiful and can be stored conveniently.

---

*Graft refers to living tissue; *transplant* is, therefore, more accurate because most bone grafts are dead. However, custom condones the use of both terms.

Recent advances in the use of large osteocartilaginous grafts obtained from fresh cadavers have opened the possibility of replacing entire joints. The bone must be removed under aseptic conditions; cartilage preservation is enhanced by immersion in glycerol, and the entire graft is then deep frozen until it is needed.

Xenografts (heterografts) Bone taken from a different species should, if treated for antigenicity, behave like an allograft; in practice, it is less effective and is little used.

Leg equalization

Inequality of leg length amounting to more than 2.5 cm needs treatment. There are three possibilities.

(1) LENGTHENING THE SHORTER LEG The simplest and safest method is a raised shoe. The alternative is operation, by which 5 or 8 cm of length can be gained in the tibia or femur. The bone is osteotomized, with minimum disturbance of periosteum, and the fragments are distracted by skeletal pins. For tibial lengthening a piece of fibula is first excised and the lower portion of the fibula is fixed to the tibia; otherwise the ankle becomes deformed. Distraction must be gradual (1 mm a day) to avoid damaging nerves or vessels. When the desired length is reached, the segment of new bone may be reinforced with a plate and thin cancellous grafts; the distraction apparatus can then be removed and partial weight-bearing allowed. The plate is removed after 1 or 2 years. The operation should be done before the age of 14; after that the chances of sound union diminish.

(2) SHORTENING THE LONGER LEG In children, epiphyseal arrest is an effective method; it can be temporary, using staples, or permanent, using bone grafts. In deciding at what age to operate,

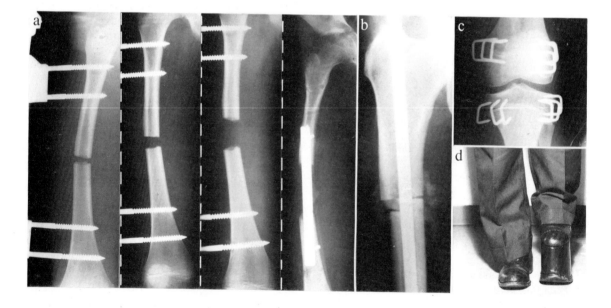

12.5 Leg equalization (a) The short leg may be lengthened by osteotomy and distraction. When maximum length has been gained, the bone is plated and the distraction pins are removed; the plate is left in position until consolidation is complete (seldom less than a year). The longer leg may be shortened by (b) excising a segment of bone, or by (c) arresting epiphyseal growth. But the simplest way to equalize length is (d) a raised shoe.

Menelaus' formula, though approximate, is useful: he assumes that each year the lower femoral and upper tibial epiphyses contribute 1.0 cm and 0.6 cm respectively to length; and that these epiphyses fuse at 16 in boys and 14 in girls. In adults a piece of bone can be excised, preferably using a step osteotomy, and the approximated ends held by internal fixation.

The danger with either method stems from the fact that the longer leg is usually the normal one; should serious complications ensue, the patient may not 'have a leg to stand on'.

(3) COMBINED METHODS Merle d'Aubigné and Dubousset (1971) advocate removing bone from the longer femur and inserting it into the shorter one. When this combination is augmented by subsequent tibial lengthening, remarkable gains can be achieved.

Internal fixation

This is dealt with on page 343.

Operations on joints

Arthrotomy

Arthrotomy (opening a joint) may be indicated: (1) to inspect the interior or perform a synovial biopsy; (2) to drain a haematoma or an abscess; (3) to remove a loose body or damaged structure (e.g. a torn meniscus); and (4) to excise inflamed synovium. The intra-articular tissues should be handled with great care, and if postoperative bleeding is expected (e.g. after synovectomy) a drain should be inserted – postoperative haemarthrosis predisposes to infection. Following the operation the joint should be rested for a few days, but thereafter movement must be encouraged.

Realignment

This is essentially an osteotomy designed to redistribute stress to a less damaged part of the joint. In early osteoarthritis of the hip or knee it is often effective in relieving pain (see pages 271 and 302).

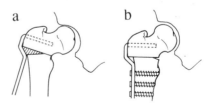

12.6 Joint realignment (a) The joint space is not congruent; (b) an osteotomy has realigned it – now it is nearly equal throughout.

Stabilization

ARTHRODESIS The most reliable operation for a painful or unstable joint is arthrodesis; where stiffness does not seriously affect function, this is often the treatment of choice. Examples are the spine, the tarsus, the ankle, the wrist and the interphalangeal joints. Arthrodesis is useful also for a knee which is already fairly stiff (provided the other knee has good movement) and for a flail shoulder.

The principles of the operation are straightforward: (1) both joint surfaces are denuded of cartilage; (2) they are apposed in the optimum position and held by some form of internal fixation; (3) bone grafts are added in the larger joints to promote osseous bridging; and (4) the limb is usually splinted until union is complete.

The main complication is non-union, with the formation of a pseudarthrosis. Rigid fixation lessens this risk, and, where feasible (e.g. the knee and ankle), the bony parts are squeezed together by compression clamps.

SOFT TISSUE STABILIZATION This is indicated for instability without pain. It can be achieved by capsular repair and reinforcement (e.g. for recurrent dislocation of the shoulder); by ligamentous reconstruction (e.g. for instability of the wrist in rheumatoid arthritis); by replacing torn ligaments with tendon and fascia (e.g. in the knee or ankle); or by musculotendinous transfer (e.g. in the paralysed hip).

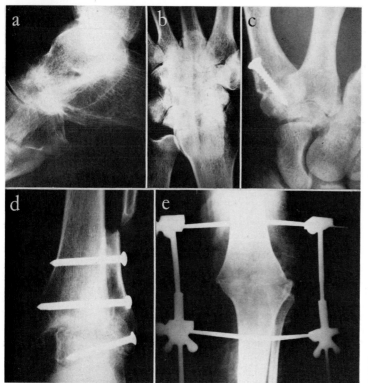

12.7 Arthrodesis In all cases the joint surfaces are first denuded of cartilage: in subtalar mid-tarsal fusion (a), no other measures are needed; at the wrist (b), bone grafts are added; at the carpometacarpal joint of the thumb (c), a screw may be inserted;

at the ankle (d), the fibula can be screwed on as a graft; at the knee (e), Charnley's compression clamps are applied.

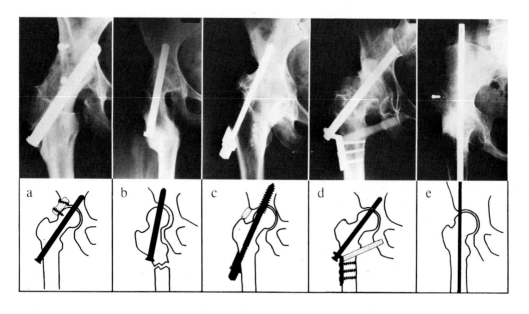

12.8 Arthrodesis of the hip   (a) Watson-Jones; (b) Pyrford; (c) compression; (d) Norwich; (e) transfixion. With (a) and (c) a long hip spica is used; with (b) a short hip spica after 6 weeks' traction; with (d) and (e) plaster can often be dispensed with.

Mobilization

Arthroplasty, the surgical refashioning of a joint, aims to relieve pain and to retain or restore movement. The following are the main varieties.

EXCISION ARTHROPLASTY Sufficient bone is excised to create a gap at which movement can occur (e.g. Girdlestone's hip arthroplasty). In some situations (e.g. after excising the trapezium) a shaped Silastic 'spacer' can be inserted.

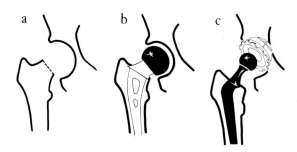

12.9 Arthroplasty The main varieties as applied to the hip joint: (a) excision arthroplasty (Girdlestone); (b) partial replacement – an Austin Moore prosthesis has been inserted after removing the femoral head; (c) total replacement.

PARTIAL REPLACEMENT One surface only is replaced (e.g. MacIntosh's hemiprosthesis for the upper tibia); or one complete bone end is replaced (e.g. Moore's prosthesis for a fractured femoral neck); or one compartment of a joint is replaced (e.g. the medial or the lateral half of the tibio-femoral joint).

TOTAL REPLACEMENT Both articular bone ends are replaced by prosthetic implants; for biomechanical reasons, the convex component is usually of metal and the concave of high-density polyethylene. As a rule both are fixed to the host bone with acrylic cement, but uncemented prostheses are being tried.

Total replacement has been spectacularly successful at the hip; at the knee, wrist and metacarpophalangeal joints results are moderate; and elsewhere the outcome is unpredictable. (For details see the appropriate chapters.)

Operations on tendons

Tendons may need to be divided (tenotomy), and to be reattached. Tendon lengthening involves both procedures: after making a long step-cut the ends are distracted and then sutured in their new position. This is done to correct joint deformity (the commonest being tendo Achillis lengthening for fixed equinus); postoperatively a plaster cast is retained for 6 weeks.

Tendon transfer

Movement lost due to paralysis can sometimes be restored by tendon transfer, using a tendon whose action can be spared. A 'balance-sheet' of what is available and what is needed should be prepared; for a radial nerve palsy it would look like this:

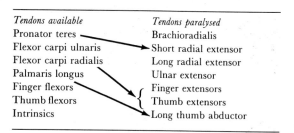

Tendons available	*Tendons paralysed*
Pronator teres	Brachioradialis
Flexor carpi ulnaris	Short radial extensor
Flexor carpi radialis	Long radial extensor
Palmaris longus	Ulnar extensor
Finger flexors	Finger extensors
Thumb flexors	Thumb extensors
Intrinsics	Long thumb abductor

Tendons which can readily be sacrificed are pronator teres and two of the three wrist flexors.

Major needs are wrist extension, finger and thumb extension, and thumb abduction. Arrows show how they can be met.

Prerequisites for successful tendon transfer are (1) stability of the proximal joints, (2) prior correction of any fixed deformity, (3) a tendon with sufficient power and excursion for its new task, (4) a direct line of pull and (5) a firm point of fixation – preferably bone. The transferred tendon should be protected by splintage for 6 weeks.

Tendon transplant

If it is impossible to substitute an active tendon for a damaged one, movement can still be restored by excising or bypassing the damaged segment and replacing it with a free tendon graft. The plantaris, palmaris longus or a toe extensor can be sacrificed for this purpose.

Microsurgery and limb replantation

Microsurgical techniques are used in repairing nerves and vessels, transplanting bone with a vascular pedicle, substituting a less essential digit (e.g. a toe) for a more essential one (e.g. a thumb) and – occasionally – for reattaching a severed limb or digit. Essential prerequisites are an operating microscope, special instruments, microsu-

tures, a chair with arm supports and – not least – a surgeon well practised in microsurgical techniques.

For replantation, the severed part should be kept cool during transport. Shortly before operation it is soaked in aqueous chlorhexidine solution. Two teams now dissect, identify and mark each artery, nerve and vein of the stump and the limb. Following careful débridement the bones are shortened to reduce tension and fixed together by wires, nails or plates. Next the vessels are sutured – veins first and (if possible) two veins for each artery. A vessel of 1 mm diameter needs seven or eight circumferential sutures! Nerves and

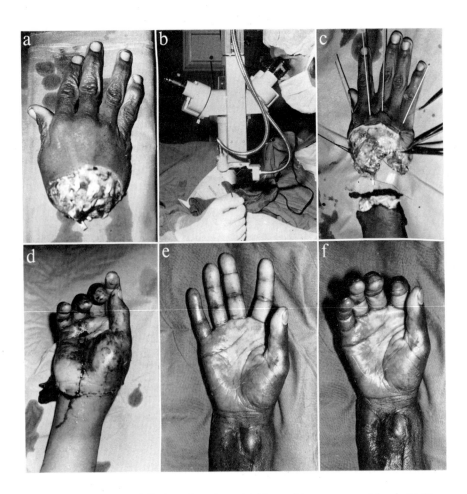

12.10 Microsurgery and limb replantation   (a) The problem – a severed hand. (b) The solution – replantation with microsurgical techniques. (c) The bones of the severed hand have been fixed with K-wires as a preliminary to suturing vessels and nerves. (d) The appearance at the end of the operation. (e) and (f) show the limb 1 year later; the fingers extend fully and bend about half-way. But the hand survived, has moderate sensation and the patient was able to return to work (as a guillotine operator in a paper works!).

tendons next need suturing; the excision of less important muscles is another way of reducing tension. Only healthy ends of approximately equal diameter should be joined; tension, kinking and torsion must be avoided. Dextran 70 (Macrodex) at the end of the operation and heparin for a few days afterwards are useful. Decompression of skin and fascia, as well as thrombectomy, may be needed in the postoperative period.

Replantation surgery is time-consuming, expensive and often unsuccessful. It should be carried out only in centres specially equipped, and by teams specially trained, for this work.

Amputations

Indications

Colloquially the indications are three Ds—Dead, Dangerous and Damn nuisance.

DEAD (OR DYING)   usually from *peripheral vascular disease*, but sometimes following *severe trauma, burns* or *frostbite*.

DANGEROUS   because it harbours a *malignant tumour*, or *potentially lethal sepsis* (especially gas gangrene), or because of a *crush injury*, where releasing the compression may result in renal failure (the crush syndrome).

DAMN NUISANCE   or worse than no limb at all – because of *pain, gross malformation, recurrent sepsis* or *severe loss of function*.

Varieties

A provisional amputation   may be necessary because primary healing is unlikely. The limb is amputated as distal as the causal condition will allow. Skin flaps sufficient to cover the deep tissues are cut and sutured loosely over a pack. Re-amputation is performed when the stump condition is favourable.

Definitive end-bearing amputation   is performed when weight is to be taken through the end of a stump. Therefore the scar must not be terminal, and the bone end must be solid, not hollow, which means it must be cut through or near a joint. Examples are through-knee and Syme's amputations.

Definitive non-end-bearing amputations   are the commonest variety. All upper limb and most lower limb amputations come into this category. Because weight is not to be taken at the end of the stump, the scar can be terminal.

Amputations at the sites of election

Most lower limb amputations (80 per cent) are for ischaemic disease and are performed through the site of election below the most distal palpable

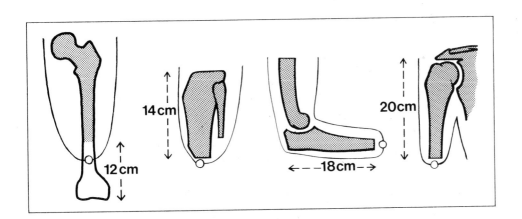

12.11 Amputations (1)   The traditional sites of election; the scar is made terminal because these are not end-bearing stumps.

pulse. The 'sites of election' are determined by the demands of prosthetic design and local function. Too short a stump may tend to slip out of the prosthesis. Too long a stump may have inadequate circulation and can become painful, or ulcerate; moreover, it complicates the incorporation of a joint in the prosthesis. For all that, the skill of the modern prosthetist has made it possible to amputate at almost any site.

Principles of technique

A tourniquet is used unless there is arterial insufficiency. Skin flaps are cut – too long at first and subsequently tailored. As a rule anterior and posterior flaps of equal length are used for the upper limb and for above-knee amputations; below the knee a long posterior flap is usual.

Muscles are divided distal to the proposed site of bone section; subsequently, opposing groups are sutured over the bone end to each other and to the periosteum, thus providing better muscle control as well as better circulation. Nerves are divided proximal to the bone cut.

The bone is sawn across at the proposed level. In below-knee amputations the front of the tibia is bevelled and the fibula cut 3 cm shorter.

The main vessels are tied, the tourniquet removed and every bleeding point meticulously ligated. The skin is sutured carefully without tension. Suction drainage is advised and the stump firmly bandaged.

After-care

If a haematoma forms, it is evacuated at 5–6 days from operation. Repeated firm bandaging or a temporary pylon helps to make the stump conical. The muscles must be exercised, the joints kept mobile and the patient taught to use his prosthesis.

Amputations other than at the sites of election

FOREQUARTER AMPUTATION This mutilating operation should be done only when there is hope of eradicating malignant disease or palliating otherwise intractable pain.

DISARTICULATION AT THE SHOULDER This is rarely indicated, and if the head of the humerus can be left, the appearance is much better. If 2.5 cm of humerus can be left below the anterior axillary fold, it is possible to hold the stump in a prosthesis.

BELOW THE ELBOW The shortest stump which will stay in a prosthesis is 2.5 cm, measured from the front of the flexed elbow. However, an even shorter stump may be useful as a hook

to hang things from. Longer stumps are an advantage only if modern prostheses, which allow pronation and supination, are available.

AMPUTATIONS IN THE HAND These are discussed on page 204.

HINDQUARTER AMPUTATION This operation is performed only for malignant disease. Sir Gordon Gordon-Taylor's technique should be followed in detail.

DISARTICULATION THROUGH THE HIP This is rarely indicated and is difficult to fit with a prosthesis. If the femoral head, neck and trochanters can be left it is possible to fit a tilting-table prosthesis in which the upper femur sits flexed; if, however, a good prosthetic service is available, a disarticulation and moulding of the torso to a wedge shape is preferable.

THIGH AMPUTATIONS A longer stump offers the patient better control of the prosthesis, but at least 12 cm must be left below the stump for the knee mechanism. With less than 18 cm from the top of the greater trochanter it is difficult to keep the stump in the socket.

AROUND THE KNEE The Stokes–Gritti operation (in which the trimmed patella is apposed to the trimmed femoral condyle) is rarely performed because the bone may not unite securely, the end-bearing stump is rarely satisfactory and there is no room for a sophisticated knee mechanism.

Amputation through the knee is becoming increasingly popular, especially for vascular insufficiency. A long anterior or equal medial and lateral flaps are used. The patella is left *in situ* and the patellar ligament sutured to the cruciate ligaments. A temporary pylon can be fitted within a few days. Through-knee amputations are also of value in children, because the lower femoral growth disc is preserved.

A very short below-knee amputation (less than 3 cm) is worse than a through-knee amputation and should be avoided.

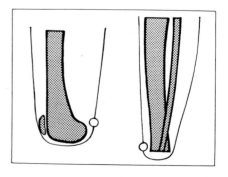

12.12 Amputations (2)   Through-knee and Syme's amputations are end-bearing; consequently the scars are not terminal.

BELOW-KNEE AMPUTATIONS Healthy below-knee stumps can be fitted with excellent prostheses allowing good function and nearly normal gait. Even a 5 or 6 cm stump may be fittable in a thin patient; more makes fitting easier, but there is no advantage in prolonging the stump beyond the conventional 14 cm. With a long posterior flap and suction drainage, healing can often be achieved even when the blood supply is impaired.

ABOVE THE ANKLE Syme's amputation is sometimes very satisfactory, provided the circulation of the limb is good. The indications are few, and the operation is difficult to do well. Because the stump is designed to be end-bearing, the scar is brought away from the end by cutting a long posterior flap. This flap must contain not only the skin of the heel but also all the fibrofatty tissue, to provide a good pad for weight-bearing, and therefore in cutting the flap the bone must be picked clean. The bones are divided just above the malleoli to provide a broad area of cancellous bone, to which the flap should stick firmly, otherwise the soft tissues tend to wobble about. Pirogoff's amputation is similar in principle to Syme's but is rarely performed. The back of the os calcis is stuck onto the cut end of the tibia and fibula.

PARTIAL FOOT AMPUTATIONS The problem is that the tendo Achillis tends to pull the foot into equinus; this can be avoided by splintage, tenotomy, or tendon transfers. The foot may be amputated at any convenient level; e.g. through the mid-tarsal joints (Chopart), through the tarsometatarsal joints (Lisfranc), through the metatarsal bones or through the metatarsophalangeal joints. It is best to disregard the classical descriptions and to leave as long a foot as possible provided it is plantigrade and that an adequate flap of plantar skin can be obtained. The only prosthesis needed is a specially moulded slipper worn inside a normal shoe.

IN THE FOOT Where feasible, it is better to amputate through the base of the proximal phalanx rather than through the metatarsophalangeal joint. With diabetic gangrene, septic arthritis of the joint is not uncommon; the entire ray (toe plus metatarsal bone) should be amputated.

Prostheses

All prostheses must fit comfortably; they should also function well and look presentable. The patient accepts and uses a prosthesis much better if it is fitted soon after operation; delay is unjustifiable now that modular components are available and only the socket need be made individually. Powered prostheses are being developed.

In the upper limb, the distal portion of the prosthesis is detachable and can be replaced by a 'dress hand' or by a variety of useful gadgets.

In the lower limb, weight can be transmitted through the ischial tuberosity, the patellar tendon, the upper tibia or the soft tissues; combinations are permissible and near-total-contact sockets are available for below-knee stumps. The prosthesis is held on by braces, or a belt or a tight thigh corset; for above-knee stumps a suction socket is available.

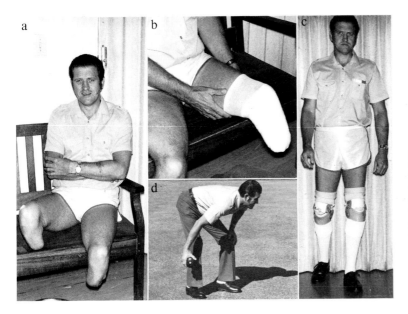

12.13 Amputations (3) – fitting the prosthesis (a) This man had severe congenital deformities which necessitated bilateral below-knee amputations. (b) A cast was made of each stump, and from this the stump socket will be fashioned and fitted into a prosthesis. (c) The prosthesis (held on in this case by straps above the knee) is called 'patellar-tendon-bearing', but most of the weight is taken on the femoral condyles. (d) After rehabilitation he has excellent balance and resumes a near-normal life.

Complications of amputation stumps

Early complications

In addition to the complications of any operation (especially secondary haemorrhage from infection), there are two special hazards.

(1) *Breakdown of skin flaps*   This may be due to ischaemia, to suturing under excessive tension or (in below-knee amputations) to an unduly long tibia pressing against the flap.

(2) *Gas gangrene*   *Clostridia* and spores from the perineum may infect a high above-knee amputation (or re-amputation), especially if performed through ischaemic tissue.

Late complications

SKIN   Eczema is common, and tender purulent lumps may develop in the groin. A rest from the prosthesis is indicated.

Ulceration is usually due to poor circulation, and re-amputation at a higher level is then necessary. If, however, the circulation is satisfactory and the skin around an ulcer is healthy, it may be sufficient merely to excise 2.5 cm of bone and resuture.

MUSCLE   If too much muscle is left at the end of the stump, the resulting unstable 'cushion' induces a feeling of insecurity which may prevent proper use of a prosthesis; if so, the excess soft tissue must be excised.

ARTERY   Poor circulation gives a cold, blue stump which is liable to ulcerate. This problem chiefly arises with below-knee amputations and often re-amputation is necessary.

NERVE   A cut nerve always forms a bulb and occasionally this is painful and tender. The treatment is to excise 3 cm of the nerve well above the nerve bulb.

'Phantom limb' is the term used to describe the feeling that the amputated limb is still present. The patient should be warned of the possibility; eventually the feeling recedes or disappears.

A painful phantom limb is very difficult to treat. Intermittent percussion to the end of the stump has been recommended both for phantom limb and for painful nerve bulb; it sounds brutal but success is claimed.

JOINT   The joint above an amputation may be stiff or deformed. A common deformity is fixed flexion and fixed abduction at the hip in above-knee stumps (because the adductors and hamstring muscles have been divided). It should be avoided by exercises. If it becomes established, subtrochanteric osteotomy may be necessary. Fixed flexion at the knee makes it difficult to walk properly and should also be avoided.

BONE   A spur often forms at the end of the bone, but is usually painless. If there has been infection, however, the spur may be large and painful and it may be necessary to excise the end of the bone with the spur.

If the bone is transmitting little weight it becomes osteoporotic and liable to fracture. Such fractures are best treated by internal fixation.

Implant materials

Metal

Metal used in implants (screws, plates, prostheses) should be tough, strong, non-corrodable, biologically inert and easily sterilizable. Those commonly used are stainless steel, cobalt-chromium alloys and titanium alloys.

No one material is ideal for all purposes. Stainless steel, because of its relative plasticity, can be cold worked; not only is it easier to manufacture such implants, but cold working is a way of hardening and strengthening the material. Moreover, its tensile plasticity (ductility) makes it possible to bend stainless steel plates to required shapes during an operation without seriously disturbing their strength.

Cobalt-based alloys (Vitallium, Vinertia) must be cast or wrought. The implants are therefore difficult to manufacture, but they are stronger, more rigid and less liable to corrosion than steel.

Titanium alloys can be worked and shaped like steel, and are corrosion-resistant; however, in metal-on-metal prostheses they are liable to adhesive wear and sludge formation.

IMPLANT FAILURE   Metal implants may not be strong enough to resist local bending forces, and fatigue fractures of plates and screws are common. In some cases, though, even strong implants fail because they are wrongly placed or inadequately fixed and cannot withstand repetitive bending movement; if used to treat a fracture, protection may be needed until the bone has joined (see page 345).

CORROSION   Corrosion is rarely a problem except with plates and screws, where it may be initiated by abrasive damage to polished oxide surfaces, or minute surface cracks due to fatigue failure. Crevice corrosion weakens the metal ('stress corrosion cracking') and may cause a local inflammatory reaction and osteoclastic bone resorption; the result is breakage or loosening of the implant.

DISSIMILAR METALS   Dissimilar metals immersed in solution in contact with one another may set up galvanic corrosion with accelerated destruction of the more reactive (or 'base') metal. In the early days of implant surgery when highly corrodible metals were used, the same thing happened in the

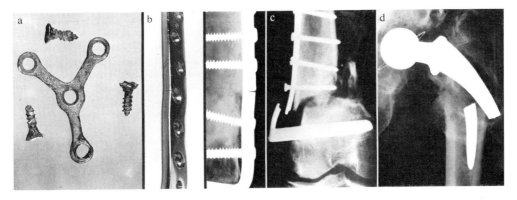

12.14 Implant failure (a) An ancient metal implant, showing corrosion of the plate and screws; (b) the tiny defect in this plate, due to stress corrosion cracking, is just visible in the x-ray; (c) complete implant failure; (d) the implant is not necessarily to blame – this man was being taken home after a small celebration; he alighted from the car, unhappily without waiting for it to stop.

body. However, the passive alloys now used for implants do not exhibit this phenomenon (titanium being particularly resistant to chemical attack), and the traditional fear of using dissimilar metals in bone implants is probably exaggerated.

FRICTION AND WEAR The coefficient of friction is constant for any two surfaces regardless of their size. However, shape has a marked influence on this property. In a ball-and-socket joint the frictional moment is related to the degree of congruity and the size of the ball (the larger the ball, the greater the frictional resistance). The type of material also is important; metal-on-metal causes adhesive wear ('seizing'), whereas metal-on-plastic has a low coefficient of friction and is therefore better for joint replacements. Metal wear particles may cause local inflammation and scarring, and occasionally a toxic or allergic reaction.

INFECTION Metal does not cause infection, but implants may encourage the persistence of infection by impeding drainage (e.g. in screw tracks).

High-density polyethylene

High-density polyethylene (HDPE) is an inert thermoplastic polymer modified to provide increased strength and wear resistance. In contact with polished metal it has a low coefficient of friction and it therefore seemed ideal for joint replacement. This has proved to be true in hip reconstruction with a simple ball-and-socket articulation. However, it has one major disadvantage – a tendency to viscoelastic deformity (stretching) and creep; this occurs particularly at the knee,

probably because of its complex and demanding load characteristics. HDPE is also easily abraded, and hard chips of bone or acrylic cement trapped on its surface cause it to disintegrate.

Silicon compounds

There is a wide variety of silicon polymers, of which silicone rubber (Silastic) is particularly useful. It is firm, tough, flexible and inert, and is used to make hinges for replacing finger and toe joints; and for spacers to replace resected bone (e.g. the head of the radius or the trapezium). Silastic wears well but may fracture if the implant surface is nicked or torn by a sharp instrument or piece of bone.

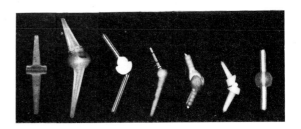

12.15 Implants Many of the implants used to replace finger joints are made partly or wholly of Silastic. A small sample of the models available is illustrated – reading from left to right: Swanson, Nicolle, Devas, St Georg, Mathys, ICLH, Helal universal.

Ceramics

Ceramic materials are being used, either alone or bonded to metal, for joint replacement prostheses. They are hard and strong, and porous ceramic implants could allow bone in-growth as a means of fixation; but they are also brittle and have not found wide acceptance.

Carbon

This eminently biocompatible material is looking for a purpose. As graphite it has wear and lubricant properties that might fit it for joint replacement. As carbon fibre it is being used to replace ligaments (e.g. cruciate ligaments); it induces the formation of longitudinally aligned fibrous tissue. Its ultimate fate is not yet known.

Acrylic cement

In joint replacements the prostheses are fixed to the bone with acrylic cement (polymethylmethacrylate), which acts as a grouting material. It is applied to the bone as a partially polymerized dough, in which the prosthesis is embedded. With sufficient pressure the pasty material is forced into the bony interstices and, when fully polymerized, the hard compound prevents all movement between prosthesis and bone. It can withstand large compressive loads but is easily broken by tensile stress.

When the partially polymerized cement is forced into the bone there is often a drop in blood pressure, which occasionally can be alarming and may even result in death. This is attributed to the uptake of residual monomer, which can cause peripheral vasodilatation.

Late complications with acrylic cement are fairly common. With time a fibrous layer forms at the cement/bone interface, its thickness depending on the degree of cement penetration into the bone crevices. In this flimsy membrane fine granulation tissue and foreign body giant cells can be seen. This relatively quiescent tissue remains unchanged under a wide range of biological and mechanical conditions, but if there is excessive movement at the cement/bone interface an aggressive reaction produces bone resorption and disintegration of the interlocking surfaces. This type of loosening may result from purely mechanical causes (inadequate cementing technique, poor prosthetic design or malposition of the prosthesis), but often it is associated with low-grade infection which can manifest for the first time 5 or 10 years after the operation; whether the infection in these cases precedes the loosening or *vice versa* is still not known for certain.

Further reading

Campbell, W. C. (1980) *Operative Orthopaedics*, 6th edn. London: Kimpton

Charnley, J. (1970) *Acrylic Cement in Orthopaedic Surgery*. Edinburgh and London: Churchill Livingstone

Gordon-Taylor, G., Wiles, P., Patey, D. H., Turner-Warwick, W. and Monro, R. S. (1952) The inter-innomino-abdominal operation. *Journal of Bone and Joint Surgery* **34B**, 14–21

Imamaliev, A. S. (1969) The preparation, preservation and transplantation of articular bone ends. In *Recent Advances in Orthopaedics*. Ed. by A. Graham Apley. London: Churchill

Klenerman, L. (1980) Tourniquet time—how long? *The Hand* **12**, 231–234

Mears, D. C. (1979) *Materials in Orthopedic Surgery*. Baltimore: Williams & Wilkins

Menelaus, M. B. (1966) Correction of leg length discrepancy by epiphyseal arrest. *Journal of Bone and Joint Surgery* **48B**, 336–339

Merle d'Aubigné, R. and Dubousset, J. (1971) Surgical correction of large length discrepancies in the lower extremities of children and adults. *Journal of Bone and Joint Surgery* **53A**, 411–430

O'Brien, B. McC. (1977) *Microvascular Reconstructive Surgery*. Edinburgh: Churchill Livingstone

Perkins, G. (1961) *Orthopaedics*. London: Athlone Press

Robinson, K. P. (1976) Amputations of the lower limb. *British Journal of Hospital Medicine* **16**, 629–637

Symposium on limb ablation and limb replacement (1967) *Annals of the Royal College of Surgeons of England* **40**, 203–288

Part 2 — Regional Orthopaedics

The Shoulder Joint

13

Examination

Symptoms

PAIN is felt anterolaterally, along the edge of the acromion, and at the insertion of the deltoid; sometimes it radiates down the arm. Pain on top of the shoulder suggests acromioclavicular dysfunction. The entire shoulder is a common site of *referred pain* from the cervical spine, heart, mediastinum and diaphragm. Cardiac ischaemia may cause localized pain in either shoulder.

STIFFNESS may be progressive and severe – so much so as to merit the term 'frozen shoulder'.

DEFORMITY may consist of prominence of the acromioclavicular joint or winging of the scapula.

LOSS OF FUNCTION is expressed as inability to reach behind the back and difficulty with combing the hair or dressing.

Signs

The patient should always be examined from in front *and from behind*. The entire upper limb, neck and chest must be included.

● LOOK

Skin Scars or sinuses are noted; don't forget the axilla!

Shape Asymmetry of the shoulders, winging of the scapula, wasting of the deltoid or short rotators and acromioclavicular dislocation are best seen from the back; joint swelling or wasting of the pectoral muscles is more obvious from in front. A joint effusion may 'point' in the axilla.

Position If the arm is held internally rotated, think of posterior dislocation of the shoulder.

● FEEL

Skin Because the joint is well covered, inflammation rarely influences skin temperature.

Soft tissues The tendons around the joint should each be palpated in turn; tenderness and crepitus should, if possible, be accurately localized. Fluid and synovial thickening are not easily detectable.

Bony points The clavicle, acromion process, acromioclavicular joint and humeral head are systematically palpated. Tenderness is sometimes difficult to localize.

● MOVE

Active movements The patient is asked to raise his arms sideways until the fingers point to the ceiling. Abduction may be (1) difficult to initiate; (2) diminished in range; (3) altered in rhythm, the scapula moving too early and creating a shrugging effect. If movement is painful, the arc of pain must be noted: pain on initiating abduction suggests a supraspinatus tear; pain in the mid-range of abduction suggests subacromial bursitis; and pain at the end of abduction is often due to acromioclavicular arthritis.

Flexion and extension are examined, asking the patient to raise his arms forwards and then backwards. To test adduction he is asked to move the arm across the front of his body. Rotation is tested in two ways: first, with the arms close to the body and the elbows flexed to 90 degrees, the

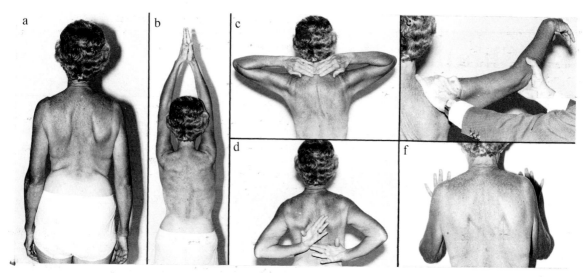

13.1 Examination Small alterations in scapulothoracic and glenohumeral rhythm are best seen from behind. (a) Symmetry of the neck, shoulders and scapulae is assessed. (b) Full abduction (or 'circumduction'), a combination of scapular and glenohumeral movements. (c) Abduction and external rotation. (d) Adduction and internal rotation (slightly limited on the right). (e) True glenohumeral movement is gauged by pressing down firmly on the scapula to stop scapulothoracic movement. (f) When the patient presses against a wall the scapula should remain flat; if serratus anterior is weak it stands out prominently ('winging').

hands are separated as widely as possible (external rotation) and brought together again across the body (internal rotation); then the patient is asked to clasp his fingers behind his neck (external rotation in abduction) and then to lower his arms and reach up his back with his fingers (internal rotation in adduction).

Passive movements With a complete tear of the supraspinatus tendon, active abduction is grossly limited but passive abduction may be full. However, passive movements can be deceptive because even with a stiff shoulder the arm can be raised to 90 degrees by scapulothoracic rotation. To test true glenohumeral abduction the scapula must first be firmly anchored; this is done by the examiner pressing firmly down on the acromion with one hand while the other hand moves the patient's arm.

Power The deltoid is examined for bulk and tautness while the patient abducts against resistance. To test serratus anterior (long thoracic nerve, C5, 6, 7) the patient is asked to push forcefully against the wall with both hands; if the

muscle is weak, the scapula is not stabilized on the thorax and stands out prominently (winged scapula). Pectoralis major is tested by having the patient thrust both hands firmly into the waist.

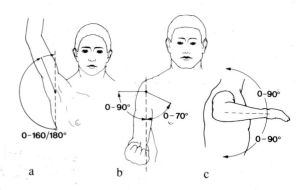

13.2 Normal range of movement (a) Abduction is from 0 to 160 (or even 180) degrees, but only 90 degrees of this takes place at the glenohumeral joint (in the plane of the scapula, 20 degrees anterior to the coronal plane); the remainder is scapular movement. (b) External rotation is usually almost 90 degrees, but internal is rather less because the trunk gets in the way. (c) With the arm abducted to a right angle internal rotation can be assessed without the trunk getting in the way.

X-RAY
At least two views should be obtained: an antero-posterior in the plane of the shoulder, and an axillary projection with the arm in abduction. The acromioclavicular joint is best shown by an anteroposterior projection with the tube tilted upwards 20–30 degrees.

Scapular disorders

Congenital undescended scapula (Sprengel's shoulder)

The scapulae normally complete their descent from the neck by the third month of fetal life; occasionally one remains unduly high. Associated deformities of the cervical spine are common and sometimes there is a family history of scapular deformity.

Deformity is the only symptom and may be noticed at birth. The shoulder on the affected side is elevated; the scapula looks and feels abnormally high, smaller than usual and somewhat prominent. Occasionally both scapulae are affected. Movements are painless but abduction may be somewhat limited by fixation of the scapula. Associated deformities such as fusion of cervical vertebrae, kyphosis or scoliosis may be present. X-rays may show such anomalies, and sometimes a bony bridge between the scapula and the cervical spine (the omovertebral bar).

In the *Klippel–Feil syndrome* there is bilateral failure of scapular descent associated with marked anomalies of the cervical spine and failure of fusion of the occipital bones. The patient looks as if he has no neck; there is a low hairline, bilateral neck webbing, and gross limitation of neck movement. (This condition should not be confused with *bilateral shortness of the sternomastoid muscle*, in which the head is poked forward and the chin thrust up; the absence of associated congenital lesions is a further distinguishing feature.)

Treatment

Mild cases are best left untreated. Marked limitation of abduction or severe deformity may necessitate operation. Excision of the omovertebral bone (when it is present) and the supraspinous part of the scapula improves both the appearance and shoulder function. The alternative is a vertical osteotomy, pulling the lateral portion downwards, then reattaching it to the rest of the scapula.

Winged scapula

Winging of the scapula causes asymmetry of the shoulders, but may not be obvious until the patient tries to contract the serratus anterior against resistance. Weakness or paralysis of the serratus anterior may arise from (1) lesions of the fifth, sixth and seventh cervical nerve roots (injury or viral neuropathy), (2) injury to the brachial plexus (a blow to the top of the shoulder, severe traction on the arm or carrying heavy loads on the shoulder), (3) direct damage to the long thoracic nerve (e.g. during radical mastectomy), and (4) in the girdle type of muscular dystrophy.

Disability is usually slight and is best accepted. However, if function is noticeably impaired, it is possible to stabilize the scapula by transferring the sternal portion of pectoralis major and attaching it via a fascia lata graft to the lower pole of the scapula; or the scapula can be fixed to the rib cage.

Grating scapula

The patient complains of grating or clicking on moving the arm. It is painless but annoying. The cause is unknown, though bony, muscular and bursal abnormalities have been blamed. No treatment is necessary.

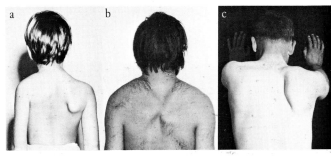

13.3 Scapular disorders (a) Sprengel shoulder; (b) Klippel–Feil syndrome; (c) winged scapula.

Rotator cuff lesions

The coraco-acromial arch consists of the acromion process posterosuperiorly, the coracoid process anteriorly and the tough coraco-acromial ligament joining them. It forms a canopy over the shoulder, beneath which run the tendons of the rotator cuff, separated from the fibro-osseous arch by the subacromial bursa. It is in this complex that the painful rotator cuff lesions arise.

Pathology

The differing clinical pictures stem from three basic pathological processes – degeneration, trauma and vascular reaction.

Degeneration   With advancing age, the cuff (especially supraspinatus) degenerates; minute tears, fibrous scarring, fibrocartilaginous metaplasia or calcification develop. The common site is the 'critical zone' of the supraspinatus, the relatively avascular region near its insertion.

Trauma   The supraspinatus tendon is liable to injury if its contraction is resisted; this may occur when lifting a weight, or when the patient uses his arm to save himself from falling. It is difficult to injure the cuff unless it is already degenerate; and the more degenerate it is the more easily it tears. An insidious type of trauma is attrition of the cuff due to impingement against the coraco-acromial arch during abduction/adduction movements. The long head of biceps also may be abraded to the point of rupture. Tears of the cuff or the long head of biceps are found at autopsy in almost everyone aged over 60.

Reaction   In an attempt to repair a torn tendon or to revascularize a degenerate area, new blood vessels grow in; calcium deposits, if they are present, are phagocytosed (Uthoff and Sarkar, 1978). This vascular reaction causes pain.

WEAR, TEAR AND REPAIR   The three pathological processes may be summed up as 'wear', 'tear' and 'repair'. In the young patient 'repair' is vigorous; consequently, healing is relatively rapid but (because the repair process itself causes pain) it is accompanied by considerable distress. The older patient has more 'wear' but less vigorous 'repair'; healing will be slower but pain less severe. Thus acute tendinitis (which affects younger patients) is intensely painful but rapidly better; chronic tendinitis (a middle group) is only moderately painful but takes many months to recover and may be complicated by partial tears or by a frozen shoulder; and a complete tear (which usually occurs in the elderly) becomes painless soon after injury, but never mends.

THE VICIOUS SPIRAL   Mild lesions presumably heal spontaneously. Chronic tendinitis may, however, lead to progressive fraying, disruption of the cuff, and upward migration of the humeral head. Abnormal movement predisposes to osteoarthritis of the acromioclavicular joint, and sometimes of the glenohumeral joint as well.

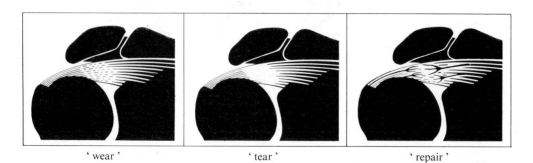

    ' wear '   ' tear '   ' repair '

13.4 The pathology of rotator cuff lesions

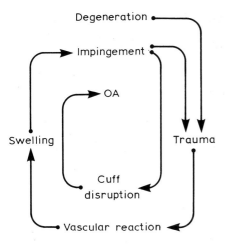

The vicious spiral of rotator cuff lesions.

Calcification itself causes little or no pain; symptoms, when they occur, are due to the florid vascular reaction which produces swelling and tension in the tendon. Resorption of the calcific material is rapid and it may soften or disappear entirely within a few weeks.

Clinical features

A young adult (usually aged 25–45, but occasionally older) complains of dull aching, sometimes following overuse. Hourly the pain increases in severity, rising to an agonizing climax. After a few days pain subsides and the shoulder gradually returns to normal. In some patients the process is less dramatic and recovery slower. During the acute stage the arm is held immobile; the joint is usually too tender to permit palpation or movement.

X-RAY Calcification just above the greater tuberosity is always present. As pain subsides the dense blotch gradually disappears.

(1) Acute tendinitis (acute calcification)

Deposits of calcium hydroxyapatite appear in the 'critical zone' of the supraspinatus tendon. The cause is unknown but it is thought that ischaemia causes the tendon to become fibrocartilaginous, and then hydroxyapatite crystals are actively shed by the chondrocytes (Uthoff and Sarkar, 1978).

Treatment

If symptoms are not very severe the arm is rested in a sling and the patient is given a short course of phenylbutazone or indomethacin. Spontaneous recovery usually ocurs within a few days and full shoulder movements return.

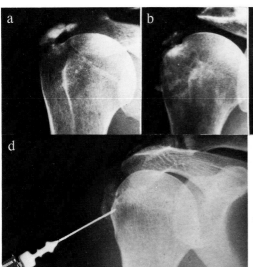

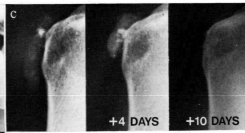

13.5 Acute calcification of supraspinatus (a) Dense mass in the tendon. (b) Following the 'reaction' some calcium has escaped into the sub-deltoid bursa; (c) spontaneous dispersal. (d) An attempt at treatment by aspiration; this procedure is much more likely to succeed if image-intensification and television control are used.

If pain is more intense a single injection of corticosteroid (methylprednisolone 40 mg) and local anaesthetic (lignocaine 1%) is given into the hypervascular area. If this is not rapidly effective, or if symptoms soon recur, relief can be obtained by operation. Through a small vertical incision just below the acromion process the deltoid fibres are separated and, on rotating the humerus, the affected area of tendon is seen. The calcific material is scooped out.

(2) Chronic tendinitis (the painful arc syndrome)

Various disorders (overuse, coraco-acromial arch impingement, minor tears or chronic calcification) may trigger a vascular response in the cuff. Swelling, though slight, may be enough to impede tendon movement between the humerus and the coraco-acromial arch.

Clinical features

The patient, usually aged 40–60 years, complains of pain in the shoulder and over the deltoid muscle. It is characteristically worse at night and may be quite severe on attempting certain activities such as putting on a jacket.

The shoulder looks normal but is tender along the edge of the acromion and anteriorly in the space between the acromion and the coracoid process. On abduction, pain is aggravated as the arm traverses an arc between 60 and 120 degrees. Often the patient negotiates this painful arc by dipping the shoulder and externally rotating the arm to allow the tendon to clear the coraco-acromial arch; beyond this point, compression of the swollen tendon is less and further abduction is painless. In long-standing cases and in those associated with a partial tear, there is also loss of power and abnormal scapulohumeral rhythm.

LOCATING THE LESION Kessel and Watson (1977) have pointed out that in one-third of patients the lesion is in the posterior part of the cuff, in one-third it is anterior (in the subscapularis) and in the remaining one-third it is in the supraspinatus. As the prognosis for the three groups differs significantly, it is important to identify the site of the lesion. Careful palpation and passive movement of the shoulder with the arm in varying degrees of rotation may pinpoint the tender spot. Confirmation is obtained by injecting the site with lignocaine, which should abolish the pain.

X-RAY There may be obvious calcification just above the greater tuberosity – a legacy of former events. In other respects the x-ray is usually normal at first; later slight erosion of the greater

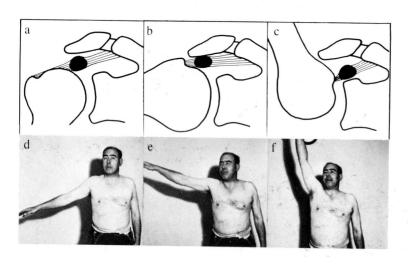

13.6 Painful arc (a–f) The patient registers pain only over a limited arc of abduction, and the diagrams show why. The middle diagram (b) explains the term 'impingement' syndrome.

tuberosity at the insertion of the rotator cuff may be seen; and in long-standing cases with cuff disruption there may be some upward luxation of the humeral head. Osteoarthritis of the acromio-clavicular joint is not uncommon. Contrast arthrography may be useful to demonstrate a cuff rupture.

NOTE: ACROMIOCLAVICULAR OSTEOARTH-RITIS This is often associated with chronic tendinitis and may be confused with it. The joint feels thick and tender; abduction is painful during the final 60 degrees. X-ray shows sclerosis and lipping. Heat and injections may help; if not, the outer end of the clavicle can be excised.

Treatment

Some patients improve with a short course of high-dosage anti-inflammatory therapy. If this fails, local injection of an anti-inflammatory 'cocktail' (a mixture of 40 mg (2 ml) methylpred-nisolone, 1 ml dilute (0.02%) nitrogen mustard and 2 ml 1% lignocaine) is tried. Anterior and posterior lesions usually respond to conservative measures; the supraspinatus lesions are more refractory.

If symptoms recur every few months, operation is advisable. Through an anterior incision the deltoid is split in the line of its fibres and part of the muscle is detached from the acromion to reveal the coraco-acromial ligament. A wedge of bone consisting of the anterior lip and undersurface of the acromion is removed together with the attached coraco-acromial ligament (Neer, 1972). This exposes the anterosuperior part of the cuff, and a tear can be repaired at the same time. If greater access is required, and especially if the acromioclavicular joint is osteoarthritic, the outer end of the clavicle is excised. Care is taken afterwards to reattach the deltoid firmly to the edge of the acromion.

(3) Adhesive capsulitis (frozen shoulder)

The process probably starts in the same way as a chronic tendinitis but it spreads to involve the entire tendinous cuff. This becomes thick, vascular and infiltrated with lymphocytes and plasma cells; it sticks to the humeral head and the infra-articular 'gusset' of capsule and synovium may be obliterated by adhesions. It has been suggested that this is an autoimmune response to the products of local tissue breakdown.

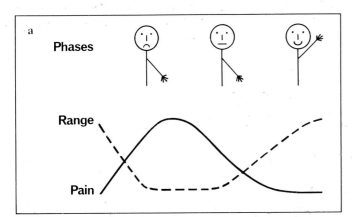

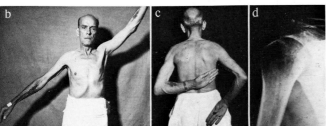

13.7 Frozen shoulder (a) Natural history of frozen shoulder. The face tells the story.

(b, c, d) Patient in phase 2: limited abduction (b); limited internal rotation (c); localized rarefaction (d).

Clinical features

The patient, aged 40–60, may give a history of trauma, often trivial, followed by pain and stiffness. The pain is felt at the deltoid insertion and radiates along the outer side of the arm to the back of the forearm and hand. Gradually it increases in severity and often prevents sleeping on the affected side. After several months it slowly subsides. Stiffness also increases in severity over the months and becomes more and more of a handicap, continuing after pain has disappeared. Gradually movement is regained, but it may not return to normal. There are thus three phases, each lasting 4–8 months: (1) increasing pain and increasing stiffness; (2) decreasing pain with persistent stiffness; (3) painless return of movement.

Usually there is nothing to see, except perhaps slight wasting; there may also be some tenderness. But movements are always limited. In a severe case the arm is held in internal rotation and movements are grossly restricted in all directions; with recovery the range slowly increases. In the mildest case there may be only slight restriction of mobility; between these extremes all grades of stiffness are seen.

X-RAY Bone density is usually decreased in the region of the greater tuberosity. Contrast arthrography shows a contracted joint.

Differential diagnosis

POST-TRAUMATIC STIFFNESS After any severe shoulder injury, stiffness may persist for some months. The stiffness is maximal at the start and gradually lessens (unlike the pattern of a frozen shoulder), and x-rays may show a fracture of the humerus or scapula.

POST-INACTIVITY STIFFNESS If the arm is nursed overcautiously (e.g. following a forearm fracture) the shoulder may stiffen. Again, the characteristic pain pattern of a frozen shoulder is absent.

REFLEX SYMPATHETIC DYSTROPHY Shoulder pain and stiffness, with fixed adduction and internal rotation deformities, may follow myocardial infarction or a stroke. The features are similar to those of a frozen shoulder (it has been suggested that the frozen shoulder syndrome may be a mild form of reflex sympathetic dystrophy). In severe cases the whole upper limb is involved, with trophic and vasomotor changes in the hand (the 'shoulder–hand syndrome').

TUBERCULOSIS Tuberculosis, like frozen shoulder, has a long history of ache and stiffness, but wasting is much more marked and x-rays show bone destruction. Caries sicca ('dry tuberculosis') is said to enjoy a good prognosis; this is readily explicable if the diagnosis is erroneously attached to cases of frozen shoulder.

Treatment

Conservative treatment aims at relieving pain and preventing further stiffening while recovery is awaited. It is important not only to administer analgesics and anti-inflammatory drugs but also to reassure the patient that recovery is certain.

Heat sometimes helps, though often ice-packs are more soothing. Exercises are encouraged, the most valuable being 'pendulum' exercises in which the patient leans forward at the hips and moves his arm as if stirring a giant pudding (this is really a form of assisted active movement, the assistance being supplied by gravity). However, the patient is warned that moderation and regularity will achieve more than sporadic masochism. Injections of corticosteroid and local anaesthetic sometimes help.

Once acute pain has subsided, manipulation under anaesthesia often hastens recovery; methylprednisolone and lignocaine are injected, then external rotation is restored, and finally abduction is gently but firmly regained. Active exercises should recommence immediately afterwards. Alternatively, movement can be increased by distending the joint with a large volume (50–200 ml) of fluid. Arthrography demonstrates that distension or manipulation achieve their effect by rupturing the capsule.

Rotator cuff tears

Rotator cuff tears may occur as a complication of chronic tendinitis,* or without any prior warning in older individuals. Except in severe athletic injuries (and possibly even there!) degeneration is a prerequisite for a tear; with gross degeneration relatively slight trauma is enough to rupture the cuff.

Most tears occur, or at any rate start, in the supraspinatus tendon. They may be *partial* (usually disrupting only the deep surface of the tendon) or *complete* (a full-thickness rent, such that the joint communicates with the subacromial bursa). With a partial tear the intact tendon fibres provide continuity and allow vascular ingrowth and repair of the damaged area. With a complete tear there is little or no reaction and no repair; the proximal fibres may retract and become stuck down. Sometimes the intra-articular portion of the long head of biceps is also frayed or completely torn.

Clinical features

The patient is usually aged 45–65; the younger he is the more likely is the tear to be partial. While lifting a weight or protecting himself from falling he 'sprains' the shoulder. Pain is felt immediately, radiating from the deltoid insertion, and he is unable to lift the arm sideways.

Often the patient seeks no advice, or is given no effective treatment. If the tear is partial, he may (1) gradually recover fully; (2) partly recover, but with a persistent painful arc of abduction; or (3) gradually develop a frozen shoulder. If the tear is

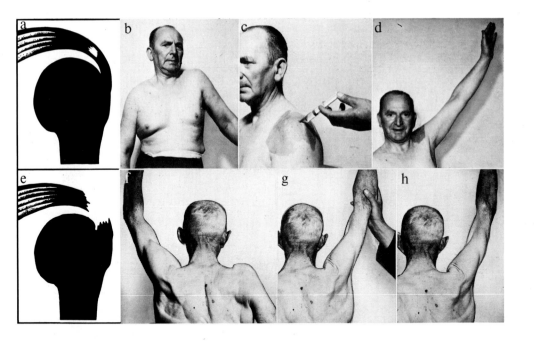

13.8 Torn supraspinatus (a–d) Partial tear of left supraspinatus: the patient can abduct actively once pain has been abolished with local anaesthetic.
(e–h) Complete tear of right supraspinatus: active abduction is impossible even when pain subsides (f), or has been abolished by injection; but once the arm is passively abducted (g), the patient can hold it up with his deltoid muscle (h).

*Refractory painful arc means the cuff is torn.

complete the pain soon subsides, but gross weakness of abduction persists; other movements return and frozen shoulder is never the sequel to a complete tear. Several years after a complete tear the power of abduction may apparently recover; possibly the teres minor hypertrophies and holds down the humeral head.

The appearance after a tear is usually normal, but in long-standing cases there may be supraspinatus wasting. Tenderness may be diffuse or may be localized to just below the tip of the acromion process.

With a recent injury, active abduction is grossly limited and painful; the scapulohumeral rhythm is reversed. Passive abduction also is limited or prevented by pain. These signs are common to both partial and complete tears; to distinguish between them, pain is abolished by injecting a local anaesthetic. If active abduction is now possible the tear must be only partial.

If some weeks have elapsed since the injury the two types are easily differentiated. With a complete tear pain has by then subsided and the clinical picture is unmistakable: active abduction is impossible and attempting it produces a characteristic shrug; but passive abduction is full and once the arm has been lifted above a right angle the patient can keep it up by using his deltoid (the 'abduction paradox'); when he lowers it sideways it suddenly drops (the 'drop arm sign').

X-rays

The presence and extent of the tear can be demonstrated by arthrography. With old tears the humeral head rides upwards in the glenoid.

Treatment

IN THE ACUTE PHASE   treatment is conservative (and in any case it is difficult to tell at that stage whether the tear is partial or complete). It consists of (1) heat, which is soothing; (2) exercises; and (3) one or two injections of local anaesthetic into the tender area.

AFTER 3 WEEKS   it is usually possible to assess the extent of the rupture. *Complete tears*, especially those in younger, active individuals, should be repaired; and the earlier the better, so as to avoid

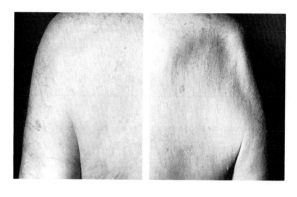

13.9 Rotator cuff tear   Some years after a tear on the right the patient regained a full range of active movement, but abduction was still weaker than normal and the muscles are wasted compared with those on the left.

retraction and fibrous adhesions. Good exposure of the cuff is obtained by the approach described earlier. Operation is contraindicated in old or sedentary individuals, and in long-standing cases that are painless. If the tendon has retracted, a muscle advancement may allow closure of the gap but the results are generally poor. If the intracapsular part of the biceps is torn it should be excised. *Partial tears* do not require operation.

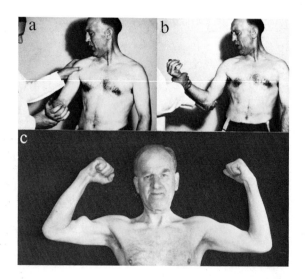

13.10 Biceps tendon   Tendinitis: localized tenderness (a), and pain on flexion against resistance (b).
(c) Ruptured long head of right biceps: compared with the normal side, the belly of biceps is lower and rounder.

Lesions of the biceps tendon

Tendinitis

Primary biceps tendinitis   may follow unaccustomed use, such as home decorating or vigorous tennis, in patients aged 30–40 years. The shoulder is normal except for pain on external rotation and tenderness in the bicipital groove. Rest and local heat are usually sufficient treatment, but if recovery is delayed local anaesthetic injections or deep transverse frictions to the tender area are useful.

Secondary tendinitis   occurs in cuff lesions when the reaction to degeneration spreads to the biceps. Signs of biceps tendinitis are added to those of the underlying lesion, and both conditions may require treatment.

Ruptured biceps tendon

It used to be thought that the tendon of the long head of the biceps ruptured because it rubbed against osteophytes in an osteoarthritic shoulder. Most orthopaedic surgeons now agree that it is simply a tear through an area of avascular degeneration, comparable to that occurring in the supraspinatus tendon.

The patient is always aged over 50. While lifting he feels something snap and the shoulder, which previously felt normal, aches for a time. Soon his ache disappears and good function returns. The clinical picture is unmistakable. The belly of the muscle is too low; and when in action it does not tauten properly and looks semi-circular instead of semi-oval. Shoulder movements are normal and no treatment is required. Occasionally the biceps insertion is avulsed; the muscle belly then retracts to a more proximal position.

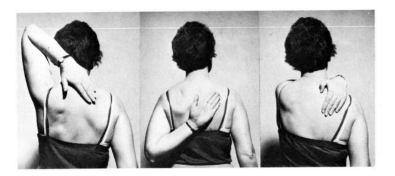

13.11 'Brachial neuralgia' – the scratch test   'Shoulder' pain may be due to disorders proximal to the joint (e.g. cervical spondylosis or cardiac ischaemia), disorders distal to the joint (e.g. arthritis of the elbow or carpal tunnel syndrome), or disorders of the shoulder itself (e.g. the rotator cuff syndromes, glenohumeral arthritis, acromioclavicular arthritis or bone disease). If the patient can scratch the opposite scapula in these three ways, the shoulder joint and its tendons are unlikely to be at fault.

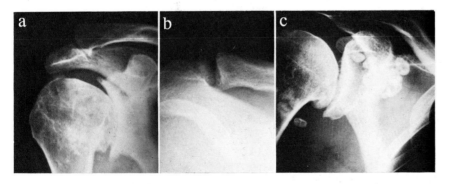

13.12   (a) Osteoarthritis of the glenohumeral joint, which is less common than (b) osteoarthritis of the acromioclavicular joint. (c) Synovial osteochondromatosis.

Tuberculosis of the shoulder
(see also page 28)

Tuberculosis of the shoulder is uncommon. It usually starts as an osteitis but is rarely diagnosed until arthritis has supervened. This may proceed to abscess and sinus formation, but in some cases the tendency is to fibrosis and ankylosis. If there is no exudate the term 'caries sicca' is used; however, one suspects that many such cases, formerly diagnosed on the basis of coexisting pulmonary tuberculosis rather than joint biopsy or bacteriological examination, are actually examples of frozen shoulder.

Symptoms and signs

Adults are mainly affected. They complain of a constant ache and stiffness lasting many months or years. The striking feature is wasting of the muscles around the shoulder, especially the deltoid. In neglected cases a sinus may be present over the shoulder or in the axilla. There is diffuse warmth and tenderness, and all movements are limited and painful. Axillary lymph nodes may be enlarged.

X-RAY   Generalized rarefaction is present, usually with some erosion of the joint surfaces. There may be abscess cavities in the humerus or glenoid, with little or no periosteal reaction.

Treatment

In addition to general treatment (page 28), the shoulder should be rested on an abduction splint until acute symptoms have settled (about 6 weeks). Thereafter movement is encouraged, and, provided the articular cartilage is not destroyed, the prognosis for painless function is good. If these measures fail, or in neglected cases, a clearance operation may be required (page 31). If there are repeated flares, or if the articular surfaces are extensively destroyed, the joint should be arthrodesed.

Rheumatoid arthritis
(see also page 35)

The acromioclavicular joint, the shoulder joint and the various synovial pouches around the shoulder are frequently involved in rheumatoid disease.

The acromioclavicular joint develops an erosive arthritis which may go on to capsular disruption and instability.

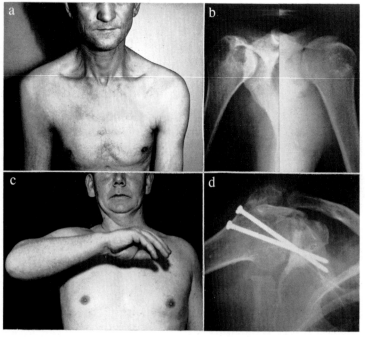

13.13 Tuberculosis   (a) Marked wasting of right deltoid. (b) Bone rarefaction and joint damage in arthritis, compared with the normal.

(c, d) After arthrodesis of the glenohumeral joint scapulothoracic movement remains, permitting useful abduction.

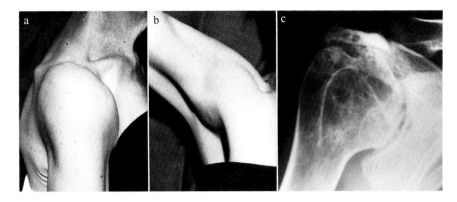

13.14 Rheumatoid arthritis   (a) Large synovial effusions cause easily visible swelling; small ones are likely to be missed – especially if they present, like this one (b), in the axilla. (c) X-rays show erosion of the joint and of the periarticular bone.

The glenohumeral joint, with its lax capsule and folds of synovium, shows marked soft-tissue inflammation. Often there is an accumulation of fluid and fibrinoid particles which may rupture the capsule and extrude into the muscle planes. Cartilage destruction and bone erosion are often severe.

The subacromial bursa and the synovial sheath of the long head of biceps become inflamed and thickened; often this leads to rupture of the rotator cuff and the biceps tendon.

Symptoms and signs

The patient may be known to have generalized rheumatoid arthritis; occasionally, however, acromioclavicular erosion discovered on an x-ray of the chest is the first clue to the diagnosis.

Pain and swelling are the usual presenting symptoms; the patient has increasing difficulty with simple tasks such as combing the hair or washing the back. Though it may start on one side, the condition usually becomes bilateral.

Synovitis of the joint results in swelling and tenderness anteriorly, superiorly or in the axilla.

Tenosynovitis produces features similar to those of cuff lesions, including tears of supraspinatus or biceps. Joint and tendon lesions usually occur together and conspire to cause the marked weakness and limitation of movement which are features of the disease.

X-ray changes are typical of rheumatoid arthritis; in addition, there may be superior subluxation of the humeral head due to complete disruption of the cuff.

Treatment

If general measures do not control the synovitis, a mixture of methylprednisolone and nitrogen mustard may be injected into the joint, the subacromial bursa and the bicipital tendon sheath; this should not be repeated more than two or three times. If synovitis persists, operative synovectomy is carried out; at the same time cuff tears may be repaired. Excision of the lateral end of the clavicle may relieve acromioclavicular pain.

In advanced cases pain and stiffness can be very disabling. Joint replacement is not very successful and alternative procedures are: (1) excision of the anterior part of the acromion and the coraco-acromial ligament (which relieves pain but does not improve mobility); (2) double osteotomy of the humeral neck and glenoid; and (3) arthrodesis of the shoulder (which, despite its apparent limitations, improves function considerably because scapulothoracic movement is usually undisturbed).

Arthrodesis of the shoulder

Apart from rheumatoid arthritis and tuberculosis, arthrodesis is indicated also for paralysis of the scapulohumeral muscles (but only if scapulothoracic movement is normal, because that is how the 'shoulder' will move after the operation). Through a posterior incision the joint is disarticulated, the surfaces are rawed, and it is then fixed by a heavy nail, or a screw or a plate. The acromion is osteotomized and hinged into a bed chiselled out of the humerus. The shoulder is held in a plaster spica for 3–6 months. The optimal position is abduction 50 degrees, flexion 25 degrees and internal rotation sufficient to allow the hand to reach the mouth.

Total replacement

Although uncertain in its results, total replacement is being tried for destructive conditions of the shoulder. A metal prosthesis is cemented into the humerus and a polyethylene socket is fixed to the scapula; because the bone around the glenoid fossa is thin, scapular fixation is somewhat insecure.

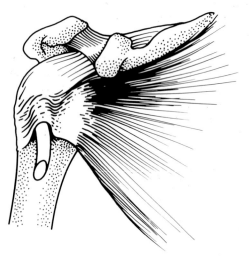

13.15 Anatomy   A tough ligament stretches from the coracoid to the acromion process; the humeral head moves beneath this arch during abduction and the rotator cuff may be irritated or damaged as it glides in this confined space.

Notes on applied anatomy

The anatomy of the shoulder is uniquely adapted to allow freedom of movement and maximum reach for the hand. Five 'articulations' are involved: (1) the true (synovial) glenohumeral joint, (2) the pseudojoint between the humerus and the coraco-acromial arch, (3) the sternoclavicular joint, (4) the acromioclavicular joint and (5) the scapulothoracic articulation.

The shallow glenohumeral joint has little inherent stability but strong muscle control makes up for this. The tendons of the short rotators – subscapularis in front, supraspinatus above, infraspinatus and teres minor behind – blend with the capsule of the shoulder to form the rotator cuff. During abduction these muscles draw the head of the humerus firmly into its socket while the deltoid elevates the arm. As abduction proceeds, the external rotators twist the arm so that the greater tuberosity clears the projecting acromion, and scapulothoracic movement permits further reach to 180 degrees. All these actions occur synchronously. The sternoclavicular joint participates in movements close to the trunk (e.g. shrugging or bracing the shoulders); the acromioclavicular joint moves in the last 60 degrees of abduction.

Further reading

Hensinger, R. N., Lang, J. E. and MacEwen, G. D. (1974) Klippel–Feil syndrome. *Journal of Bone and Joint Surgery* **56A,** 1246–1253
Kessel, L. and Watson, M. (1977) The painful arc syndrome. *Journal of Bone and Joint Surgery* **59B,** 166–172
McLaughlin, H. L. (1962) Rupture of the rotator cuff. (an Instructional Course Lecture) *Journal of Bone and Joint Surgery* **44A,** 979–983
MacNab, I. (1973) Rotator cuff tendinitis. *Annals of the Royal College of Surgeons of England* **53,** 271–287
Mosely, H. F. (1969) *Shoulder Lesions,* 3rd edn. Edinburgh: Livingstone
Neer, C. S. (1972) Anterior acromioplasty for the chronic impingement syndrome in the shoulder. *Journal of Bone and Joint Surgery* **54A,** 41–50
Richardson, A. T. (1975) The painful shoulder. *Proceedings of the Royal Society of Medicine* **68,** 731–736
Uthoff, H. K. and Sarkar, S. D. (1978) Calcifying tendinitis – its pathogenetic mechanism and rationale for its treatment. *International Orthopaedics* **2,** 187–194
Wolfgang, G. L. (1974) Surgical repair of tears of the rotator cuff of the shoulder. *Journal of Bone and Joint Surgery* **56A,** 14–26

The Elbow Joint 14

Examination

Symptoms

Pain sharply localized to the lateral condyle and worse on pronation is usually due to tennis elbow. Pain arising in the joint itself also is felt locally. *Referred pain* (from the neck or shoulder) is more diffuse.

Because of the close anatomical relationship *ulnar nerve symptoms* (tingling, numbness and weakness of the hand) are common in elbow disorders.

Stiffness, especially loss of extension, though also common, is not necessarily much of a disability. *Swelling* (from injury or inflammation) and *locking* (from a loose body) are occasional symptoms.

Signs

● LOOK
The patient holds his arms alongside his body with palms forwards. Varus or valgus deformity is then obvious, but it cannot be accurately assessed unless the elbow is straight. He then holds his arms out sideways at right angles to the body with palms upwards and elbows straight. In this position, wasting or lumps are easily seen.

● FEEL
The back of the joint is palpated for warmth, subcutaneous nodules, synovial thickening and fluid (fluctuation on each side of the olecranon); the back and sides are felt for tenderness (which should be located precisely) and to determine whether the bony points are correctly located.

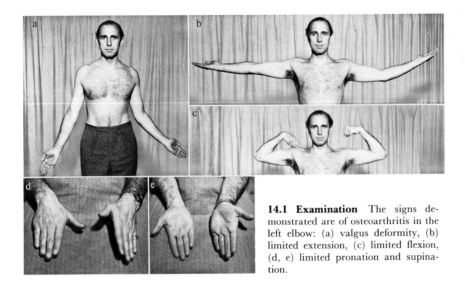

14.1 Examination The signs demonstrated are of osteoarthritis in the left elbow: (a) valgus deformity, (b) limited extension, (c) limited flexion, (d, e) limited pronation and supination.

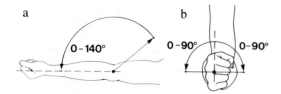

14.2 Normal range of movement   (a) The extended position is recorded as 0 degrees and any hyperextension as a minus quantity; flexion is full when the arm and forearm make contact. (b) From the neutral position the radioulnar joint rotates 90 degrees into pronation and 90 into supination.

- MOVE
Flexion and extension are compared on the two sides. Then, with the elbows tucked into the sides and flexed to a right angle, the radioulnar joints are tested for pronation and supination.

- X-RAY
The position of each bone is noted, then the joint line and space. Next, the individual bones are inspected for evidence of old injury or bone destruction. Finally, loose bodies are sought.

NOTE   Where appropriate, other parts are examined: the neck (for cervical disc lesions), the shoulder (for cuff lesions) and the hand (for nerve lesions).

Elbow deformities

Cubitus varus ('gun-stock' deformity)

The commonest cause is malunion of a supracondylar fracture. The deformity is obvious only when the elbow is extended, but it looks rather ugly and the hand brushes against the body in walking. The deformity can be corrected by a wedge osteotomy of the lower humerus, after which the arm is held in plaster in full extension and slight valgus; alternatively, internal fixation may be used.

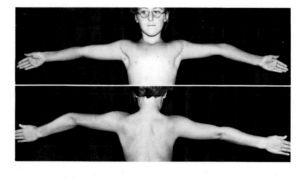

14.3 Cubitus varus   This ugly deformity, the sequel to a supracondylar fracture, was later corrected by osteotomy.

Cubitus valgus

The commonest cause is non-union of a fractured lateral condyle; this may give gross deformity and a bony knob on the inner side of the joint. The importance of valgus deformity is the liability for

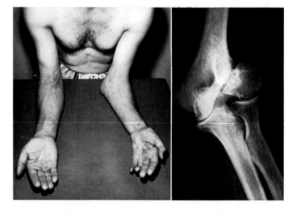

14.4 Cubitus valgus   This man's valgus deformity, the sequel to an un-united fracture of the lateral condyle, has resulted in ulnar nerve palsy.

delayed ulnar palsy to develop; years after the causal injury the patient notices weakness of the hand with numbness and tingling of the ulnar fingers. The deformity itself needs no treatment but for delayed ulnar palsy the nerve should be transposed to the front of the elbow.

Dislocated head of radius

Congenital dislocation of the radial head may be anterior or posterior and is usually bilateral. The patient may notice the lump, which is easily palpable and can be felt to move when the forearm is rotated. X-rays show that the dislocated head is dome-shaped. If the lump limits elbow flexion it can be excised (beware of the posterior interosseous nerve).

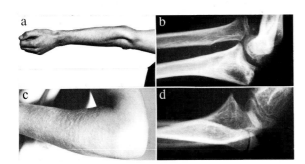

14.5 Dislocated head of radius   (a, b) Anterior dislocation, from an old Monteggia fracture; (c, d) posterior dislocation – the radial head is dome-shaped, suggesting that the dislocation was congenital.

Unilateral anterior dislocation may be acquired (if a Monteggia fracture-dislocation was left unreduced) and in time the head becomes dome-shaped. Open reduction and stabilization with a Kirschner wire is worth considering.

Congenital subluxation of the radial head, usually lateral, is commonly associated with a wide variety of bone dysplasias.

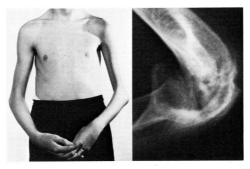

14.6 Tuberculosis of the elbow   Muscle wasting is marked and bone destruction extensive.

accompanied by pain and spasm. X-rays show generalized rarefaction, and often an apparent increase of joint space because of bone erosion. With healing a little movement returns, but the arm remains thin.

In addition to general treatment (page 28), the the elbow is rested. At first, it may be held in a plaster gutter flexed more acutely than a right angle and in mid-rotation. Later a removable polythene splint, or collar and cuff, is sufficient and even these are sometimes discarded. Healing is by fibrosis. The fibrous tissue gradually elongates because of the weight of the arm; hence the need to splint the elbow well above the right angle during the acute stage.

Tuberculosis
(see also page 28)

Although the disease begins as synovitis or osteomyelitis, tuberculosis of the elbow is rarely seen until arthritis supervenes, by which time complete resolution cannot occur. Because the elbow is a superficial joint, sinus formation is common.

The onset of symptoms is insidious and the patient gives a long history of aching and stiffness. The most striking physical sign is the marked wasting. While the disease is active the joint is held flexed, looks swollen, feels warm and diffusely tender; movement is considerably limited and

Rheumatoid arthritis
(see also page 35)

The elbow is involved in more than 50 per cent of patients with polyarticular rheumatoid arthritis. In the early stages the synovitis causes pain and tenderness, especially over the radiohumeral joint line. Later, the whole elbow may become swollen and stiff. If, however, bone destruction is severe, instability and capsular rupture are more frequent sequels. X-rays show bone erosion, with gradual destruction of the radial head and widening of the trochlear notch of the ulna. Sometimes large synovial extensions penetrate the articular surface and appear as cysts in the proximal radius or ulna.

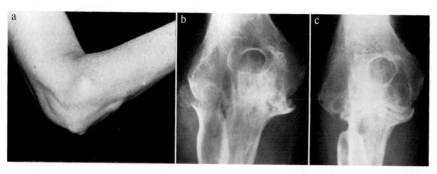

14.7 Rheumatoid arthritis   (a) This rheumatoid patient has nodules over the olecranon and a bulge over the radiohumeral joint; (b) his x-rays show deformity of the radial head and marked erosion of the rest of the elbow. (c) Excision of the radial head combined with synovectomy relieved the pain and the joint looks much healthier.

Treatment

In addition to general treatment, the elbow should be splinted during periods of active synovitis. For chronic, painful arthritis with x-ray signs of bone destruction, resection of the radial head and partial synovectomy from the lateral side gives good results. If the joint is completely unstable, long-term splintage may be preferable to the uncertain results of total joint replacement.

ARTHROPLASTY

Many methods have been tried; none has been very successful. Skin, fascia, Silastic or polyethylene interposed between the joint surfaces may allow a certain amount of painless movement, provided the patient accepts some loss of power and stability. Total replacement, with prostheses cemented to the humerus and ulna, often fails after a few years because of loosening, but may nevertheless be worth trying if disability is severe.

Osteoarthritis

Osteoarthritis may result from articular damage when the joint contains a loose body (especially with osteochondritis dissecans) or multiple loose bodies (synovial chondromatosis), or it may follow severe fractures.

The symptoms are slight. Until stiffness is considerable it often passes unnoticed. There is rarely much pain; occasionally the joint may lock. Symptoms of ulnar palsy may be the presenting feature. Apart from limited movement the signs are few: the joint may look and feel somewhat enlarged, but there is no wasting or tenderness. X-rays show diminution of the joint space with bone sclerosis and osteophytes; one or more loose bodies may be seen.

The osteoarthritis itself rarely requires treatment. Loose bodies, however, if they cause locking, should be removed; and if there are signs of ulnar neuritis, the nerve should be transposed.

Stiffness of the elbow

BOTH ELBOWS

The commonest cause of bilateral stiffness is rheumatoid arthritis; other causes include arthrogryposis and ankylosing spondylitis. If both elbows are completely stiff at impractical angles, disability is severe; arthroplasty or joint replacement, to enable at least one hand to reach the mouth, may be needed.

ONE ELBOW

Congenital synostosis of the superior radioulnar joint (with loss of rotation) is only moderately inconvenient, but if the humerus shares in the synostosis the disability is considerable; a more useful angle can be achieved by osteotomy, although the stiffness is of course unaffected.

Post-traumatic stiffness

Temporary stiffness may follow any elbow injury; although manipulation under anaesthesia may improve movement at other joints, at the elbow it often makes matters worse and should not be attempted. Permanent limitation of movement is likely after severe fractures into the joint in adults, or when injury has been complicated by myositis ossificans.

To minimize post-traumatic stiffness, an injured elbow should be rested and forced movements absolutely prohibited. At the first suggestion of myositis ossificans, complete rest in a plaster gutter is imperative; later, when the calcified area has become well-defined, it may be removed, sometimes with benefit.

Flailness of the elbow

A flail elbow often causes surprisingly little disability, though a removable leather or polythene splint is usually helpful. There are three causes.

GUNSHOT WOUND
There is a scar, the elbow is flail, and often there is ulnar nerve palsy. X-rays show that the bones have been shot away.

CHARCOT'S DISEASE
There is flailness, but no scar and no ulnar palsy. The joint is enlarged and can be moved painlessly in any direction. X-rays show dislocation, bone destruction and calcification in the capsule.

POLIOMYELITIS
With a balanced paralysis the elbow may be flail, but flailness is not a presenting symptom.

Tennis elbow

The cause of this common elbow disorder is unknown but it is seldom due to tennis. Most cases probably follow unrecognized minor trauma to the origin of the wrist extensors, with subsequent adhesions. Other alleged causes include tendinitis, epicondylitis, fibrillation of the radial head and entrapment of a branch of the radial nerve.

Clinical features

The onset is commonly gradual, rarely sudden, and hardly ever at tennis. The patient complains of pain on certain movements such as pouring out tea, turning a stiff door-handle, shaking hands or lifting with the forearm pronated. The pain in severe cases may radiate widely.

The elbow looks normal, and flexion and extension are full and painless (though extension is sometimes temporarily painful). The x-ray appearance is normal.

There are three positive physical signs: (1) localized tenderness (over the lateral epicondyle);

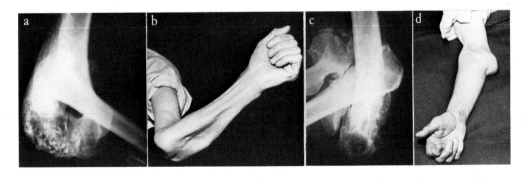

14.8 Flail elbow   (a, b) Following gun-shot wound; (c, d) Charcot's disease.

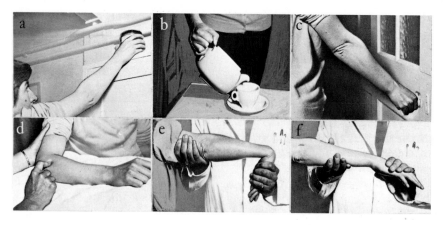

14.9 Tennis elbow   Symptoms: (a, b, c) movements which cause pain – in all three the extensor carpi radialis brevis is in action.
Signs: (d) localized tenderness; (e) pain on passive stretching; (f) pain on resisted dorsiflexion.

(2) pain on passive stretching (the wrist extensors are stretched by holding the elbow straight, the forearm prone and the wrist palmarflexed); and (3) pain on active contraction against resistance (the elbow is held straight and the forearm prone and the patient is prevented from dorsiflexing his wrist).

Treatment

Many methods of treatment are available; a useful sequence is as follows.

(1) INJECTION   The tender area is injected with a mixture of 1 per cent lignocaine and methylprednisolone. If the condition is improved, but not cured, the injection is repeated 3 weeks later.

(2) PHYSIOTHERAPY   Deep transverse frictions, though sometimes effective, are painful; a more comfortable alternative is ultrasound.

(3) MANIPULATIONS   The elbow is forcibly extended with the forearm prone and the wrist fully palmarflexed.

(4) REST   If the patient will submit to resting the arm in a sling or, better still, in plaster, for several weeks recovery is usual.

(5) OPERATION   A few cases are sufficiently persistent or recurrent for operation to be indicated. The origin of the common extensor muscle is detached from the lateral epicondyle and the orbicular ligament divided.

Variants

Golfer's elbow is comparable to tennis elbow except that the flexor origin (not the extensor) is affected. Treatment is similar.

Javelin throwers using the over-arm action may avulse the tip of the olecranon; with the round-arm action the medial ligament may be avulsed.

Baseball pitchers may suffer extensive elbow damage with hypertrophy of the lower humerus which no longer fits into the olecranon, and loose-body formation. The junior equivalent (little leaguer's elbow) is partial avulsion of the medial epicondyle.

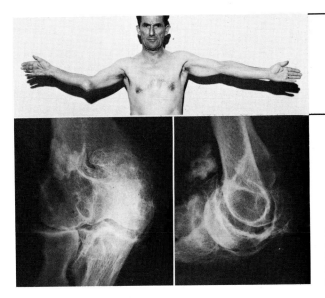

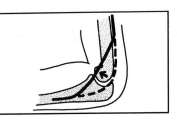

14.10 Loose bodies This patient had osteoarthritis and loose bodies in the elbow; the associated ulnar palsy was treated by transposing the nerve (diagram).

Loose bodies

Possible causes include the following.

INJURY
A fracture, dislocation or repeated minor injury may break off a piece of bone into the joint. Osteochondritis dissecans, in which a piece of bone becomes detached from the capitulum, is possibly traumatic in origin.

DEGENERATION
In osteoarthritis small osteophytes may break off, and in Charcot's disease large pieces of bone are found in the joint.

INFLAMMATION
Small fibrinous loose bodies may occur in inflammatory disease, but the inflammatory process overshadows the loose bodies.

IDIOPATHIC
Synovial chondromatosis occasionally occurs, producing many loose bodies.

The patient may complain of sudden locking and unlocking of the joint. Symptoms of osteoarthritis may coexist.

A loose body is rarely palpable. When degenerative changes have occurred, extremes of movement are limited. X-rays nearly always reveal the loose body or bodies; and in the special case of osteochondritis dissecans there is a rarefied cystic area in the capitulum and enlargement of the radial head.

If loose bodies are troublesome they can be removed.

Nerve lesions

Ulnar nerve

Ulnar palsy is often the sequel to elbow disorders such as osteoarthritis, valgus deformity or constriction of the nerve by a fibrous band at the proximal end of the flexor carpi ulnaris muscle (ulnar tunnel). Occasionally the nerve repeatedly dislocates forwards.

There may be no pain. The usual presenting symptom is numbness or weakness in the hand. The hand becomes clawed and the interossei (especially the first) are wasted. The nerve may be tender in the region of the elbow.

The nerve can be freed by dividing the roof of the ulnar tunnel if this is the cause; but transposition to the front of the elbow is more reliable.

Ulnar nerve transposition The nerve is exposed by a long incision centred over the medial epicondyle. It is freed upwards for several centimetres; the medial intermuscular septum in this area is excised to prevent kinking of the transposed nerve. Mobilization of the distal portion is facilitated by careful stripping of the branches. A bed is prepared in the flexor muscles and, when the nerve can lie easily in it without tension, one or two catgut sutures are placed to hold the nerve in its new bed. Alternatively, the common flexor origin is detached, the nerve placed deep to the muscle belly, and the divided tendon reattached.

Posterior interosseous nerve

Posterior interosseous nerve lesions just below the elbow can give rise to palsy. Tumour (e.g. lipoma), ganglion, fibrosis and traumatic neuritis have all been described. The treatment is operative decompression.

Bursae

The olecranon bursa sometimes becomes enlarged as a result of pressure or friction, and if the enlargement is a nuisance the fluid may be aspirated. The commonest non-traumatic cause is gout; there may be a sizeable lump with calcification on x-ray. A chronically enlarged bursa may need excision. In rheumatoid arthritis, also, the bursa may become enlarged, but more often subcutaneous nodules develop just distal to the olecranon process.

Notes on applied anatomy

The elbow needs to be able to convey the hand upwards to the head and mouth, downwards to the perineum and legs, and also to a wide variety of working positions at bench, desk, wall or table. A varied combination of flexion and extension with pronation and supination is clearly needed.

The hinge at which flexion and extension take place is a complex one. The humeroulnar component needs not only flexibility, but also stability, for pushing (or using crutches); this combination is provided by the conformity of the pulley (the trochlea) with the olecranon. The humeroradial component is held in position by the strong orbicular ligament; the circular and slightly concave upper surface of the radius ensures that in all positions of rotation it retains adequate contact with the capitulum.

In the coronal plane the axis of the hinge is tilted so that, in full extension, the elbow is in a few degrees of valgus. This 'carrying' angle may be altered by malunion of a fracture or by epiphyseal damage; increased valgus is likely to stretch the ulnar nerve as it passes behind the medial condyle. Distal to the condyle the nerve is closely applied to the elbow capsule, and there also it may be affected if the joint is osteoarthritic. If transposition of the ulnar nerve to the front is needed, it is important to divide the lower end of the medial intermuscular septum, otherwise the nerve may be kinked.

On the lateral side of the elbow the posterior interosseous nerve passes between the two parts of the supinator muscle; there it is vulnerable when the head of the radius is being approached surgically. In front of the elbow lies the brachialis muscle and also the median nerve in company with the great vessels; these relationships make an anterior approach to the elbow somewhat uninviting.

Elbow injuries are common in children, and a knowledge of the ossific centres is important. That for the capitulum appears at the age of 2 years, the medial epicondylar epiphysis appears at 5 and the trochlear epiphysis at 10. The centre for the lateral condyle does not appear until the age of 12, so that avulsion before that age will not show on x-ray. Any doubts as to whether these centres are normal on an x-ray are best resolved by comparison with a film of the uninjured elbow.

Further reading

Capener, N. (1966) The vulnerability of the posterior interosseous nerve of the forearm. *Journal of Bone and Joint Surgery* **48B,** 770–773 (see also 3 following articles)

Godshall, R. W. and Hansen, C. A. (1971) Traumatic ulnar neuropathy in adolescent baseball pitchers. *Journal of Bone and Joint Surgery* **53A,** 359–361

MacNicol, M. F. (1979) The results of operation for ulnar neuritis. *Journal of Bone and Joint Surgery* **61B,** 159–164

Roles, N. C. and Maudsley, R. H. (1972) Radial tunnel syndrome. *Journal of Bone and Joint Surgery* **54B,** 499–508

The Wrist Joint

15

Examination

Symptoms

Pain may be localized to the radial side (especially in tenovaginitis of the thumb tendons), to the ulnar side (possibly from the radioulnar joint) or to the dorsum (the usual site in disorders of the carpus). *Stiffness* is often not noticed until it is severe. *Swelling* may signify involvement of either the joint or the tendon sheaths. *Deformity* is a late symptom except after trauma.

After pain, the commonest symptom is loss of function in the hand – a firm grip is possible only with a strong, stable, painless wrist.

Signs

Examination of the wrist is not complete without also examining the elbow, forearm and hand.

● LOOK
The skin is inspected for scars. Both wrists and forearms are compared to see if there is deformity. Swelling, lumps and wasting of the forearm are noted.

● FEEL
Undue warmth is noted. Tender areas must be accurately localized, and the bony landmarks compared with those of the normal wrist.

● MOVE
To compare passive dorsiflexion of the wrists the patient places his palms together in a position of prayer, then elevates his elbows. Palmarflexion is examined in a similar way. With the elbows at right angles and tucked in to the sides, radial and ulnar deviation are next examined, then pronation and supination. Active movements should be tested against resistance; loss of power may be due to pain, tendon rupture or muscle weakness.

● X-RAY
Anteroposterior and lateral views are necessary, and often both wrists must be x-rayed for comparison. General rarefaction, alteration of joint spaces (in the radiocarpal or intercarpal joints) and abnormalities in shape or density of the individual bones are noted.

Wrist deformities

RADIAL CLUB HAND
The whole or part of the radius is missing. The wrist is palmarflexed and radially deviated, the hand lacks a thumb, and other anomalies of the fingers and of the elbow usually coexist.

Operations to stabilize and centralize the carpus may be cosmetically attractive, but they seldom improve function; the untreated deformity may already be in the hand-to-mouth position. Function usually diminishes as the child grows older, and centralization of the carpus over the ulna is recommended at about the age of 3 years.

MADELUNG'S DEFORMITY
This disorder of the lower radial growth disc may result from trauma, but most cases are bilateral and associated with a

177

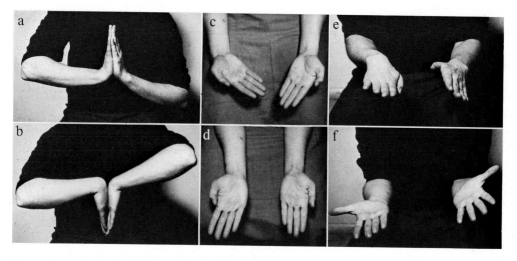

15.1 Examination   All movements of the left wrist are limited: (a) dorsiflexion, (b) palmarflexion, (c) ulnar deviation, (d) radial deviation, (e) pronation, (f) supination.

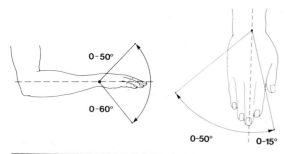

15.2 Normal range of movement   From the neutral position dorsiflexion is slightly less than palmarflexion. Most hand functions are performed with the wrist in ulnar deviation; normal radial deviation is only about 15 degrees.

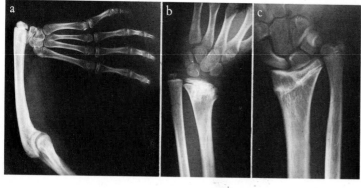

15.3 Deformities   (a) Absent radius and first ray. (b) Damage to radial growth disc; this type of injury might cause (c) Madelung's deformity.

general dysplasia (dyschondrosteosis); in these, girls are more severely affected. The deformity is rarely seen before the age of 10 years and increases until growth is complete. The lower radius curves forwards, carrying with it the carpus and hand, but leaving the lower ulna sticking out as a lump on the back of the wrist. If deformity is severe the lower ulna may be excised (Darrach's procedure), or osteotomy of the lower radius may be combined with shortening of the ulna.

POST-TRAUMATIC

After a Colles' fracture radial deviation and posterior angulation are common. These deformities cause little disability but may look ugly.

POST-INFLAMMATORY

After rheumatoid arthritis or tuberculosis forward subluxation at the radiocarpal joint commonly develops.

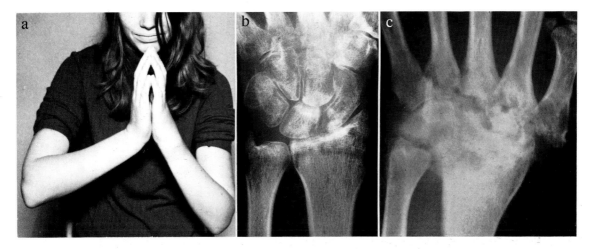

15.4 Tuberculosis (a) This girl presented with chronic ache and swelling of her left wrist; the forearm was wasted and extension absent; (b) her x-ray shows the washed-out appearance of osteoporosis around the wrist. (c) A different patient who had severe tuberculous arthritis; the disease is no longer active (hence the dense appearance), but destruction has been extensive.

Tuberculosis
(see also page 28)

At the wrist, tuberculosis is rarely seen until it has progressed to a true arthritis. Pain and stiffness come on gradually and the hand feels weak.

The forearm looks wasted, the wrist is swollen, the carpus subluxed forwards, and there may be a sinus. Movements are restricted and painful. The x-ray looks hazy, with narrowing and irregularity of the radiocarpal and intercarpal joints, and sometimes bone erosion.

The condition must be differentiated from rheumatoid arthritis. Bilateral arthritis of the wrist is nearly always rheumatoid in origin, but when only one wrist is affected the signs strongly resemble those of tuberculosis; serological tests may establish the diagnosis, but often a biopsy is necessary.

Anti-tuberculous drugs are given and the wrist is rested in plaster which extends from the upper forearm to the proximal palm crease (permitting finger flexion) and holds the wrist 20 degrees dorsiflexed. Later a removable splint is used. Only rarely is arthrodesis necessary.

Rheumatoid arthritis

Clinical features

After the metacarpophalangeal joints, the wrist is the commonest site of rheumatoid disease. Pain, swelling and tenderness usually start on the ulnar side and are due either to tenosynovitis of the extensor carpi ulnaris or to erosion of the radioulnar joint. With extension to the radiocarpal joint, the wrist gradually drifts into radial deviation and volar subluxation. X-rays show osteoporosis and erosion of the ulnar styloid, the radiocarpal and the intercarpal joints. Pain and instability at the wrist contribute signficantly to the loss of power grip in the hand, and radial deviation of the carpus may predispose to 'compensatory' ulnar drift of the fingers.

Treatment

In the early stage (synovitis or tenosynovitis) splintage and intrasynovial injection of hydrocortisone and nitrogen mustard are usually effective. In the second stage (early joint erosion with minimal instability) synovectomy and soft-tissue

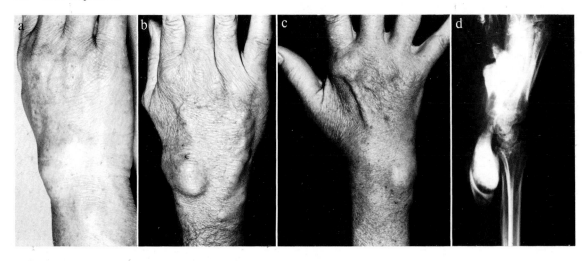

15.5 Rheumatoid arthritis (1)   (a) Synovitis of the wrist; (b) here there is also tenosynovitis of the extensor carpi ulnaris; (c) synovitis of the inferior radioulnar joint; (d) contrast radiography showing a large protrusion from the flexor sheath.

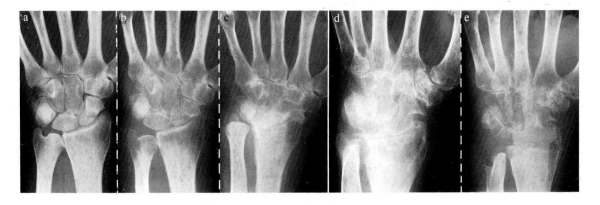

15.6 Rheumatoid arthritis (2)   (a) At first the x-rays show only soft-tissue swelling; (b) 7 years later, this patient shows early bone changes – periarticular osteoporosis and diminution of the joint space; (c) 5 years later still, bony erosions and joint destruction are marked. (d) Shows another patient with severe disease, who has been treated by (e) excising the diseased surfaces and inserting a Silastic spacer – reasonable stability was restored; this can be done only if the joint has not been too severely distorted.

stabilization may prevent further destruction and deformity; this may be combined with excision of the ulnar head and transposition of the extensor carpi radialis longus to the ulnar side of the wrist (to counteract its tendency to radial drift). In stage 3, articular destruction and radiocarpal dislocation may require either arthrodesis or an arthroplasty with a Silastic prosthesis.

ARTHRODESIS
Through a dorsal incision the radiocarpal and intercarpal joints are exposed; the head of the ulna is excised. A bed is cut into the bony mosaic, extending from the distal end of the radius to the proximal ends of the second and third metacarpals; into this trough is slotted a corticocancellous graft taken from the ilium. If the joint is very unstable it may be held by a Rush nail passing from the metacarpals up the radius; a dorsal staple can be added. The wrist is then immobilized in plaster

for 8 weeks. The optimal position is 10 degrees of dorsiflexion and slight ulnar deviation.

ARTHROPLASTY

This has not yet stood the test of time. The simplest of several available methods is to expose the wrist as for arthrodesis and then hollow out the distal radius and the carpus to receive the limbs of a flexible Silastic hinge.

Warning After either arthrodesis or arthroplasty the skin on the dorsum may slough; great care is required in handling the tissues and ensuring complete haemostasis.

Osteoarthritis

Osteoarthritis of the wrist is uncommon except as the sequel to injury. Any fracture into the joint may predispose to degeneration, but the commonest is a fractured scaphoid, especially with non-union or avascular necrosis. Kienböck's disease is a less frequent cause.

The patient may have forgotten the original injury. Years later he complains of pain and stiffness. At first these occur intermittently after use; later they become more constant, and recurrent 'wrist sprains' are common.

The appearance is usually normal and there is no wasting. Movements at the wrist and radio-ulnar joints are limited and painful. X-rays show irregular narrowing at the radiocarpal joint, with bone sclerosis; the proximal portion of the scaphoid or the lunate may be irregular and dense.

Rest, in a polythene splint, is often sufficient treatment. Excision of the radial styloid process is helpful when osteoarthritis has followed scaphoid injury. Arthrodesis of the wrist is rarely necessary.

Note At the carpometacarpal joint of the thumb osteoarthritis is much commoner than at the wrist. The joint is painful and tender, and full extension and adduction are painful. X-rays show narrowing of the space between the trapezium and first metacarpal, often with sclerosis. If short-wave diathermy and restriction of activity do not give relief, operation may be advisable. Excision of the trapezium (possibly with a Silastic replacement) gives relief of pain and often rapid return of full function; arthrodesis may also give a good result, but involves 3 months in plaster.

Kienböck's disease

The name refers to avascular necrosis of the carpal lunate. Trauma (a single definite injury or repeated minor ones) may be the precipitating cause. Often the ulna is short relative to the radius, so that the lunate is compressed against the edge of the radius. The condition is not uncommon in cerebral palsy.

The patient, often a young adult, complains of ache and stiffness. Localized tenderness and limited dorsiflexion are

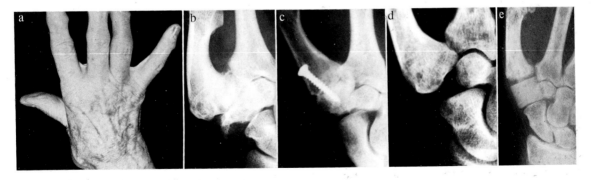

15.7 Osteoarthritis of the carpometacarpal thumb joint (a) Typical deformity in an advanced case, with (b) narrow joint space and osteophytes. If operation is needed, the possibilities are (c) arthrodesis, (d) excision of the trapezium, or (e) replacement arthroplasty using a Silastic spacer.

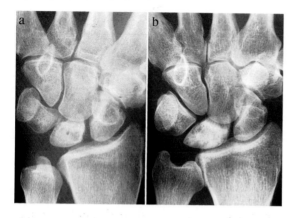

15.8 Kienböck's disease (osteochondritis)   (a) Early – the lunate looks mottled and slightly dense. (b) Later – not only is the lunate dense, but the radiocarpal joint is narrowed. In both these patients the ulna looks slightly short.

usual. X-rays at first show increased density and perhaps slight mottling of the lunate; later the bone looks squashed and irregular; still later the wrist may become osteoarthritic.

In early cases, shortening the radius or lengthening the ulna, to 'decompress' the lunate, may lead to improvement. Later, replacing the lunate with a prosthesis (made of plastic or Silastic) has been advocated. Once osteoarthritis has supervened the alternatives are splintage, excision of the proximal row of the carpus, or arthrodesis of the wrist.

Carpal tunnel syndrome

There is insufficient space for the median nerve beneath the anterior carpal ligament. In the normal carpal tunnel there is barely room for all the tendons and the median nerve; consequently any swelling is likely to result in compression. Usually the cause eludes detection; the syndrome is, however, common in menopausal women, in rheumatoid arthritis and in pregnancy. Computerized tomography has shown that women have smaller tunnels than men, and those with carpal tunnel syndrome have the smallest tunnels of all.

Symptoms

Pain and paraesthesia occur in the distribution of the median nerve in the hand. Night after night the patient is woken in the early hours with burning pain, tingling and numbness; the fingers may feel swollen and the whole arm heavy. Hanging the arm over the side of the bed, or getting up and walking about may, after an hour or so, relieve the pain. During the day little pain is felt except with such activities as knitting or holding a newspaper. The pain may radiate up the arm. There is often clumsiness and difficulty in fine movements such as sewing.

Signs

The condition is eight times more common in women than men. The usual age group is 40–50 years; in younger patients it is not uncommon to find related factors such as pregnancy, rheumatoid disease or tenosynovitis.

Both hands, or only the dominant hand, may be involved. Abnormal physical signs are usually

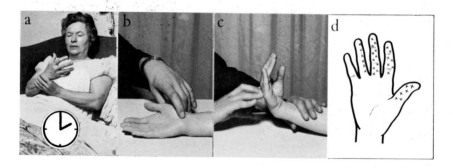

15.9 Carpal tunnel syndrome   (a) The patient is woken in the early hours. (b, c) Pressure on the tunnel, or forced palmarflexion, may reproduce pain or tingling. (d) A positive 'map test'.

absent and indeed the condition should be diagnosed before signs are obvious. The pattern of sensory changes can sometimes be reproduced by holding the wrist fully palmarflexed for 1 minute, by tapping the front of the wrist, or by compressing the arm with a sphygmomanometer cuff. The patient is often unsure of the precise distribution of paraesthesia, and it is helpful to ask her to return after a few days when she has mapped it out. The diagnosis can be confirmed by nerve conduction studies.

In late cases there is wasting of the thenar muscles with altered sensation in the median area.

Treatment

Conservative treatment consists of injecting methylprednisolone into the flexor sheath or wearing a cock-up splint. If these fail, or if there is already clinically detectable neurological deficit, operation is advised. The anterior carpal ligament is divided. The patient wakes up relieved of pain and from then on is not disturbed at night; but neurological deficit may not recover fully.

Swellings around the wrist

Ganglion

It seems that ganglia arise not by synovial herniation from a joint or tendon sheath, but from small bursae within the substance of the joint capsule or the fibrous tendon sheath. These bursae become distended, possibly following trauma, giving rise to a main 'cyst' containing viscous fluid and smaller pseudopodia.

The patient, often a young adult, presents with a painless lump, though occasionally there is slight ache and weakness. The lump is well-defined, cystic and not tender; it can sometimes

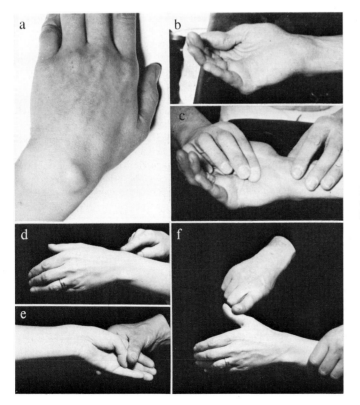

15.10 Wrist swellings (a) Simple ganglion; (b, c) compound palmar ganglion with cross-fluctuation.

de Quervain's disease: (d) the patient can point to the painful area; (e) forced adduction is painful; (f) pain on active extension against resistance.

be transilluminated and may feel more tense when the tendons are put into action. The back of the wrist is the commonest site, but ganglia in front may compress a nerve or penetrate between the fibres, causing numbness or weakness.

Squashing the lump may disperse it, but recurrence is common. If it recurs and is troublesome the best treatment is operative excision. A tourniquet is used; the ganglion is removed together with all the pseudopodia and the fibrous layer from which they arise.

Note Ganglia occasionally occur in the palm or fingers. They are then small, hard and tender, so that diagnosis is not easy until the lump is exposed.

Compound palmar ganglion

Chronic inflammation distends the common sheath of the flexor tendons both above and below the flexor retinaculum. Rheumatoid arthritis and tuberculosis are the commonest causes. The synovial membrane becomes thick and villous. The amount of fluid is increased and it may contain fibrin particles moulded by repeated movement to the shape of melon seeds. The tendons may eventually fray and rupture.

Pain is unusual, but paraesthesia due to median nerve compression may occur. The swelling is hourglass in shape, bulging above and below the flexor retinaculum; it is not warm or tender; fluid can be pushed from one part to the other (cross-fluctuation).

If the condition is tuberculous, general treatment is begun (page 28). The contents of the ganglion are evacuated, streptomycin instilled, and the wrist is rested in a splint. If these measures fail the entire flexor sheath is dissected out. Complete excision is also the best treatment when the cause is rheumatoid disease.

Stenosing tenovaginitis (de Quervain's disease)

Like trigger finger and thumb, this is a tendon tunnel syndrome. The sheath containing the extensor pollicis brevis and abductor pollicis longus tendons becomes thickened. There may be an underlying abnormality in the number of tendons.

The condition is commonest in women aged 40–50 years, who complain of pain on the radial side of the wrist, worse after such actions as wringing clothes. A small lump is visible on the radial side 2 cm above the wrist. The lump feels almost bony hard, so that it is frequently mistaken for an exostosis (but the x-ray appearance is always normal); tenderness is precisely localized to the lump. Pain is felt if the patient extends the thumb against resistance, or if it is passively adducted across the palm.

The early case can be relieved by hydrocortisone injections into the tendon sheath. More resistant cases may benefit from prolonged splintage combined with injection. But operation, which consists of slitting the sheath, is uniformly successful and the patient wakes up cured.

Notes on applied anatomy

The styloid process of the ulna normally extends further distally than that of the radius, though this relationship may be altered as a result of injury or with Kienböck's disease. Just distal to the radial styloid is the scaphoid, immediately beneath the anatomical snuffbox, which is one of the key areas for localizing tenderness.

Tenderness at the distal end of the snuffbox may incriminate the carpometacarpal joint of the thumb. More proximal tenderness may be from tenovaginitis of the extensor pollicis brevis and abductor pollicis longus; within their fibrous sheath these tendons may be duplicated or triplicated, and, unless this is appreciated, surgical decompression may be inadequate. Dorsal to the snuffbox the oblique course of extensor pollicis longus exposes it to damage by a careless incision.

The mosaic of the carpal bones is arranged in two rows, with the pisiform as the odd man out. The scaphoid, trapezium and thumb combine to function almost as a separate entity, a 'jointed strut', with independent movement; degenerative arthritis of the wrist occurs almost exclusively in the joints of this strut (Fisk, 1970).

Wrist dorsiflexion takes place at both the radiocarpal joint (the first two-thirds) and at the midcarpal joint (the final third). When the wrist is fully dorsiflexed the scaphoid, which straddles the midcarpal joint, swivels backwards. Even so it is vulnerable and liable to fracture. When it does so, the more ulnar deviated the wrist, the more proximal is the fracture.

Stability of the carpus depends not only upon bony conformity, joint capsules and overlying tendons, but also upon a series of tough ligaments. The volar radiocarpal ligament is the most important of these and, if torn, leads to carpal instability. It is precisely when a scaphoid fracture is associated with carpal instability that complications, such as non-union, are likely to occur.

On their volar aspect the carpal bones form a concavity roofed over by the carpal ligament; in the tunnel lie the flexor tendons and sheath together with the median nerve. The palmar branch of the nerve (supplying the all-important thenar muscles) is in danger if, during a decompression operation, the carpal ligament is divided too far radially. On the radial side of the wrist, branches of the radial nerve are vulnerable; and on the ulnar side, the close relationship of the ulnar nerve to the pisiform must be borne in mind.

Further reading

Andren, L. and Eiken, O. (1971) Arthrographic studies of wrist ganglions. *Journal of Bone and Joint Surgery* **53A,** 299–302

Fisk, G. R. (1970) Carpal instability and the fractured scaphoid. *Annals of the Royal College of Surgeons of England* **46,** 63–76

Lamb, D. W. (1972) The treatment of radial club hand. *The Hand* **4,** 22–30

Ranawat, C. S., DeFiore, J. and Straub, L. R. (1975) Madelung's deformity. *Journal of Bone and Joint Surgery* **57A,** 772–775

Roca, J., Beltran, J. E., Fairen, M. F. and Alvarez, A. (1976) Treatment of Kienböck's disease using a silicone rubber implant. *Journal of Bone and Joint Surgery* **58A,** 373–376

The Hand

16

Examination

Symptoms

The common symptoms are pain, paraesthesia, deformity, stiffness and weakness. *Pain* may be local or referred from the neck, thoracobrachial junction, shoulder, elbow or wrist. *Abnormal sensation* usually follows the distribution of a peripheral nerve or root, but with reflex sympathetic dystrophy the sensory symptoms are not segmental. Even minor *deformities* are quickly noticed (and often bitterly resented). Complaints of joint *swelling* and unsightly deformity in Heberden's arthropathy may seem out of proportion to the functional loss, but they should be taken seriously; the hand is (in more senses than one) the medium of introduction to the outside world.

Signs

Both upper limbs should be bared for comparison.

● LOOK
The skin may be scarred, altered in colour, dry or moist, and hairy or smooth.* Wasting and deformity, and the presence of any lumps, should be noted. The resting posture is an important index of nerve or tendon damage. Swelling may be in the subcutaneous tissue (oedema or pus), in a tendon sheath (tenosynovitis) or in a joint (arthritis).

● FEEL
The skin temperature is noted and sensation assessed, testing for touch, pinprick and two-point discrimination if a nerve lesion is suspected. If a nodule is felt in the palm, the corresponding finger should be passively moved, to discover if the nodule is in a tendon.

● MOVE
Active movements are tested by examining the motor functions of the hand as pincers (e.g. in writing), as a vice (e.g. in holding a hammer), as a hook (e.g. in carrying a bag) and for tapping (e.g. typewriting). With palms facing upwards the patient is asked to curl the fingers into full flexion; a 'lagging finger' (from tendon thickening, tendon rupture or joint stiffness) is immediately obvious. Individual finger and thumb movements must be examined when a nerve or tendon is suspect. The range of passive movement for each digit is recorded. Overall grip strength is then rapidly assessed by asking the patient to squeeze the examiner's fingers; it may be diminished because of muscle weakness, finger stiffness or wrist instability. Grip strength can be measured more accurately by rolling up a sphygmomanometer cuff, inflating it to 30 mmHg, and seeing to what pressure the patient can squeeze it (normally 150 mmHg can be achieved easily).

*A scar on the surface means damage below.

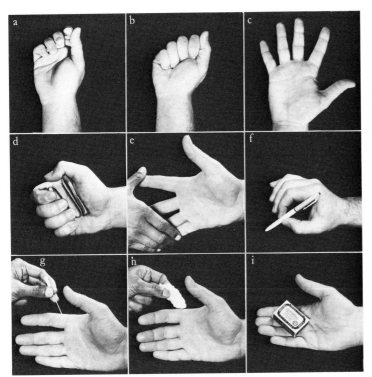

16.1 Examination Positions: (a) resting position, (b) full flexion, (c) full extension.

Strength: (d) power grip, (e) finger abduction, (f) pinch grip.

Sensation: (g) pin prick, (h) light touch, (i) stereognosis.

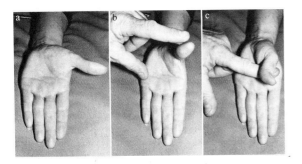

16.2 Movements of the thumb With the hand held flat on the table and palm upwards, the patient is asked (a) to stretch the thumb away from the hand (extension), (b) to lift it towards the ceiling (abduction) and (c) to squeeze down onto the examiner's finger (adduction).

The examination is not complete until the wrist, elbow, shoulder and neck have been examined as well.

Congenital deformities

The hand and foot are much the commonest sites of congenital deformities of the locomotor system; the incidence is no less than 1 in 2500 live births. Early recognition is important, and definitive treatment should be timed to fit in with the functional demands of the child. There are five types of malformation.

(1) Failure of development

Total or partial absence of parts may be transverse ('congenital amputations') or axial.

Lobster hand is a congenital absence of the middle rays. Function is usually good, but a deep cleft may need closing.

Radial club hand is due to partial or complete absence of the radius and thumb. The wrist falls into marked radial deviation. During infancy the hand should be splinted, with the intention of operating by the age of 3 years; the carpus is then centralized over the ulna.

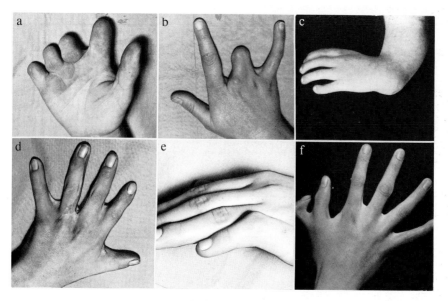

16.3 Congenital deformities   (a) Congenital amputations; (b) missing digits; (c) radial club hand; (d) syndactyly; (e) camptodactyly; (f) extra digits.

(2) Failure of differentiation

Syndactyly (congenital webbing)   may be corrected by separating the fingers and repairing the defects with skin grafts.

Camptodactyly   is a fixed flexion deformity of the proximal interphalangeal joint (usually of the little finger). It is hereditary and often bilateral, but deformity is rarely obvious before the age of 10 years.

(3) Focal defects

Polydactyly (extra digits)   is the commonest hand malformation. The extra finger should be amputated, if only for cosmetic reasons.

Constriction bands   may occur in the fingers (as elsewhere in the limbs). Distal oedema may be severe. The constricted skin is excised and repaired by Z-plasty or grafting.

(4) Overgrowth

A giant finger is unsightly, but attempts at operative reduction are fraught with complications.

(5) Generalized malformations

The hand may be involved in generalized disorders such as Marfan's syndrome ('spider hands') or achondroplasia ('trident hand').

Acquired deformities

Deformity of the hand may be due to disorders of the skin, subcutaneous tissues, muscles, tendons, joints, bones or neuromuscular function. Often there is a history of trauma, or infection or concomitant disease; at other times the patient is unaware of any cause.

(1) Skin contracture

Cuts and burns of the palmar skin are liable to heal with contracture. Surgical incisions should never cross skin creases; they should be parallel with them or in the mid-axial line of the fingers. Established contractures may require excision and Z-plasty.

(2) Subcutaneous contracture (Dupuytren's contracture)

This is a nodular hypertrophy and contracture of the palmar aponeurosis. The condition is inherited as an autosomal dominant and is most

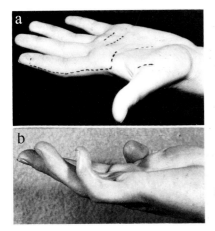

16.4 Deformities – skin   (a) Skin incisions should never cross the creases on the flexor surface; those shown are safe; (b) postoperative contracture of a badly placed scar.

common in people of European (especially Anglo-Saxon) descent. There is a high incidence in epileptics receiving phenytoin therapy; associations with alcoholic cirrhosis, diabetes and pulmonary tuberculosis have also been described.

Pathology

The palmar aponeurosis thickens, usually opposite the ring finger. Early on, there is proliferation of immature fibroblasts; later the fascia thickens and shrinks, its distal prolongations pulling the fingers into flexion and its cutaneous attachments puckering the palmar skin.

Clinical features

The patient – usually a middle-aged man – may complain of pain on grasping, or of a nodule in the palm. Later the condition is painless, but deformity may slowly develop with increasing impairment of grip. The bent finger becomes a nuisance and there is difficulty in letting objects go.

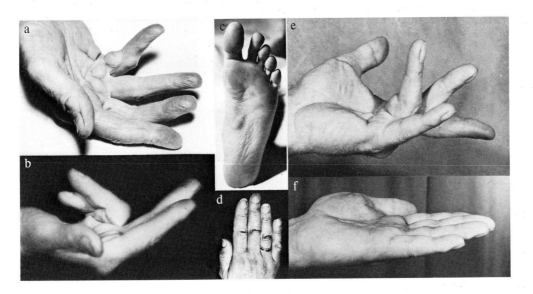

16.5 Dupuytren's contracture   (a) Moderately severe, with diagnostic nodules and pits; (b) severe contracture. (c) Dupuytren's nodule in the sole; (d) Garrod's pads. (e, f) Before and after subcutaneous fasciotomy.

Nearly always, both hands are involved, one more than the other. The palm is puckered, nodular and thick. There may be obvious subcutaneous cords, and if these extend into the fingers the metacarpophalangeal and proximal interphalangeal joints are held in flexion. In the most severe cases the finger tips dig into the palm and smelly sebaceous material collects in the skin folds.

Thickening of the dorsal skin of the proximal interphalangeal joints (Garrod's pads) may be seen, and puckering comparable to that in the palm may occur on the soles of the feet. There is a rare association with fibrosis of the corpus cavernosum (Peyronie's disease).

Treatment

Operation is indicated if the deformity is a nuisance or rapidly progressing. The aim is reasonable, not complete, correction.

Closed fasciotomy   A tenotome is inserted subcutaneously and the deforming bands are carefully divided. This is repeated at several points until passive correction is obtained. In experienced hands this is a good procedure, but there is a danger of injuring nerves or vessels.

Limited fasciectomy   This is the operation of choice, but in severe deformities it may have to be preceded by fasciotomy to obtain some corection and permit adequate skin toilet. The affected area is approached through a longitudinal or a Z-shaped incision and, after carefully freeing the nerves, the hypertrophic cords are excised. The skin can be elongated by multiple Z-plasties or the wound can be left open.

Total fasciectomy   has many complications, including haematoma, skin necrosis and infection; it is not recommended.

Amputation   is occasionally advisable if there is severe contraction of the joint capsule.

After operative correction a splint is applied, and removed daily for wax baths and exercises. After 6 weeks it is used only as a night splint for a further 6 months.

(3) Muscle contracture

Ischaemic contracture of the forearm or hand muscles may follow circulatory insufficiency due to injuries at or below the elbow (see pages 355–357). In forearm contracture there is shortening of the long flexors; the fingers are held

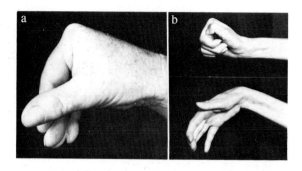

16.6 Deformities – muscle   (a) Flexion deformity due to ischaemic contracture of the intrinsic hand muscles (the 'intrinsic-plus' hand); (b) ischaemic contracture of the long flexors in the forearm; with the wrist in extension, the fingers involuntarily curl into flexion; when the wrist flexes, the pull on the finger flexors is released.

in flexion and can be straightened only when the wrist is flexed. In distal ischaemia there is contracture of the intrinsic muscles.

INTRINSIC CONTRACTURE (THE 'INTRINSIC-PLUS' HAND)   Shortening of the interossei and lumbricals results in metacarpophalangeal flexion, interphalangeal extension and thumb adduction with interphalangeal extension. Slight degrees of deformity may not be obvious, but can be diagnosed by the 'intrinsic-plus test': with the metacarpophalangeal joints pushed passively into hyperextension (thus putting the intrinsics on stretch), it is difficult or impossible to flex the interphalangeal joints passively. The causes of intrinsic shortening or contracture are: (1) spasm (e.g. in cerebral palsy); (2) volar subluxation of the metacarpophalangeal joints (e.g. in rheumatoid arthritis); (3) scarring after trauma or infection; and (4) shrinkage due to distal ischaemia. Moderate contracture can be treated by resecting a triangular segment of the intrinsic 'aponeurosis' at the base of the proximal phalanx (Littler's operation).

(4) Tendon lesions

MALLET FINGER   This results from injury to the extensor tendon of the terminal phalanx. It occurs if the finger tip is forcibly bent during active extension, as in making a bed or catching a ball.

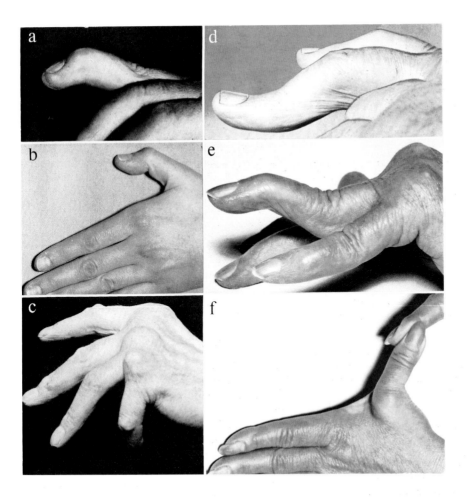

16.7 Deformities – tendons   (a) Mallet finger. (b) Mallet thumb. (c) Dropped fingers due to rupture of extensor tendons. (d) Boutonnière. (e) Swan-neck deformity. (f) Game-keeper's thumb (rupture of the medial collateral metacarpophalangeal ligament).

The terminal joint is flexed and the patient cannot straighten it, though the surgeon can. The finger should be held for 6 weeks in a splint with the distal joint extended (see also page 414).

MALLET THUMB   The extensor pollicis longus tendon usually ruptures at the wrist after a fracture (page 405) or following invasion by rheumatoid granulations, but it may be accidentally cut anywhere. The distal phalanx can be passively but not actively extended and thumb pinch is weakened. Except after an open cut, direct repair is not advisable because the ends are ragged.

A tendon transfer, using the extensor to the index finger, is preferable. However, this tendon (or any other tendon in the vicinity) only reaches as far as the neck of the first metacarpal, so a transfer is suitable only for division proximal to that level; for secondary repair of a ragged rupture beyond this level a free tendon graft is necessary.

DROPPED FINGER   Sudden loss of finger extension at the metacarpophalangeal joint is usually due to rupture of a long extensor tendon at the wrist (e.g. in rheumatoid arthritis). If direct repair is not possible, the distal portion can be attached to an adjacent finger extensor.

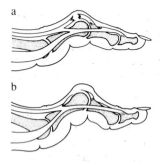

16.8 Deformities – boutonnière (a) When the middle slip of the extensor tendon first ruptures there is no more than an inability to extend the proximal interphalangeal joint. If it is not repaired, (b) the lateral slips slide towards the volar surface, the knuckle 'buttonholes' the extensor hood, and the distal joint is drawn into hyperextension.

BOUTONNIÈRE This lesion (which the French call 'le buttonhole') presents as a flexion deformity of the proximal interphalangeal joint. It is due to interruption or stretching of the central slip of the extensor tendon where it inserts into the base of the middle phalanx. The lateral slips separate and the head of a proximal phalanx thrusts through the gap like a finger through a buttonhole. Initially deformity is slight and passively correctible; later the soft tissues contract, resulting in fixed flexion of the proximal and hyperextension of the distal interphalangeal joint. (If caused by a small cut on the dorsum the injury is often missed.)

In the early post-traumatic case, splinting the proximal interphalangeal joint in full extension for 3 weeks usually leads to union; the alternative is direct suture.

In later cases where the joint is still passively correctible, one lateral slip can be transposed to the base of the middle phalanx, or the healthy portion of the middle slip can be lengthened and reattached, the joint being held straight with a Kirschner wire for 4 weeks. Long-standing fixed deformities are extremely difficult to correct and may be better left alone.

Boutonnière deformity of the thumb metacarpophalangeal joint is common in rheumatoid arthritis (see page 195).

SWAN-NECK DEFORMITY This is the reverse of boutonnière deformity; the proximal interphalangeal joint is hyperextended and the distal interphalangeal joint flexed. The deformity can be reproduced voluntarily by lax-jointed individuals. The clinical disorder has many causes, with one thing in common: imbalance of extensor versus flexor action at the proximal interphalangeal joint. Thus it may occur (1) *if the proximal interphalangeal extensors overact* (e.g. due to intrinsic muscle spasm or contracture, or after disruption of the distal extensor attachment or volar subluxation of the metacarpophalangeal joint, both of which cause extensor force to be concentrated on the proximal interphalangeal joint); or (2) *if the proximal interphalangeal flexors are inadequate* (paralysis or division of the flexor sublimis). If the deformity is allowed to persist, secondary contracture of the intrinsic muscles, and eventually of the proximal interphalangeal joint itself, make correction increasingly difficult and ultimately impossible.

While the deformity is still correctible, the cause can usually be established by three simple manoeuvres: (1) test for isolated sublimis action (Fig. 16.9); (2) test for intrinsic contracture (page 190); (3) stabilize the metacarpophalangeal joint and see if this corrects the deformity. Treatment depends on the cause, and may involve operative release of shrunken intrinsics, reduction and stabilization of the metacarpophalangeal joint, and tightening of the volar proximal interphalangeal structures. An isolated injury or rupture of the sublimis tendon seldom warrants repair.

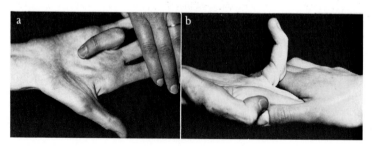

16.9 Testing sublimis To detect sublimis competence, first anchor the profundus, which is a 'mass action' muscle. In (a) the sublimis is normal; it alone is flexing the annularis – the tip is flail. In (b) sublimis is not working; only by using profundus (with difficulty) can the annularis be flexed, consequently the tip is not flail (Apley, 1956).

(5) Joint disorders

RHEUMATOID ARTHRITIS causes multiple deformities of both hands. The most typical is ulnar deviation of the fingers, but this may be combined with boutonnière and swan-neck deformities (see page 195).

OSTEOARTHRITIS Osteoarthritis of the distal and middle finger joints is common in postmenopausal women and may cause deformity. If disability is severe the joint may be arthrodesed. Osteoarthritis of the thumb carpometacarpal joint may result in subluxation, with adduction of the first metacarpal and hyperextension of the thumb metacarpophalangeal joint. Treatment is essentially that of the underlying disorder, but if metacarpal adduction is severe the thenar muscles may have to be released.

GOUT produces large tophi and severe joint deformity. In addition to systemic treatment, evacuation of tophaceous material is sometimes advisable.

TRAUMA may result in recurrent or persistent dislocation or subluxation. The best known, '*game-keeper's*' thumb, is due to disruption of the ulnar collateral ligament of the thumb metacarpophalangeal joint with instability (see page 415).

STIFF JOINTS may follow trauma, infection or injudicious splintage. A stiff finger, whether bent or straight, is a nuisance. Physiotherapy may help, but in long-standing cases, if operative release is unsuccessful, the finger may have to be amputated.

(6) Bone lesions

A variety of bone lesions (acute infection, tuberculosis, malunited fractures, infantile rickets, tumours) may cause metacarpal or phalangeal deformity. X-rays usually show the abnormality. In addition to treating the pathological lesion, deformity may need correction by osteotomy with internal fixation.

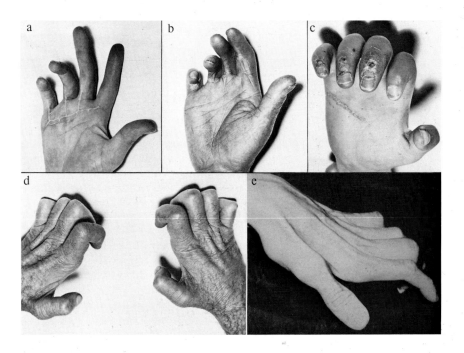

16.10 Examples of claw hand   (a) Following badly placed incisions; (b) ulnar nerve palsy. (c) Volkmann's contracture. (d) Bilateral clawing in peroneal muscular atrophy; (e) associated with the nerve lesions of leprosy.

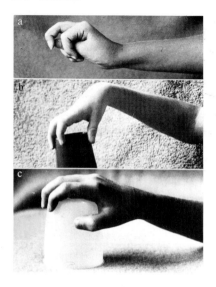

16.11 The hand in cerebral palsy (a) Typically, when the wrist is extended the fingers flex and the thumb tucks into the palm; the hand unclasps only (b) when the wrist is flexed. After muscle release (c) the hand may be able to open with the wrist in a functional position.

pointing index finger of median nerve palsy, and the claw hand of ulnar nerve palsy (pages 132 –134).

INTRINSIC PARALYSIS (THE 'INTRINSIC-MINUS' HAND) Weakness or paralysis of the intrinsics results in metacarpophalangeal extension and partial flexion of the interphalangeal joints of the fingers and thumb (a type of 'claw hand'); finger abduction and adduction are impossible. If all the intrinsics are affected (e.g. after poliomyelitis) the thumb lies flat at the side of the hand and cannot be opposed. In ulnar nerve palsy only the ring and little fingers are clawed, because the index and middle lumbricals are supplied by the median nerve; thumb opposition is retained but thumb pinch is unstable because index-finger abduction is weak, and loss of thumb adduction is compensated by exaggerated interphalangeal flexion during strong pinch (Froment's sign). The objectives of treatment are: (1) stabilization of the metacarpophalangeal joints in flexion; this can be achieved by a many-tailed tendon transfer (splitting a flexor sublimis tendon) or, if a suitable motor is not available, by tightening the volar metacarpophalangeal capsules; (2) restoration of index abduction to provide stable pinch (e.g. by extensor tendon transfer to the first dorsal interosseous); and (3) restoration of thumb opposition (if it is lost) by a tendon transfer looped around a pisiform pulley and attached to the proximal phalanx of the thumb. *Before any of these operations, stiff finger joints must be made mobile.*

(7) Neuromuscular disorders

CEREBRAL PALSY AND STROKE may cause spastic paresis with severe hand deformities. The 'intrinsic-plus' posture is easily recognized. Another common disability is 'thumb-in-palm'; the tendency to adduct and flex the thumb into the palm is increased by activity, especially finger flexion. Releasing the adductor pollicis from the third metacarpal may improve the appearance, but normal thumb pinch is rarely restored.

OTHER NEUROLOGICAL DISORDERS such as poliomyelitis, leprosy, syringomyelia and peroneal muscular atrophy may cause hand deformities. If there is only partial involvement, tendon transfer may be feasible.

PERIPHERAL NERVE LESIONS cause characteristic deformities: the drop wrist and drop fingers of radial nerve palsy, the flat simian thumb and

Trigger finger

A flexor tendon may become trapped at the entrance to its sheath and, on forced extension, pass the constriction with a snap (trigger effect). Causes are tenosynovitis (traumatic or rheumatoid), nodular thickening of the tendon or thickening of the fibrous sheath (stenosing tenovaginitis).

In adults any digit may be affected, but the ring and middle fingers most commonly. The patient notices that the finger clicks, often painfully, when he bends it. Later, when the hand is unclenched, the affected finger remains bent; with further effort it may suddenly straighten with a snap, or it may remain flexed until forced straight with the other hand. A tender nodule can be felt in front of the affected metacarpophalangeal joint, and there is a palpable click when the finger or thumb is moved.

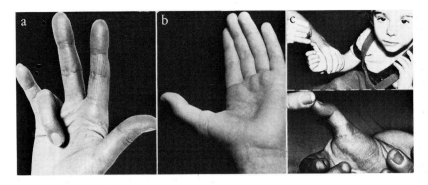

16.12 Stenosing tenovaginitis   (a) Trigger finger; (b) trigger thumb – the only variety which occurs in children, in whom (c) the thumb may be stuck bent.

In babies only the thumb is affected; the mother notices that it remains bent and often dislocation is wrongly diagnosed.

Treatment

Early cases may be cured by an injection of methylprednisolone carefully placed at the entrance of the tendon sheath. Refractory cases need operation: through a transverse incision in the distal palmar crease, or in the metacarpophalangeal crease of the thumb, the fibrous sheath is incised until the tendon moves freely. In babies it is worth waiting a few months, as spontaneous recovery may occur.

The rheumatoid hand

The hand, more than any other region, is where rheumatoid arthritis carves its story. In *stage 1* there is synovitis of joints (metacarpophalangeal and proximal interphalangeal) and of tendon sheaths (flexor and extensor). In *stage 2*, joint and tendon erosions prepare the ground for mechanical derangement. And in *stage 3*, joint instability and tendon rupture cause progressive deformity and loss of function.

Clinical features (see also page 36)

STAGE 1   Pain, stiffness and swelling of the fingers are early symptoms; often the wrist also is painful and swollen. Carpal tunnel compression from flexor tenosynovitis sometimes causes the first symptom. Examination may show swelling of the metacarpophalangeal joints, the proximal interphalangeal joints (giving the fingers a spindle shape) or the wrists; both hands are affected, more or less symmetrically. Swelling of tendon sheaths is usually seen on the dorsum of the wrist, on its ulnar side (extensor carpi ulnaris) and on the volar aspect of the proximal phalanges. The joints are tender and crepitus may be felt on moving the tendons. Joint mobility and grip strength are diminished.

STAGE 2   As the disease progresses, early deformities make their appearance: slight radial deviation of the wrist and ulnar deviation of the fingers; correctible swan-necking; an isolated boutonnière; the sudden appearance of a drop finger or mallet thumb (from extensor tendon rupture).

STAGE 3   In the late stage, long after inflammation may have subsided, established deformities are the rule: the carpus settles into radial tilt and volar subluxation; there is marked ulnar drift of

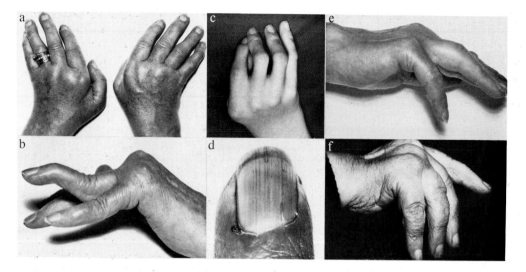

16.13 Rheumatoid arthritis – hands   (a) Ulnar drift; (b) swan-neck deformity; (c) boutonnière deformities; (d) 'nail-fold lesion' due to arteritis; (e) dropped finger; (f) three dropped fingers.

the fingers and volar dislocation of the metacarpophalangeal joints, often associated with multiple swan-neck and boutonnière deformities. When these abnormalities become fixed, functional loss may be so severe that the patient can no longer dress or feed herself.

X-rays

During *stage 1* the x-rays show only soft-tissue swelling and osteoporosis around the joints. In *stage 2* joint 'space' narrowing and small periarticular erosions appear; these are commonest at the metacarpophalangeal joints and in the styloid process of the ulna. In *stage 3* articular destruction may be marked, affecting the metacarpophalangeal, proximal interphalangeal and wrist joints almost equally. Joint deformity and dislocation are common.

Treatment

IN STAGE 1   treatment is directed essentially at controlling the systemic disease and the local synovitis. In addition to general measures (page 39), splints may reduce pain and swelling and improve mobility. *These splints are not corrective but are designed to rest inflamed joints and tendons*; in mild

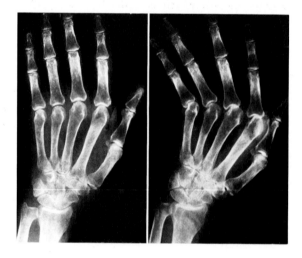

16.14 Rheumatoid arthritis – ulnar drift   These x-rays were taken 2 years apart; they show how the progressive finger deformity is accompanied by (perhaps preceded by) an equal and opposite wrist deformity, in which the entire carpus moves ulnarwards and rotates radialwards.

cases they are worn only at night, in more active cases during the day as well. Persistent synovitis of a few joints or tendon sheaths may benefit from local injections of the 'anti-inflammatory cocktail' containing methylprednisolone (40 mg), nitrogen mustard (1 ml of a 0.02% solution) and 1%

lignocaine (1 ml); only small quantities are injected (e.g. 0.5 ml for a metacarpophalangeal joint or flexor tendon sheath, and 1 ml for the wrist). This should not be repeated more than two or three times. A boggy flexor tenosynovitis may not respond to this limited therapeutic assault; operative synovectomy may be needed. If carpal tunnel symptoms are present, the transverse carpal ligament is divided.

IN STAGE 2   it becomes increasingly important to prevent deformity. Uncontrolled synovitis of joints or tendons requires operative synovectomy followed by physiotherapy. Excision of the distal end of the ulna, synovectomy of the common extensor sheath and the wrist, and reconstruction of the soft tissues on the ulnar side of the wrist may arrest joint destruction and progressive deformity. Early instability and ulnar drift at the metacarpophalangeal joints can be corrected by excising the inflamed synovium, tightening the capsular structures, releasing the ulnar pull of the

intrinsic tendons and hitching the proximal phalanx back into position by reinforcing the extensor attachment to the base of the finger. A mobile boutonnière also can be treated operatively (page 192). Isolated tendon ruptures are repaired or bypassed by appropriate tendon transfers. All these procedures are followed by dynamic splintage and physiotherapy.

IN STAGE 3   deformity is combined with articular destruction; soft-tissue correction alone will not suffice. For the metacarpophalangeal and interphalangeal joints of the thumb, arthrodesis gives predictable pain relief, stability and functional improvement. The metacarpophalangeal joints of the fingers can be excised and replaced with Silastic 'spacers', which improve stability and correct deformity. Replacement of interphalangeal joints gives less predictable results; if deformity is very disabling (e.g. a fixed swan-neck) it may be better to settle for arthrodesis in a more functional position. At the wrist, painless

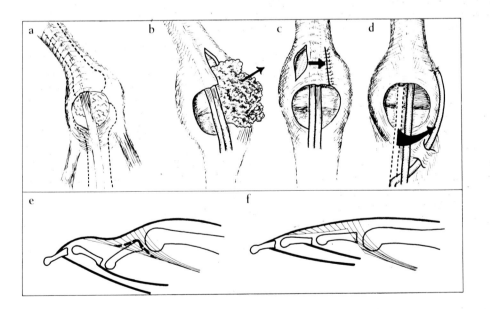

16.15 Rheumatoid arthritis – treatment   (a)Synovial hypertrophy has 'shouldered' the extensor tendon out of its groove: the resulting ulnar drift may be treated by synovectomy (b), followed by dividing the capsule on the ulnar side and reefing it on the radial side (c), and by rerouting the extensor indicis proprius (d). Swan-neck deformity (e). Littler's release (f) is useful before stiffness develops.

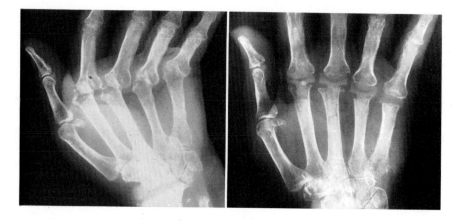

16.16 Rheumatoid arthritis – treatment   In advanced rheumatoid arthritis the metacarpophalangeal joints may be completely dislocated, as they were in this patient; joint replacement with flexible Silastic spacers corrected her deformity and restored stability.

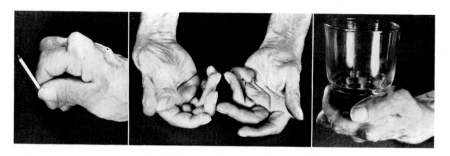

16.17 Rheumatoid arthritis – does it need treatment?   Not always. Why interfere if deformities have been present for years and the hand still works? Despite gross deformity this patient can manipulate tiny objects and large ones.

stability can be regained by replacing the joint with a Silastic prosthesis or, if need be, by arthrodesis in slight flexion and ulnar deviation.

When planning these procedures the golden rule is: *stabilize proximal joints before tackling distal joints.*

Acute infections of the hand

Almost invariably, staphylococci have been implanted by trivial or unobserved injury. Streptococcal infections occasionally occur and cause widespread disturbance.

Clinical features

Usually there is a history of trauma, but it may have been so trivial as to pass unnoticed. A few hours or days later the finger becomes painful and swollen. The patient may be ill and pyrexial. The local signs are as follows.

● LOOK   The finger may be red and swollen. Oedema of the dorsum of the hand is common in any infection. Red streaks on the forearm indicate lymphangitis.

- FEEL   Palpation must be gentle, but the site of maximal tenderness is important for diagnosis and treatment, and must be carefully pinpointed. Sometimes fluctuation can be elicited. Enlarged axillary lymph nodes may be palpable.

- MOVE   With superficial infections the patient can move his finger, though he may be unwilling to do so. With deep infections the finger is immobile.

- X-RAY   Severe pulp infections may lead to bone necrosis which is shown by x-ray.

Treatment

Superficial hand infections are common; if their treatment is delayed or inadequate, infection may rapidly extend, with serious consequences.

The essentials of treatment are as follows.

PENICILLIN   Penicillin must be given in large doses immediately a hand infection is seen, and suitable antibiotic therapy continued until there is healing.

DRAINAGE   Drainage is essential as soon as pus forms or its presence is suspected. A tourniquet and adequate anaesthesia are necessary. There are no standard incisions, but no incision should cross a skin crease. Nearly always the incision should be small and at the site of maximal tenderness. (With the use of antibiotics, the old-fashioned long incisions are hardly ever necessary.) When pus is encountered it must be carefully mopped away and a search made for deeper pockets of infection. It may be necessary to snip away necrotic skin. A drain is unnecessary, and only dry dressings are used. The pus obtained is sent for culture.

REST AND ELEVATION   Rest and elevation are important in all hand infections. Once the acute inflammation has subsided, gentle movements are begun.

Infections at special sites

Subcutaneous tissues

NAIL BED (PARONYCHIA)   Infection beneath the horny layer of skin at the nail base or edge is common. The infected area is slightly swollen, red or purulent, and locally tender. Finger movements are full.

Unless discharge is already free, a portion of the nail may need to be excised.

PULP (WHITLOW)   Pulp infection is common. Swelling is resisted by the fibrous bands connecting bone to skin, so that pain is severe and bone necrosis may occur. The finger tip is swollen, red and locally very tender. The patient guards the finger against contact; he is unwilling but able to move the finger.

Early drainage is essential. Under antibiotic cover a small incision over the site of maximal tenderness is usually sufficient, but the incision may need to be enlarged in late cases when the pus has extended. If healing is delayed, x-rays may show a sequestrum which should be removed.

ELSEWHERE IN THE HAND   Anywhere in the hand a blister or superficial cut may become infected, causing local redness, swelling and tenderness. A local collection of pus should be drained through a small incision over the site of maximal tenderness. It is important to exclude a deeper pocket of pus.

Subcutaneous infection over the front of the middle phalanx carries the risk of involving a tendon sheath. Infection in a web space may also extend, usually along the lumbrical canal and thence either forwards through the palmar fascia or backwards between the metacarpal bones. In all these instances the importance of seeking a deeper pocket of pus is obvious.

Erysipeloid   Erysipeloid is a specific infection of one finger in meat or fish porters. It is rapidly cured by penicillin.

Tendon sheaths (suppurative tenosynovitis)

Pus in a tendon sheath is uncommon but dangerous and painful. It is liable to leave a stiff finger because of synovial adhesions.

MIDDLE THREE FINGERS   The affected finger is swollen and looks like a sausage. It is held bent, is very tender and the patient will not move it or permit it to be moved.

Usually two transverse incisions are necessary, one near the distal end of the sheath and one near the proximal end; using a ureteric catheter the

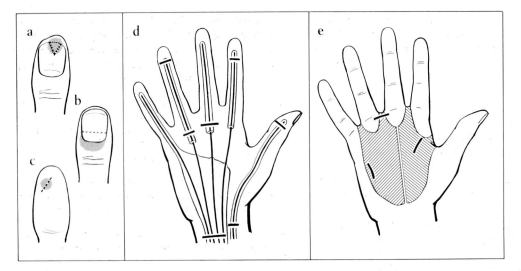

16.18 Infections (a) To drain an apical abscess it is often best to excise a triangle of nail. (b) Acute paronychia is most efficiently drained by excising the proximal part of the nail. (c) A pulp abscess should be drained over the point of maximal tenderness. (d) Synovial sheath infections can be drained by incisions near their proximal or distal ends, or both. (e) Incisions for web abscess and for the rare infections of the mid-palmar and thenar spaces (partly redrawn from *Infections of the Hand* by D. N. Bailey, published by H. K. Lewis, London).

sheath is then irrigated with penicillin; with localized infections one incision is sometimes sufficient. Delayed healing may be caused by necrosis of tendon, and if so the tendon should be removed or the finger amputated.

THUMB AND LITTLE FINGER   Tendon-sheath infection in the thumb may spread to the radial bursa, and in the little finger to the ulnar bursa. The affected digit is swollen, bent, tender and held still, and swelling and tenderness extend proximally.

In addition to draining the digital portion of the sheath the ulnar or radial bursa may need to be drained through transverse incisions just above the wrist; the sheath is then irrigated with penicillin.

Fascial spaces

Infection from a web space or from an infected tendon sheath may spread to either of the deep fascial spaces of the palm.

MEDIAL SPACE (MIDPALMAR)   The palm is ballooned so that its normal concavity is lost. There is extensive tenderness and the whole hand is held still. For drainage an incision is made directly over the abscess, and sinus forceps inserted; if the web space also is infected it too should be incised.

LATERAL SPACE (THENAR)   The palm is flat, there is deep tenderness, and the thumb and index finger are held still. For drainage the skin is incised in the first web and the abscess opened with sinus forceps.

PROXIMAL EXTENSIONS   From medial or lateral space infections, pus may track up the forearm where it can be drained by anteromedial or anterolateral incisions.

Open injuries of the hand

In the USA, 2 million disabling work injuries occur annually; 75 per cent affect the hand. In Britain the problem is equally serious. Early and expert surgery is essential to minimize disability; the care of the injured hand is no job for the junior casualty officer. He should, however, be cautioned to avoid irritants such as iodine or spirit; only bland substances (e.g. cetrimide) should be applied.

Signs

Detailed examination may have to await exploration, but careful preoperative assessment is important if needless groping is to be avoided. The spectrum of open injuries embraces tidy or 'clean' cuts, lacerations, crushing and injection injuries, burns and pulp defects. The patient's occupation and social status are important.

Skin damage is the dominant factor. 'Untidy' wounds, degloving and crushed skin are all serious, but even a tiny clean cut may conceal nerve or tendon damage. Localized swelling may suggest an injection injury or a traumatic aneurysm. Sensation is tested and retested several times. Active movements are tested to assess tendon damage, but if this is too painful the resting attitude of the fingers is a useful guide.

X-RAY   Fractures, dislocations or foreign bodies may be seen by x-ray.

Primary treatment

Preoperative procedures

PROPHYLAXIS   Antibiotics, if indicated, are given as soon as possible, and suitable prophylactics against tetanus and gas-gangrene.

ANAESTHETIC   General anaesthesia is preferable, though brachial or axillary block can be used, or even digital block for finger-tip injuries.

TOURNIQUET   A high pneumatic tourniquet, applied after elevating the limb, is helpful but not essential. It should certainly not be used with crush injuries, where muscle viability is in doubt.

CLEANING   The wound is covered with a sterile pack while the neighbouring skin is cleaned with cetrimide.

POSITION   The hand must be placed on an arm table in a good light. The sterile pack is removed, the wound itself gently cleaned with cetrimide and towelled off.

Wound excision and deep repair

SKIN   Do not excise a strip of skin around the wound – skin is too precious to waste. Only

obviously dead skin should be removed. For adequate exposure the wound may need enlarging, but incisions must not cross a skin crease, nor an interdigital web. Through the enlarged wound, loose débris is picked out.

Burns   with only partial skin loss are cleaned, and covered with non-stick dressings backed by wool; the limb is elevated. The dressing is left undisturbed for 10–14 days, but finger movements are encouraged. (Treatment by exposure, practised in some burns units, demands a specially clean environment.) With whole-thickness skin loss, devitalized tissue is excised, the wound cleaned and dressed, and 5 days later skin-grafted. Electric burns may cause extensive damage and thrombosis which become apparent only after several days.

SUBCUTANEOUS TISSUES   *Injection injuries* of oil or paint under pressure are damaging because of tension, toxicity or both. Immediate decompression and removal of the foreign substance offers the best hope, but most reported series feature a high incidence of finger or partial hand amputation.

EXTENSOR TENDONS   Primary repair is easy and safe; the only contraindication is a dirty wound.

FLEXOR TENDONS   Repair must not be attempted if the wound is grossly contaminated, or if the ends can be found only by extensive dissection. With cuts proximal to the vincula, the profundus tendon may retract high into the palm.

Division of the sublimis tendon alone causes little disability and does not require repair. All other lacerations of one or both tendons at any level should ideally be treated by primary suture – but only if the cut is clean, operation is early and the surgeon sufficiently expert. Otherwise only cuts proximal to the flexor sheath or distal to the sublimis insertion should be sutured directly. Those within the flexor sheath (between the distal palmar crease and the proximal interphalangeal joint) are liable to form adhesions if sutured, and are therefore best left alone; the wound is closed and secondary suture or grafting carried out 3–6 weeks later.

Technique of primary suture   The cut tendon is exposed through a mid-axial incision in the finger or a zig-zag extension of the skin wound. Proximal to the flexor sheath repair is easy and the suture line can be covered by one of the lumbrical muscles. Distal to the sublimis insertion only the profundus will be divided; it can be sutured to the stump or reattached to the bone without disturbing the sublimis. Cuts within the flexor sheath are meticulously repaired by the Kleinert technique (Kleinert *et al.*, 1973); if both tendons are divided, both are sutured. As much of the tendon sheath as possible is preserved. The finger is held in flexion by an elastic splint which

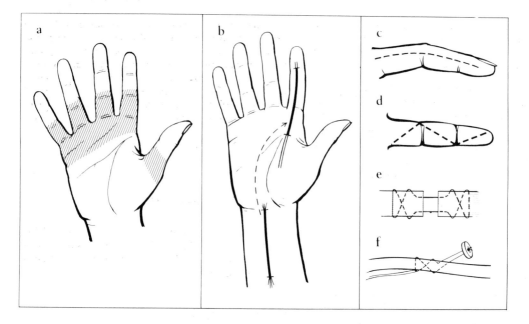

16.19 Tendon injuries   (a) Zones of the hand (redrawn from *Injuries of the Hand* by R. J. Furlong, published by Churchill, London). The intermediate zone (shaded) contains two tendons and two sheaths; primary suture usually fails. (b) The principle of tendon grafting to replace a cut profundus. (c) Mid-axial incision. (d) Bruner's zig-zag incision. (e) One method of tendon suture. (f) Bunnell's pull-out technique.

allows active extension; after 3 weeks the splint is removed and exercises are begun.

MUSCLE   Muscle damage occurs only in the palm and mainly in the thenar and hypothenar eminences. Dead or doubtfully viable muscle is excised with meticulous care to avoid nerves.

NERVE   Digital nerves are best repaired at the primary operation, provided the wound is not too dirty and no extensive dissection is needed.

JOINTS   Suture of torn capsule and ligaments helps to restore stability and permit early movement.

BONES   Fractures are reduced and subsequently treated as described in Chapter 24. If the fracture is unstable, internal fixation is sometimes employed. The risk is worth taking because stiffness in the hand from prolonged external splintage is so disabling; percutaneous pinning techniques are used.

Amputation   Amputation of a finger as a primary procedure should be avoided unless the damage involves many tissues and is clearly irreparable. Even when a finger has been amputated by the injury, the possibility of reattachment should be considered.

Wound closure

HAEMOSTASIS   The tourniquet is removed and meticulous haemostasis obtained. The success of the operation depends largely upon this and skin healing.

SKIN CLOSURE   Only if the wound is grossly contaminated is closure delayed for a few days. Nearly always immediate closure is carried out by one of three methods.

Direct suture   This method is preferred if it can be achieved without tension and with only slight undercutting of skin edges.

Free skin grafts   These are often useful as temporary cover. They are usually taken from the front of the forearm and stitched into place. Partial-thickness grafts take better, though it may be necessary later to replace them with full-thickness grafts.

Flap grafts   Flap grafts are necessary if tendon or bare bone is exposed, for thin grafts do not take on these tissues. Flap grafts may be taken from local or distant sites. Sometimes a severely mutilated finger is sacrificed and its skin used as a rotation flap. A skin graft must be fixed securely and without dead space.

Pulp and finger-tip injuries   Split-skin or full-thickness grafts are conventional, but in most children and selected adults spontaneous healing (carefully supervised) offers an equally good appearance, with better sensation.

DRESSING   The wound is covered with several thicknesses of dry gauze, and ample wool soaked in flavine–paraffin emulsion. A firm crêpe bandage ensures even pressure, and a light plaster slab holds the wrist and hand with the metacarpophalangeal joints in flexion and the interphalangeal joints in extension. If possible, the finger tips are left visible.

Postoperative plan

IMMEDIATE AFTER-CARE   The hand is kept elevated and at rest. Antibiotics are continued as necessary. For the first 3 weeks the dressing is not disturbed unless the fingers become unduly swollen or blue or numb.

ASSESSMENT   At 3 weeks the dressings are taken off. It is now possible to estimate, from the state of healing and a knowledge of the operative findings, what the future function of the hand is likely to be.

The sensory and the various motor functions (see page 186) are separately assessed. With this information, and a knowledge of the patient's work and hobbies, the nature of further treatment can be decided; it may be conservative (rehabilitation) or operative.

REHABILITATION   When the wound has healed, active exercises and wax baths are started. The hand is increasingly used for more and more arduous and complex tasks, especially those which resemble the patient's normal job, until he is fit to start work; if necessary, his work is modified temporarily. Even if further surgery is required, tendon or nerve repair is postponed until the skin is healthy, there is no oedema and the joints have regained a normal range of passive movement.

Secondary operations

One of three procedures may be necessary: secondary repair or replacement of damaged structures, amputation of fingers, or reconstruction of a mutilated hand.

Secondary repair

SKIN   If the skin cover has broken down or is unsuitable for surgery it is replaced by a graft. As always, the skin creases must be respected. Contractures are dealt with by Z-plasty or skin replacement. When important volar surfaces are insensitive, a flap of skin complete with its nerve supply may be transposed (sensory flap).

TENDONS   Primary suture may have been contraindicated by wound contamination, undue delay between injury and repair, or inadequate operating facilities. In these circumstances secondary repair or tendon grafting is necessary.

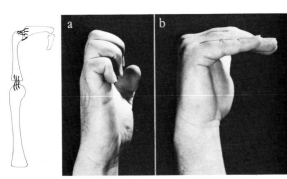 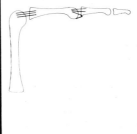

16.20 Position for splintage   Fingers must not be splinted in position (a). The ligaments must be kept taut, otherwise they contract, causing stiffness. At the metacarpophalangeal joints the collateral ligaments are taut at 90 degrees; at the interphalangeal joints the important ligaments linking the volar plate to the collaterals are taut when the joint is fully straight. This is why James (1970) rightly insists on position (b) as the only safe one for splintage.

Cuts proximal to the flexor sheath   can be treated by direct suture as a secondary procedure; the suture line is protected by wrapping the lumbrical muscle round it.

Cuts in the flexor sheath   If the sublimis tendon alone is cut and the proximal end forms an uncomfortable lump, it should be excised. A cut profundus may be left if the patient is willing to accept the disability; otherwise a tendon graft is necessary.

Technique of tendon graft   Three donor sites can be used: (1) sublimis tendon from the injured finger (but this has no paratenon); (2), the fourth toe extensor (but this is rather thin, and the foot operation keeps the patient in bed); (3) palmaris longus tendon (the best) which must be excised with a wide margin of paratenon. It is absent in some people and its presence must be confirmed before operation.

The cut tendon is exposed by a longitudinal incision just behind the flexor finger creases (mid-axial), or by a zig-zag incision (Fig. 16.19, page 202).

The fibrous sheath is next excised, leaving a pulley opposite the proximal phalanx and one opposite the middle phalanx. Through a separate incision in the proximal palmar crease the sublimis tendon is excised and the profundus tendon trimmed. The graft is then sutured to the proximal profundus stump, threaded through the pulleys and sutured to the distal profundus stump with the finger flexed. (In difficult situations a Silastic 'tendon' is used as a spacer at this stage; 10 weeks later it is replaced by the tendon graft.)

Distal zone   Only the profundus tendon can have been cut. The disability of a flail terminal phalanx may require surgery. Possible procedures are: (1) a tenodesis to stabilize the joint in 30 degrees of flexion; (2) an arthrodesis in the same position; (3) a tendon graft as described above, which is capable of restoring normal function but necessitates excision of an undamaged sublimis tendon, thus entailing a risk of leaving the finger worse than before operation; or (4) advancing the profundus tendon and reattaching it to the terminal phalanx.

NERVES   Cut median or ulnar nerves are repaired in the usual way. Digital nerves also are sutured if the finger has satisfactory motor function, but suture distal to the knuckle often fails. Useful sensation can sometimes be restored by using a sensory cross-finger pedicle graft.

JOINTS   Joint stiffness is best treated by active exercises. Stiff knuckle joints are sometimes helped by capsulotomy. Flail joints are stabilized by tenodesis or arthrodesis.

BONES   Malunion hardly ever requires treatment. Non-union is exceedingly rare, but grafting may be required.

Amputation

INDICATIONS   A finger is amputated only if it remains painful or unhealed, or is a nuisance (that is, if the patient cannot flex it, or cannot straighten it or cannot feel with it) and then only if repair is impossible or uneconomic.

TECHNIQUE   The aim is a mobile digit covered by healthy skin with normal sensation. A palmar flap is best and must always be ample in size; a tight flap usually gives pain.*

In the thumb every millimetre is worth preserving; even a stiff or deformed thumb is worth keeping. The index and little fingers are amputated as distally as possible, provided there is voluntary control of the proximal phalanx; if not, oblique amputation through the metacarpal shaft gives a good cosmetic result.

The middle and ring fingers should not be amputated through the knuckle joint, or the hand will be ugly and coins fall through it. If the proximal phalanx can be left, the hand is still ugly but stronger. Alternatively, the entire finger with most of its metacarpal may be amputated; the hand is weakened but the amputation is less noticeable.

Late reconstruction

A severely mutilated hand should be dealt with by a hand expert. Three possibilities may be considered in exceptional cases.

(1)   If all the fingers have been lost but the thumb is present, a new finger can sometimes be constructed with cancellous bone, covered by a tube flap of skin.
(2)   If the thumb has been lost the three possibilities are: pollicization (rotating a finger to oppose the other fingers); osteoplastic reconstruction (which requires several operations but may provide a good grip); and toe transplant (usually from the hallux).
(3)   If the thumb and all the fingers have been lost, making a cleft between two metacarpal bones may permit pincer action.

Notes on applied anatomy

The hand serves three basic functions: *sensory perception, precise manipulation* and *power grip*. The first two involve the thumb, index and middle fingers; without normal sensation and the ability to oppose these three digits, manipulative precision will be lost. The ring and little fingers provide power grip, for which they need full flexion though sensation is less important.

*Unless the flap seems too loose it is too tight

With the wrist flexed the fingers and thumb fall naturally into extension. With the wrist extended the fingers curl into flexion and the tips of the thumb, index and middle fingers form a functional tripod; this is the *position of function*, because it is best suited to the actions of prehension.

Finger flexion is strongest when the wrist is powerfully extended; normal grasp is possible only with a painless, stable wrist. Spreading the fingers produces abduction to either side of the middle finger; bringing them together, adduction. Abduction and adduction of the thumb occur in a plane at right angles to the palm (i.e. with the hand lying palm upwards, abduction points the thumb to the ceiling). By a combination of movements the thumb can also be opposed to each of the other fingers. Functionally, the thumb is 40 per cent of the hand.

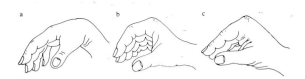

16.21 Three positions of the hand The hand in (a) the position of relaxation, (b) the position of function ('ready for action') and (c) the position of splintage ('ligaments taut').

JOINTS *The carpometacarpal joints* The second and third metacarpals have very little independent movement; the fourth and fifth have more, allowing greater closure of the ulnar part of the hand during power grip. The metacarpal of the thumb is the most mobile and the first carpometacarpal joint is a frequent target for degenerative arthritis.

The metacarpophalangeal joints flex to about 90 degrees, the range increasing progressively from the index to the little finger. The collateral ligaments are lax in extension (permitting abduction) and tight in flexion (preventing abduction). *If these joints are immobilized they should always be in flexion, so that the ligaments are at full stretch and therefore less likely to shorten if they should fibrose.*

The interphalangeal joints are simple hinges, each flexing to about 90 degrees. Their collateral ligaments send attachments to the volar plate and these fibres are tight in extension and lax in flexion; *immobilization of the interphalangeal joints, therefore, should always be in extension.*

MUSCLES AND TENDONS Two sets of muscles control finger movements: the long extrinsic muscles (extensors, deep flexors and superficial flexors), and the short intrinsic muscles (interossei, lumbricals and the short thenar muscles). The extrinsics act synergistically, extending the metacarpophalangeal and flexing the interphalangeal joints; the intrinsics do the

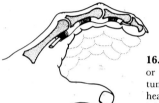

16.22 Anatomy The flexor tendons run in fibrous tunnels from the metacarpal heads to the distal finger joints.

reverse – they flex the metacarpophalangeal and extend the interphalangeal joints. The intrinsics also abduct and adduct the fingers and oppose the thumb. Spasm or contracture of the intrinsics produces the *intrinsic-plus* posture – flexion at the metacarpophalangeal joints, extension at the interphalangeal joints and adduction of the thumb. Paralysis of the intrinsics produces the *intrinsic-minus* posture – hyperextension of the metacarpophalangeal and flexion of the interphalangeal joints ('claw hand').

Tough fibrous sheaths enclose the flexor tendons as they traverse the fingers; starting just proximal to the metacarpophalangeal joints (level with the distal palmar crease) they extend to the distal interphalangeal joints. They serve as runners and pulleys, so preventing the tendons from bowstringing during flexion. Scarring within the fibro-osseous tunnel prevents normal flexion.

The long extensor tendons are prevented from bowstringing at the wrist by the extensor retinaculum; here they are liable to frictional trauma. Over the metacarpophalangeal joints each extensor tendon widens into an expansion which inserts into the proximal phalanx and then splits in three; a central slip inserts into the middle phalanx, the two lateral slips continue distally, join and end in the distal phalanx. Division of the middle slip causes a flexion deformity of the proximal interphalangeal joint (boutonnière); rupture of the distal conjoined slip causes flexion deformity of the distal interphalangeal joint (mallet finger).

NERVES Most of the muscles and the palmar skin of the first three digits (which work together as a functional tripod) are supplied by the median nerve, the muscles and palmar skin of the ring and little fingers by the ulnar nerve, and the long extensors and dorsal skin by the radial nerve. The ulnar nerve also supplies the intrinsics.

SKIN The palmar skin is relatively tight and inelastic; skin loss can be ill-afforded and wounds sutured under tension are liable to break down. The acute sensibility of the digital palmar skin cannot be achieved by any skin graft. By contrast, dorsal skin is lax and mobile, skin wounds are easier to close and skin loss can be readily made good by grafts.

Just deep to the palmar skin is the superficial aponeurosis, which thickens in Dupuytren's contracture. Incisions on the palmar surface are also liable to contracture unless they are placed in the line of the skin creases or along the mid-lateral borders of the fingers.

Further reading

Apley, A. Graham (1956) Test for the power of flexor digitorum sublimis. *British Medical Journal* **1,** 25–26

Boyes, J. H. (Ed.) (1971) *Bunnell's Surgery of the Hand,* 5th edn. Philadelphia: Lippincott

James, J. I. P. (1970) The assessment and mangement of the injured hand. *The Hand* **2,** 97–105

Kleinert, H. E., Kutz, J. E., Atasoy, E. and Stormo, A. (1973) Primary repair of flexor tendons. *Orthopedic Clincis of North America* **4,** 865–876

Lamb, D. W. (1977) Radial club hand. *Journal of Bone and Joint Surgery* **59A,** 1–13

Miura, T., Kino, Y. and Nakamura, R. (1976) Reconstruction of the mutilated hand. *The Hand* **8,** 78–85

Pulvertaft, R. G. (1973) Twenty-five years of hand surgery. *Journal of Bone and Joint Surgery* **55B,** 32–55

Rank, B. K., Wakefield, A. R. and Hueston, J. J. (1973) *Surgery of Repair as Applied to Hand Injuries,* 4th edn. Edinburgh: Churchill Livingstone

Stack, H. G. (1973) *The Palmar Fascia.* Edinburgh: Churchill Livingstone

Wynn Parry, C. B. (1981) *Rehabilitation of the Hand,* 4th edn. London: Butterworths

The Neck

17

Examination

Symptoms

The common symptoms of neck disorder are *pain* in the neck, scapular region or upper limbs; *stiffness* either intermittent or constant; *deformity*, especially wry neck; and *tingling, numbness* or *weakness* in the upper limbs.* Weakness of the lower limbs may result from cord compression.

Headache, especially over the occipitoparietal region, may emanate from the neck, but if this is the only symptom other causes should be suspected. Occasionally facial paraesthesia (and even pain) may be due to cervical pathology.

Signs

No examination of the neck is complete without examination of both upper limbs.

- LOOK
Any deformity is noted; the neck may be flexed forward, tilted sideways or twisted. From the back, skin blemishes, scapular abnormalities or muscular asymmetry can be seen. One shoulder may be higher and there may be muscle wasting in the arm or hand.

- FEEL
The neck is examined for tender areas or lumps. Muscle spasm may be felt. The anterior structures (trachea, thyroid, oesophagus) should be carefully palpated.

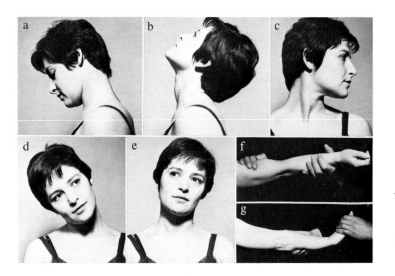

17.1 Examination (a) Flexion, (b) extension, (c) rotation, (d, e) sideways tilt; (f, g) testing power in the elbow and wrist extensors. In this patient with signs of a prolapsed disc, flexion and tilting to the left are limited.

*2 arms = 1 neck; if both arms are affected, suspect the neck.

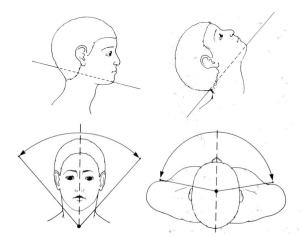

17.2 Normal range of movement   In full flexion the chin normally touches the chest; in full extension the imaginary line joining the chin to the posterior occipital protuberance (the occipitomental line) forms an angle of at least 45 degrees with the horizontal, and usually over 60 degrees in young people. Lateral flexion and rotation are equal in both directions.

● MOVE

Forward flexion, extension, lateral flexion and rotation are tested, and then shoulder movements.

NEUROLOGICAL EXAMINATION

Neurological examination of the upper limbs is mandatory in all cases; in some the lower limbs should be examined as well.

PULSES

The radial pulse is felt with the arm at rest and on traction; it may weaken or disappear if the thoracic outlet is abnormally tight. The subclavian artery also is palpated; it is much easier to feel if a cervical rib is present.

● X-RAY

The anteroposterior view should show the regular, undulating outline of the lateral masses; their symmetry may be disturbed by destructive lesions or fractures. A projection through the mouth is required to show the upper two vertebrae. In the lateral view the cervical curve shows four parallel lines: one along the anterior surfaces of the vertebral bodies, one along their posterior surfaces, one along the posterior borders of the lateral masses and one along the bases of the spinous processes; any malalignment suggests subluxation (see Fig. 25.4, page 418). The disc spaces are

inspected and the posterior interspinous spaces compared; if one is wider than the rest, it suggests subluxation or vertebral tilting. Osteophytes are sought; in oblique views their relationship to the intervertebral foramina can be seen. Flexion and extension views are required to demonstrate instability.

COMPUTERIZED TOMOGRAPHY

In the cervical spine, computerized tomography may be invaluable; it shows the shape of the spinal canal and the integrity of the bony structures.

Infantile torticollis (congenital muscular torticollis)

The sternomastoid muscle on one side is fibrous and fails to elongate as the child grows; consequently progressive deformity develops. The cause is unknown; the muscle may have suffered ischaemia from a distorted position *in utero* (the association with breech presentation and hip dysplasia is supporting evidence), or it may have been injured at birth.

Clinical features

A history of difficult labour or breech delivery is common. In 20 per cent of patients a lump is noticed in the first few weeks of life; it is well-defined and involves one or both heads of the sternomastoid. At this stage there is neither deformity nor obvious limitation of movement and within a few months the lump has disappeared.

Deformity does not become apparent until the child is 3 or 4 years old. During growth, as the normal sternomastoid gradually elongates, discrepancy becomes more obvious. It is as though, on the affected side, the mastoid process were growing closer to the sternal notch; consequently, the ear becomes lower and further forward. In fact, on the affected side the entire face is tilted downwards, twisted forwards and is shorter than on the normal side. The sternomastoid tendon feels tight and cord-like, restricting movements away from the affected side. Secondary facial deformities may occur. X-rays are normal.

Treatment

PROPHYLAXIS   If a child has had a sternomastoid 'tumour' every effort should be made to prevent torticollis from developing. Each day a physiotherapist or the mother manipulates the neck into a position which elongates the affected sternomastoid to the full. The baby is laid to sleep on alternate sides.

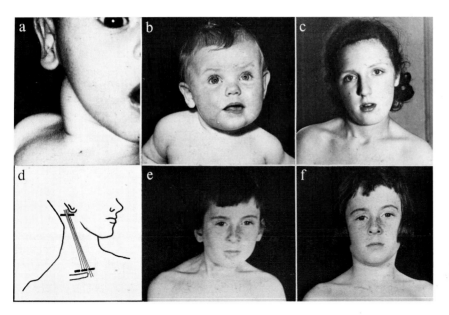

17.3 Torticollis   Natural history: (a) sternomastoid tumour in a young baby, (b) early wry neck, (c) deformity with facial hemiatrophy in the adolescent.
Surgical treatment: (d) two sites at which the sternomastoid may be divided; (e, f) before and a few months after operation.

STRETCHING AND SPLINTAGE   If, when the child is first seen, the head cannot be tilted fully in the direction opposite to that of the deformity, daily stretching is followed by the application of a splint or a linen skull-cap attached by tapes tied under the axilla. This treatment is continued until the child naturally comes to hold its head correctly and the cap is worn at night for a further 6 months at least. A careful watch is kept for recurrence of the deformity.

OPERATIONS   One of three procedures designed to elongate the sternomastoid is indicated if stretching fails or the deformity is not seen until the age of 3–4 years.

Subcutaneous tenotomy at the lower end   This must be carefully performed if the vessels are to be avoided, but leaves no visible scar – an important consideration in an operation which is performed mainly for cosmetic reasons.

Open division of the lower end   A transverse incision is used, and the tendon divided. The anaesthetist then twists the child's head so as to obtain further correction of the deformity, and tight fascial bands are divided; this must be repeated until complete overcorrection is achieved. The operation is completely safe and the scar hardly visible.

Division of the upper end   This procedure may be performed alone, or may be combined with either of the above methods, the advantage being that the scar is hidden by the hair.

After operation correction must be maintained, at first by a skull-cap tied under the axilla, then by a polythene collar which holds the head over and is worn for several months until the child has learnt to hold his head correctly.

Secondary torticollis

A tilt or twist of the neck may develop as a result of acute disc prolapse (the commonest cause in adults), so-called fibrositis (usually a prolapsed cervical disc), skin scarring (especially after burns), inflamed neck glands, vertebral tuberculosis, ocular disorders or injuries of the cervical spine. In all these the diagnosis is usually obvious; the condition does not necessarily date from infancy and there is no facial asymmetry.

'Spasmodic torticollis' is also a secondary deformity, and is thought to be due to a neurological or psychological disorder. The sternomastoid muscle is in marked spasm, and the head grossly twisted. Sometimes violent jerking movements occur or are provoked by attempted correction.

The treatment of secondary torticollis is that of the primary cause.

Prolapsed cervical disc

Cause and pathology

The factors responsible for a prolapsed cervical disc are the same as those for lumbar disc prolapse: injury (especially sudden unguarded movements), absorption of fluid causing nuclear tension to increase, and degenerative changes in the annulus (see page 231).

Prolapsed material may press on (1) the dura mater, causing neck pain and stiffness; or (2) the nerve roots, causing pain and paraesthesia in one or both arms. Prolapse usually occurs immediately above or below the sixth cervical vertebra, so that the nerve roots affected are C6 or C7.

Clinical features

The original attack, unlike that of lumbar disc prolapse, can seldom be related to definite and severe strain. It often occurs when a patient stretches himself on waking.

Subsequent attacks may be sudden or gradual in onset, and with trivial cause. The patient may complain of:

(1) Pain and stiffness of the neck; the pain often radiates to the scapular region and sometimes to the occiput.
(2) Pain and paraesthesia in one upper limb (rarely both), often radiating to the outer elbow, back of the wrist and to the index and middle fingers. Weakness is rare.

Between attacks the patient feels well. There are no general signs and the patient is a fit adult.

NECK SIGNS (DURING AN ATTACK)
The neck may be tilted forwards and may also be tilted sideways. Tender areas are felt in the posterior neck muscles, the trapezius and the scapular region. Some movements are restricted and painful, but at least one movement is full and painless unless the attack is very severe. Shoulder movements are full.

X-RAY At the affected level the normal lordosis is interrupted and the disc space is often narrowed.

ARM SIGNS
The arms should be examined for neurological deficit. The C6 root innervates the biceps jerk, the biceps muscle and wrist dorsiflexors, and

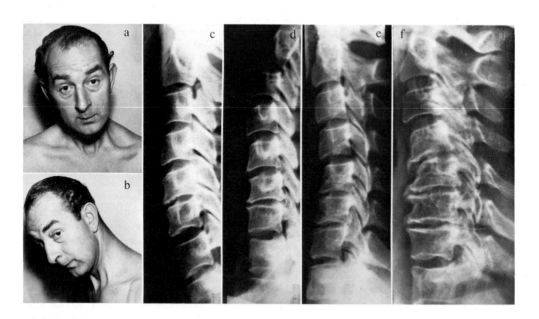

17.4 Cervical disc lesions (a, b) Acute wry neck due to prolapsed disc. (c) A reduced disc space at C5/6 is not necessarily significant when the cervical lordosis is normal; in (d) the lordosis is obliterated, and in (e) it is reversed – both strongly suggest a prolapsed disc. (f) Spondylosis, with multiple disc degeneration.

sensation of the lateral forearm, thumb and index finger; C7 innervates the triceps and radial jerks, the triceps muscle, wrist palmarflexors and finger extensors, and sensation in the middle finger.

Differential diagnosis

CERVICAL RIB SYNDROME Pain is felt usually in the ulnar forearm and hand, a lump may be palpable in the neck and the rib may show on x-ray.

CARPAL TUNNEL SYNDROME Neck movements are painless, and the pain in the hand is felt on the palmar surface in the distribution of the median nerve. Nerve conduction is slowed across the wrist.

SUPRASPINATUS TENDON LESIONS Although the distribution of pain may resemble that of a prolapsed cervical disc, movements at the shoulder joint are abnormal.

CERVICAL TUMOURS With tumours of the spinal cord, nerve roots or cervical lymph nodes, the symptoms are not intermittent and the x-ray picture may be abnormal. Tumours of the cervical vertebrae are seen on x-ray.

CERVICAL SPINE INFECTIONS The symptoms do not occur in attacks, there may be an abscess, and x-rays show narrowing of a disc space and bone destruction.

NEURALGIC AMYOTROPHY Pain is sudden and severe; multiple neurological levels are involved.

Treatment

Heat and analgesics are soothing but, as with lumbar disc prolapse, there are only three satisfactory ways of treating the prolapse itself.

REST A collar is comforting and prevents unguarded movement; it may be made of cardboard and felt, stiff sponge-rubber, polythene or metal.

REDUCE Traction may enlarge the disc space, thus permitting the disc to slip back into place. The head of the couch is raised and weights are tied to a harness fitting under the chin and occiput. Up to 7 kg may be used for 6 hours daily. Continuous traction using up to 5 kg for 48 hours is more effective but the patient must be in hospital and sedated. Rapid reduction by manipulation (without anaesthetic) can be effective, and is probably safe provided the neck is first pulled in the extended position.

REMOVE If symptoms are refractory and severe enough for operation, the disc is removed through an anterior approach; bone grafts are inserted to fuse the affected area and to restore the normal intervertebral height.

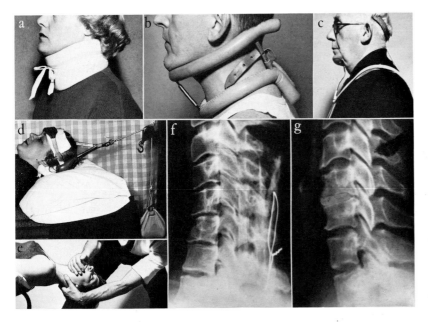

17.5 Cervical disc treatment (a, b, c) Varieties of collar; (d) outpatient traction; (e) manipulation. Operation is rarely needed; grafting from the back (f) is being superseded by anterior fusion (g), which necessarily includes disc removal.

Cervical spondylosis

Spondylosis is the commonest disorder of the cervical spine. The lower cervical discs degenerate and disc material extrudes; surrounding fibrosis may spread to the root sleeves. The edges of the vertebral bodies hypertrophy (lipping) and later the intervertebral joints degenerate.

Symptoms

The patient, aged over 40, complains of neck pain which comes on gradually and is often worse on first getting up. The pain may radiate widely: to the occiput and frontal region; to the scapular muscles; and down one or both arms. Paraesthesia, weakness and clumsiness are occasionally symptoms.

Signs

The appearance is normal. Tenderness in the posterior neck muscles and scapular region is common, and all movements are slightly limited by pain at their extremes.

LIMB SIGNS   In one or both upper limbs numbness or weakness may occasionally be found. Very rarely, the lower limbs may have increased tone and brisk reflexes from upper motor neuron pressure.

X-RAY   Several disc spaces are diminished, and the corners of the vertebrae show lipping. (Identical x-ray changes may be present in a patient with no symptoms.)

NOTE   When a normal neck is moved the vertebral and basilar arteries have a considerable excursion. If the fibrosis associated with spondylosis sufficiently restricts this excursion the patient, on twisting his neck, may feel dizzy or even black out and fall. Angiography demonstrates the lesion.

Treatment

Heat and massage are often soothing, but restricting neck movements in a collar is the most effective treatment during painful periods.

Operation is sometimes indicated. If severe symptoms are relieved only by a rigid and irksome support, anterior spinal fusion is valuable. Very rarely, when abnormal signs in upper and lower limbs are not abolished by splintage or traction, decompression by laminectomy is performed.

Technique of anterior cervical fusion   The patient lies supine with the neck supported on a sandbag and the head turned to one side. At the appropriate disc level a transverse incision is made to one side of the midline. The plane between the trachea and the carotid sheath leads to the anterior surface of the spine. The central portion of the affected disc together with the adjacent bone is excised; the gap is filled with a corticocancellous bone graft. After the operation the patient wears a brace for 3–4 months.

Tuberculosis of the cervical spine

Cervical spine tuberculosis is very rare. The presenting symptoms may vary from trivial neck pain to tetraplegia. Deformity is usually slight, though the normal cervical lordosis may be lost and there may be torticollis. Movements are limited, provoking pain and spasm when attempted. X-rays usually show bone destruction with a narrowed disc space and forward angulation. If there is an abscess it may be retropharyngeal, or present behind the sternomastoid muscle.

Anti-tuberculous drugs are given (page 28). The neck must be held still, but this is so irksome that, when the general condition permits, operation is advised. Through an anterior approach caseous material is evacuated and bone grafts are used to fix the diseased vertebrae together.

Rheumatoid arthritis

The cervical spine is severely affected in 30 per cent of patients with rheumatoid arthritis. Three types of lesion are common: (1) erosion of the atlantoaxial joints and the transverse ligament, with resulting instability; (2) erosion of the atlanto-occipital articulations, allowing the odontoid peg to ride up into the foramen magnum; and (3) erosion of the facet joints in the mid-cervical region, sometimes ending in fusion but more often leading to subluxation.

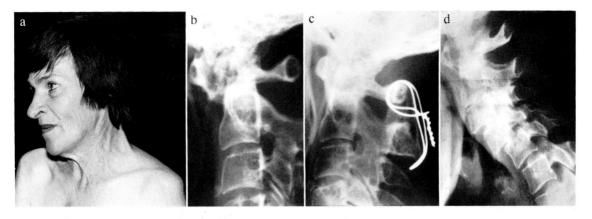

17.6 Rheumatoid arthritis (a) Movement is severely restricted; attempted rotation causes pain and muscle spasm. (b) Atlantoaxial subluxation is common; erosion of the joints and the transverse ligament has allowed the atlas to slip forward about 2 cm; (c) reduction and posterior fusion with wire fixation. (d) This patient has subluxation not only at the atlantoaxial joint, but also at two levels in the mid-cervical region.

Symptoms and signs

The patient is usually a woman with advanced rheumatoid disease. She has neck pain and may support her head in her hands. Movements are markedly restricted.

X-rays, if carefully done, show the abnormality. (1) Atlantoaxial instability is visible in lateral films taken in flexion and extension; in flexion the anterior arch of the atlas rides forwards leaving a gap of 5 mm or more between the back of the anterior arch and the odontoid process; on extension the subluxation is reduced. (2) Atlanto-occipital erosion is more difficult to see, but a lateral tomograph shows the relationship of the odontoid to the foramen magnum. (3) Flexion views show anterior subluxation in the mid-cervical region.

Symptoms and signs of root compression may appear in the upper limbs; less often there is lower limb weakness and upper motor neuron signs due to cord compression.

Treatment

Despite the startling x-ray appearances, serious neurological complications are uncommon. Pain can usually be relieved by wearing a collar. Only if it is persistent and severe, or associated with increasing neurological deficit, is posterior spinal fusion advised.

Neuralgic amyotrophy (acute brachial neuritis)

This unusual cause of severe shoulder pain and weakness is believed to be a viral infection of the cervical nerve roots; there is often a history of an antecedent viral infection and sometimes a small epidemic occurs among inmates of an institution.

The history alone often suggests the diagnosis. Pain in the shoulder and arm is intense and sudden in onset. It may extend into the neck and down as far as the hand; usually it lasts a few days but may continue for weeks. Other symptoms are paraesthesia in the arm or hand, and weakness of the muscles of the shoulder, forearm and hand.

Wasting of the deltoid or the small muscles of the hand may be obvious after only a few days, and winging of the scapula is common. Shoulder

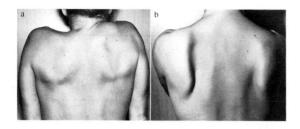

17.7 Neuralgic amyotrophy   (a, b) This young nurse complained of acute neck and shoulder pain on the left. She has weakness of levator scapulae and slight winging of the left scapula. The neurological defect usually returns to normal but occasionally wasting and weakness are permanent.

movement is limited by pain but this is invariably transient. Sensory loss in one or more of the cervical dermatomes is not uncommon. The feature that distinguishes neuralgic amyotrophy from an acute cervical disc herniation is the involvement of multiple nerve root levels.

There is no specific treatment; pain is controlled with analgesics. The prognosis is usually good but full neurological recovery may take months or years (Bacevich, 1976).

Cervical rib syndrome

The subclavian artery and first thoracic nerve pass through a triangle based on the first rib and bordered by scalenus anterior and medius. Even under normal circumstances these structures bend acutely when the arm rests by the side; an extra rib (or its fibrous equivalent extending from a large costal process), or an anomalous scalene muscle, sharpens the angle by forcing the vessel and nerve still higher. Even with normal ribs and muscles a post-fixed brachial plexus is excessively angulated.

These anomalies are all congenital; yet symptoms are rare before the age of 30. This is probably because, with declining youth, the shoulders sag, increasing the angulation; indeed drooping shoulders alone may cause the syndrome.

As a result of increased angulation the first thoracic nerve may be stretched or compressed, causing sensory changes along the post-axial forearm and hand, with weakness of the intrinsic hand muscles. The subclavian artery is rarely compressed but may be narrowed by irritation of its sympathetic supply, or its wall damaged leading to the formation of small emboli.

Clinical features

There are no general symptoms or neck symptoms. The patient, usually a female in her thirties, may complain of: (1) pain in the ulnar forearm and hand, worse after household chores or after carrying parcels; (2) weakness or clumsiness; and (3) excessive sweating, or blueness and coldness of the fingers.

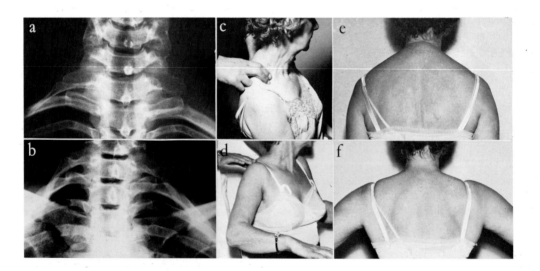

17.8 Cervical ribs   (a) Unilateral; (b) bilateral. (c) A pulsating lump (the elevated subclavian artery) is usually palpable. (d) Teaching the patient shrugging exercises; before exercises the shoulders sag (e) – the aim is to restore the posture shown in (f).

NECK SIGNS

The shoulder on the affected side may be lower, or both may sag. A lump (the abnormally elevated subclavian artery) may be palpable above the clavicle. It pulsates, is tender, and pressure on it may increase symptoms. Neck and shoulder movements are normal, but pulling the arm downwards while pushing the neck away may obliterate the pulse too readily.

X-RAY Occasionally a well-formed rib is seen, but more often there is merely enlargement of the transverse process of the seventh cervical vertebra.

ARM SIGNS

The small muscles of the hand may be wasted: thenar, hypothenar and interosseous muscles are affected because all are supplied by the first thoracic nerve. Occasionally increased sweating or cyanosis is seen. If there are sensory changes, they occur in the distribution of the first thoracic nerve root and are not confined to the distribution of a single peripheral nerve. If there is wasting, muscle power is reduced.

Differential diagnosis

Many disorders resemble cervical rib syndrome.

CARPAL TUNNEL SYNDROME Until this common disorder was widely recognized many cases were wrongly called cervical rib syndrome. Even when x-rays show a rib, the symptoms may still be due to median nerve compression in the carpal tunnel. The nocturnal pain and its distribution are characteristic.

ULNAR TUNNEL SYNDROME The symptoms and signs are sharply confined to the distribution of the ulnar nerve, and the neck is unaffected.

ACROPARAESTHESIA There is sensory disturbance in both hands and sometimes the feet. When only the hands are affected the diagnosis is usually wrong, and the patient is probably suffering from a carpal tunnel syndrome.

PANCOAST SYNDROME Apical carcinoma of the bronchus may infiltrate the structures at the root of the neck, causing pain, numbness and weakness of the hand. A hard mass may be palpable in the neck and x-ray of the chest shows a characteristic opacity.

CERVICAL SPINE LESIONS In disc prolapse or spondylosis, pain is not postaxial in distribution and neck movements are limited. In tuberculosis and secondary deposits the x-ray appearance is characteristic.

SPINAL CORD LESIONS Syringomyelia or other spinal cord lesions may cause wasting of the hand, but other neurological features establish the diagnosis.

CUFF LESIONS With supraspinatus tendon lesions pain sometimes radiates to the arm and hand but shoulder movement is limited and painful.

Treatment

CONSERVATIVE The patient is taught exercises to strengthen the shrugging muscles. She is given analgesics, and advised to reduce her own weight and that of her shopping basket. These measures are usually adequate.

OPERATIVE Operation is indicated if pain is severe, if muscle wasting is obvious or if there are vascular disturbances.

Technique The neurovascular bundle is exposed through a transverse incision 1.3 cm above the clavicle. The scalenus anterior muscle is identified, the phrenic nerve retracted and the muscle cut across. The rib (or its fibrous counterpart) also is divided; if none is present, 2.5 cm of the first rib is excised.

Notes on applied anatomy

In the upright posture the neck has a gentle anterior convexity; this natural lordosis may straighten but is never quite reversed, even in flexion, unless it is abnormal.

Eight pairs of nerve roots from the cervical cord pass through the relatively narrow intervertebral foramina, the first between the occiput and C1, and the eighth between C7 and the first thoracic (T1) vertebra; thus each segmental root from the first to the seventh lies above the vertebra of the same number. Thus a lesion between C5 and C6 might compress the sixth root.

The intervertebral discs lie close to the nerve roots as they emerge through the foramina; even a small herniation often causes root symptoms rather than neck pain. Moreover, disc degeneration is associated with spur formation on both the posterior aspect of the vertebral body and the associated facet joint; the resulting encroachment on the intervertebral foramen traps the nerve root. It is important to remember, however, that 'root pain' alone (i.e. pain in the shoulder and arm) does not necessarily signify nerve-root irritation; it may be referred from the facet joint or the soft structures around it. Only paraesthesiae and sensory or motor loss are unequivocal evidence of nerve root compression.

Further reading

Bacevich, B. B. (1976) Paralytic brachial neuritis. *Journal of Bone and Joint Surgery* **58A,** 262–263
Editorial (1972) Signs and symptoms in cervical spondylosis. *Lancet* **ii,** 70–72
LaRocca, H. (1978) Survey of current concepts in the evaluation and treatment of common cervical spine disorders. *Instructional Course Lectures* **27,** 144

The Back

18

Examination

Symptoms

The most common presenting symptoms of back disorders are pain, stiffness, deformity or a lump in the back; and pain, paraesthesia or weakness of the legs.

PAIN felt simultaneously in the buttock, the back of the thigh and the calf, though called *sciatica*, is rarely due to sciatic nerve disorder; it is referred, usually from a single nerve root or a facet joint.

STIFFNESS may be transient and recurrent (the common pattern in disc disorders), or continuous and predictably worse in the mornings (suggesting arthritis or ankylosing spondylitis).

DEFORMITY is usually noticed by others, but the patient may become aware of shoulder asymmetry or of clothes not fitting well.

NUMBNESS OR PARAESTHESIA may be related to a particular posture or activity (e.g. standing or walking), and may be consistently relieved by a change in position (e.g. sitting or squatting).

OTHER SYMPTOMS important in back disorders are urethral discharge, diarrhoea and sore eyes – the classic triad of Reiter's disease.

Signs with the patient standing

Adequate exposure is essential; patients must strip to pants and bra.

● LOOK
Skin Scars, pigmentation, abnormal hair or unusual skin creases may be seen.

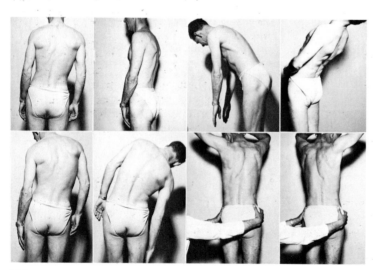

18.1 Examination (1) This patient has a prolapsed lumbar disc. He stands with a tilt. Forward flexion and tilting to the left are limited – other movements full.

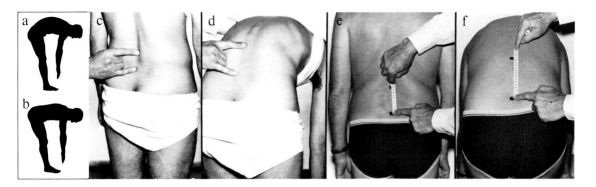

18.2 Examination (2) In both diagrams the hands nearly reach the toes; to distinguish spine flexion (a) from hip flexion (b), watch the lumbar lordosis undoing as the patient bends. Alternatively (c, d) note the separation of fingers placed on the spinous processes. Better still (e, f) *measure* the lumbar excursion; with the patient upright, two bony points 10 cm apart are selected – in full flexion they should separate by at least a further 5 cm.

Shape and posture Asymmetry of the chest, trunk or pelvis may be obvious, or may appear only when the patient bends forwards. Lateral deviation of the spine is described as a list to one or other side; lateral curvature is scoliosis.

Seen from the side the thoracic spine may seem unduly bent (kyphosis); if it is sharply angulated the prominence is called a kyphos. The lumbar spine may be unusually flat or excessively lordosed.

● FEEL
The spinous processes and the interspinous ligaments are palpated, noting any prominence (e.g. a small kyphos) or a 'step'.

● MOVE
Forward flexion is tested by asking the patient to try to touch his toes. Even with a stiff back he may be able to do this by flexing the hips; so watch the lumbar spine to see if it really moves, or, better still, measure the spinal excursion. To test extension ask the patient to lean backwards; with a stiff spine he may cheat by bending the knees. The 'wall test' will unmask a minor flexion deformity; standing with the back flush against a wall, the heels, buttocks, shoulders and occiput should all make contact with the surface. Lateral flexion is tested by asking the patient to bend sideways, sliding his hand down the outer side of his leg; the two sides are compared. Rotation is examined by asking him to twist the trunk to each side in turn while the pelvis is anchored by the surgeon's hands; this is essentially a thoracic movement and is not limited in lumbosacral disease. Finally, rib excursion must be assessed by measuring the chest circumference in full expiration and then inspiration.

Signs with the patient lying face downwards

Bony outlines and small lumps can be felt more easily with the patient lying face down. Deep tenderness is easy to localize, but difficult to ascribe to a particular structure. The tone and bulk of the back and buttock muscles are examined and the hips tested for full extension.

The popliteal and posterior tibial pulses are felt, hamstring power is tested and sensation on the back of the limbs assessed. The femoral stretch test (for lumbar root tension) is carried out by flexing the patient's knee and lifting the hip into extension; pain may be felt in the front of the thigh and the back.

Signs with the patient lying on his back

The patient is observed as he turns – is there pain or stiffness? Hip and knee mobility are examined before testing for cord or root involvement. *The straight leg raising test* discloses lumbosacral root tension. With the knee held absolutely straight,

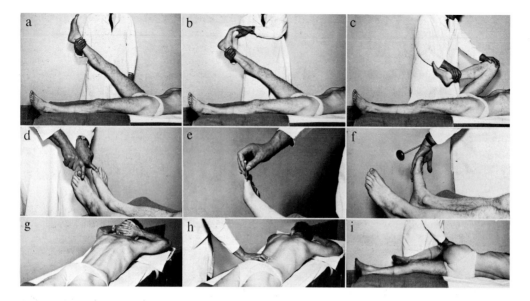

18.3 Examination (3) The legs are examined for nerve root involvement. (a) Straight leg raising is limited, and (b) the sciatic stretch is positive; but (c) flexion of the hip with the knee bent is painless, demonstrating that the hip is not at fault. (d) Muscle power, (e) skin sensation, and (f) the tendon reflexes are tested. With the patient prone he is examined for (g) muscle power and (h) tenderness; (i) the sacroiliac joints also may be examined.

the leg is lifted from the couch until the patient experiences pain – not merely in the thigh (which is common and not significant) but in the buttock and back; the angle at which this occurs is noted. At this point passive dorsiflexion of the foot may cause an additional stab of pain. If the knee is slightly flexed, buttock pain is suddenly relieved. Pain may then be reinduced without extending the knee by simply pressing on the lateral popliteal nerve, to tighten it like a bowstring.

Muscle bulk and tone, reflexes and sensation are then assessed. The pedal and femoral pulses are felt. If infection is suspected, the groin and abdomen are examined for an abscess. If the diagnosis is still uncertain, a full thoracic, abdominal, rectal and vaginal examination is mandatory.

SACROILIAC JOINTS The sacroiliac joints are difficult to examine because they are too deep to feel. The iliac crests may be squeezed together, pushed apart or forcibly rotated to one or other side in an attempt to jog the sacroiliac joint, but it is almost impossible to be sure that movement is not occurring at the lumbar spine or hips.

X-ray

In the anteroposterior view the spine should look perfectly straight and the soft-tissue shadows should outline the normal muscle planes. Curvature (scoliosis) is obvious, and bulging of the psoas muscle plane may indicate a paravertebral abscess. Individual vertebrae may show alterations in structure (e.g. asymmetry or collapse) and the intervertebral spaces may be edged by bony spurs (suggesting disc degeneration) or bridged by fine bony syndesmophytes. The sacroiliac joints may show erosion or ankylosis.

In the lateral view the normal thoracic kyphosis and lumbar lordosis should be regular and uninterrupted. Anterior shift of an upper segment upon a lower (spondylolisthesis) may be associated with defects of the posterior arch which show best in oblique views. Individual vertebrae, which should be rectangular, may be wedged or biconcave. Bone density and trabecular markings also are best seen in lateral films.

Special techniques such as tomography, radionuclide imaging, contrast myelography and computerized tomography are sometimes needed.

Scoliosis

Seen from behind, the normal spine is straight; lateral curvature constitutes scoliosis. Two main types are recognized: mobile and fixed.

Mobile scoliosis

There is no structural abnormality, the vertebrae are not rotated and the curve is always reversible. There are three varieties – *postural*, *compensatory* and *sciatic*.

POSTURAL   This is common, especially in adolescent girls. The curve is mild, usually convex to the left, and it disappears when the child bends forwards. Spontaneous recovery is invariable and exercises serve only to placate the parents.

COMPENSATORY   The most important causes are (1) a short leg, and (2) pelvic tilt due to abduction or adduction contracture of the hip. When the patient sits (thereby cancelling leg asymmetry) the curve disappears.

SCIATIC   A lateral tilt or list may accompany a prolapsed lumbar disc. The clinical features of the underlying condition are manifest and the tilt disappears when the cause is remedied.

Fixed scoliosis (structural)

Structural scoliosis is always accompanied by vertebral rotation; the bodies rotate towards the convexity and the spinous processes towards the concavity of the curve. The deformity is fixed and does not disappear with changes in posture. Secondary curves nearly always develop to counterbalance the primary deformity; they, too, may later become fixed. The primary curve is fixed from the start and for a long time is less correctible than the secondary curves; if there are three curves, the middle one is the primary (or 'major') curve.

Once established, the deformity is liable to increase throughout the growth period. A reliable x-ray guide to spinal maturity is ossification of the full extent of the iliac apophysis (Risser's sign), which occurs at around 14 years in girls and 16 in boys. Thereafter, further deterioration is slight, though curves greater than 50 degrees may go on increasing by 1 degree per year.

Most cases have no obvious cause (*idiopathic scoliosis*); other varieties are *osteopathic* (due to bony anomalies), *neuropathic* (often due to asymmetrical paresis), *myopathic* (associated with some muscle dystrophies) and a *miscellaneous* group of connective-tissue disorders.

Clinical features

Deformity is usually the presenting symptom. The age of onset is important: high curves are noticed early; lumbar curves and balanced double curves may pass unnoticed until an adult presents with backache. There may be a family history.

General examination includes a search for the possible cause and an assessment of cardiopulmonary function (which is reduced in severe curves). The local signs are as follows.

● LOOK   Skin pigmentation and congenital anomalies such as sacral dimples or hair tufts are sought. The spine may be obviously deviated from the midline, or this may become apparent only when the patient bends forward. The level and direction of the major curve convexity are noted (e.g. 'right thoracic' means a curve in the thoracic spine and convex to the right). In balanced deformities the occiput is over the midline; in unbalanced curves it is not. The hip sticks out on the concave side and the scapula on the convex The breasts and shoulders also may be asymmetrical. With thoracic scoliosis, rotation causes the rib angles to protrude; these may be sufficiently prominent to justify the term 'razorback'.

● FEEL   There is nothing particular to feel, and tenderness is not a feature. However, leg length and pelvic tilt should be assessed.

● MOVE   The diagnostic feature of fixed (as distinct from mobile) scoliosis is that forward bending makes the curve more obvious. Spinal mobility should be assessed and the effect of lateral bending on the curve noted.

● X-RAY   Full length anteroposterior and lateral films of the spine and iliac crests must be taken in the erect position. The angle of curvature (i.e. the angle between unwedged discs at each end of the

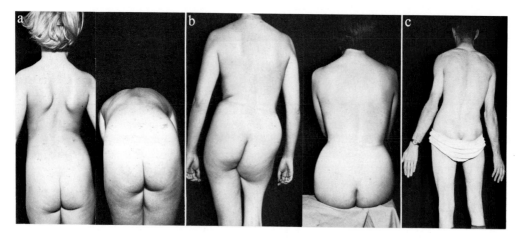

18.4 Mobile scoliosis (a) Postural scoliosis disappears on flexion. (b) Short leg scoliosis disappears when the patient sits. (c) Sciatic scoliosis disappears when the underlying cause (a prolapsed disc) has been treated.

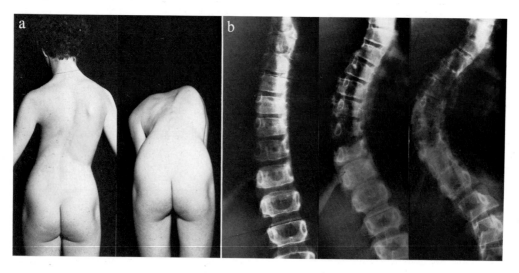

18.5 Fixed scoliosis (a) A fixed (structural) curve is more obvious on flexion. (b) Over a period of 4 years this curve has increased – most rapidly in the last 12 months, during the prepubertal spurt of growth.

primary curve) is measured. The iliac apophyses are sought; about a year elapses between their appearance and their complete ossification. Congenital bony anomalies may be present.

Treatment

Prognosis is the key to treatment: the aim is to prevent severe deformity. Generally speaking, the younger the child and the higher the curve the worse is the prognosis. A period of preliminary observation may be needed before deciding between conservative and operative treatment. At 3-monthly intervals the patient is examined, photographed and x-rayed so that the curves can be measured.

CONSERVATIVE TREATMENT

Exercises alone have no effect on the curve, but they are useful to maintain muscle tone and to 'stretch' the spine while it is held in a support.

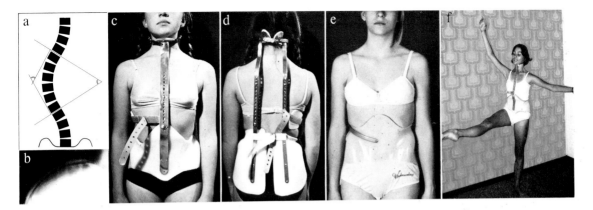

18.6 Fixed scoliosis – conservative treatment   (a) Measuring the primary curve; the disc spaces are wider on the convex side – at each end of the primary curve, lines are drawn to show the angle of curvature. (b) The iliac apophysis is visible throughout its length – Risser's sign of spinal maturity. (c, d) The Milwaukee brace fits snugly over the pelvis below; chin and head pads promote active postural correction; a thoracic pad presses on the ribs at the apex of the curve. (e) The Boston brace is used for low curves. All braces are cumbersome, but (f) if they are well made they need not interfere much with activity.

Supports are used (1) for all progressive curves over 20 degrees but less than 50 degrees; (2) for well-balanced double primary curves; (3) with younger children needing operation, to hold the curve stationary until aged 10, when fusion is more likely to succeed; and (4) to prevent recurrence after spinal fusion in young children.

Three kinds of support are available. (1) The Milwaukee brace has a snugly fitting pelvic corset connected by adjustable steel supports to a cervical ring carrying an occipital pad posteriorly and a throat pad anteriorly; extending the steels straightens the curve. (2) The Boston brace (for lumbar and thoracolumbar curves) is a rigid, padded body-corset extending from the pelvis to the thorax. A well-made brace can be worn 23 hours out of 24 and does not preclude full daily activities, including sport and exercises. (3) A distraction plaster jacket is applied with the patient on a Risser frame receiving traction to the head and pelvis and local pressure to the rib hump.

Unless the curve is reduced by more than 50 per cent, relapse is likely when the brace is discontinued. Weaning from a brace must be gradual (6–12 months).

Electrical stimulation of muscles on the convex side is being tried.

OPERATIVE TREATMENT

Operation is indicated for curves of more than 50 degrees, or for milder deformity that deteriorates in spite of conservative treatment. High curves, paralytic curves and those associated with neurofibromatosis usually need operative treatment; so do curves in younger patients, but below the age of 10 preliminary treatment in a brace is usually wise.

Correction and fusion The deformity is corrected as well as possible and the spine is then fused. With mobile curves the correction is achieved by a brace or a Risser cast. With severe curves or particularly rigid deformities (e.g. neurofibromatosis), more powerful correction can be obtained by halo-pelvic traction. A metal hoop (the halo) is screwed to the outer table of the skull and a second hoop is anchored by transfixing screws to the pelvis; the two hoops are gradually racked apart via connecting steel rods. The child walks about in this apparatus and it is retained for the first few postoperative weeks until replaced by plaster. Alternatively, halo-femoral traction may be used with the patient lying on a Stryker bed.

At operation the laminae and transverse processes are rawed, the facet joints excised and the area is packed with autogenous bone grafts. A Harrington rod is applied to the top and bottom vertebrae, extended to separate them (thereby further reducing the curve) and left *in situ* as internal fixation. Fusion extends from one vertebra above to one vertebra below the primary curve; with lumbar paralytic curves it should extend to the sacrum. After a few days the patient is allowed up in the halo-pelvic apparatus, or in a well-fitting plaster which is worn for at least 6 months.

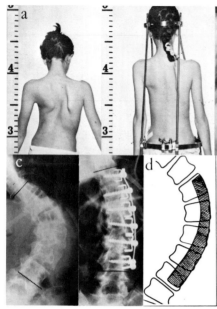

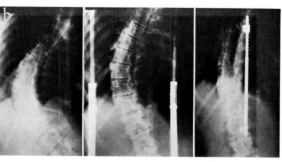

18.7 Fixed scoliosis – operative treatment   (a) Halo-pelvic traction is very effective, though seldom necessary; (b) here it was followed by fusion with Harrington rod instrumentation. (c) Dwyer's technique is valuable for lumbar curves. (d) Growth control has been largely abandoned.

Dwyer's anterior fusion is useful for lumbar and thoracolumbar curves, especially paralytic. A series of wedges is excised, each including an intervertebral disc and the adjoining vertebral end plates. Staples and screws are fixed to the vertebral bodies and through the screw heads a cable is threaded. Tightening the cable closes the vertebral wedges and straightens the curve.

Varieties of scoliosis

IDIOPATHIC   About 80 per cent of all scoliosis is idiopathic. The deformity is often familial, and the population incidence of serious curves (over 20 degrees and therefore needing treatment) is 3 per 1000, though trivial curves are very much more common. The age of onset defines three groups.

(1) *Adolescent* (presenting aged 10 or over)   This, the commonest group, occurs mostly (90 per cent) in girls. Primary thoracic curves are usually convex to the right, lumbar curves to the left; intermediate (thoracolumbar) and combined (double primary) curves also occur.

(2) *Infantile* (aged 3 or under)   This variety is rare in North America, perhaps because most babies there sleep prone. Boys predominate and most curves are thoracic with convexity to the left. Although most infantile curves resolve spontaneously, progressive curves can become very severe; those in which the rib–vertebra angle at the apex of the curve differs on the two sides by more than 20 degrees are likely to deteriorate (Mehta,

1972). Progressive curves should be treated with a Milwaukee brace, which can be fitted even to an infant.

(3) *Juvenile* (aged 4 to 9)   The characteristics of this group are similar to those of the adolescent group, but the prognosis is worse and fusion may be necessary before puberty.

OSTEOPATHIC (INCLUDING CONGENITAL)   Although fractures and bone softening (as in rickets or osteogenesis imperfecta) may lead to scoliosis, the commonest bony cause is congenital. The anomalies include hemivertebrae, fused vertebrae and absent or fused ribs; the overlying tissues often show angiomas, naevi, excess hair, dimples or a pad of fat; spina bifida may be associated. Although congenital scoliosis may remain mild, some cases progress to severe deformity; before operation is undertaken myelography is essential, to exclude diastematomyelia.

NEUROPATHIC (INCLUDING PARALYTIC)   Neuropathic conditions associated with scoliosis include poliomyelitis, cerebral palsy, syringomyelia, Friedreich's ataxia and the rarer lower motor neuron disorders; the curve may take some years to develop. The typical paralytic curve is long, convex towards the side with weaker muscles (spinal, abdominal or intercostal), and at first is mobile. Correction can be held in a brace until the child is old enough for spinal fusion.

MYOPATHIC   Patients with muscle dystrophy may have no supporting trunk muscles; they develop a floppy, unstable spine which may require fusion.

Infantile thoracic

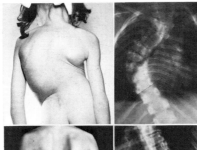

60% male.
90% convex to left.
Associated with ipsilateral plagiocephaly. May be resolving or progressive.
Progressive variety becomes severe.

Adolescent thoracic

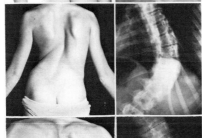

90% female.
90% convex to right.
Rib rotation exaggerates the deformity.
50% develop curves of greater than 70 degrees.

Thoracolumbar

Slightly commoner in females.
Slightly commoner to right.
Features mid-way between adolescent thoracic and lumbar.

Lumbar

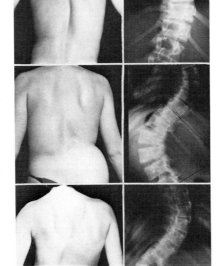

Commoner in females.
80% convex to left.
One hip prominent but no ribs to accentuate deformity.
Therefore not noticed early, but backache in adult life.

Combined

Two primary curves, one in each direction.
Even when radiologically severe, clinical deformity relatively slight because always well balanced.

18.8 Fixed scoliosis – idiopathic curve patterns

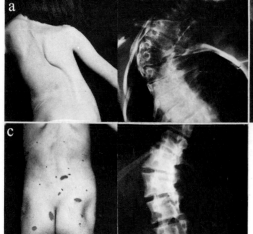
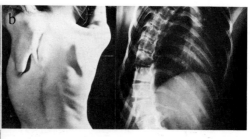

18.9 Fixed scoliosis – non-idiopathic (a) Congenital – a curve as high as this is not 'idiopathic'; (b) paralytic – a characteristic long C curve, following polio; (c) with neurofibromatosis – a short sharp curve is not uncommon.

MISCELLANEOUS   A variety of connective tissue disorders may be associated with scoliosis. In neurofibromatosis 30 per cent of patients develop scoliosis, often a short sharp thoracic curve which is liable to become severe and usually needs open correction and fusion. Other conditions include Marfan's syndrome, Ehlers–Danlos syndrome and the mucopolysaccharidoses. In juvenile chronic polyarthritis, asymmetrical joint involvement may be a factor in causing scoliosis. Congenital cardiothoracic anomalies also are sometimes associated with scoliosis.

Kyphosis

Classification

MOBILE KYPHOSIS   Mobile kyphosis may be (1) postural, (2) associated with muscle weakness or (3) compensatory to lumbar lordosis. Mobile deformities are not in themselves important, though they may in later life cause backache. They are correctable either by the patient's own muscular efforts or by the surgeon.

Postural Postural kyphosis is common, and associated with other postural defects such as flat feet. It occurs most often in adolescents, in women after childbirth and with obesity. The treatment is posture training, exercises and dieting.

Muscle weakness Weakness of the trunk muscles, as in muscle dystrophies and poliomyelitis, is often associated with lumbar lordosis and thoracic kyphosis.

Compensatory Gross hip deformity, such as congenital dislocation or fixed flexion, is accompanied by excessive lumbar lordosis which is balanced by thoracic kyphosis.

FIXED KYPHOSIS   The following varieties occur; (1) Scheuermann's disease (page 225); (2) ankylosing spondylitis (page 41); and (3) senile kyphosis (page 227). Some bone dystrophies are associated with kyphosis, but this is not the presenting feature (see Chapter 8).

A fixed kyphosis cannot be corrected by the patient or the surgeon; it is balanced by a lumbar lordosis unless the lumbar spine also is stiff, as in ankylosing spondylitis.

ANGULAR KYPHOSIS (KYPHOS)   Forward angulation may be (1) congenital; (2) tuberculous; (3) the result of a fracture (which may be pathological); or (4) due to Calvé's disease. A kyphos is always fixed. The distinction between a sharp angular kyphos and a smooth kyphosis is of the utmost help in diagnosis.

In congenital kyphos vertebral bodies are partly missing or fused anteriorly. Progressive deformity is inevitable and operative correction (from the front or the back) is needed.

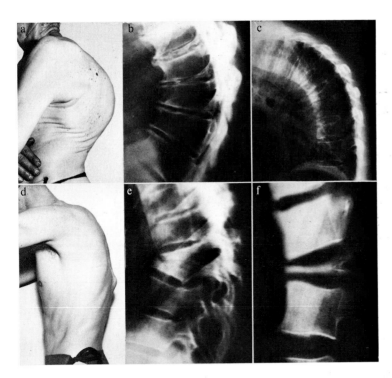

18.10 Kyphosis and kyphos   (a, b) Old Scheuermann's disease; (c) senile kyphosis.

(d, e) Small kyphos due to tuberculosis; (f) Calvé's disease.

In Calvé's disease, a rare condition which is probably the sequel to an eosinophilic granuloma, one vertebral body becomes flattened but the disc spaces remain normal. A child develops back pain and an angular kyphos. Clinical recovery occurs after a few months' rest.

Age of onset

In children, a congenital cause is likely; in adolescents, kyphosis is usually postural or due to Scheuermann's disease; in young adults, ankylosing spondylitis is an important cause; in the elderly, senile kyphosis, pathological fractures and Paget's disease must be considered; at all ages, tuberculosis must be excluded.

Adolescent kyphosis (Scheuermann's disease)

The cause of this condition is unknown. Scheuermann used the term 'osteochondritis' because the epiphyseal plates are irregularly ossified. Schmorl drew attention to the function of the cartilage plates in transmitting pressure evenly and suggested that a defect in them threw undue strain on the anterior portion of the vertebral bodies. More recently it has been postulated that a traumatic infraction of the epiphyseal plates occurs in children who outgrow their bone strength during the pubertal growth spurt; there may also be vertebral osteoporosis and the discs herniate into the fragile bone.

Clinical features

The condition starts at puberty and is twice as common in girls as in boys. The parents notice that the child, an otherwise fit teenager, is becoming increasingly round-shouldered. The patient may complain of backache and fatigue; this sometimes increases after the end of growth and may become severe.

A smooth thoracic kyphosis is seen; it may produce a distinct hump. Below it is a compensatory lumbar lordosis. The deformity cannot be corrected by changes in posture. Movements are normal but tight hamstrings often limit straight leg raising. Rarely, a spastic paresis is found. In later life cardiopulmonary failure may occur.

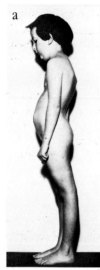

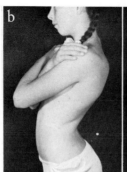

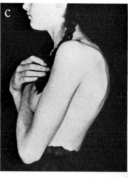

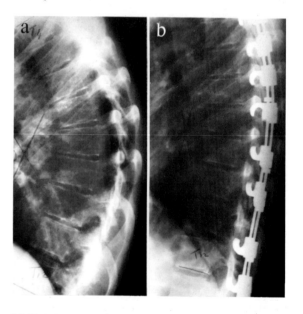

18.11 Kyphosis (continued) (a) Postural kyphosis and (b) kyphosis compensatory to a lumbar 'sway-back'. Unlike these two varieties, the deformity in Scheuermann's disease (c, d) is fixed.

X-RAY   The bodies of several adjacent vertebrae, usually T 6–10, are wedged; that is, narrower in front. They may contain small translucent areas (Schmorl's nodes). The epiphyseal plates appear fragmented, especially anteriorly. The angle of deformity should be measured (normal kyphosis varies from 20 to 40 degrees).

Differential diagnosis

Postural kyphosis is common in adolescence. It is painless, and the deformity is correctable by the patient's own efforts if properly instructed. The curve is a long one and other postural defects are common. The x-ray appearance is normal.

Tuberculosis produces an angular kyphos. X-rays show destruction of at least two adjacent vertebrae with narrowing of the intervening disc and often a paravertebral abscess.

Treatment

Curves around 40 degrees require only back-strengthening exercises and postural training. More severe curvature in a child who still has some years of growth ahead responds well to a period of 12–24 months in a Milwaukee brace.

The older adolescent or young adult with a rigid curve of more than 60 degrees may need operative correction and fusion using Harrington compression rods. In severe cases this can be a massive undertaking, carried out in stages: anterior release by multiple disc excision and fusion, followed by traction for 2 weeks, and then posterior fusion and Harrington rod fixation; the patient remains in a Risser cast for 9–12 months (Bradford *et al.*, 1980). Indications are a painful kyphosis of more than 60 degrees in a skeletally mature patient, or impending spastic paresis.

18.12 Scheuermann's disease – operative treatment A severe curve may need operation especially if, as in this girl (a), it is associated with chronic pain; (b) the same girl after operative correction and fixation with Harrington rods; bone grafts were added and can be expected to produce fusion after a year or two.

Kyphosis in the elderly

TRUE SENILE KYPHOSIS Degeneration of intervertebral discs probably produces the gradually increasing stoop characteristic of the aged. The disc spaces become narrowed and the vertebrae slightly wedged. There is little pain unless osteoarthritis of the facet joints is also present.

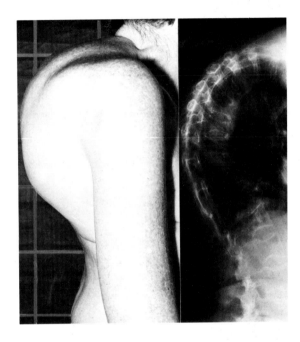

18.13 Senile kyphosis Progressive kyphosis in the elderly can occur because of collapse and wedging of osteoporotic vertebrae. Typically the x-ray shows only faint bony outlines. In a case as severe as this, some pre-existing deformity or long-standing metabolic bone disease was probably present.

SENILE OSTEOPOROSIS The patients, usually women, are thin and kyphotic ('dowager's hump'). There is widespread osteoporosis and the discs indent the soft vertebral bodies, which become biconcave. There may be pain, and pathological fractures are common (see page 77). In very severe cases there is always a history of some kyphosis in early adult life. Often the main complaint is of lumbosacral pain, which results from the compensatory lumbar lordosis in an ageing, osteoarthritic spine.

PAGET'S DISEASE Considerable kyphosis occurs because of bone softening. There is usually evidence of Paget's disease (such as thick bent bones) elsewhere. The affected vertebrae are enlarged and show coarse trabeculation.

PATHOLOGICAL FRACTURE IN MALIGNANT DISEASE Usually the affected vertebra is the site of a secondary deposit and collapses with slight trauma. There is a kyphos and x-rays show that only the vertebral body (or bodies) is affected.

Treatment

The deformity itself requires treatment only if it is painful. A walking-stick relieves the patient from the strain of forcing himself to stand upright. Heat and analgesics are soothing. A corset is often prescribed but is either too short to be effective or too high to be tolerated.

Senile osteoporosis may benefit from dietary treatment (page 78), and pain due to a carcinomatous deposit is often relieved by radiotherapy.

Tuberculosis of the spine

The spine is the commonest site of skeletal tuberculosis, and also the most dangerous.

Pathology

OSTEOMYELITIS Blood-borne infection settles in a single vertebra which squashes down into the one below and infects it; or two neighbouring vertebrae are infected simultaneously. The neural arches are usually unaffected so that, as the bodies collapse, forward angulation (kyphos) develops.

SPREAD The collapse squeezes out caseous material which may infect neighbouring vertebrae, or press on the cord, or escape into the soft tissues as a cold abscess. As the disease progresses, destruction, wedging and forward angulation increase and may, in the thoracic spine, become severe.

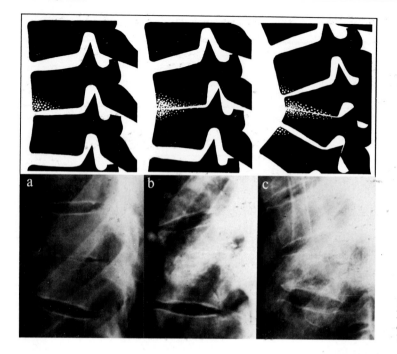

18.14 Spine tuberculosis – pathology (a, b, c) Progressively increasing destruction of the front of the vertebral bodies leads to forward collapse.

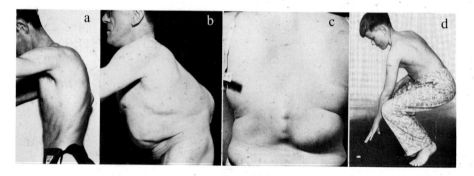

18.15 Spine tuberculosis – clinical features   (a) This kyphos is slight but diagnostic. If collapse continues (b) kyphos becomes severe. (c) Large lumbar abscess. (d) The coin test – he bends his hips and knees rather than bending his back.

HEALING   With healing, the vertebrae recalcify and bony fusion may occur between them. Nevertheless, if there has been much forward angulation, the spine is usually 'unsound', and flares are common, with further illness and further collapse.

Clinical features

There is a long history with insidious onset and vague ill health. Pain is usually slight, often only a dull ache, worse after standing or jolting. Sometimes a lump (the kyphos or an abscess) is the presenting symptom; occasionally paraesthesia or weakness of the legs (due to paraplegia).

In the active stage   the local signs are as follows.

● LOOK   A characteristic feature in the thoracic spine is an angular kyphos, best seen from the side. In advanced cases the patient is a hunchback. In the lumbar spine the kyphos is scarcely visible, but an abscess in the loin or groin may be obvious. If the cervical spine is affected, the neck may be stiff.

FEEL   The fingers can detect a kyphos, however slight; one need only run the hand down the spinous processes. Abscesses are fluctuant and the skin over them slightly warm (the term 'cold abscess' is merely a reminder that they lack the heat of a pyogenic abscess).

MOVE   Diminished movement is undetectable in the thoracic region, but easy to observe in the lumbar spine; the back should be carefully watched while movements are attempted. Usually all are limited and the attempt provokes muscle spasm. Formerly the coin test was used; a child with lumbar spasm prefers bending at the hips and knees rather than at the spine when picking a coin up from the floor.

The legs also must be examined for neurological deficit, which may be very slight.

X-RAY   In lateral films two adjacent bodies show destruction and the intervening disc space is narrowed; a characteristic feature in the antero-posterior view with thoracic disease is a paraver-tebral abscess. It is important to x-ray the whole spine, as in 20 per cent of patients there is more than one lesion; neural arches and processes also may, very occasionally, be involved.

In the healing stage   pain vanishes and the patient is fit again. The bones recalcify and look 'harder' on x-ray; even the abscesses may become calcified. Deformity is permanent, and with an exaggerated thoracic kyphos the spine remains 'unsound' and liable to flare (see page 32).

Differential diagnosis

Thoracic tuberculosis must be differentiated from other causes of kyphosis (page 224): the diagnostic x-ray features are the narrowed disc space between two affected vertebrae and the tell-tale shadow of a paravertebral abscess.

Lumbar tuberculosis must be differentiated from other causes of backache in a slightly unfit patient. Confusion sometimes arises with Scheuermann's disease which, in the lumbar spine, usually presents in adolescence: x-rays show the anterior corner of one (or two) vertebra(e) eroded and slight narrowing of the disc space; but the erosion has a sclerosed margin, the vertebra below the narrow disc looks bigger from the side and, of course, the patient is not ill. A brief period of rest settles the problem.

Treatment

The objectives of treatment are (1) to eradicate or at least arrest the disease, (2) to prevent or correct deformity and (3) to prevent the major complica-tion – paraplegia. The first objective can be achieved with drugs alone (combined with bed rest for children), which must be continued for at least a year.

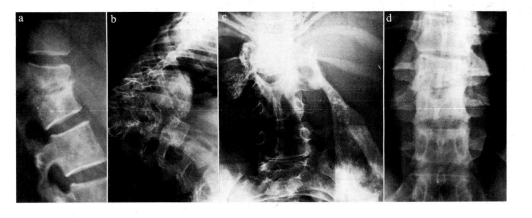

18.16 Spine tuberculosis – x-rays   (a) Early disease with loss of the disc space. (b) If several vertebrae are involved forward collapse is severe – this patient did not, however, have any signs of paraplegia. (c) Psoas abscesses often calcify during the healing stage. (d) A paravertebral abscess is a fairly constant finding with thoracic disease.

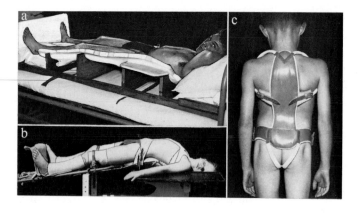

18.17 Spine tuberculosis – conservative treatment Splintage is sometimes used. (a) Adult on plaster bed; (b) child on hyperextension frame; (c) Jones' back brace.

The deformity In a child a kyphos involving two or more vertebrae will almost certainly increase with time; to prevent this, spinal fusion is advisable. If the kyphotic angle is less than 40 degrees, posterior fusion will suffice; if more than 40 degrees, anterior and posterior fusion is better. Postoperatively the child remains in a plaster jacket for 6 months and then wears a spinal brace for a year. In adults, operation is indicated mainly for cosmesis; again, anterior plus posterior fusion is the most effective procedure. It should be emphasized that operation is by no means essential, and should be undertaken only if sufficient expertise is available.

Pott's paraplegia

The spinal cord may be compressed by soft inflammatory material (an abscess, a caseous mass or granulation tissue) or by hard solid material (a bony sequestrum, a sequestrated disc or the ridge of bone at the kyphos). Occasionally fibrous tissue is the compressing agent.

Clinically the patient presents with signs of paraplegia added to those of spine tuberculosis. Clumsiness, inco-ordination and weakness are early symptoms; later, voluntary power is reduced, muscle tone increased and the tendon reflexes are brisk; clonus and extensor plantar

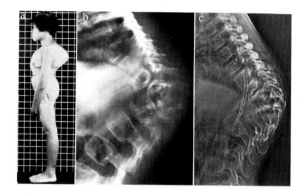

18.18 Spine tuberculosis – operative treatment A severe kyphos (a) may benefit from operation. This curve (b) has been partially corrected and held (c) by both anterior strut grafts and posterior fusion (this film is a xerographic tomograph – the best way of showing these grafts).

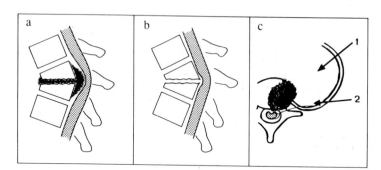

18.19 Spine tuberculosis – paraplegia In Pott's paraplegia the cord may be compressed by an abscess (a) which may resolve with effective conservative treatment; or (b) by a hard knuckle of bone which clearly needs operation. (c) Shows the routes most often used for decompressing the cord: 1, transthoracic; 2, anterolateral.

responses may occur. Paraesthesia, or numbness, and disturbance of bladder control are common.

Early-onset paresis is due to pressure by an abscess or bony sequestration. It usually produces a block on myelography. It is treated by early anterior decompression and débridement followed by spinal fusion. About 80 per cent recover, usually within a few weeks.

Late-onset paresis is due to increasing deformity, or reactivation of disease or vascular insufficiency of the cord. Investigations should be carried out to establish the precise diagnosis. If the myelogram shows a block, operative débridement is still worth while even in late cases. If there is no block, operation is unlikely to be of use.

Disc degeneration and prolapse

It has been estimated that each year in Great Britain almost 2 million people aged over 15 consult their doctor because of back pain; of these, 1 in 20 are referred for further help; of these, 1 in 10 are admitted to hospital, and of the hospital patients about 1 in 10 have an operation. In the vast majority of cases the problem arises in the lower two lumbar discs and their surrounding structures.

Pathology

With *normal ageing* the disc gradually dries out: the nucleus pulposus changes from a turgid, gelatinous bulb to a brownish, desiccated structure, and the annulus fibrosus develops fissures parallel to the vertebral end plates running mainly posteriorly. Small herniations of nuclear material squeeze through the annulus in all directions and frequently perforate the vertebral end plates to produce the Schmorl's nodes which are found in over 75 per cent of autopsies.

Disc degeneration is therefore a common expression of senescence. Chronic herniation causes reactive bone formation around the Schmorl's

nodes and where the discs protrude at the vertebral margins. The flattening of the disc and the marginal osteophytes are readily seen on x-ray and are referred to as *spondylosis*.

Displacement of the facet joints is an inevitable consequence of disc space collapse, and this in turn leads to *osteoarthritis*; if this is severe, osteophytes may narrow the lateral recesses of the spinal canal and the intervertebral foramina.

*Acute disc rupture** is less common (but more dramatic). Physical stress is a factor but, even at L4/5 or L5/S1 (where stress is most severe), it

Normal disc

Increased nuclear pressure causes bulging

Ruptured annulus and ligament

Degeneration + joint displacement

18.20 Disc pathology (1) From above, downwards: an abnormal increase in pressure within the nucleus causes splitting and bulging of the annulus; the posterior ligament may rupture, allowing disc material to extrude into the spinal canal; with chronic degeneration (lowest level) the disc space narrows and the posterior facet joints are displaced, giving rise to osteoarthritis.

---

*The terms 'rupture', 'prolapse', 'protrusion' and 'herniation' can be used interchangeably.

seems unlikely that a disc would rupture unless there were also some disturbance of the hydrophilic properties of the nucleus. When rupture does occur, fibrocartilaginous material is extruded posteriorly and the annulus usually bulges to one side of the posterior longitudinal ligament. With a complete rupture, part of the nucleus may sequestrate and lie free in the spinal canal or work its way into the intervertebral foramen. A large central rupture may cause compression of the cauda equina. A posterolateral rupture presses on the nerve root proximal to its point of exit through the intervertebral foramen; thus a herniation at L4/5 will compress the fifth lumbar nerve root, and a herniation at L5/S1 the first sacral root. Sometimes a local inflammatory response with oedema aggravates the symptoms.

The pain of disc herniation is referred pain.   Irritation of the dura causes widespread backache but fairly localized tenderness at the affected level; irritation of a nerve root (or, rather, its dural sleeve) causes pain and muscle tenderness in the buttock, thigh and calf (sciatica). Nerve pressure causes paraesthesia, loss of sensation, weakness and depressed reflexes.

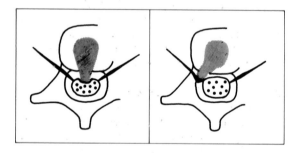

18.21 Disc pathology (2)   A prolapsed disc may press on the dura or on the nerve roots.

Repeated disc rupture   leads to rapid degeneration, with the features of spondylosis appearing at a younger age than usual.

Acute disc rupture (prolapse)

Symptoms

The first severe attack may be preceded by minor episodes of backache. Then one day, while lifting or stooping, the patient has severe back pain and may be unable to straighten up; occasionally the initial pain is slight but increases over the next few hours. During the first attack, or with a subsequent attack, pain is felt in the buttock and lower limb (sciatica). Both backache and sciatica are made worse by coughing or straining. Later there may be paraesthesia or numbness in the leg or foot, and occasionally muscle weakness. Cauda equina compression is rare but may cause urinary retention.

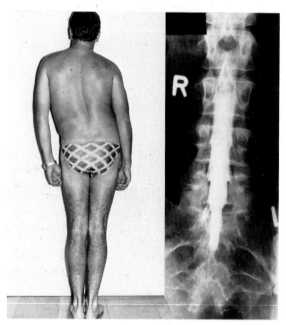

18.22 Lumbar disc – signs   The patient (seen from behind) has a sideways list or tilt; his x-ray (seen from in front) confirms the list, and the contrast medium shows a cut-off of the nerve root at the lumbosacral level.

Usually the acute symptoms subside in a few days or weeks, but recurrent attacks are common and between severe episodes some backache or sciatica may persist.

Signs

The patient is usually a healthy adult, though children can be affected. When standing there is a typical deformity: slight forward tilt obliterating the lumbar lordosis, and a lateral list or 'sciatic scoliosis'. Sometimes the knee on the painful side is held bent to relax tension on the sciatic nerve; straightening the knee makes the list more obvious. All back movements are limited, and during forward flexion the list may increase.

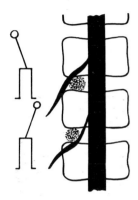

18.23 Lumbar disc prolapse – explanation of tilt   If the disc protrudes medial to the nerve root, the patient lists towards the painful side (to relieve pressure on the nerve); with a far lateral prolapse (lower level) the spinal tilt is away from the painful side.

There is often tenderness in the midline of the low back, and paravertebral muscle spasm. Straight leg raising is limited and painful on the affected side; dorsiflexion of the foot and bowstringing of the lateral popliteal nerve may accentuate the pain. In young adults (or adolescents) these signs are particularly marked. Sometimes raising the unaffected leg causes acute sciatic tension on the painful side (the 'crossed leg raising sign'). With a high or mid-lumbar prolapse the femoral stretch test may be positive.

NEUROLOGICAL EXAMINATION may show muscle weakness (and later wasting), loss of reflexes and sensory diminution corresponding to the affected level. S1 impairment causes weak eversion of the foot, a depressed ankle jerk and sensory loss along the lateral border of the foot. L5 impairment causes weakness of big-toe extension and knee flexion, an *increased* knee jerk (because of the weak antagonists) and sensory loss on the outer aspect of the leg and the dorsomedial side of the foot. Occasionally an L4/5 disc prolapse may compress both L5 and S1. Cauda equina compression causes urinary retention and sensory loss over the sacrum.

X-RAYS are essential, not to show an abnormal disc space but to exclude bone disease. After several attacks the disc space may be narrowed and small osteophytes appear.

Myelography (radiculography) using metrizamide is a reliable method of confirming disc protrusion, localizing it, and excluding intrathecal tumours, though occasionally it fails to show a far lateral prolapse.

Computerized tomography may then be helpful; it has none of the disadvantages of myelography and for many is now the preferred method of spinal imaging.

Differential diagnosis

The full-blown syndrome is unlikely to be misdiagnosed, but with repeated attacks and with lumbar spondylosis gradually supervening the features often become atypical. Diagnostically there are three guidelines, three warnings and three major disorders to exclude.

The guidelines (1) Old people with desiccated discs do not sustain acute ruptures. (2) An ill patient probably has a more serious disorder. (3) In disc rupture the episodes of pain are punctuated by intervals of normality.

The warnings (1) Sciatica is referred pain and occurs also in disorders of the facet joints, the sacroiliac joints or with vertebral infections. (2) Disc rupture affects at most two neurological levels; if multiple levels are involved, suspect a neurological disorder. (3) Severe, unrelenting pain is not characteristic of a ruptured disc; suspect a tumour or infection.

The differential diagnosis (1) Inflammatory disorders, such as tuberculosis or ankylosing spondylitis, cause severe stiffness, a raised ESR and erosive changes on x-ray. (2) Vertebral tumours cause severe pain and marked spasm. With metastases the patient is ill, the ESR raised and the x-ray shows bone destruction or sclerosis. (3) Nerve tumours, such as neurofibromata of the cauda equina, may cause 'sciatica', but pain is continuous, and myelography may show the defects.

Acute pyogenic osteomyelitis is quite different from disc rupture. The patient becomes rapidly ill with high fever, severe back pain and often severe root pain. The x-rays at first show no abnormality; after 2–3 weeks bone destruction is seen. If antibiotic treatment is prompt and effective, the patient recovers and the x-rays show sclerosis.

Discitis   In children, this presents with backache or leg pain. The child is unwell and has limited back movement. X-rays at first show narrowing of the disc space, then scalloping of bone on each side and finally obliteration of the space with bony fusion. Bed rest and antibiotics are effective. In adults, paraplegia may occur, necessitating operative decompression.

Treatment

Heat and analgesics soothe, and exercises strengthen muscles; but there are only three ways of treating the prolapse itself – *rest*, *reduction* and *removal*.

REST   With a severe attack the patient should be kept in bed for 2–3 weeks, with hips and knees slightly flexed and 10 kg traction to the legs or pelvis. An anti-inflammatory drug such as indomethacin is useful. For mild attacks a spinal corset and reduced activity may suffice.

REDUCTION   Manipulation may move a small disc herniation away from the nerve, but it should be avoided if there is sciatica. An epidural injection of corticosteroid and local anaesthetic may help. The injection of chymopapain, a proteolytic enzyme, directly into the disc is still regarded as experimental.

REMOVAL   The indications for operative removal of a disc are: (1) a cauda equina compression syndrome which does not clear up within 6 hours of starting bed rest and traction – this is an emergency; (2) persistent pain and severely limited leg raising after 2 weeks of conservative treatment; (3) neurological deterioration while under conservative treatment; and (4) frequently recurring attacks.

METHODS OF DISC REMOVAL
Partial laminectomy   The lamina and ligamentum flavum on one side are removed, taking great care not to damage the facet joint. The dura and nerve root are then gently retracted towards the midline and the pea-like bulge is displayed. This is incised and the mushy disc material plucked out piecemeal with pituitary forceps. The nerve is traced to its point of exit in order to exclude other pathology. A sequestrated disc may require further exploration.

Fenestration   This is an interlaminar approach with removal of the ligamentum flavum and perhaps the edge of the lamina above. There is no sound evidence of any advantage over partial laminectomy.

Total laminectomy   Removal of the spinous process and both laminae may be necessary if there is severe spinal stenosis, or a massive central rupture or suspicion of other pathology.

Disc removal and spine fusion   If there is marked lumbar spondylosis and instability, disc removal should be followed by spine fusion. Some surgeons prefer to do the combined procedure through an anterior approach.

COMPLICATIONS   The main intraoperative complication is bleeding from epidural veins. This is less likely to occur if the patient is placed on his side or in the kneeling position, thus minimizing the rise in venous pressure. The major postoperative complication is disc space infection, but fortunately this is rare. It causes severe pain and muscle spasm and is treated by rest and antibiotics.

REHABILITATION   After recovery from an acute disc rupture, or disc removal, the patient is taught isometric exercises and how to lie, sit, bend and lift with the least strain. Light work is resumed after a month and heavy work after 3 months. At that stage, if recovery is anything but total, the patient should be advised to avoid heavy lifting tasks altogether.

Persistent postoperative backache and sciatica

Persistent symptoms after operation may be due to: (1) residual disc material in the spinal canal; (2) disc prolapse at another level; or (3) nerve root pressure by a hypertrophic facet joint or a narrow lateral recess ('root canal stenosis'). After careful investigation, any of these may call for re-operation; but second procedures do not have a high success rate – third and fourth procedures still less.

Lumbar instability and spondylosis

With disc degeneration, and especially after recurrent disc prolapse, there may be gradual flattening of the disc and displacement of the posterior facet joints. The disturbed movement in flexion and extension constitutes a type of instability which produces well-recognized symptoms.

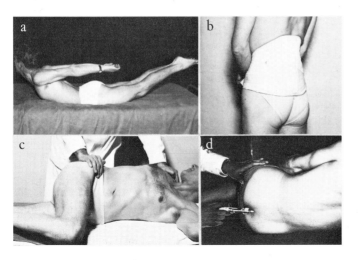

18.24 Lumbar disc – treatment   (a) Exercises; (b) corset; (c) manipulation; (d) epidural injection.

This may continue until the disc has completely collapsed, but the marginal osteophytes and progressive osteoarthritis of the facet joints eventually stabilize that level and the symptom pattern changes.

Clinical features

The patient with lumbar instability often gives a history of acute disc rupture and recurrent attacks of pain over several years. Backache may be intermittent and related to spells of hard work, standing or walking a lot, or sitting in one position during a long journey; it is relieved by lying down. Pain is often referred to the buttock and the back of the greater trochanter; sometimes it extends down the leg like sciatica. There may be acute incidents of 'locking' or 'giving way'.

As the condition modulates from instability to osteoarthritis of the facet joints, pain is more constant but can sometimes be temporarily re-lieved by manipulation, local warmth and anti-inflammatory drugs.

The patient is usually over 40 and otherwise fit. Often, tender areas are felt in the back and buttocks. Lumbar movements are limited and may be painful at their extremes. With instability there may be a typical 'heave' or 'jerk' as the patient straightens up after bending forward. Neurological examination may show residual signs of an old disc prolapse (e.g. an absent ankle jerk). In the very late stages, symptoms and signs of spinal stenosis or of unilateral root canal stenosis may supervene.

X-RAYS   Early signs are slight narrowing of the anterior half of the disc space and retrolisthesis (posterior displacement of the upper vertebra) at L4/5 or L5/S1 in the lateral views.

Later there is more marked flattening of the disc and marginal osteophytes which vary from very small to very large. MacNab (1977) has referred to the 'traction spur' which arises a few

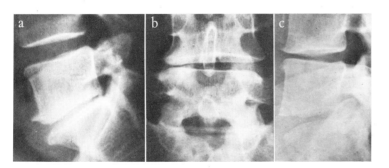

18.25 Spondylosis   (a) With chronic disc degeneration the space at L5/S1 has become narrow. (b, c) A similar disorder at L4/5 has caused lateral and forward tilting. Anterior 'traction spurs' in (a) and (c) suggest local instability.

millimetres away from the vertebral margin and is said to be characteristic of instability. With advanced degeneration the disc space may show increased radiolucency (the 'vacuum sign'), and oblique views may show facet joint malalignment and osteoarthritis.

Myelography is indicated only if neurological symptoms and signs are marked. *Discography* and *facet joint arthrography* are useful if the diagnosis is in doubt, or before spinal fusion in order to establish the condition of the upper level discs; in the presence of degeneration the contrast medium leaks into the surrounding tissues and its injection may reproduce the symptoms.

Treatment

As the disability is seldom severe, and may even decrease with time (as the spine stabilizes itself), conservative measures are encouraged for as long as possible. These consist of instruction in modified activities, isometric exercises, manipulation during acute episodes, the wearing of a lumbar corset and small doses of anti-inflammatory drugs. Psychotherapy may be helpful for pain control. If these measures cannot control pain,

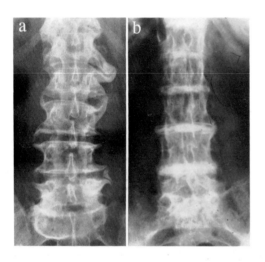

18.26 Other causes of 'spondylosis' (a) In Forestier's disease (see page 43) there are large spurs at multiple levels, often worse on the right side; (b) in ochronosis (see page 50) intervertebral calcification is characteristic.

spinal fusion is indicated. The choice of method depends on the associated pathology (Newman, 1973).

Spinal stenosis

One of the long-term consequences of disc degeneration and osteoarthritis is narrowing of the spinal canal due to hypertrophy at the posterior disc margin and the facet joints. This is more likely if the canal was always small, or if a spondylolisthesis decreases its anteroposterior diameter.

The following classification (based on that of Arnoldi *et al.*, 1976) may be useful.

(1) *Congenital stenosis* This occurs in achondroplasia and hypochondroplasia, but usually is a developmental variant.

(2) *Post-degenerative stenosis* As described above, this is more likely if spondylosis is superimposed on developmental narrowing.

(3) *Post-spondylolisthetic stenosis* A degenerative spondylolisthesis at L4/5 quite often produces stenosis and is the commonest cause in elderly patients.

(4) *Miscellaneous* Paget's disease, a spinal tumour or even tuberculosis may present with features of spinal stenosis. Rarely, the condition follows trauma or operation.

Clinical features

Typically, the patient complains of aching, heaviness, numbness and paraesthesia in the thighs and legs; it comes on only after standing upright or walking for 5 or 10 minutes, and is consistently relieved by sitting, squatting or leaning against a wall to flex the spine (hence the confusing term 'spinal claudication'). Symptoms are often unilateral, suggesting an asymmetrical stenosis ('root canal stenosis').

Examination, especially after getting the patient to reproduce the symptoms by walking, may show neurological deficit in the lower limbs. Electromyography may be helpful if the clinical findings are equivocal.

X-RAYS Lateral views may show degenerative spondylolisthesis or advanced disc degeneration and osteoarthritis. Measurement of the spinal

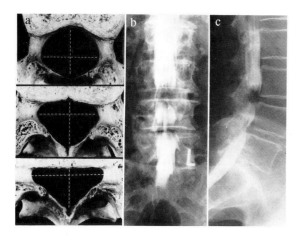

18.27 Spinal stenosis   (a) The shape of the lumbar spinal canal varies from oval (with a large capacity) to trefoil (with narrow lateral recesses); further encroachment on an already narrow canal can cause an ischaemic neuropathy and 'spinal claudication'. (b, c) Myelogram showing marked narrowing of the radio-opaque column at the level of stenosis.

canal may be carried out on plain films, but more reliable information is obtained from *ultrasound* or from *computerized tomography*. *Myelography* is done if operation is planned; it shows the level of the block and the effect of spinal extension and flexion.

Treatment

Conservative measures, including instruction in spinal posture, may suffice. If they fail, operative decompression is almost always successful. A wide laminectomy is performed, if necessary extending over several levels and outwards to clear the nerve root canals. This relieves the leg pain, but not the back pain, and occasionally it actually increases instability; consequently, in patients under 60 the operation is sometimes combined with spinal fusion.

Spondylolisthesis

Spondylolisthesis means forward shift of the spine. The shift is nearly always between L4 and L5, or between L5 and the sacrum. Normal laminae and facets constitute a locking mechanism which prevents each vertebra from moving forwards on the one below. Forward shift (or slip) occurs only when this mechanism has failed. Three varieties are described.

Dysplastic (20 per cent)   The superior sacral facets are congenitally defective; slow but inexorable forward slip leads to severe displacement.

Degenerative (25 per cent)   Degenerative changes in the facet joints and the discs permit forward slip (nearly always at L4/5) despite intact laminae.

Isthmic (50 per cent)   Usually the posterior arch is in two pieces (spondylolytic) with a gap in the pars interarticularis; repeated breaking and healing may lead to elongation of the pars. It is difficult to exclude a genetic factor because spondylolisthesis often runs in families, and is commoner in certain races, notably Eskimos; but the incidence increases with age, so an acquired factor probably supervenes to produce what is essentially a stress fracture. The condition is more common than usual in those whose spines are subjected to extraordinary stresses (e.g. competitive gymnasts).

The remaining 5 per cent of cases comprise traumatic spondylolisthesis following a single major injury, and pathological spondylolisthesis due to bone disease or neoplasm.

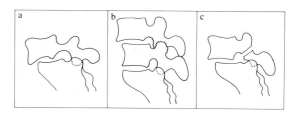

18.28 Spondylolisthesis – varieties   (a) The pars interarticularis may be long and attenuated, with forward shift of the upper vertebra on the lower; (b) degeneration of the facet joints (usually at L4/5) may allow slipping of the upper vertebra; or (c) there may be a break in the pars interarticularis – a type of stress fracture.

Pathology

When the pars interarticularis is in two pieces (spondylolysis) the gap is occupied by fibrous tissue; behind the gap the spinous process, laminae and inferior articular facets remain as an isolated segment. With stress, the vertebral body and superior facets in front of the gap may

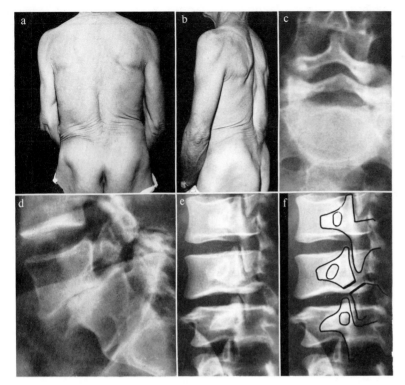

18.29 Spondylolisthesis – clinical and x-ray   (a, b) The transverse loin creases, short lumbar spine and long sacrum are characteristic. (c) In the AP x-ray the 'slipped' vertebral body may be seen obliquely as an oval shadow. In the lateral x-ray (d) the slip may be obvious, but the defect in the pars interarticularis is better seen in the oblique view (e, f) where it is likened to a 'collar' around the 'neck' of an illusory 'dog'.

subluxate or dislocate forwards, carrying the superimposed vertebral column; the isolated segment maintains its normal relationship to the sacral facets. When there is no gap, the pars interarticularis is elongated or the facets are defective.

With forward slipping there may be pressure on the dura mater and cauda equina, or on the emerging nerve roots; these roots may also be compressed in the narrowed intervertebral foramina. Disc prolapse is liable to occur.

Clinical features

In children the condition is painless but the mother may notice the unduly protruding abdomen. In adolescents and adults backache is the usual presenting symptom; it is often intermittent, coming on after exercise or strain. Sciatic pain may occur in one or both legs.

Spondylolysis, and even a well-marked spondylolisthesis, may be discovered incidentally during routine x-ray examination.

Degenerative spondylolisthesis usually occurs in women over 40 years; the other varieties may occur at any age, but the dysplastic type is commoner in girls and the isthmic type in males.

On examination the buttocks look curiously flat, the sacrum appears to extend to the waist and transverse loin creases are seen. The lumbar spine is on a plane in front of the sacrum and is too short. Sometimes there is a scoliosis.

A 'step' can often be felt when the fingers are run down the spine. Movements are usually normal in younger patients; in the degenerative group the spine is often stiff.

X-RAYS show the forward shift of the upper part of the spinal column on the stable vertebra below; elongation of the arch or defective facets may be seen. The gap in the pars interarticularis is best seen in the oblique views.

Treatment

CONSERVATIVE TREATMENT is indicated (1) if the patient is no longer young and symptoms are not disabling, or (2) if there is doubt whether the symptoms arise from the slip or from an associated disc prolapse. It consists of bed rest during an acute attack and a supporting corset between attacks.

OPERATIVE TREATMENT is indicated (1) at any age if the symptoms are disabling, (2) in the young adult with even moderate symptoms, and (3) if neurological compression is marked. Four methods are available.

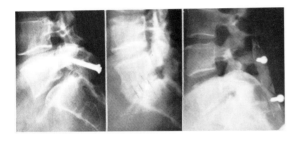

18.30 Spondylolisthesis – treatment (left) Stability may be regained by fixing only the bony defect; or (centre) by fusing the vertebral bodies anteriorly; or (right) by fusing the posterolateral elements of the spine.

(1) *Direct repair* Buck (1970), who regards the bony gap as a fatigue fracture, advises direct repair. Through a posterior approach the gap is thoroughly rawed, then fixed by chip grafts and a screw; both sides are fixed. The method applies only where there is a gap and slipping is not severe; its advantage is that no movement whatsoever is sacrificed.

(2) *Posterior fusion* To prevent further slipping of the fifth lumbar body on the sacrum, a posterolateral fusion between the fifth transverse process and the ala of the sacrum is usually successful. For a slip at L4/5, intertransverse fusion has a significant failure rate, especially if compared with posterior decompression.

(3) *Anterior fusion* The disc between the forwardly slipped vertebra and the one below is removed and one or more bone grafts used to fix the bodies together. Freebody *et al.* (1971), who report excellent results, advise a transperitoneal approach with careful dissection of the presacral nerve.

(4) *Laminectomy* If the operation is indicated chiefly for spinal stenosis or nerve compression, laminectomy will relieve the symptoms and fusion may be unnecessary.

Note on post-traumatic spondylolisthesis

The patient found to have spondylolysis or spondylolisthesis after recent back injury (usually hyperextension) may have fractured a lamina, or merely have strained the fibrous tissue of a pre-existing lesion. If doubt exists (and it usually does) a plaster jacket is worn for 3 months; the recent fracture may join spontaneously. If union does not occur the assumption is that spondylolisthesis was present before injury and treatment is along the lines already indicated.

Causes of backache

There are many causes of backache and it is useful to group them.

Injury

(1) *Twisting forces*, causing muscle injury (sometimes with a fractured transverse process).
(2) *Lifting strain*, causing ligament injury ('sprung back') or disc prolapse.
(3) *Crushing force*, causing bony injury (compression fracture).

In all these the onset is sudden, after strain or violence; the patient is otherwise fit, and the x-ray appearance is normal or shows a fracture.

Degeneration

The back is mechanically unsound and joint degeneration develops because of some underlying structural fault.

(1) *Lumbar instability* and spondylosis following previous disc prolapse.
(2) *Lumbar strain* due to spinal deformity (thoracic kyphosis often gives lumbar pain because this area is constantly under strain to keep the patient upright).
(3) *Osteoarthritis* of the facet joints.

In all these conditions the onset is gradual, though often there is a history of previous back trouble; the pain is worse after strain and better after rest; the patient has no general illness; and x-rays show lipping of the vertebral bodies and may reveal the deformity.

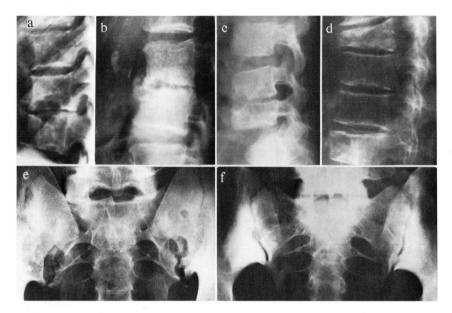

18.31 Some causes of chronic backache   (a) Tuberculosis; (b) acute osteomyelitis – note the sclerosis which developed within a few weeks; (c) discitis. (d) Here, unlike the previous three, the disc spaces are normal – the bodies are not – these are secondary deposits. (e) Bilateral sacroiliac tuberculosis; (f) osteitis condensans ilii, which is probably symptomless.

Spinal disease

(1) *Inflammation*   The most important chronic inflammatory conditions are tuberculosis and ankylosing spondylitis. Pyogenic osteomyelitis is rare but may present acutely.
(2) *Tumours*   The most common tumour is a secondary vertebral deposit. Other tumours may involve the cord, meninges or nerve roots. Vertebral haemangioma is often symptomless.
(3) *Paget's disease.*

In all these conditions the onset is not sudden or with violence; the patient may have other evidence of disease, the ESR may be raised and x-rays often reveal the cause.

Sacroiliac disease

Sacroiliac disease, especially if bilateral, causes backache indistinguishable from that of lumbosacral disease. The common causes are:

(1) Ankylosing spondylitis.
(2) Reiter's disease.

Other features (such as urogenital infection and conjunctivitis) may be present and the ESR is often raised.

Disease elsewhere

Backache occurs in non-spinal conditions as follows.

(1) *Any acute febrile illness* – e.g. influenza.
(2) *Disorders of abdominal viscera* – e.g. the stomach, duodenum, pancreas and urogenital tract.
(3) *Disorders, including carcinoma and presacral malignant deposits, of the pelvic viscera* – e.g. the uterus, ovaries, bladder and rectum. (Hence the importance of rectal and vaginal examination.)

In all these conditions the onset is not sudden or with violence; there is other evidence of disease; and x-rays of the spine itself are normal.

Idiopathic

In many patients the cause of backache is never found. It is attributed to the following.

(1) *Poor posture.*
(2) *Overwork.*
(3) *Mental depression.*

These are grist to the mill of the osteopath.

Causes of sciatica

Inflammation

(1) Rarely, in sciatica, there is a true neuritis (e.g. diabetic or alcoholic).
(2) Arachnoiditis may follow repeated surgery or myelography.

In these conditions the onset is not sudden, the patient is unfit, the nerve itself is tender and peripheral neurological signs are present.

Compression of a nerve

(1) *In the vertebral canal* compression is usually due to a prolapsed disc, occasionally to tuberculous material or to a tumour of the cauda equina or meninges.
(2) *In the intervertebral foramen* compression may arise from a tumour of the root, a lymphadenomatous deposit or because of narrowing of the foramen in spondylolisthesis.
(3) *In the pelvis or buttock* compression may arise from an abscess, a haematoma or a tumour if impacted or adherent to the nerve.

In all these stretching the nerve is painful. A prolapsed disc is much the most common cause, and also the most innocuous. A mass in the buttock shows on computerized tomography.

Referred

Pain may be referred from spinal ligaments or unstable facet joints. 'Fibrositic' pain is probably of this nature.

In this condition there are tender areas on which pressure may also provoke sciatic pain; local anaesthesia abolishes both the local and the referred pain. The patient is otherwise fit. The x-ray appearance of the spine is often normal.

Notes on applied anatomy

THE SPINE AS A WHOLE   The spine has to move, to transmit weight and to protect the spinal cord. In upright man the lumbar segment is lordotic and the column acts like a crane; the paravertebral muscles are the cables which counterbalance any weight carried anteriorly. The resultant force, which passes through the nucleus pulposus of the lowest lumbar disc, is therefore much greater than if the column were loaded directly over its centre; even at rest, tonic contraction of the posterior muscles balances the trunk, so that the lumbar spine is always loaded. Nachemson and Morris (1964) measured the intradiscal pressure in volunteers during various activities and found it as high as $10–15\,\text{kg/cm}^2$ while sitting, about 30 per

cent less on standing upright and 50 per cent less on lying down. Leaning forward or carrying a weight produces much higher pressures, though when a heavy weight is lifted breathing stops and the abdominal muscles contract, turning the trunk into a tightly inflated bag which cushions the force anteriorly against the pelvis. (Could it be that champion weight-lifters benefit in this way from having voluminous bodies?)

Seen from the side, the dorsal spine is concave forwards (kyphosis); the cervical and lumbar regions are concave backwards (lordosis). In forward flexion the lordotic curves straighten out. Lying supine with the legs straight tilts the pelvic brim forwards; the lumbar spine compensates by increasing its lordosis. If the hips are unable to extend fully (fixed flexion deformity), the lumbar lordosis increases still more until the lower limbs lie flat and the flexion deformity is masked.

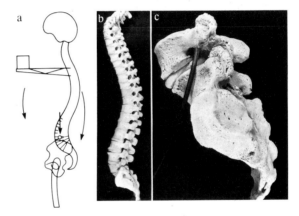

18.32 Anatomy (a, b) The vertebral column has a series of gentle curves which produce lordosis in the cervical and lumbar regions and kyphosis in the dorsal segment. The column functions like a crane, the weight in front of the spine being counterbalanced by contraction of the posterior muscles. (c) Relationship of nerve root to disc and facet joint.

THE VERTEBRAL COMPONENTS   Each segment of the vertebral column transmits weight through the vertebral body anteriorly and the facet joints posteriorly. Between adjacent bodies (and firmly attached to them) lie the intervertebral discs. These compressible 'cushions', and the surrounding ligaments and muscles, act as shock-absorbers; if they are degenerate or weak their ability to absorb some of the force is diminished and the bones and joints suffer the consequences.

The vertebral body is cancellous, but the upper and lower surfaces are condensed to form sclerotic end plates. In childhood these are covered by cartilage, which contributes to vertebral growth. Later the peripheral rim ossifies and fuses with the body, but the central area remains as a thin layer of cartilage adherent to the intervertebral disc. The epiphyseal end plates may be damaged by disc pressure during childhood, giving rise to irregular ossification and abnormal vertebral growth (Scheuermann's disease).

THE INTERVERTEBRAL DISC   The disc consists of a central avascular *nucleus pulposus* – a hydrophilic gel made of protein-polysaccharide, collagen fibres, sparse chondroid cells and water (88 per cent) – surrounded by concentric layers of fibrous tissue, the *annulus fibrosus*. If the physicochemical state of the nucleus pulposus is normal, the disc can withstand almost any load that the muscles can support; if it is abnormal, even small increases in force can produce sufficient stress to rupture the annulus.

THE SPINAL CANAL   The shape of the canal changes from ovoid in the upper part of the spine to triangular in the lower. Variations are common and include the trefoil canal whose shape is mainly due to thickening of the laminae posteriorly (Eisenstein, 1980). This shape is harmless in itself, but further encroachment on the canal (e.g. by a bulging disc or hypertrophic facet joints) may cause compression of the spinal contents (spinal stenosis).

THE SPINAL CORD   The spinal cord ends at about L1 in the conus medullaris, but lumbosacral nerve roots continue in the spinal canal as the cauda equina and leave at appropriate levels lower down. The dural sac continues as far as S2, and whenever a nerve root leaves the spine it takes with it a dural sleeve as far as the exit from the intervertebral foramen. These dural sleeves can be outlined by contrast medium radiography ('radiculography').

THE INTERVERTEBRAL FORAMINA AND NERVE ROOTS   Each intervertebral foramen is bounded anteriorly by the disc and adjoining vertebral bodies, posteriorly by the facet joint, and superiorly and inferiorly by the pedicles of adjacent vertebrae. It can therefore be narrowed by a bulging disc or by joint osteophytes. The segmental nerve roots leave the spinal canal through the intervertebral foramina, each pair below the vertebra of the same number (thus, the fourth lumbar root runs between L4 and L5). The segmental blood vessels to and from the cord also pass through the intervertebral foramen. Occlusion of this little passage may occasionally compress the nerve root directly or may cause nerve root ischaemia (especially when the spine is held in extension).

NERVE SUPPLY OF THE SPINE   The spine and its contents (including the dural sleeves of the nerve roots themselves) are supplied by small branches from the anterior and posterior primary rami of the segmental nerve roots. Lesions of different structures (e.g. the posterior longitudinal ligament, the dural sleeve or the facet joint) may therefore cause pain of similar distribution. *Pain down the thigh and leg ('sciatica') does not necessarily signify root pressure; it may equally well be referred from a facet joint.*

BLOOD SUPPLY   In addition to the spinal arteries, which run the length of the cord, segmental arteries from the aorta send branches through the intervertebral foramina at each level. Accompanying veins drain into the azygos system and inferior vena cava, and anastomose profusely with the extradural plexus which extends throughout the length of the spinal canal (Batson's plexus).

Further reading

Arnoldi, C. C., Brodsky, A. E., Cauchoix, J., Crock, H. V., Dommisse, G. F., Edgar, M. A. *et al.* (1976) Lumbar spinal stenosis and nerve root entrapment. *Clinical Orthopaedics* **115,** 4–5

Benson, M. K. D. and Byrnes, D. P. (1975) The clinical syndromes and surgical treatment of thoracic intervertebral disc prolapse. *Journal of Bone and Joint Surgery* **57B,** 471–477

Bradford, D. S., Khalid, B. A., Moe, J. H., Winter, R. B. and Lonstein, J. E. (1980) The surgical management of patients with Scheuermann's disease. *Journal of Bone and Joint Surgery* **62A,** 705–712

Buck, J. E. (1970) Direct repair of the defect in spondylolisthesis. *Journal of Bone and Joint Surgery* **52B,** 432–437

Eisenstein, S. (1980) The trefoil configuration of the lumbar vertebral canal. *Journal of Bone and Joint Surgery* **62B,** 73–77

Freebody, D., Bendall, R. and Taylor, R. D. (1971) Anterior transperitoneal lumbar fusion. *Journal of Bone and Joint Surgery* **53B,** 617–627

Hodgson, A. R. and Yau, A. (1969) Surgical approaches to the spinal column. In *Recent Advances in Orthopaedics.* Ed. by A. Graham Apley. London: Churchill

James, J. I. P. (1976) *Scoliosis,* 2nd edn. Edinburgh: Churchill Livingstone.

Journal of Bone and Joint Surgery (1968) Symposium: Low Back and Sciatic Pain (by various authors). Instructional Course Lectures. **50A,** 167–210

Kemp, H. B. S., Jackson, J. W., Jeremiah, J. D. and Hall, A. J. (1973) Pyogenic infections occurring primarily in intervertebral discs. *Journal of Bone and Joint Surgery* **55B,** 698–714

McCullough, J. A. (1977) Chemonucleolysis. *Journal of Bone and Joint Surgery* **59B,** 45–52

MacNab, I. (1977) *Backache.* Baltimore: Williams & Wilkins

Mehta, M. H. (1972) The rib–vertebra angle in the early diagnosis between resolving and progressive infantile scoliosis. *Journal of Bone and Joint Surgery* **54B,** 230–243

Moll, J. M. H. (Ed.) (1980) *Ankylosing Spondylitis.* Edinburgh: Churchill Livingstone

Nachemson, A. and Morris, J. M. (1964) *In vivo* measurements of intradiscal pressure. *Journal of Bone and Joint Surgery* **46A,** 1077–1092

Newman, P. H. (1973) Surgical treatment for derangement of the lumbar spine. *Journal of Bone and Joint Surgery* **55B,** 7–19

Newman, P. H. with Stone, K. H. (1963) The etiology of spondylolisthesis. *Journal of Bone and Joint Surgery* **45B,** 39–59

Seddon, H. J. (1976) The choice of treatment in Pott's disease. *Journal of Bone and Joint Surgery* **58B,** 395–397

Winter, R. B., Moe, J. H. and Wang, J. D. (1973) Congenital kyphosis. *Journal of Bone and Joint Surgery* **55A,** 223–256

The Hip Joint

19

Examination

Symptoms

The patient who speaks of 'hip' pain often means buttock pain, which usually derives from the lumbar spine. *Pain* arising in the hip joint itself is more often felt in front, or in the groin; it radiates to the thigh and knee, which sometimes are the only painful sites. *Limp* is equally common, but *stiffness* is seldom complained of directly; instead, the patient speaks of difficulty in putting on his socks or cutting his toenails.

Signs with the patient upright

The gait is noted, and also whether the patient uses any form of support. If there is a limp it may be possible to attribute it to pain (the antalgic gait), to shortening (the short-leg limp) or to abductor weakness (the Trendelenburg gait).

The patient is then asked to lift his bad leg by bending his knee behind him (keeping the hip extended); the weight-bearing hip, which is the normal one, abducts and the pelvis therefore rises on the unsupported side. Next he lowers the bad leg and lifts the good one; he is now taking weight through the affected hip and, if Trendelenburg's sign is positive, the pelvis drops on the unsupported side ('sound side sags').

The lumbar spine is examined and any deformity or limitation of movement is noted.

TRENDELENBURG'S SIGN
Normally each leg bears half the body weight. When one leg is lifted (as in normal walking) the other takes the entire weight.

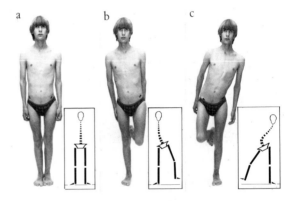

19.1 Trendelenburg's sign (a) Standing normally on two legs. (b) Standing on the right leg which has a normal hip whose abductor muscles ensure correct weight transference. (c) Standing on the left leg whose hip is faulty, so that abduction cannot be achieved; the pelvis drops on the unsupported side and the shoulder swings over to the left.

As a result the trunk has to incline towards the weight-bearing leg. This is achieved by the hip abductors; their insertion is fixed and the pull is exerted on their origin (the ilium). Consequently the pelvis tilts, rising on the side not taking weight. When this mechanism fails Trendelenburg's sign is positive. The pelvis drops instead of rising on the unsupported side, and this occurs if (1) the abductors are weak, as in poliomyelitis or muscle dystrophies; (2) there is insufficient room for abduction, as in coxa vara where the trochanter meets the pelvic wall before the pelvis can tilt sufficiently; (3) the hip is dislocated so that the muscles have no stable fulcrum, as in congenital or pathological dislocations; (4) the femoral neck is fractured so that the lever system is not intact; or (5) if it hurts the patient to put the abductors into action, as in inflammatory conditions.

Signs with the patient lying on his back

● LOOK

Skin   Scars or sinuses may be seen.

Shape   Asymmetry, swelling or wasting is observed.

Position   There may be deformity or shortening.

● FEEL

Skin   The joint is too deep for excessive warmth to be detected.

Soft tissues   Synovial thickening and fluid are not detectable in the hip. Muscle bulk and tautness should be tested; but this is best done with the patient prone.

Bones   With the thumbs anchored against the anterior superior iliac spines, the middle fingers palpate each greater trochanter; while the fingers maintain pressure on the trochanters, the thumbs are moved medially in an attempt to feel the head of the femur – if the head is not in its socket, the thumb sinks in too far. Occasionally tenderness is elicited.

● MOVE

To test extension the sound hip is flexed until any lumbar lordosis is obliterated (Thomas' test); if by this manoeuvre the affected thigh is raised from the couch, then extension is shown to be limited (this is called 'fixed flexion'). Flexion of the hips is compared by bending both simultaneously to their limit.

To test abduction both anterior superior iliac spines must first be level. The sound hip is then abducted until the pelvis starts to move; it is left in the abducted position while the affected hip in turn is abducted until the pelvis starts to move. In this way the difference in abduction of the two hips is easily seen. Adduction is compared by moving each hip in turn and watching the pelvis for movement. Alternatively, the surgeon tests abduction and adduction while one hand on the ilium detects when the pelvis starts to move.

To test rotation both legs, lifted by the ankles, are rotated first internally then externally; the patellae are watched to estimate the amount of rotation. Rotation in flexion is tested with the hip and knee each flexed 90 degrees.

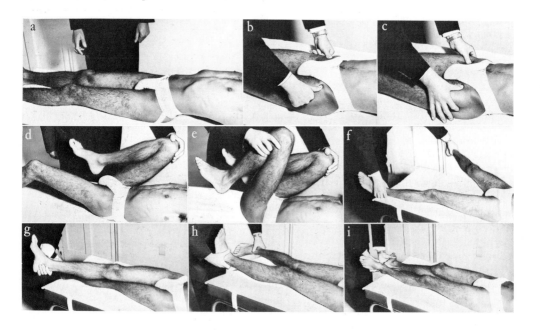

19.2 Signs with patient supine   (a) Looking at the patient: his legs and pelvis are square with the couch; the lordosis indicates fixed flexion of the hip. (b) Feeling the anterior superior iliac spine. (c) Locating the top of the greater trochanter. (d) Flexing the right hip causes the left to lift off the couch (fixed flexion). The left hip also has limitation of (e) flexion, (f) abduction, (g) adduction, (h) internal rotation, and (i) external rotation.

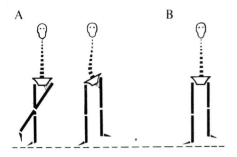

19.3 Shortening (1) – real or apparent?   A leg may look short without actually being short. Thus A, with adduction of his left hip, has to hitch up his pelvis in order to uncross his legs; this makes the leg *appear* short.

B has no hip deformity; unlike A he is able to stand (or lie) with his legs at right angles to his pelvis. His leg really *is* short.

SHORTENING

Shortening of the lower limb is analysed as follows.

Is it real or apparent? The words 'real' and 'apparent' mean precisely what they say. Real shortening means that the distance from the top of the femoral head to the heel (or the medial malleolus) is shorter on one side than the other. But clinically we cannot measure that length because the top of the femoral head is inaccessible; instead, we measure from the anterior superior iliac spine. Consequently the position of the hip influences our measurement; adduction makes the limb appear shorter – each 10 degrees of fixed adduction adds a further 3 cm of apparent shortening to any real shortening which the disorder may have caused (Ireland and Kessel, 1980).

Shortening is measured with the patient lying flat and, if possible, with the legs at right angles to a line joining both anterior superior iliac spines. If this position is possible, there can be no fixed adduction or abduction deformity and any shortening is real. It is measured from the anterior superior iliac spine to the bottom of the medial malleolus. If there is fixed deformity creating an illusion of difference, the good leg must be placed in a comparably deformed position before measurements can be compared. Apparent shortening is measured from any point in the midline (e.g. the xiphisternum).

Is it above or below the knee? Both knees are flexed while the heels remain together on the couch. It is then obvious whether shortening is in the femur or the tibia.

Is it above or below the greater trochanter? With a thumb pressed firmly against each anterior superior iliac spine, the surgeon gropes with his middle fingers for the top of each greater trochanter. With the hands in this position, it is easy to estimate elevation of one trochanter. More formal methods of estimation are: (1) to draw Nélaton's line, which runs from the anterior superior iliac spine by the shortest route to the ischial tuberosity – with the hip flexed and adducted the line normally crosses the top of the greater trochanter; or (2) to construct Bryant's triangle, in which a vertical line is drawn from the anterior superior

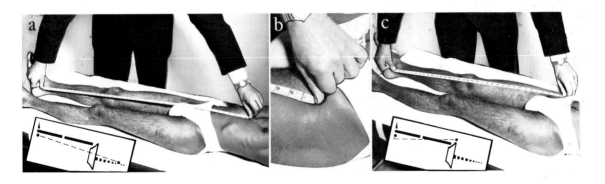

19.4 Shortening (2) – measurements   Apparent length (a) is measured from a fixed point in the midline (e.g. the xiphisternum) to the bottom of the medial malleolus. Real length is measured from the anterior superior iliac spine; note how the thumb is pressed hard up against it (b) – also to the medial malleolus (c).

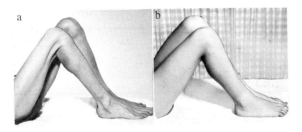

19.5 Shortening (3) Provided the backs of both heels are exactly level, bending the knees immediately shows whether shortening is above or below the knee.

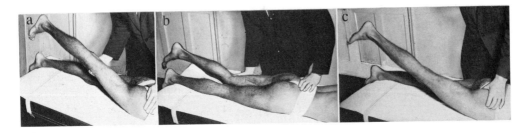

19.6 Signs with patient prone (a) Extension of the good hip is full; (b) in the affected leg it is limited. (c) Testing power in the glutei.

iliac spine to the couch, and a perpendicular drawn from this line to the top of the trochanter – by comparing the length of the perpendicular at each hip, trochanteric elevation can be measured.

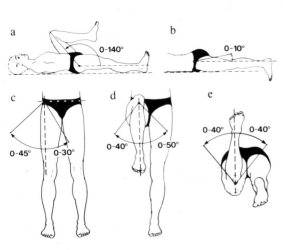

19.7 Normal range of movements (a) The hip should flex until the thigh meets the abdomen, but (b) only extends a few degrees. (c) Abduction is usually greater than adduction. The relative amounts of internal and external rotation vary according to whether the hip is in (d) flexion or (e) extension; in flexion the unwary may confuse internal with external rotation, but a hand on the thigh resolves the difficulty.

Signs with the patient lying on his face

● LOOK   Scars, sinuses or wasting are noted.

● FEEL   Muscle bulk and tautness are most easily assessed when the patient is prone.

● MOVE   Extension of the two hips is most accurately compared with the patient lying on his face. Rotation also can be assessed prone by first flexing both knees.

X-ray

With the anteroposterior view it is always an advantage to have both hips on the same film. The bone density and architecture on the two sides can be compared, as well as the hip joints themselves; any difference in the size, shape or position of the two femoral heads is important. With a normal hip Shenton's line, which continues from the inferior border of the femoral neck to the inferior border of the pubic ramus, looks smooth; any interruption in the line suggests a mechanical disorder.

Lateral films are important in nearly all juvenile disorders and in some adult ones; they are more difficult to read and it helps in orientation to remember that the lesser trochanter projects posteriorly.

THE DIAGNOSTIC CALENDAR

Age of onset (years)	Probable diagnosis
0 (birth)	Congenital dislocation
0–5	Infections
5–10	Perthes' disease
10–15	Slipped epiphysis
Adults	Osteoarthritis

It is surprising how often these approximations are correct, though infections can occasionally occur at any age.

Congenital dislocation of the hip

Causal factors

GENETIC

The familial tendency of congenital hip dislocation is well known; this may explain the relatively high incidence in certain geographic areas (e.g. North Italy). Two genetic factors are involved: (1) joint laxity (of dominant inheritance) which accounts for most of the cases diagnosed in the first week of life; and (2) acetabular dysplasia (of polygenic inheritance) which accounts for those diagnosed late. Probably three-quarters of the early cases with lax joints recover spontaneously; that is, hips which were dislocatable do not remain so.

ENVIRONMENTAL

Shortly before delivery the mother secretes a ligament-relaxing hormone. If this crosses the placental barrier, any tendency to joint laxity is enhanced. This accounts for the rarity of dislocation in premature babies (born before the hormones reach their peak) and possibly for the relative infrequency in boys (in whom male hormones counteract the female).

Intrauterine malposition (especially a breech position with extended legs) favours dislocation; this is linked with the higher incidence in first-born babies, because in them spontaneous version is less likely.

In the postnatal period racial customs influence the frequency. Dislocation is commoner in Lapps and North American Indians who swaddle their babies tightly with the hips fully extended; and is rare in Hong Kong Chinese and in some African groups where the baby's hips are not extended and may indeed be kept abducted.

Pathology

With a dislocated hip, the acetabular roof is defective. On its lateral aspect the acetabulum is underdeveloped; it is too shallow and its roof slopes too steeply. After weight-bearing a false acetabulum develops above the original fossa. The bony nucleus of the femoral head appears later than on the normal side and remains smaller; the cartilaginous head, however, is large. The dislocation is always posterior and, as the head rides upwards, the slope of the pelvis pushes it laterally. The femoral neck is usually short and is often excessively anteverted.

The capsule, unlike that in traumatic dislocation, remains intact. In time it becomes hourglass in shape, developing an isthmus where it is crossed by the psoas muscle. The cartilaginous labrum is often unduly large and folded into the acetabulum; the infolded portion (the limbus) constitutes an obstacle to reduction. The ligamentum teres is often unduly thick. In time the muscles arising from the pelvis become adaptively shortened.

Symptoms

Before the baby starts walking an observant mother may spot asymmetry, a clicking hip, or difficulty in applying the napkin because of limited abduction. Contrary to popular belief, late walking is not a marked feature; nevertheless, in children who do not walk by the age of 18 months, dislocation must be excluded. After walking starts, asymmetry is more obvious and now limp also becomes apparent.

Nearly all the above symptoms refer to unilateral dislocation. Bilateral dislocation rarely presents early, because there is no asymmetry and the characteristic waddling gait is mistaken by the parents for normal toddling.

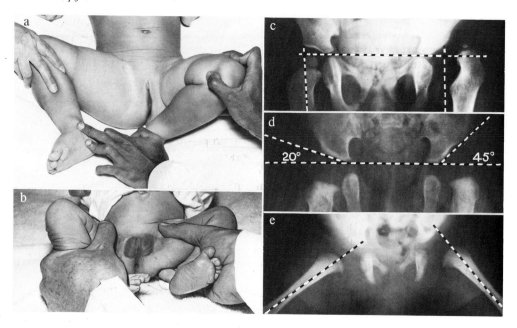

19.8 Congenital hip dislocation – early signs   (a) Ortolani's test; (b) Barlow's test; (c) Perkins' lines; (d) acetabular angle; (e) Von Rosen's lines.

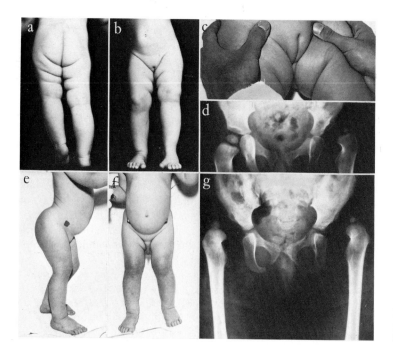

19.9 Congenital hip dislocation – late signs   Unilateral dislocation of left hip: (a, b) asymmetry, (c, d) the head is not in the socket.

Bilateral dislocation: (e, f) lordosis and a perineal gap, (g) both hips obviously dislocated.

Signs

Dislocation is much more common in girls than in boys, the left hip is more often affected than the right, and occasionally there are other congenital anomalies, such as a calcaneovalgus foot.

With unilateral dislocation the skin creases look asymmetrical and the leg slightly short and rotated externally; with bilateral dislocation there is an abnormally wide perineal gap. Too little resistance is encountered when the thumb is pressed over the front of the joint.

Abduction is decreased; this is most obvious in flexion. The flexed hip of a young baby should abduct almost to a right angle. In congenital dislocation it often stops halfway; but if pressure is then applied to it there is a clunk as the dislocation reduces and then the hip abducts fully (Ortolani's 'jerk of entry'). Another valuable test is Barlow's: the surgeon holds the upper femur between his middle finger on the greater trochanter and his thumb in the groin; by levering the femoral head in and out of the acetabulum dislocation is demonstrated. These important signs indicate a reducible dislocation and should be sought in every newborn baby; later they are not obtainable. Obviously decreased abduction without a clunk suggests irreducible dislocation.

When the child can stand, a positive Trendelenburg sign and gait are detectable.

X-RAY   Dislocation may be displayed by drawing Perkins' lines (a horizontal through the triradiate cartilages and verticals from the outer edge of each acetabulum; the head normally lies medial to the vertical and below the horizontal lines). Alternatively, the increased acetabular angle due to the defective roof can be measured. In newborn babies Von Rosen's method is probably the best: a film is taken with both hips abducted 45 degrees and internally rotated; the line of the femoral shaft is produced upwards and on the dislocated side strikes the pelvis above the top of the acetabulum.

Differential diagnosis

OTHER CAUSES OF LATE WALKING
These include mental backwardness, spina bifida and cerebral palsy. Many late walkers are otherwise normal and do later walk normally. Nevertheless the hip should be x-rayed if walking has been unduly delayed.

OTHER CAUSES OF A PAINLESS LIMP SINCE INFANCY
The most important are as follows.

Infantile coxa vara   Congenital dislocation is simulated except that the head can be felt in its socket and the x-ray appearance is distinctive.

Pathological dislocation   There is a history of illness in infancy and a scar; x-rays show that the femoral head is not merely small, it is totally absent.

Poliomyelitis   Trophic changes are present and evidence of paralysis. Moreover the head is in its socket, although paralytic dislocation can occur.

Treatment before weight-bearing

Weight-bearing begins long before walking; it begins with crawling when the baby is only a few months old. Before then, treatment is simple and the prognosis excellent. Von Rosen and Barlow convincingly demonstrated that routine postnatal examination enables dislocation to be diagnosed, and that treatment at this early age gives consistently excellent results. Much unnecessary disability could be prevented if their methods were followed everywhere.

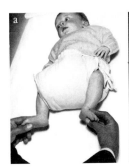 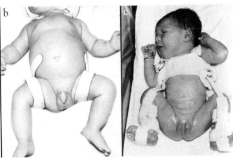

19.10 Congenital hip dislocation – treatment before weight-bearing Reduction is usually easy and can be held by (a) an abduction pillow, (b) Von Rosen's malleable splint, or – best of all – by (c) the Pavlik harness. The hips should not be more than about 60 degrees abducted, though flexion sometimes needs to be well beyond a right angle.

The hip with a positive Barlow or Ortolani sign is dislocatable, but may become normal without treatment. To avoid unnecessary splintage many surgeons (by no means all) advocate waiting 3 weeks. If either sign is then still positive the hip is abducted widely (no anaesthetic is needed) and so reduced. Both hips are held in abduction by means of a polyurethane foam pillow or a pliable aluminium splint until, after a few months, x-rays show a good acetabular roof. If the hip is irreducible the treatment advocated in the next group is applied.

Treatment after weight-bearing but below the age limit

The prognosis in this group is less satisfactory but the principle does not vary – the hip must be reduced and held reduced until it is stable.

Closed reduction This is the ideal, but risks damaging the blood supply to the femoral head and causing necrosis. To minimize this risk traction is applied to both legs, preferably on a vertical frame. Abduction is gradually increased until, by 3 weeks, the legs are widely separated. This manoeuvre alone (aided if necessary by adductor tenotomy), may achieve stable, concentric reduction. If not, the gentlest manipulation under anaesthesia may now succeed and is probably not harmful.

If reduction feels unstable, or x-ray shows that it is not concentric, an arthrogram is performed. This may reveal an infolded limbus; if so, open reduction is advisable. But if no obstruction is revealed the hip is splinted and reassessed after a few weeks; by then it may have become concentric.

Splintage The concentrically reduced hip is held in plaster for 6 weeks; both hips are included. Salter and Kostuik (1969) have shown that the frog position (90 degrees abduction, 90 degrees flexion) may cause necrosis* (epiphysitis); they advocate the 'human position' with the hips only 60 degrees abducted. After 6 weeks the plaster is replaced by a splint which prevents adduction but allows movement (the Pavlik harness and the Denis Browne splint are popular models). Within 12 months (often less) x-rays may show a concentric femoral head with a normal acetabular roof; if so, splintage is discarded.

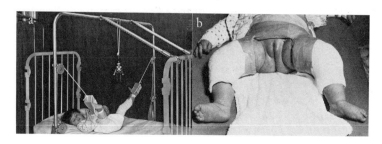

19.11 Congenital hip dislocation – treatment after weight-bearing (a) Vertical traction with abduction gradually increased; (b) plaster.

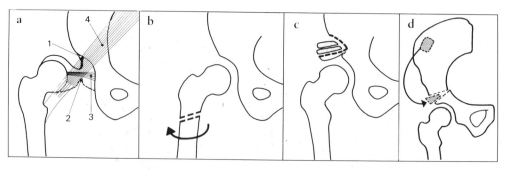

19.12 Congenital hip dislocation – operative treatment (1) (a) Obstructions to closed reduction: 1, inverted limbus; 2, hourglass constriction of capsule; 3, thick ligamentum teres; 4, tight psoas. (b) Rotation osteotomy. (c) Shelf operation. (d) Innominate osteotomy.

*The frog position should only be used for frogs (Salter).

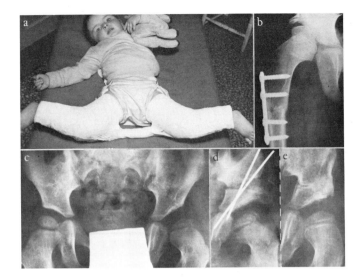

19.13 Congenital hip dislocation – operative treatment (2) (a) Reduced open, but stable only in medial rotation – 6 weeks later (b) derotation osteotomy.

(c) Reduced open, but head poorly covered; (d, e) innominate osteotomy.

Operation If, at any stage, concentric reduction has not been achieved, then open operation is needed. Any obstruction, such as an inverted limbus, is dealt with, and the hip reduced. Reduction may look satisfactory only when the hip is rotated medially; it is held in this reduced position in plaster for 6 weeks. Then a subtrochanteric osteotomy is performed. The hip is left pointing in its stable direction, but the leg below the osteotomy is derotated until the foot points forward; internal fixation is reinforced by plaster.

If the medially rotated hip does not look satisfactory on x-ray, osteotomy alone is of no value. If the head, though reduced, is still poorly covered, it should be provided with a bony roof; a shelf operation is one method, but innominate osteotomy (Salter, 1961) is better. Whatever operation is needed, the hip is subsequently held in plaster until radiologically satisfactory.

Treatment above the age limit

The term 'age limit' implies that above a certain age reduction of the dislocation is unwise. The force needed for reduction damages the hip so much that pain and stiffness are likely to develop within a few years.

With unilateral dislocation the age limit is about 6 years. The untreated hip is mobile; the patient limps but has no pain until middle life. This is the justification for non-intervention. A contrary view advocates reduction (aided if necessary by shortening the femoral neck), even above the age limit; the possible techniques include

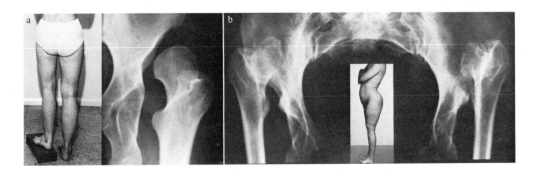

19.14 Congenital hip dislocation – above the age limit (a) Unilateral dislocation in a young adult. (b) Bilateral dislocation – this patient had no symptoms till aged 40 when she presented with backache.

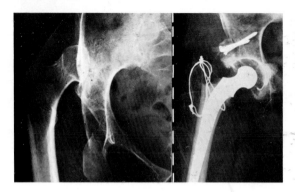

19.15 Congenital hip dislocation – hip replacement   Old congenital dislocation treated by total hip replacement; the femoral head has been used as a graft to augment the acetabular margin.

capsular arthroplasty (Colonna), innominate osteotomy (Salter) and pelvic osteotomy (Chiari). Should pain subsequently develop, joint replacement, though undesirable in the young, is at least feasible; the excised femoral head can be used to augment the defective acetabular roof.

With bilateral dislocation the age limit is about 4. It is lower because the risk of intervention is doubled, and because partial failure leads to asymmetry.* The untreated patient waddles through life until, at the age of 40 or 50, she develops backache (a sequel to the lumbar lordosis). Unhappily this is difficult to manage; a corset is a placebo, but bilateral total hip replacement in the absence of reasonable acetabula is a formidable undertaking.

Subluxation of the hip

For normal weight transmission the femoral head must be well contained within the socket. If the 'roof' is defective the acetabulum is said to be dysplastic. It is too shallow and faces too laterally; on x-ray the centre–edge angle is less than 20

degrees. Containment is inadequate and the hip is liable to subluxate. When this happens the femoral head (which is often too big) is not displaced upwards like a dislocation, but stands away too far laterally.

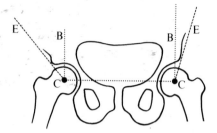

19.16 The centre–edge (CE) angle   The line C–C joins the centre of each femoral head; CB is perpendicular to this, and CE cuts the superior edge of the acetabulum. The angle BCE is normally 30 degrees or more, as in the right hip; an angle of less than 20 degrees, as in the left hip, suggests dysplasia.

Subluxation may follow unsuccessful treatment of congenital dislocation, or it may occur without any preceding disorder. In either case, weight transmission is faulty and early degeneration follows. These patients develop painful and progressive osteoarthritis in their twenties; the first step towards remedy is early diagnosis.

Clinical features

All hips should be examined soon after birth. Subluxation is less obvious than dislocation because there is neither shortening nor a click; but abduction in flexion is limited and this should always alert suspicion. The same sign is detected when an observant mother brings the child because she has noticed asymmetrical creases or difficulty in applying napkins. X-rays at this age are not easy to read; the bony nucleus of the femoral head does not appear before the age of about 6 months, but the acetabular angle shows that the roof is too sloping.

Bilateral subluxation is even more likely to be missed. Napkin difficulty is greater but there is no

---

*One short leg is worse than two.

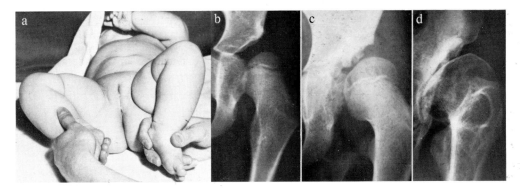

19.17 Congenital subluxation　(a) The cardinal physical sign; (b) x-ray in childhood; (c) in adolescence; (d) degeneration in early adult life.

asymmetry. Clinical experience is needed to appreciate that both hips have limited abduction in flexion, and radiological awareness to notice that both acetabula are too sloping.

Treatment

The infant under a year old often responds to closed treatment similar to that for dislocation. A vertical frame is used; skin traction is applied to both legs, which are gradually separated. When abduction is full a splint is applied; it is worn until, after a few months, the acetabular roof looks normal.

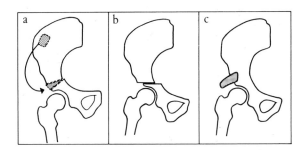

19.18 Congenital subluxation – treatment　(a) Salter's innominate osteotomy; (b) Chiari's pelvic osteotomy; (c) giant shelf.

If the femoral head remains poorly covered, or if the child is more than a year old, operation is needed. A varus femoral osteotomy may be enough to produce a congruent joint under the age of about 2. In the older child it is better to provide a good acetabular roof by Salter's innominate osteotomy or Chiari's pelvic osteotomy, or by constructing a massive shelf.

Acquired dislocation of the hip

Following sepsis

In infancy the femur may be infected via the umbilicus or via femoral vein puncture; at this age the growth disc is no barrier and infection readily involves the femoral head and the joint. In older children acute osteomyelitis usually affects the metaphysis; but since this is intracapsular again the joint is readily attacked. If the infection is unchecked the head and neck of the femur may be destroyed and a pathological dislocation result. The pus may escape and, when the child recovers, the sinus heals. The hip signs then resemble those of a congenital dislocation, but the tell-tale scar remains and on x-ray the femoral head is completely absent.

Even in the acute stage diagnosis is not easy. The ill child who cries when the hip is moved presents little problem; but some of these children have immunodeficiency and in them the signs are deceptively slight despite severe bone destruction. Aspiration under anaesthesia is often necessary. Even if pus is withdrawn, immediate arthrotomy is still advisable (Paterson, 1970); a piece of capsule and synovium is excised, antibiotic instilled and the wound closed without drainage. Systemic antibiotics are given and the hip is splinted in abduction until all evidence of activity has disappeared.

Persistent dislocation after infection has totally settled can be treated by traction, followed by open 'reduction' (in the absence of a femoral head the greater trochanter can be placed in the acetabulum); varus osteotomy of the upper femur helps to achieve stability.

Other acquired dislocations

Traumatic dislocations, which may be posterior, central or anterior, are described on page 436. Even without trauma a hip is liable to dislocate if, because of unbalanced paralysis, the adductor muscles are stronger than the abductors, notably in cerebral palsy, in myelomeningocele and after

poliomyelitis (see Chapter 10). Rare causes of acquired dislocation include tuberculosis and Charcot's disease.

Intoe gait

A familiar sight at every paediatric orthopaedic clinic is the child brought because of intoe gait. The child walks awkwardly and trips over his feet when running. The cause is rarely serious but a bland assurance that 'he will grow out of it' is not enough; the parents are genuinely distressed and the grandparents invariably fussed.

The commonest cause of intoe gait is excessive anteversion of the femoral neck, so that internal rotation of the hip is increased and external rotation diminished. The gait may look clumsy, but is no bar to athletic prowess and usually improves with growth. These children often sit on the floor in the 'television position' (with the knees facing each other) but should be encouraged to adopt the 'Buddha position'. Correction by osteotomy is feasible, but seldom indicated, and certainly not before the age of 8.

To measure anteversion the child lies prone on an x-ray table with the knee flexed to a right

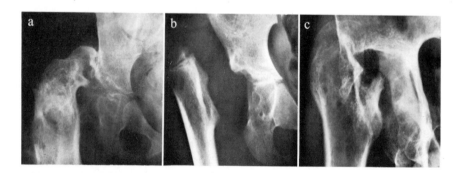

19.19 Acquired dislocation (non-traumatic)   (a) Acute suppurative arthritis following osteomyelitis of the femoral neck in a child. (b) Acute suppurative arthritis in infancy has resulted in complete disappearance of the femoral head and neck. (c) Pathological dislocation in tuberculosis.

angle; the leg is externally rotated and when, on the fluoroscope, the neck is seen to be in line with the shaft of the femur, the angle of rotation of the leg is measured.

Other causes of intoe gait include femoral torsion, tibial torsion and forefoot adduction. To differentiate these the child is examined first with hips and knees extended, then with both flexed to a right angle; finally the position of the foot is inspected.

Below the age of about 18 months, the commonest cause is forefoot adduction; from then to the age of 3 years tibial torsion is the usual cause and above that age femoral torsion (of the shaft or neck).

The irritable hip

The patient with an irritable hip (the term 'irritable' is non-specific) presents with pain and limp. Both are usually intermittent, following activity. The pain is felt in the groin or front of the thigh, sometimes reaching as far as the knee. Slight wasting may be detectable, but the cardinal sign is that the extremes of all movements are limited, and the attempt to produce them is painful.

A thorough general examination and x-rays are the first steps in management. The patient is put to bed without delay, and skin traction applied to the affected leg. Blood investigations are instituted and every effort is made to establish the diagnosis. The following conditions must be considered.

TRANSIENT SYNOVITIS　The cause is unknown and the irritability subsides quickly. X-rays are normal and investigations negative.

EARLY TUBERCULOSIS　The patient may be unwell, the sedimentation rate raised and the Heaf test positive; however, sometimes systemic features are minimal and the diagnosis hinges on a positive biopsy or bacteriological culture.

CHRONIC SYNOVITIS　Monarticular rheumatoid disease may be undiagnosable without a biopsy. Other joints usually become affected later.

PERTHES' DISEASE　The child is aged 4 to 10 years, is well, and the irritability subsides fairly quickly. Abduction in flexion is the movement most restricted, and x-rays show increased density of the head with an increased joint space.

SLIPPED EPIPHYSIS　The gradual type may present with an irritable hip. Age and build are characteristic and the x-ray appearance is diagnostic, provided a lateral view also is taken.

Tuberculosis of the hip

The disease process may start as a synovitis, or as an osteomyelitis in the bone of the acetabulum, femoral head or neck. Once arthritis develops, destruction is rapid. Muscle spasm presses the femoral head against the acetabulum, which is eroded and appears to enlarge upwards (wandering acetabulum). The femoral head also may be destroyed, permitting pathological dislocation. Healing usually leaves a long unsound fibrous joint with considerable limb shortening and deformity.

Clinical features

The patient, usually a child, limps a little and complains of slight ache in the groin or thigh; later, pain is more severe and may wake the child from sleep.

With early disease (synovitis or osteomyelitis) the joint is held slightly flexed and abducted, and extremes of movement are a little limited and painful; but until x-ray changes appear the hip is merely 'irritable' and diagnosis is difficult. If arthritis supervenes the hip becomes flexed, adducted and medially rotated, muscle wasting becomes obvious, and all movements are grossly limited by pain and spasm.

The first x-ray change is general rarefaction but with a normal joint space and line; the femoral epiphysis may be enlarged or a bone abscess visible; with arthritis, in addition to the general rarefaction, there is destruction of the acetabular

19.20 Hip tuberculosis – active   (a) Apparent lengthening in early disease of the left hip. (b) Synovitis of left hip. (c) Osteomyelitis of the femoral neck. (d) Florid arthritis. (e) Trochanteric infection – this rarely extends to the joint.

roof or the femoral head, usually both; the joint may be subluxed or even dislocated. With healing the bones recalcify.

Early disease may heal leaving a normal or almost normal hip; but if there has been arthritis the usual result is an unsound fibrous joint. The leg is scarred and thin; shortening is often severe because many factors contribute – adduction deformity, bone destruction, damage to the upper femoral epiphysis and occasionally premature fusion of the lower femoral epiphysis.

Treatment

Anti-tuberculous drugs are, of course, essential (page 28). Skin traction is applied and, for a child, a double abduction frame may be used. An abscess in the femoral neck is best evacuated; if, after 6–8 weeks, an arthritis is not settling, joint 'débridement' is performed.

As the disease settles, traction is discontinued and the patient is got up: non-weight-bearing with crutches if the joint has been preserved, weight-bearing in an abduction plaster if it has been destroyed.

For the aftermath of tuberculous arthritis a raised shoe and a removable splint may be useful; in addition three operative procedures are available.

Osteotomy   Subtrochanteric osteotomy is useful to correct deformity and to increase apparent length; a full-length hip spica is needed for at least 3 months (unless internal fixation has been used). Sometimes an unsound hip becomes sound after osteotomy.

Arthrodesis   Formerly, because of the fear of reactivating infection, extra-articular arthrodesis was favoured; bone grafts were used to bypass the joint and bridge the gap between femur and ilium or femur and ischium. With modern chemotherapy, however, direct impaction of the joint surfaces and internal fixation is usually preferred.

Arthroplasty   In older patients with residual pain and deformity, if the disease has clearly been inactive for a considerable time, total joint replacement is feasible.

In countries where squatting and sitting cross-legged are essential, Girdlestone's excision arthroplasty is sometimes used.

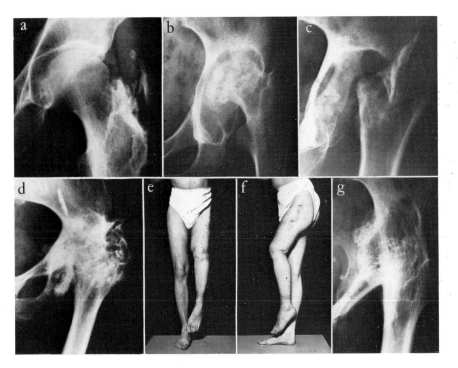

19.21 Hip tuberculosis – healing and aftermath   (a) Healed trochanteric disease with the hip joint still normal. (b) Healing arthritis with gross enlargement of the acetabulum. (c) Healing arthritis with large acetabulum and destruction of the head. (d) Joint destruction with considerable calcification in the aftermath stage; and (e, f) appearance of the hip in this patient – note the gross shortening. (g) A patient in whom secondary infection was followed by bony ankylosis.

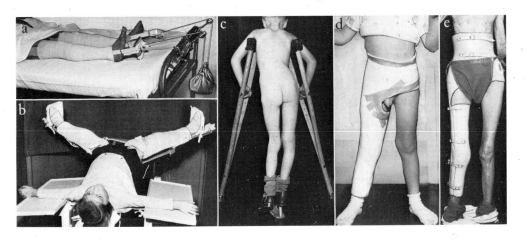

19.22 Hip tuberculosis – closed treatment   (a) In the active stage the adult is usually treated with skin traction; (b) a child being treated on a Pyrford double abduction frame. (c) The disease has been arrested early – weight-bearing is avoided by using a patten and crutches. (d) The disease has been arrested late – weight-bearing is permitted but the hip held in plaster; (e) later, a removable polythene spica may be sufficient.

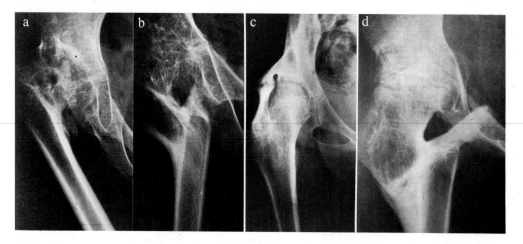

19.23 Hip tuberculosis – operative treatment   (a, b) Before and after osteotomy in the late healing stage. (c) Attempted iliofemoral arthrodesis has failed – the graft is not in compression. (d) Brittain's combined osteotomy and arthrodesis has succeeded (the Norwich V-arthrodesis is sometimes preferred).

Perthes' disease (coxa plana; pseudocoxalgia)

Cause

The femoral head becomes partly or wholly avascular. The cause is not definitely known, but a logical explanation is emerging; the picture is of a precipitating cause operating against an anatomical background.

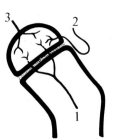

19.24 Perthes' disease – the background 1, Metaphyseal vessels; 2, lateral epiphyseal vessels; 3, vessels in the ligamentum teres.

THE BACKGROUND

In the fetus and up to the age of 4 months, the femoral head derives its blood supply from: (1) metaphyseal vessels which penetrate the area of the growth disc; (2) lateral epiphyseal vessels running in the retinacula; and (3) very slightly from vessels in the ligamentum teres. The metaphyseal supply gradually declines until, by the age of 4 years, it has virtually disappeared; by the age of 7, however, the vessels in the ligamentum teres have developed fully. Between 4 and 7 the femoral head may depend for its blood supply almost entirely on the lateral epiphyseal vessels whose situation in the retinacula makes them susceptible to pressure from an effusion.

THE PRECIPITATING CAUSE

Probably this is an effusion into the hip joint; Kemp *et al.* (1971) have shown experimentally that ischaemia can be produced in this way. The effusion could follow trauma, of which there is a history in over half the cases; a non-specific infection, or transient synovitis, could explain others. Recent studies strongly suggest that one incident of ischaemia (infarction) is not enough to cause Perthes' disease; two or more are needed.

Pathology

The pathological process takes 2–4 years to complete and can be conveniently considered in stages.

Stage 1 All or part of the bony femoral head is dead. It still looks normal on x-ray but it stops enlarging; its cartilaginous envelope, being nourished by synovial fluid, continues to grow, consequently the joint 'space' increases.

Stage 2 Trabeculae in the dead bone fracture; sometimes a subchondral fracture is large enough to show up as a tangential line on x-ray. New blood vessels enter the head and, as new bone is laid down on the dead trabeculae, the ossific nucleus becomes denser. The metaphysis becomes hyperaemic and on x-ray looks rarefied or cystic.

Stage 3 Once new bone has been laid down, dead bone is resorbed. Provided the repair process has been rapid and complete, the femoral head may keep its shape. But the bone may collapse, causing further flattening and fragmentation. Excessive stress is then transmitted to the growth plate; this may distort, or temporarily halt, epiphyseal growth. The epiphysis is often displaced so that the lateral portion of the head is no longer covered by the acetabulum. Eventually the normal density and architecture of the head are restored, but flattening and displacement remain, and predispose to later degeneration.

Clinical features

The only symptoms are limp and ache, often slight and intermittent; and, once the irritable stage has passed, pain is distinctly unusual. The contrast between paucity of symptoms and gross x-ray changes is striking.

The child is usually aged 4–8 years (rarely, 2–14), but the bone age may be less. The condition is four times commoner in boys and may be bilateral. The children are quite well, though they tend to be undersized; 4 per cent have an associated urogenital anomaly.

The hip looks deceptively normal, though there may be a little wasting. Early on, the joint is irritable, so that all movements are diminished and their extremes painful. Often the child is not seen till later, when most movements are full; but abduction (especially in flexion) is nearly always limited and usually internal rotation also.

X-RAY Even before x-ray changes appear, the ischaemic area can sometimes be demonstrated as a 'void' on scanning. The earliest x-ray changes are slight granular increase in density and an increased joint space. Flattening, fragmentation and lateral displacement of the epiphysis follow, with rarefaction and widening of the metaphysis.

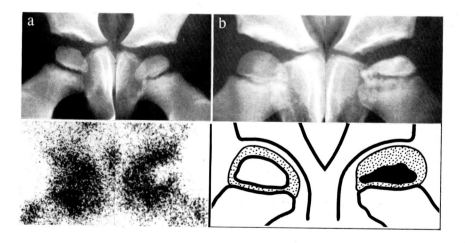

19.25 Perthes' disease – early features (a) This boy had an irritable left hip; his x-ray is virtually normal, but a scan on the same day shows a void in the lateral portion of the femoral head. (b) Later the head becomes radiologically dense; it stops growing but the cartilage does not – the diagram shows how this results in an increased 'joint space'.

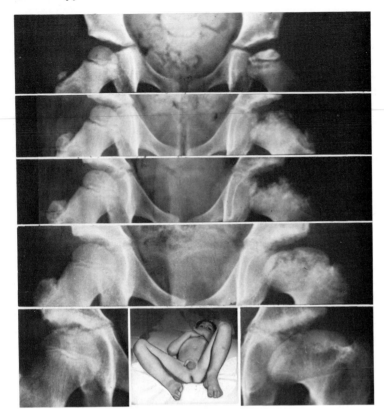

19.26 Perthes' disease Serial x-rays over a period of 5 years. Despite radiological severity the clinical signs are usually slight, but abduction in flexion is nearly always limited (inset).

The picture varies with the age of the child, the stage of the disease and the amount of head which has been ischaemic. Four groups are described (Catterall, 1972). In group 1 only half the head is necrotic and no collapse occurs; in group 2 more is involved but enough remains viable to prevent collapse; in group 3 most, and in group 4 all of the head is ischaemic, so that collapse is severe. Adverse prognostic signs (the *head at risk*) are: (1) lateral subluxation leaving the head partly uncovered; (2) a translucent area in the lateral part of the epiphysis (Gage's sign); (3) specks of calcification lateral to the epiphysis; and (4) a severe metaphyseal reaction.

The 'sagging rope sign' refers to a line which remains permanently after severe Perthes' disease; it serves as a diagnostic fingerprint (Apley and Weintroub, 1981).

Differential diagnosis

The irritable hip of early Perthes' disease must be differentiated from other causes of irritability; the child's fitness, the increased joint space and the patchy bone density are characteristic. In transient synovitis the x-ray is normal.

Morquio–Brailsford disease, cretinism, multiple epiphyseal dysplasia, sickle-cell disease and Gaucher's disease may resemble Perthes' disease radiologically, but other diagnostic features are apparent.

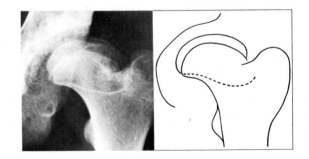

19.27 Perthes' disease The 'sagging rope sign' – the radiological relic of former Perthes' disease.

Treatment

As long as the hip is irritable the child should be in bed with skin traction applied to the affected leg. Once irritability has subsided, which usually takes about 3 weeks, there is a choice of treatments between 'supervised neglect' and 'containment'.

'Supervised neglect' This somewhat flippant term implies that treatment is abandoned; the child resumes normal activities but is checked regularly. If symptoms recur or signs increase, treatment by containment is instituted.

'Containment' The aim is to counteract lateral displacement and to contain the head within the acetabulum. Containment can be achieved: (1) by holding the hips widely abducted, in plaster or in a removable splint (ambulation, though awkward, is just possible, but the position must be maintained for at least a year); or (2) by operation, either a varus osteotomy of the femur (which may give a little shortening) or by an innominate osteotomy of the pelvis; plaster is worn until the osteotomy has united (6–8 weeks), after which the child is allowed free.

Choice of method

The objectives of treatment are (1) to alleviate symptoms, and (2) to restore or maintain the shape of the femoral head, expecting thereby to postpone or prevent the development of osteoarthritis. But (1) once irritability has subsided the child rarely has any symptoms; and (2) even with considerable radiological deformity significant symptoms of osteoarthritis are seldom seen before middle life. Consequently, since any form of treatment has disadvantages or dangers, a case can be made out for treating all patients by 'supervised neglect' – except, of course, those in whom symptoms fail to subside with rest or recur when activity is resumed.

Most surgeons, however, believe that the choice between containment and doing nothing should not be decided purely by symptoms and clinical signs; they maintain that it should depend upon the age of onset and the radiological severity of the disease. Patients classified as Catterall group 1 need no treatment. Nor do patients in groups 2 and 3 if aged less than 7, unless the head is at risk; those aged over 7 or with a head at risk need containment. Group 4 patients of any age

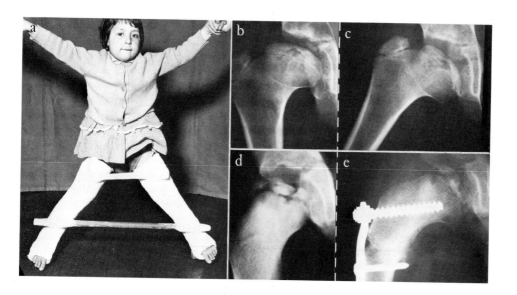

19.28 Perthes' disease – treatment (a) So-called 'broomstick' plaster; (b) shows this girl's x-ray with her hip in the neutral position; when her hip is abducted (c) containment is achieved. (d, e) Show similar containment in another patient, achieved by femoral osteotomy.

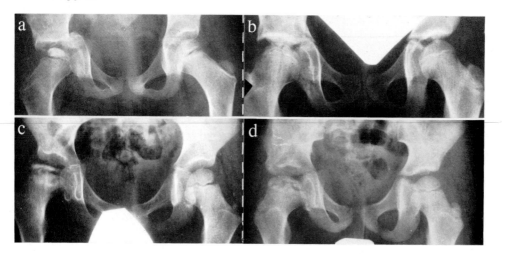

19.29 Perthes' disease – treatment (continued)   Pelvic osteotomy also can achieve containment: (a, b) shows the effect of a Chiari osteomy, and (c, d) of an innominate osteotomy.

also need containment; but if deformity is very severe this may be unattainable, and the attempt to force it is then harmful.

Even in patients selected for containment, there is still a choice, between splintage and operation. Surgery is not devoid of risk but has the great merit of achieving containment rapidly, so that the child's social development is less affected; the two operations (femoral osteotomy and pelvic osteotomy) give similar results.

Slipped epiphysis

In adolescents the upper femoral epiphysis may become displaced at the growth disc, resulting in coxa vara. This condition, termed 'slipped epiphysis', occurs gradually in 70 per cent of cases, and suddenly in 30 per cent. The cause and pathology are similar in both varieties.

Cause and pathology

A slipped epiphysis resembles a pathological fracture. Trauma may be the precipitating cause, but an underlying abnormality predisposes to slipping.

TRAUMA
This is undoubtedly a factor because (1) there is often a history of hip 'sprains'; (2) sometimes a gross slip is seen immediately following a fall; and (3) during growth the femoral growth disc becomes increasingly oblique, and is thus more liable to displacement with injury.

UNDERLYING ABNORMALITY
An underlying abnormality is strongly suggested because (1) the slipping occurs gradually in 70 per cent of cases; (2) it often becomes bilateral and the second side may slip even while the patient is in bed undergoing treatment for the first; and (3) the disorder occurs just before puberty, many of the patients show evidence of endocrine imbalance and the pituitary fossa on x-ray is sometimes small.

The nature of the underlying abnormality is not known, but the following hypothesis, based on animal experiments, is plausible.

Shortly before puberty, growth hormones stimulate the growth disc to produce much additional cartilage in preparation for the prepuberty growth spurt. The sex hormones normally play a part in converting this additional cartilage to bone; if they fail to keep pace, there is too much unossified cartilage which is unable to resist the stress imposed by the increase in body weight. Consequently, during walking and standing the shaft of the femur will tend to drive upwards, and when the patient is lying in bed, the weight of the leg will tend to make the shaft roll outwards.

Gradual slip

Clinical features

Even with 'gradual slip' there is a history of injury in half the cases. Pain, sometimes in the groin, but often only in the thigh or knee, is the presenting symptom. It may be called a 'sprain'; often, and unfortunately, it is disregarded. It soon disappears only to recur with further exercise. Limp also occurs early and is more constant.

The disorder is slightly commoner in boys than in girls. In boys the average age of onset is 15; in girls it is 12 and is rare after menstruation has started. Two-thirds of the patients are unduly fat and sexually underdeveloped; the other third may be tall, thin and sexually normal. The local signs are as follows.

● LOOK   In the earliest stage the appearance is normal, but the patient is rarely seen until significant slipping has occurred and deformity is perceptible. The leg then is externally rotated and is 1 or 2 cm short. Slight wasting is not uncommon.

● FEEL   The greater trochanter may be higher and more posterior than that of the unaffected hip.

● MOVE   The joint is sometimes irritable with a little diminution of movement in all directions, but the most constant and diagnostic limitations are of abduction and internal rotation. The more definite the slip, the more are these two movements limited.

Muscle bulk is often reduced and a Trendelenburg sign and limp may be present.

● X-RAY   In the anteroposterior view, even when slipping is trivial, changes are apparent. The growth disc is too wide and too 'woolly' on its metaphyseal side. A line drawn along the superior surface of the neck remains superior to the head instead of passing through it (Trethowan's sign). In a normal hip the posterior acetabular margin cuts across the medial corner of the upper femoral metaphysis; with slipping the entire metaphysis is lateral to the posterior acetabular margin (Capener's sign). With further slipping, the upward displacement of the shaft and neck becomes more apparent.

In the lateral view, deformity is usually obvious from the beginning. The head and neck are angulated on each other so that there is a forward bow.

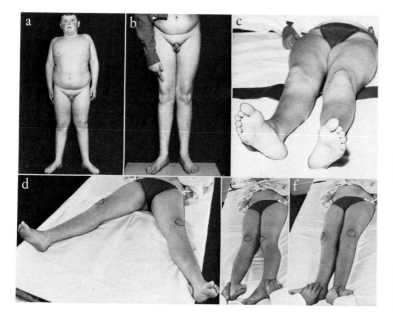

19.30 Slipped epiphysis – clinical features (a) The build is unmistakable; (b) this boy complained of pain only in the knee; (c) the leg lies in external rotation.

Another patient, showing (d) diminished abduction of the right hip; (e) diminished internal rotation; and (f) increased external rotation.

![figure 19.31]

19.31 Slipped epiphysis – x-rays   (a) Anteroposterior and (b) lateral views of early slipped epiphysis of right hip. The upper diagrams show Trethowan's line passing just above the head on the affected side, but cutting through it on the normal. The lower diagrams show Capener's sign: the femoral head is apparently extruded from the acetabulum on the affected side, but contained within it on the normal.

Pre-slipping stage   A pre-slipping stage has been postulated. However, it seems unlikely that the condition could present clinically without slight displacement, and a lateral x-ray shows even the smallest slip.

Treatment

With modest displacement (less than a third) reduction is not attempted. Under x-ray control the epiphysis is fixed where it is, using at least three threaded pins. If operation is to be delayed, traction may prevent further slip.

With unacceptable displacement reduction is desirable, but traction is ineffective and manipulation is dangerous (the blood supply to the femoral head, already reduced by the slip, may be still further impaired). Open reduction is theoretically ideal, but unless Dunn's technique (1978) is followed meticulously, the complication rate (from avascular necrosis or from chondrolysis) is unacceptably high. The safest procedure is to fix the head in its displaced position with three pins and to compensate for the displacement by an osteotomy when the epiphysis has joined (usually within a few months). Griffith (1976) has shown that the epiphysis rotates downwards and backwards around the curved upper surface of the metaphysis: he has designed an ingenious 'geometric flexion osteotomy' to correct the deformity. The alternative is an

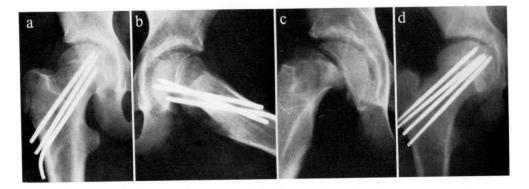

19.32 Slipped epiphysis – treatment   (a, b) Minimal slip – no reduction has been attempted, but further slip prevented by three Moore's pins. (c, d) A sudden slip has been reduced by manipulation, and fixed in position.

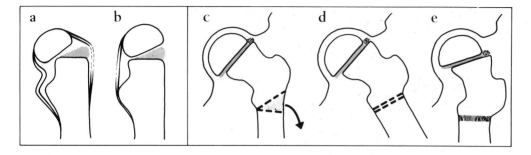

19.33 Slipped epiphysis – treatment (continued)   (a) Diagram of lateral view of the hip, showing that the head has slipped backwards off the neck, new bone has formed and the anterior blood vessels are stretched or torn; (b) if the head is dragged into position over this bone, the remaining posterior vessels are endangered. In (c) – an AP view – the deformity has been left but a lateral wedge of bone has been excised lower down; (d) the leg is then held abducted until the osteotomy joins; (e) when the leg returns to its correct position the growth disc becomes more horizontal.

immediate subtrochanteric osteotomy, designed to make the growth disc more horizontal; a laterally based wedge of bone is excised, rotation also is corrected and the new position held in an abduction plaster or by internal fixation.

Sudden slip

The term is misleading. Almost certainly gradual slipping occurs first; then, following a fall, there is severe displacement or even complete separation. The signs are those of a fractured neck of femur. Traction or gentle manipulation, though ineffective with gradual slip, may restore a sudden slip to the pre-injury position. If so, the epiphysis is fixed with threaded pins. But reduction may be spurious (an illusion created by altered rotation of the limb), and even gentle manipulation may be hazardous; consequently some surgeons advocate the same treatment as for a gradual slip: namely, immediate fixation without attempted reduction, followed by subtrochanteric osteotomy (if needed) when the epiphysis has closed.

Sequels to slipped epiphysis

COXA VARA   If displacement has not been reduced, the epiphysis fuses in its deformed position. The patient limps, but the condition is painless until osteoarthritis later develops.

Osteotomy should be performed to relieve symptoms and in the hope of preventing osteoarthritis.

AVASCULAR NECROSIS   Death of the femoral head is an important complication. Formerly common, the incidence has been reduced by : (1) avoiding forcible manipulation; and (2) using threaded pins in preference to a bulky trifin nail.

CHONDROLYSIS   The femoral head is not dense but rarefied, and the joint space becomes much narrower. The hip becomes very stiff. Relief of weight-bearing may lead to restoration of the joint space, but movement does not often return.

OSTEOARTHRITIS   Early osteoarthritis is a likely sequel if displacement has not been reduced, and inevitable if there has been avascular necrosis.

BILATERAL SLIPPING   The parents should be warned that, up to 2 years after a slipped epiphysis, slipping may occur at the other hip. This happens in 15–30 per cent of cases and is commoner in patients with endocrine abnormality.

Coxa vara

In coxa vara the angle between the neck and shaft of the femur is diminished. The normal is 160 degrees in a child, decreasing to 125 degrees in adult life.

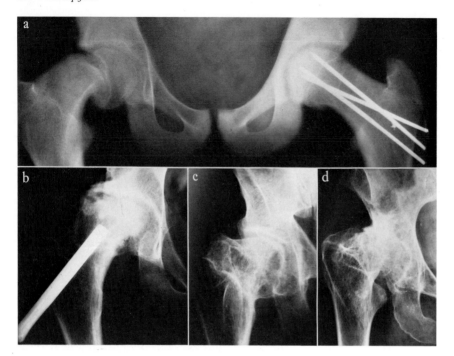

19.34 Slipped epiphysis – sequels   (a) The left side had been pinned; now the right has slipped – the patient should be warned of this possibility. (b) Avascular necrosis after trifin nailing – this type of fixation has now been abandoned. (c) Malunion in an untreated patient. (d) Osteoarthritis at age 45 followed malunion.

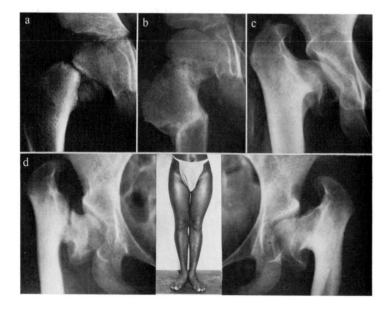

19.35 Infantile coxa vara   (a) Growth disc too vertical and triangle of bone on undersurface of neck; (b) abduction osteotomy should be performed early; otherwise (c) the shaft migrates upwards. (d) Bilateral infantile coxa vara – untreated; only some 30 cm of ankle separation was possible.

CONGENITAL (INFANTILE)

The epiphyseal line is too vertical; with stress the shaft is gradually but inevitably pushed upwards. The condition is painless and presents as a short leg in infancy. X-ray shows that the epiphyseal line is too vertical, and in the infant there is also a separate triangle of bone in the inferior portion of the metaphysis (Fairbank's triangle). Subtrochanteric osteotomy is necessary. If bilateral, the condition may not be seen until a young adult presents with osteoarthritis. Sometimes congenital coxa vara is associated with a congenitally short or bowed proximal shaft of femur (page 95).

ACQUIRED

Coxa vara can develop only if the neck bends (because it is soft) or if it breaks.

Bone softening Bone softening may produce coxa vara in children (rickets, bone dystrophies and possibly Perthes' disease), in adults (osteomalacia) and in the elderly (osteoporosis and Paget's disease).

At any age, tuberculosis or pyogenic infection may soften bone and lead to coxa vara, but the deformity is overshadowed by the causal condition.

Fracture Fracture may produce coxa vara in children (through a solitary cyst), in adolescents (slipped epiphysis) and in the elderly (malunion of a trochanteric fracture).

Rheumatoid arthritis

The hip joint is frequently affected in rheumatoid arthritis; occasionally the disease remains monar-ticular for several years, but eventually other sites are affected. Persistent synovitis in a joint with so little room for expansion soon leads to cartilage destruction; the acetabulum is eroded and eventually the femoral head may perforate its floor. The hallmark of the disease is progressive bone destruction on both sides of the joint without any reactive osteophyte formation.

Clinical features

Usually the patient already has rheumatoid disease affecting many joints. Pain in the groin comes on insidiously; limp, though common, may be ascribed to pre-existing arthritis of the foot or knee. When both hips are affected the patient has difficulty getting into or out of a low chair, and in negotiating stairs.

Wasting of the buttock and thigh is often marked and the limb is usually held in external rotation and fixed flexion. All movements are restricted and painful.

X-RAYS During the early stages there is a concentric diminution of the joint space, and osteoporosis. Later, the acetabulum deepens and the femoral head sinks medially. In the worst cases (and especially in patients on corticosteroids) there is gross destruction of the acetabulum or the femoral head, or both.

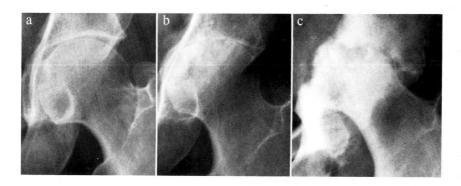

19.36 Rheumatoid arthritis   Three stages in the development of rheumatoid arthritis: (a) loss of joint space; (b) erosion of bone after cartilage has disappeared; (c) perforation of the acetabular floor – such marked destruction is more likely to occur if the patient is having corticosteroids.

...disease can be arrested by general treat-
..., hip deterioration may be slowed down. But
... .ce cartilage and bone are eroded no treatment
is likely to influence the progression to joint
destruction. Total joint replacement is then the
best answer. It relieves pain and restores a useful
range of movement. It is advocated even in
younger patients, because the polyarthritis so
limits activity that the implants are not unduly
stressed.

Osteoarthritis
(see also Chapter 5)

Cause

Osteoarthritis of the hip is liable to develop in a
relatively young adult as the sequel to congenital
subluxation or dysplasia, Perthes' disease, coxa
vara or following injury. In the older patient
osteoarthritis may supervene on rheumatoid
arthritis, or following injury (fracture or dislocation), especially when the femoral head becomes
avascular. Avascular necrosis also occurs without
injury (page 64).

Another precursor of osteoarthritis is protrusio
acetabuli (Otto pelvis). This usually affects
females and develops soon after puberty; at this
stage there are often no symptoms though move-

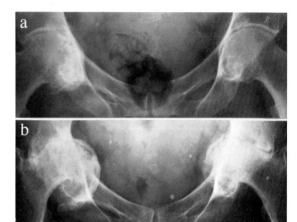

19.37 Osteoarthritis – causal factors Protrusio acetabuli
is one of the many predisposing causes of osteoarthritis of the
hip. When first seen (a) this woman of 42 had symptoms
only in the right hip; 4 years later (b) both show advanced
degeneration.

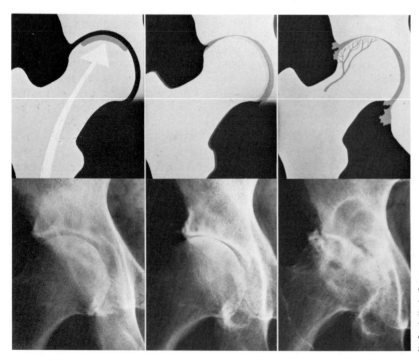

**19.38 Osteoarthritis – path-
ology** Where stress is taken the
cartilage is abraded and the joint
space becomes narrower. The
vascular reaction is followed by
osteophyte formation. Cysts form
at high spots of pressure.

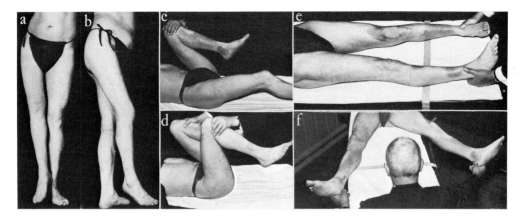

19.39 Osteoarthritis – signs The right hip is osteoarthritic and shows: (a, b) apparent shortening, with adduction and flexion deformity; (c) demonstrating fixed flexion; (d, e, f) limitation of flexion, internal rotation and abduction.

ments are limited. X-rays show the sunken acetabulum which may form as much as two-thirds of a sphere instead of the normal half.

Even when no cause is apparent it should be sought; minor abnormalities probably account for some cases previously labelled 'primary'.

Causes of osteoarthritis of the hip

Abnormal stress	Defective cartilage	Abnormal bone
Subluxation	Infection	Fracture
Coxa magna	Rheumatoid	Necrosis
Coxa vara	Calcinosis	Paget's
Minor deformities	Traumatic chondrolysis	Other causes of sclerosis

Pathology

CARTILAGE AND BONE
The articular cartilage becomes soft and fibrillated. Where subjected to most pressure (chiefly the top of the femoral head) it becomes worn and thin; the underlying bone becomes dense, hard and sometimes cystic; areas of necrotic bone may collapse. Where pressure is less, the cartilage proliferates, then ossifies producing osteophytes.

SYNOVIUM AND CAPSULE
Irritated by flakes of cartilage and bone, the synovium hypertrophies; flakes probably also penetrate the synovium and stimulate capsular fibrosis. As the fibrous tissue matures it shrinks, thus limiting movement.

Clinical features

Pain radiates from the groin to the knee. At first it occurs when movement follows a period of rest; later it is more constant, more severe and sometimes disturbs sleep. Stiffness at first is also noticed only after rest; later it increases progressively until putting on socks and shoes becomes difficult. Limp is often noticed early and the patient may say his leg is getting shorter.

The patient is usually fit and, unless there has been previous hip disorder, is aged over 50. There may be an obvious limp and, except in early cases, a positive Trendelenburg sign. The affected leg usually lies in external rotation and adduction, so that it appears short; there is nearly always some fixed flexion, though this may only be revealed by Thomas' test. Muscle wasting is detectable but rarely severe. Deep pressure may elicit tenderness and the greater trochanter is somewhat high and posterior. Movements, though often painless within a limited range, are restricted; internal rotation, abduction and extension are the first to be lost, but in advanced cases all movements are limited.

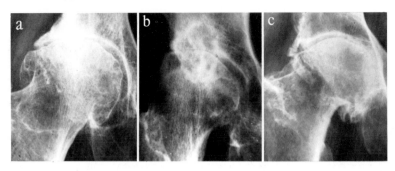

19.40 Osteoarthritis – x-rays (a) The most common variety, with 'eccentric' loss of joint space; (b) cysts like these are often associated with pain; (c) 'concentric' type of degeneration.

X-RAY   The earliest sign is a decreased joint space, usually maximal in the superior weight-bearing region but sometimes affecting the entire joint. Later signs are subarticular sclerosis, cyst formation and osteophytes.

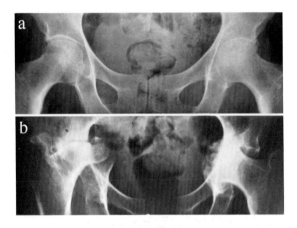

19.41 Osteoarthritis – conservative treatment   This patient with only mild osteoarthritis (a) was given anti-inflammatory drugs in such high doses that her pain was totally abolished – but (b) her hips have been totally destroyed.

Conservative treatment (see also page 55)

Warmth is soothing and may be applied by using a hot-water bottle or electric pad at night, by radiant heat or by short-wave diathermy. The patient is encouraged to use a walking-stick and to try to preserve movement by non-weight-bearing exercises. In early cases a manipulation under anaesthesia (accompanied by a hydrocortisone injection) is often useful; the patient should try to preserve the increased range obtained.

If conservative methods fail, operation is indicated.

Operative treatment

There are three main operations: osteotomy, arthrodesis and arthroplasty. Osteotomy, if performed early, can arrest the degenerative process, or may even reverse it so that the joint space re-forms and cysts heal. Arthrodesis is now rarely performed; the tide of opinion is against it, despite its advantages in the young. Arthroplasty (joint replacement) is much the most popular operation for patients over 55. These operations are described below.

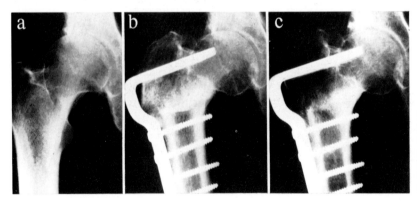

19.42 Osteoarthritis – treatment by osteotomy   Following a varus type of osteotomy this patient lost most of her pain and the x-rays suggest articular cartilage regeneration (would 'rejuvenation' be too strong a word?).

Hip operations

Osteotomy

When performed for osteoarthritis, osteotomy is best done early, before collapse of the head, in the hope that the disease will regress. Even when performed late, it often reduces pain (especially pain at rest) and it allows deformity to be corrected. Movement is usually retained or even increased, and its arc is more useful; but if movement was considerably limited before operation then the joint may become even stiffer afterwards. Some years after osteotomy, pain sometimes returns; by then the patient may be old enough for hip replacement to be a satisfactory option.*

Technique

Preoperative tracings of the hip in abduction and in adduction are useful in deciding whether the femoral head should be moved into a more varus or a more valgus position; the aim is to take weight through an undamaged area. An appropriate wedge of bone is removed from just above the lesser trochanter and the gap closed; alternatively, the bone can be divided and wedged open by a bone graft. Fixed flexion and malrotation are corrected and the new position is held by internal fixation. Weight-bearing should be deferred for at least 3 months.

Arthrodesis

This is unpopular today because the stiffness is said to interfere with function, to throw excessive strain on the unaffected hip and, most of all, to cause backache. There is some truth in all these reasons, but they should not be overemphasized. Arthrodesis remains the only certain way of achieving total and permanent freedom from hip pain, as well as stability. Provided the 'compensating joints' (lumbar spine, knee and opposite hip) are completely normal, the patient can look forward to many years of comfort with only a slight limp, and with the ability to walk long distances, run and play vigorous games. If, eventually, significant disability develops, the patient may well be old enough for replacement to be satisfactory; the hip can (with a little difficulty) be 'unpicked' and a prosthesis inserted.

Technique

When arthrodesing a hip it is wise to remove the articular cartilage unless it has already been destroyed by disease. The bones are coapted as closely as possible and held together with internal fixation (see Fig. 19.43). The optimum position is 20 degrees of flexion, neutral rotation (up to 5 degrees of external rotation is acceptable) and neither adducted nor abducted (though if there was much shortening a little abduction is permissible).

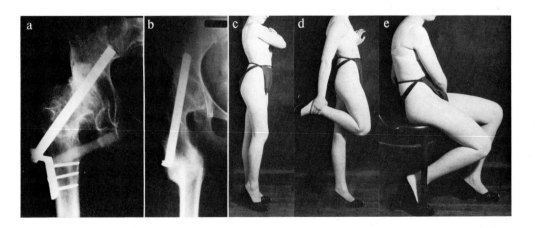

19.43 Osteoarthritis – treatment by arthrodesis (a) Norwich V technique. (b) Pyrford arthrodesis with osteotomy; (c–e) patient after Pyrford arthrodesis; (c) standing posture; (d, e) show why it is important for the lumbar spine and knee to be fully mobile with an arthrodesed hip.

*Osteotomy is not the end of the line; arthroplasty may be.

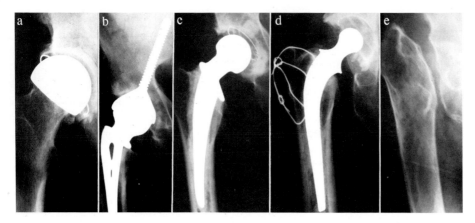

19.44 Osteoarthritis – treatment by hip replacement   (a) Surface replacement by a double cup – the patient was aged 45; (b) Ring's uncemented prosthesis; (c) McKee–Arden model; (d) Charnley's prosthesis – the greater trochanter was lifted off and has been wired back in position; (e) Girdlestone's operation – originally designed as a primary operation for osteoarthritis, but now used only when replacement has failed.

Total hip replacement

Indications

These are difficult to define but can be considered under the following headings.

Pain   especially if severe enough to interfere with sleep or work.

Stiffness   especially of both hips, but even of one hip if associated with ipsilateral knee stiffness, back stiffness or sexual problems.

Age   is important. Below the age of (say) 55, osteotomy or arthrodesis should be considered. Replacement is indicated, however, if these have already failed or if any of the following special circumstances prevail: (1) the expectation of life is short (e.g. with patients who are necessarily having steroid therapy); (2) the quality of life is poor (e.g. the young woman with advanced osteoarthritis of both hips hoping to have children and to bring them up); (3) the amount of activity is limited (e.g. the patient with widespread rheumatoid arthritis has a built-in limitation of activity which will prevent excessive wear or stress of the prosthesis).

Essentials of technique

The approach must adequately display the upper femur and the entire acetabulum. The femoral head is excised; the synovium is then removed and (except in Charnley's operation) the entire capsule also. The acetabulum is deepened, shaped to fit the acetabular prosthesis, and holes are gouged or drilled in it to augment subsequent fixation. The acetabular prosthesis is now fixed in position with cement (methylmethacrylate).

Attention is then turned to the femur; the upper shaft is reamed and cancellous bone scraped away. After a trial of reduction the femoral component also is cemented in position. The joint is now reduced, its mobility and stability are tested and the wound is closed in layers with suction drainage.

VARIANTS
(1) For younger patients surface replacement, where feasible, is preferred; a hemispherical metal cup cemented onto the femoral head fits into a polyethylene socket which is cemented into the acetabulum. (2) Ring's prosthesis is uncemented; the acetabular component has a long screw for fixation. (3) In other models (e.g. Müller's) a femoral component which does not need cement is available; revision, if needed, is much easier. (4) Ceramic screw-threaded acetabular components are being tried; they are almost frictionless and are used without cement. (5) Different varieties of cement are available, some of which can be 'injected' into the femur; the cement can be compacted into the bone with special instruments; and sometimes a plug is inserted into the femoral shaft before the cement, to allow greater compaction.

Complications

Hip replacements are often performed on patients who are somewhat elderly; some are rheumatoid and may be having steroid therapy. Consequently the general complication rate is by no means trivial; deep vein thrombosis in particular is common.

The remaining complications are more likely to occur with this particular operation, or are peculiar to it. Factors which may contribute to their development include previous hip operations, severe deformity, inadequate 'bone stock', an insufficiently sterile operating environment, and lack of experience or expertise on the part of the surgeon or his team.

OPERATIVE COMPLICATIONS

(1) *Exposure* An inappropriate or inaccurately placed incision may lead to major nerve or vessel damage, either by direct injury or by forcible retraction.

(2) *Acetabulum* Unless the new acetabulum is positioned with meticulous accuracy the hip may subsequently dislocate. A thin medial wall may fracture.

(3) *Femur* While reaming the femur or driving hom prosthesis the femoral shaft may be penetrated or fract ̣ːu. Great care is needed if the medullary canal is narrow or the bone osteoporotic.

(4) *Cement* If the cement is inserted too soon after mixing, especially into the femur, absorption of the monomer may cause a considerable drop in blood pressure.

(5) *Closure* Blood goes on oozing after the operation; a suction drain is used to minimize the haematoma.

POSTOPERATIVE COMPLICATIONS

(1) *Dislocation* (see above) This is most likely to occur soon after operation. Reduction is not difficult and traction or a hip spica usually allows the hip to stabilize; but re-operation may be needed for gross errors.

(2) *Infection* The large bulk of foreign material restricts the access of the body's normal defence mechanism; consequently even slight wound contamination may be serious. Organisms may multiply in the postoperative haematoma to cause early infection, and, even many years later, haematogenous spread from a distant site may cause late infection.

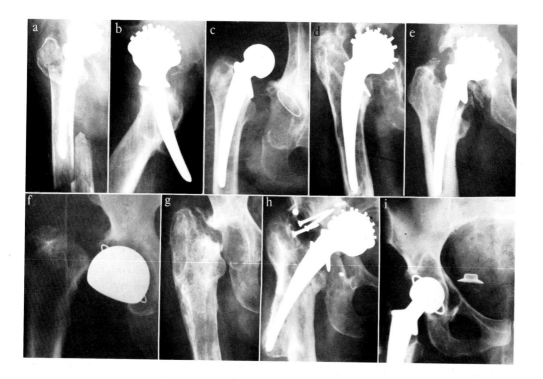

19.45 Complications of hip replacement (a) Fracture; (b) penetration; (c) dislocation; (d) loosening; (e) infection; (f) fractured femoral neck beneath a double cup. (g) Girdlestone excision – the universal salvage – but salvage is not always needed – this patient (h) requested the same operation to her other hip; and (i) – well, we take our hats off to this one! (With acknowledgements to St Elsewhere's Hospital.)

Prophylaxis is the key. The wound should not be open for too long, the tissues should be handled gently and haematoma formation minimized. The asepsis required is of an even higher order than with other surgical procedures. Special operating enclosures are on trial; powerful filtration and careful aerodynamic design (e.g. laminar air-flow) minimize the chances of contamination. The instillation of antibiotics such as polymyxin is a further wise precaution.

Early wound infection sometimes responds to antibiotics. Later infection does so less often and may need operative 'débridement' followed by the continuous instillation of antibiotic solution combined with continuous drainage for 2 or 3 weeks. If all else fails the prosthesis and cement may have to be removed, a procedure euphemistically called 'conversion to a Girdlestone operation'; once the wound is sterile a new prosthesis may be inserted.

An alternative, still experimental, is 'immediate exchange replacement'; all foreign material and all infected tissue are removed and a new prosthesis is fixed in position with cement containing gentamicin.

(3) *Loosening*   Infection or major trauma may cause loosening; but even without either, torque forces may be great enough to break the bond between cement and bone; hence the importance of low friction at the artificial joint interface. Metal sensitivity, especially to cobalt, is another cause of loosening and another reason for preferring metal-on-plastic joints. If loosening causes sufficient pain, the operation needs 'revision'.

(4) *Periarticular ossification*   Masses of new bone occasionally develop round the new joint and lead to considerable stiffness. The cause is unknown. Usually the patient's disposition is blamed, perhaps rightly, for if the second hip is operated on or the first is revised, the same complication is apt to occur.

(5) *Long-term effects*   Between two moving surfaces friction, however slight, is inevitable; one or other surface wears. With metal-to-metal joints the abraded particles form a sludge; but absorption also occurs, for metallic traces can be detected in, for example, hair and nails. With plastic-to-metal joints the abraded particles are of plastic, whose fate is uncertain.

Exposure of the hip

Anterior (Smith-Petersen) approach

The patient lies on his back with a small sandbag under the affected buttock and a large one under the knee. The skin is incised from the anterior superior iliac spine upwards along the iliac crest for one-third of its length, and downwards for 12 cm towards the lateral side of the patella. The deep fascia is incised in the same line. The abductor muscles are detached from the lateral aspect of the iliac crest and the abdominal muscles from its medial aspect. From both aspects the muscles are separated subperiosteally by gauze dissection and a pack is left in to control oozing. The plane between the sartorius muscle medially and the tensor fascia lata laterally is deepened, preserving the lateral cutaneous nerve of the thigh. Retracting these muscles exposes the rectus femoris, on the lateral side of which a leash of circumflex vessels is divided between ligatures. The rectus is then detached from the anterior inferior iliac spine and retracted medially with the psoas, exposing the hip capsule. To expose the femoral head, the capsule is incised parallel to the neck. To dislocate the hip, the capsule is divided in front and the femur rotated laterally.

Lateral approaches

Charnley, for his low-friction arthroplasty, advocates a lateral approach with the patient supine. A 25 cm skin incision is made in the line of the femur, one-third above the trochanter and two-thirds below. The deep fascia and iliotibial tract are divided, exposing the greater trochanter. The anterior capsule of the hip is exposed by defining the interval between tensor fascia lata and the gluteus medius and minimus. The capsule is incised in the line of the femoral neck, but not excised. The greater trochanter is osteotomized and turned upwards with its attached muscle and capsule. The hip is now dislocated by adduction, flexion and lateral rotation.

For the Müller hip replacement an anterolateral approach is used. The patient is supine and the skin incision runs from the iliac crest downwards and backwards to the greater trochanter, and then along the line of the upper femoral shaft. The interval between tensor fascia lata and the gluteus medius and minimus is developed, and by retraction the anterior hip capsule is exposed. It is thoroughly excised and the femoral neck is then divided with a motor saw. The head and neck can now be removed from the acetabulum to leave a wide exposure.

Posterior approach

The patient lies slightly prone of the full lateral position. The curved incision is centred over the greater trochanter, extending down the line of the femur for 10 cm, and for the same distance upwards and backwards towards the posterior superior iliac spine. In the line of the incision, the sheet composed above of gluteus maximus fibres and below of the iliotibial band is split: the posterior flap of this layer overlies the sciatic nerve. The small lateral rotators of the hip (pyriformis, obturators, gemelli and, if necessary, quadratus femoris) are divided near their insertions into the femur, turned back to expose the posterior part of the hip capsule, and used to protect the sciatic nerve. After capsulectomy, the hip may be dislocated by medially rotating the thigh.

Notes on applied anatomy

The ball-and-socket arrangement of the hip combines stability for weight-bearing with freedom of movement for locomotion. A deeper acetabulum would confer greater stability but would limit the range of movement. Even with the fibrocartilaginous labrum the socket is not deep enough to accommodate the whole of the femoral head, whose articular surface extends considerably beyond a hemisphere.

The opening of the acetabulum faces downwards and forwards (about 30 degrees in each direction); the neck of the femur points upwards and forwards. Consequently, in the neutral position, the anterior portion of the head is not 'contained'. The amount of forward inclination of the neck relative to the shaft (the angle of anteversion) varies from 10 to 30 degrees in the adult. The upward inclination of the neck is such that the neck–shaft angle is 125 degrees.

A neck–shaft angle of less than 125 degrees is referred to as 'coxa vara' because, were the neck normally aligned relative to the pelvis, the limb would be deviated towards the midline of the body – in varus; a neck–shaft angle greater than 125 degrees (i.e. with the neck unduly vertical) is coxa valga. The angle is mechanically important because the further away the abductor muscles are from the hip, the greater is their leverage and their efficiency.

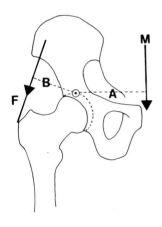

During standing and walking, the femoral neck acts as a cantilever; the line of body weight passes medial to the hip joint and is balanced laterally by the abductors (especially gluteus medius). The combination of body weight, leverage effect and muscle action means that the resultant force transmitted through the femoral head can be very great – about five times the body weight when walking slowly and much more when running or jumping. It is easy to see why the hip is so liable to suffer from cartilage failure – the essential feature of osteoarthritis.

The ligaments of the hip, though very strong in front, are weak posteriorly; consequently posterior dislocation is much commoner than anterior. When the hip is adducted and medially rotated it is particularly vulnerable, and when this position results from unbalanced paralysis, the hip can slip unobtrusively out of position.

During the swing phase of walking not only does the hip flex, it also rotates; this is because the pelvis swivels forwards. As weight comes onto the leg, the abductor muscles contract, causing the pelvis to tilt downwards on the weight-bearing side; it is failure of this abductor mechanism which causes the Trendelenburg lurch.

The femoral head receives its arterial blood supply from three sources: (1) intraosseous vessels running up the neck, which are inevitably damaged with a displaced cervical fracture; (2) vessels in the retinacula reflected from capsule to neck, which may be damaged in a fracture, or compressed by an effusion; and (3) vessels in the ligamentum teres, which are undeveloped in the early years of life and even later convey only a meagre blood supply. The relative importance of these vessels varies with age, but at all ages avascular necrosis is a potential hazard.

The nerve supply of the hip, unlike the blood supply, is plentiful. Sensory fibres, conveying proprioception as well as pain, abound in the capsule and ligaments. But the venous sinusoids of the bones also are supplied with sensory fibres; a rise in the intraosseous venous pressure accounts for some of the pain in osteoarthritis, and a reduction of this pressure for some of the relief which may follow osteotomy.

19.46 Forces around the hip
When standing on one leg the pelvis is balanced on the femoral head. The vertical force due to the body weight (M) is counterbalanced by contraction of the lateral muscles (F). The force borne by the femoral head at ⊙ is produced by the combined moments M×A and F×B.

Further reading

Apley, A. Graham and Weintroub, S. (1981) The sagging rope sign in Perthes' disease and allied disorders. *Journal of Bone and Joint Surgery* **63B,** 43–47
Catterall, A. (1972) Coxa vara. In *Modern Trends in Orthopaedics – 6*. Ed. by A. Graham Apley. London: Butterworths
Charnley, Sir J. (1979) *Low Friction Arthroplasty of the Hip*. Berlin, Heidelberg, New York: Springer-Verlag

Colton, C. L. (1972) Chiari osteotomy for acetabular dysplasia in young subjects. *Journal of Bone and Joint Surgery* **54B,** 578–589

Dunn, D. M. and Angel, J. C. (1978) Replacement of the femoral head by open operation in severe adolescent slipping of the upper femoral epiphysis. *Journal of Bone and Joint Surgery* **60B,** 394–403

Griffith, M. J. (1976) Slipping of the capital femoral epiphysis. *Annals of the Royal College of Surgeons of England* **58,** 34–42

Ireland, J. and Kessel, L. (1980) Hip abduction/adduction deformity and apparent leg-length inequality. *Clinical Orthopaedics* **153,** 156–157

Kemp, H. B. S., Cholmeley, J. A. and Baijens, J. K. (1971) Recurrent Perthes' disease. *British Journal of Radiology* **44,** 675–681

Langlais, F., Roure, J.-L. and Maquet, P. (1979) Valgus osteotomy in severe osteoarthritis of the hip. *Journal of Bone and Joint Surgery* **61B,** 424–431

Lloyd-Roberts, G. C. and Ratliff, A. H. C. (1978) *Hip Disorders in Children.* (Postgraduate Orthopaedics series. Ed. by A. Graham Apley.) London: Butterworths

Maurer, R. C. and Larsen, I. J. (1970) Acute necrosis of cartilage in slipped capital femoral epiphysis. *Journal of Bone and Joint Surgery* **52A,** 39–50

Paterson, D. C. (1970) Acute suppurative arthritis in infancy and childhood. *Journal of Bone and Joint Surgery,* **52B,** 474–482

Salter, R. B. (1961) Innominate osteotomy in the treatment of congenital dislocation and subluxation. *Journal of Bone and Joint Surgery* **43B,** 518–539

Salter, R. B. and Kostuik, J. (1969) Avascular necrosis of the femoral head as a complication of treatment for congenital dislocation of the hip in young children. *Canadian Journal of Surgery* **12,** 44–49

Solomon, L. (1976) Patterns of osteoarthritis of the hip. *Journal of Bone and Joint Surgery* **58B,** 176–183

The Knee Joint

20

Examination

Symptoms

Pain, the commonest knee symptom, is felt locally; with inflammatory or degenerative disorders it is usually diffuse, but with mechanical disorders and especially after injury it is often localized – the patient can, and should, point to the painful spot.

Stiffness also is common and, like pain, may result in a limp.

Swelling is almost always noticed above the knee (in the suprapatellar pouch) and is diffuse; by contrast, swellings (note the plural) are localized lumps and situated anywhere round the knee.

Locking is an ambiguous term: patients often use it to describe marked restriction of movement; to surgeons it means loss of full extension and nothing more. Sudden unlocking is a more reliable indication of mechanical disorder.

Giving way also suggests a mechanical disorder, though it can result from muscle weakness; when it occurs particularly on stairs, the patellofemoral joint is suspect. Instability sufficient for the patient to fall suggests patellar dislocation.

Signs with the patient upright

Valgus or varus deformity is best observed with the patient standing.* Then he should be observed walking: in the stance phase note whether the knee extends fully and if there is any lateral instability; in the swing phase note whether the knee is held rigid or moves freely.

Signs with the patient lying on his back

(1) The tibiofemoral joint

● LOOK
Skin The colour of the skin and any sinuses or scars are noted.

Shape Wasting, swelling or lumps are observed.

Position The knee may be held flexed, hyperextended, valgus or varus.

● FEEL
Skin Increased warmth is detected either by comparing the two knees or, better, by noting the temperature gradient of the affected limb.

*A straight knee is crooked – this paradox emphasizes that the normal knee is valgus (about 7 degrees).

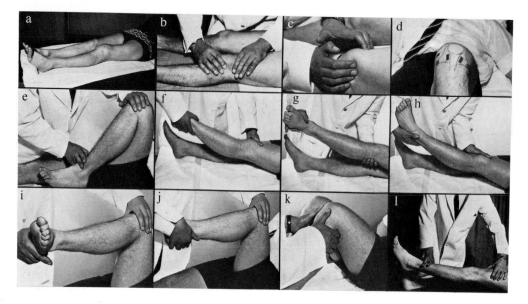

20.1 Examination – supine   (a) Looking at both knees – the left is swollen and the thigh wasted; (b) testing for fluid by cross-fluctuation; (c) feeling for synovial thickening; (d) the points which should be palpated for tenderness.
Testing movements: (e) flexion, (f) extension, (g) abduction, (h) adduction. Lateral rotation (i), medial rotation (j) and anteroposterior glide (k) are tested with the knee bent; (l) testing quadriceps power. (Alternative methods are shown in Fig. 20.15 on page 290, and Fig. 27.21 on page 457.)

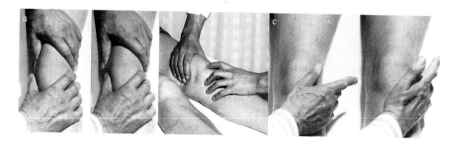

20.2 Tests for fluid   (a) Cross-fluctuation, the easiest test for large quantities of fluid; (b) the patellar tap, most likely to be positive with a moderate amount of fluid; and (c) the bulge test, with which small quantities can be detected.

Soft tissues   With careful palpation a thickened synovium can be felt, and occasionally also a displaced meniscus.

Three tests for fluid are available. (1) Cross-fluctuation: the left hand, with thumb and index finger apart, compresses the suprapatellar pouch, while the right hand (held similarly) straddles the lower part of the patella; squeezing either hand transmits pressure to the other. (2) The patellar tap: again the suprapatellar pouch is compressed with the left hand, while the index finger of the right pushes the patella sharply backwards; with a positive test the patella can be felt striking the femur and bouncing off again. (3) The bulge test: the thumb strokes fluid away from one side of the patella and is lifted away as the fingers of the same hand press on the other side; even a small quantity of fluid, insufficient for a positive patellar tap, can be seen to ripple across and bulge the hollow which the thumb created.

Bones   To identify the bony points and to localize tenderness, the knees should be flexed, if possible to 90 degrees. The joint is then palpated systematically with both thumbs: first the femoral condyles, then the tibial condyles and joint line, and finally the ligamentous attachments.

MOVE
As usual, the range of movement should be recorded in degrees.

Flexion and extension   Normally the knee flexes until the calf meets the ham, and extends completely with a snap; even slight loss of extension, or 'springiness' on attempting it, is important.

Abduction and adduction   These movements are virtually absent with the knee straight. Any laxity or pain on attempting angulation is important.

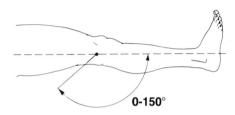

0-150°

20.3 Normal range of movements   Full extension is recorded as 0 degrees. Flexion is usually from 0 to about 150 degrees.

Rotation   This is tested first with the patient's hip and knee flexed to 90 degrees; one hand steadies and feels the knee, the other hand rotates the foot; rotation is then repeated with the knee in varying degrees of flexion. In McMurray's test, the knee is rotated in varying degrees of flexion while being subjected to an abduction force. There may be pain, or a click, or the meniscus may be felt to protrude.

Anteroposterior glide   The patient's hips are flexed 45 degrees and his knees 90 degrees. The surgeon sits on the patient's feet and with both hands rocks the tibia backwards and forwards; this test is repeated at different angles and with the leg rotated in both directions.

Power   The quadriceps muscle is tested and, if necessary, the girth of the two thighs is measured (both must be measured at precisely the same level).

(2) The patellofemoral joint

With the patient still lying on his back, the patellofemoral joint should be examined – separately, otherwise disorders of that joint (which are common) may be missed.

● LOOK
The size, shape and position of the patella are noted.

● FEEL
Much of the posterior (articular) surface is accessible to palpation if the patella is pushed first to one side, then to the other; tenderness suggests degeneration of its articular cartilage.

● MOVE
Moving the patella up and down while pressing it lightly against the femur (the 'friction test') causes painful grating if the central portion of the articular cartilage has degenerated. Pressing the patella laterally with the thumb while flexing the knee slightly may induce anxiety and resistance to further movement; this, the 'apprehension test', is diagnostic of recurrent patellar dislocation.

Signs with the patient lying on his face

● LOOK   Scars or swellings are noted.

● FEEL   Any posterior lump is carefully palpated – does it pulsate? and can it be emptied into the joint?

● MOVE   The knee is flexed to 90 degrees and rotated while a compression force is applied; this, the grinding test, reproduces symptoms if a meniscus is torn. Rotation is then repeated while the leg is pulled upwards with the surgeon's knee holding the thigh down; this, the distraction test, produces increased pain only if there is ligament damage (Apley, 1947).

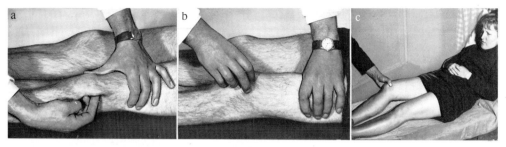

20.4 Examination of patella   (a) Feeling for tenderness behind the patella; (b) the patellar friction test; (c) the apprehension test.

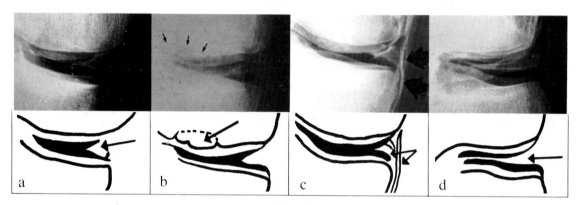

20.5 Arthrography   (a) Left knee – torn medial meniscus; (b) left knee – osteochondritis dissecans of medial femoral condyle; (c) left knee – torn medial meniscus with tear of medial collateral ligament; (d) right knee – discoid lateral meniscus. (By courtesy of Dr J. Pemberton and Dr M. J. Simmons)

X-ray

Anteroposterior, lateral and sometimes patellofemoral (or skyline) and intercondylar (or tunnel) views are needed. The anteroposterior view should be taken with the patient standing. It is worth while inspecting the tibiofemoral joint first, then the patellofemoral joint as a separate entity. When a loose body is seen, its origin should be sought; it should not be confused with a fabella, which lies on the lateral side and behind the line joining the femur to the tibia. If valgus or varus has to be measured, a long film (from hip to ankle) is needed. Arthrography is useful in doubtful meniscal or ligament injuries.

Arthroscopy

Arthroscopy is useful: (1) to establish or refine the accuracy of diagnosis; (2) to help in deciding whether to operate, or to plan the operative approach with more precision; (3) to observe and record photographically the progress of a knee disorder; (4) to perform certain operative procedures. Arthroscopy is not a substitute for clinical examination; a detailed history and meticulous assessment of the physical signs are indispensable preliminaries and remain the sheet anchor of diagnosis. Full asepsis in an operating theatre is essential. One technique is as follows.

The patient is anaesthetized and a thigh tourniquet applied. Saline is injected into the joint and, through a tiny incision, a trocar and cannula introduced. Penetration of synovium is recognized by the flow of saline when the trocar is withdrawn. A fibreoptic viewer, light source and irrigation system are attached. All compartments of the joint are now systematically inspected; with special instruments biopsy, partial meniscectomy, patellar shaving and other procedures are possible. Before withdrawing the instrument, saline is squeezed out. A skin stitch is inserted and a firm bandage applied. The postoperative recovery is remarkably rapid.

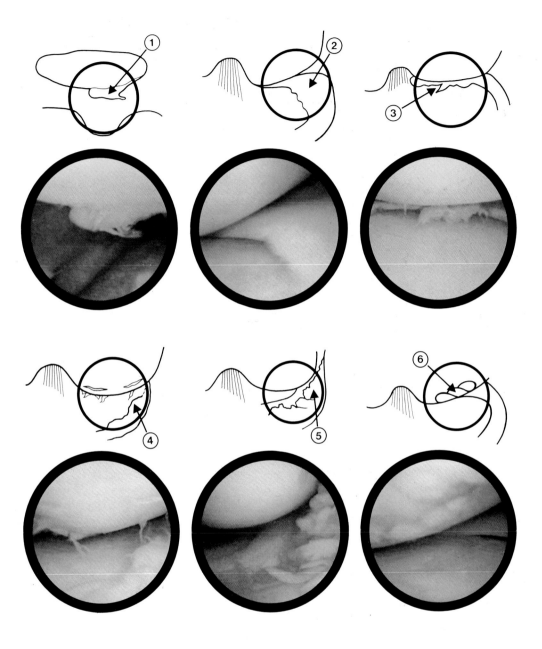

20.6 Arthroscopy In each case the view is of the right knee from the lateral side. (1) Chondromalacia patellae; (2) normal medial meniscus; (3) torn medial meniscus; (4) degenerate medial meniscus and osteoarthritic femoral condyle; (5) rheumatoid synovium; (6) osteochondritis dissecans medial femoral condyle.

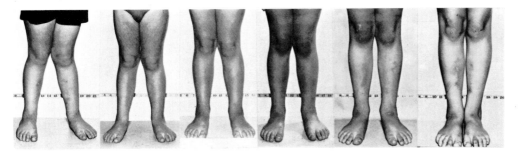

20.7 Genu valgum (1)   Idiopathic knock knee – natural history without treatment. Age: 3 years   3½   4   5   6   7.

Deformities of the knee

Knock knee (genu valgum)

Causes

IDIOPATHIC

This is much the commonest. It is almost invariably bilateral and is so common in young children that it may almost be considered normal.

OTHER VARIETIES

Many other conditions may be associated with knock knee. These include: (1) *bone softening*, occurring in rickets, in bone dysplasias and with rheumatoid arthritis; (2) *bone injury*, with epiphyseal damage, or following a fractured lateral tibial condyle; (3) *thinned cartilage*, when osteoarthritis predominantly affects the lateral half of the joint; and (4) *stretched ligaments*, in association with Charcot's disease, with paralytic deformities, and when a patient walks on a fixed adducted hip.

Clinical features

With idiopathic knock knee, deformity is the only symptom. In the other varieties there may also be symptoms of the underlying cause.

IDIOPATHIC

Idiopathic knock knee usually appears at the age of 2–3 years and nearly always recovers by the age of 6. Other postural deformities such as flat foot may coexist but these children are normal in all other respects.

To estimate the amount of deformity, the surgeon holds the legs with the knees straight and the patellae facing the ceiling. The knees are brought together till their medial sides are touching, then the distance between the medial malleoli is measured. Except for the deformity, the knees are normal both clinically and radiologically; unless deformity is severe, x-rays are unnecessary.

OTHER VARIETIES

In these there may be general or local signs of the underlying abnormality. Thus with renal rickets the child is usually anaemic and the knee deformity often develops rapidly in adolescence; with bone dysplasias other deformities may coexist; with osteoarthritis movements are limited and painful; and with Charcot's disease there is joint laxity.

Treatment

IDIOPATHIC

The child is seen at intervals of 3 months and progress recorded. The parents should be told that the legs will grow straight; almost invariably the condition requires no treatment. Raising the inner side of the heels by 4–5 mm may possibly relieve strain on the ankles; it certainly helps to set the mother's fears at rest. Splints, used extensively in the past, are ineffective and psychologically harmful.

If, by the age of 4, the intermalleolar distance is 10 cm or more, the parents should be told that operation may become necessary. Unless deformity is increasing rapidly, however, operation is best postponed till the child is aged at least 10. The alternative procedures are: (1) stapling the inner side of the knee epiphyses (the staples are removed when the knee has grown slightly varus); or (2) supracondylar osteotomy after growth is complete.

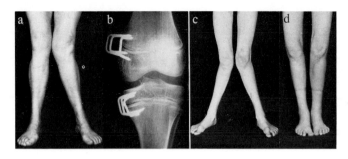

20.8 Genu valgum (2)   Only rarely does knock knee persist: (a, b) an adolescent treated by stapling; (c, d) before and after bilateral osteotomy for severe deformity.

OTHER VARIETIES

Knock knee due to rickets or dystrophy may require osteotomy but it is important first to exclude renal rickets because operation may provoke a uraemic crisis. Knock knee following a fractured lateral tibial condyle seldom needs treatment; surprisingly, osteoarthritis rarely follows. Following epiphyseal damage osteotomy may be necessary, and when knock knee is associated with osteoarthritis the pain and deformity can be treated by low femoral osteotomy. With Charcot's disease a caliper is usually necessary.

Bow legs (genu varum)

Causes

IDIOPATHIC

Some babies are born with slight bow legs, or develop the deformity while wearing napkins. These children nearly all grow straight.

OTHER VARIETIES

Other conditions which may be associated with bow legs include: (1) *bone softening*, occurring in rickets, and with Paget's disease; (2) *bone injury*, with epiphyseal injuries, and sometimes following fractures of the upper tibia; (3) *thinned cartilage*, in association with osteoarthritis; and (4) *stretched ligaments*, which may account for the bow legs of jockeys. (5) A special variety, common in the West Indies and in Africa, is tibia vara (*Blount's disease*) in which the posteromedial part of the proximal tibial epiphysis fails to grow normally during the first 3 years of life.

20.9 Bow legs (1)   (a) Infantile, which usually recovers spontaneously. (b) In this older child, deformity persisted and osteotomy was performed (c).

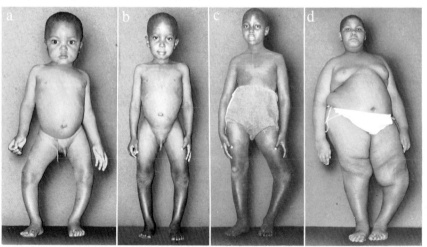

20.10 Bow legs (2) (a) Blount's disease; (b) healed rickets; (c) trauma has damaged the upper tibial epiphysis; (d) this patient has an endocrine disorder and her upper tibial epiphysis has slipped.

Clinical features

The child may be brought because of the deformity, or because of an intoe gait. Older patients may complain that bow legs are ugly.

The patient should be examined supine, the knees extended, the patellae facing the ceiling and the medial malleoli touching each other. The distance between the knees can then be measured; if more than 8 cm, further investigation is needed.

With idiopathic bow legs the only abnormal feature is the deformity, but it is important to be sure that this is 'real' and not merely 'apparent'; the child with anteversion of the femoral neck may look bow-legged as a consequence of the medial rotation of the femora – but with the patellae facing forwards the 'varus' deformity disappears.

With the non-idiopathic varieties of bow legs, there may be clinical or radiological signs of the underlying disorder.

Treatment

The idiopathic deformity usually recovers spontaneously; in any case splints are probably of no value. If bow legs persist beyond childhood operation is desirable, both for cosmetic reasons and to prevent osteoarthritis. The alternative methods are stapling the lateral side of the lower femoral epiphysis, and upper tibial osteotomy. If operation is contemplated, x-rays taken standing are essential for precise measurement.

Hyperextension of the knee (genu recurvatum)

Causes

CONGENITAL
A child may be born with considerable hyperextension of the knee due to abnormal intrauterine posture; spontaneous recovery usually occurs. Very rarely, gross hyperextension is the precursor of true congenital dislocation of the knee.

LAX LIGAMENTS
Prolonged traction, especially on a frame, or holding the knee hyperextended in plaster, may overstretch ligaments, leading to permanent hyperextension deformity. Ligaments may also become overstretched following chronic or recurrent synovitis (especially in rheumatoid arthritis), the hypotonia of rickets, the flailness of poliomyelitis or the insensitivity of Charcot's disease. Generalized laxity of ligaments is described on page 10.

BONE INJURY
Epiphyseal injury may result in faulty growth; a malunited fracture also may lead to hyperextension deformity.

Clinical features and treatment

The symptoms and signs depend largely upon the underlying condition. In itself, the hyperextension may be symptomless and may be accompanied by no other abnormal signs; but other evidence of ligamentous laxity should be sought, the patellofemoral joint examined for recurrent dislocation and the knees x-rayed for bony abnormality. If treatment is needed the possibilities are a caliper, soft-tissue reconstruction or bone carpentry.

Swelling of the knee

Traumatic synovitis

Injury stimulates the synovial membrane to produce excess fluid. When the fluid is synovial, with little or no blood, swelling is rarely obvious until several hours after injury. The patient complains, not only of swelling, but of pain and weakness.

Signs

The swelling obliterates the hollows on each side of the patella; it extends up into the suprapatellar pouch, but not beyond it. It feels cold and fluctuant; a patellar tap can usually be elicited. Movements are limited by the bulk of fluid. On x-ray the patella is displaced forwards.

Treatment

Quadriceps exercises are essential. If the muscles are allowed to waste, the knee loses stability and is easily resprained; a vicious circle is thereby set up. A crêpe bandage helps to control the swelling and is comforting.

The patient should be up and walking, but may need a back splint until he has regained muscle control; that is, until he can lift the straight leg against resistance.

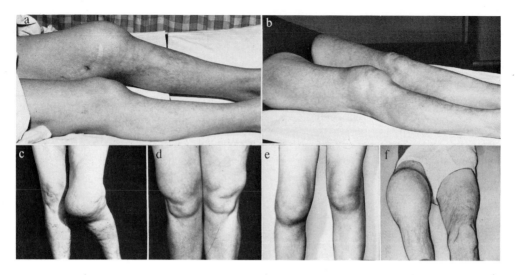

20.11 Swollen knees   Some causes of chronic swelling in the absence of trauma: (a) tuberculous arthritis; (b) rheumatoid arthritis; (c) Charcot's disease; (d) villous synovitis; (e) haemophilia; (f) malignant synovioma.

Non-traumatic synovitis

A synovial effusion or swelling without injury may be due to any of the following.

INFLAMMATION (1) Acute (from gout, pseudogout or pyogenic arthritis); (2) chronic (rheumatoid or tuberculous).

DEGENERATION   Osteoarthritis or Charcot's disease.

DOUBTFUL CAUSES   Pigmented villonodular synovitis and recurrent synovitis.

Signs

There may be general signs of the underlying cause. The local signs, other than swelling in the suprapatellar pouch, vary with the cause.

In acute suppurative arthritis the joint is held flexed, and feels hot and tender; movement is prevented by spasm, and the x-ray appearance is at first normal.

Acute gout resembles infection, but clears up promptly with indomethacin or colchicine.

In chronic inflammation due to tuberculosis or rheumatoid arthritis wasting is marked, there may be warmth and tenderness, movement is restricted and x-rays show generalized rarefaction.

In osteoarthritis wasting is slight, the joint is not warm, tenderness is usually localized, movement limited at extremes, and x-rays show diminution of joint space at the pressure area, with underlying sclerosis and often lipping.

In Charcot's disease the joint is grossly swollen and deformed, neither warm nor tender, has abnormal painless mobility and x-rays show bone destruction and calcification in the capsule.

In villous synovitis there is gross synovial thickening, but often no warmth or tenderness, a surprisingly good range of movement and a normal x-ray appearance. Middle-aged women are particularly affected and sometimes both knees are swollen. Only rarely is synovectomy indicated.

Pigmented villonodular synovitis grows progressively and the bones look cystic on x-ray (page 111).

Haemarthrosis

In the absence of injury haemarthrosis is rare: it occurs in haemophilia (page 59) and occasionally in osteochondritis dissecans (page 67).

Following severe injury the joint may rapidly fill with blood and synovial fluid. The swelling becomes obvious within an hour or two and pain is often considerable.

Signs

The joint is held flexed and the suprapatellar pouch is swollen. The knee feels warm, tense and tender; later there may be a 'doughy' feel. Movements are painful and restricted. X-rays are essential to see if there is a fracture into the joint.

Treatment

The joint should be aspirated under aseptic conditions. If a ligament injury is suspected, examination under anaesthesia is helpful and may indicate the need for operation; otherwise a crêpe bandage is applied and the leg cradled in a back splint.

Quadriceps exercises are practised from the start. The patient may get up when he is comfortable, retaining the back splint until muscle control returns.

Tuberculosis of the knee
(see also Chapter 3)

The blood-borne infection settles in synovium or in bone; the metaphysis or epiphysis of the femur or tibia may be affected, very rarely the patella. This early stage may heal by resolution or may progress to arthritis. After arthritis, healing can only occur by fibrosis, and a fairly short fibrous ankylosis is common. As the joint is superficial, sinuses are likely to develop.

Clinical features

Limp and ache are early symptoms; later there is swelling and stiffness with night cries and increasing deformity.

With early active disease the joint is held slightly flexed and is a little swollen; muscle wasting highlights the swelling. The skin feels warm and synovial fluid may be detectable; the synovium may feel thickened or the bone tender. Movement is slightly limited in all directions, and the attempt to force an extreme of movement causes pain. If arthritis supervenes, flexion is more marked, wasting is severe and movements are grossly restricted by spasm.

X-RAY There is general rarefaction, but so long as the articular cartilage is undamaged the joint space and line remain normal. With synovial infection the epiphyses may be enlarged, and with osteomyelitis a bone focus is seen. Once arthritis has developed the joint space is reduced and the line irregular.

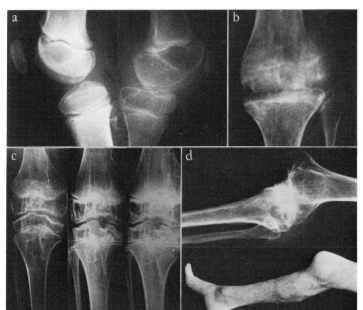

20.12 Tuberculosis – clinical and x-ray In synovitis (a) the bones are rare and the epiphyses enlarged compared with the normal side; (b) arthritis.

(c) Series showing healing with recalcification, but with joint destruction. (d) The aftermath of arthritis.

As the disease heals, any pain subsides; the patient looks and feels well, and the joint is no longer warm or tender. X-rays show recalcification. If the disease is arrested early, movement gradually returns; otherwise a varying degree of stiffness remains, and the fibrous joint, being unsound, may increasingly deform, and may give pain.

Differential diagnosis

If treatment is to be effective, tuberculous synovitis must be diagnosed promptly; the most important conditions from which it must be distinguished are transient synovitis, and chronic synovitis of rheumatoid type presenting at a single joint. Both are common at the knee; whenever synovitis persists despite rest, or recurs with activity, further investigations are needed, including a full blood count, chest x-ray, tests for rheumatoid factor and, if necessary, a synovial biopsy.

Treatment

ACTIVE STAGE

Apart from general treatment (see page 28), the essentials are as follows.

Rest   A Thomas' bed knee splint is used.

Traction   Skin traction is applied and the tapes are tied to the foot of the Thomas' splint.

Clearance   A bone abscess in the tibia should be evacuated. In the femur this is less advisable because the joint may become infected by the operation. With synovitis or arthritis a clearance operation should be considered if, after 4–6 weeks of rest and chemotherapy, progress is not satisfactory; the careful evacuation of dead and diseased material often accelerates healing.

HEALING STAGE

If the disease is arrested early, the patient is gradually allowed free, and got up wearing a weight-relieving caliper during the day. Gradually the caliper is left off, but frequent observation is essential. If the disease is arrested late, the aim is stiffness in the straight position. The patient is got up in a plaster tube or weight-bearing caliper, for which a removable polythene splint is later substituted.

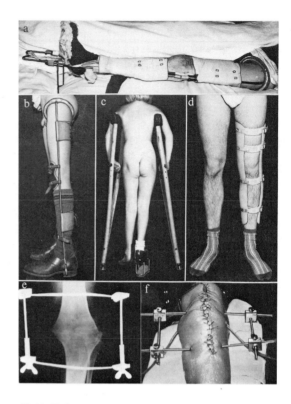

20.13 Tuberculosis – treatment   (a) Active disease – traction on a Thomas' splint.
Healing disease: (b) weight-relieving caliper; (c) patten and crutches; (d) removable polythene splint.
(e, f) Arthrodesis in the aftermath stage (Charnley's method).

AFTERMATH

An unsound joint is best arthrodesed. In children the operation is usually postponed until growth is almost completed.

Meniscus lesions

Torn medial meniscus

The meniscus is split along its substance by a force grinding it between the femur and the tibia. In the young, this can occur only when (1) weight is being taken; (2) the knee is flexed; and (3) there is a twisting strain; hence the frequency in footballers and miners. In middle life, when fibrosis

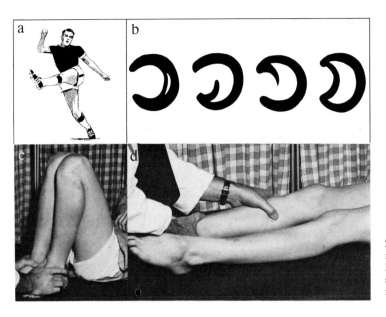

20.14 Torn medial meniscus (a) The meniscus is torn by a twisting force with the knee bent and taking weight; (b) the initial split may extend; (c) a locked knee flexes fully but (d) lacks full extension.

has restricted mobility of the meniscus, tears occur with relatively little force.

The initial split may be in the anterior horn, or posterior horn, or both (bucket-handle type). The torn portion may displace and become jammed between femur and tibia, blocking extension. Further injuries may extend the tear or cause secondary tears. Recurrent displacement leads to osteoarthritis.

A meniscus is avascular and is incapable of repair (unless the tear is peripheral). After excision, partial regeneration may occur, but years later osteoarthritis may develop.

Symptoms

An accurate history is all-important.

THE ORIGINAL INJURY

Following injury, there is pain on the inner side, sometimes locking and, within a few hours, swelling. Apparent recovery may occur. It is important to realize that, in patients aged 40 or more, the original injury may be apparently trivial.

FURTHER INCIDENTS

With relatively little force, the knee periodically gives trouble. With each attack, the patient may complain of locking (an unreliable symptom), unlocking (sudden unlocking is pathognomonic of a mechanical block), 'something moving', a click, or pain on the inner side, often with a click.

Locking The term 'locking' is unfortunate, because a locked door is immovable, whereas a locked knee will flex but not extend. Moreover, the patient speaks of 'locking' when his knee is too painful to move, whereas to the surgeon locking means that extension is blocked mechanically. With a torn meniscus, usually only the last few degrees of extension (or, rarely, only of flexion) are prevented.

BETWEEN INCIDENTS

Between incidents, the knee is normal, unless the quadriceps muscle is wasted or a bucket-handle tear is in the intercondylar fossa.

Signs

Most patients are fit young men (or athletic women); the remainder, in whom the injury is often trivial, are aged 40 or more. The local signs depend upon when the joint is examined and whether it is still locked.

IF THE JOINT IS LOCKED The joint is held flexed, but usually only 10–20 degrees. The medial joint line is tender and there is some fluid. Full extension is impossible; the attempt provokes pain and the surgeon feels an elastic resistance. Flexion is almost full and usually painless. Lateral rotation with the knee flexed may hurt.

IF THE JOINT IS NOT LOCKED Soon after an attack the signs are the same as when the joint is locked except that extension is full.

ONCE AN ATTACK HAS SUBSIDED Tenderness and pain on rotation may completely disappear. Diagnosis rests upon the history, aided by special tests; namely, McMurray's test and the grinding test.

POSTERIOR HORN TEAR A torn posterior horn rarely causes locking, and presents with a less definite history and less definite signs. Tenderness is more posterior and the special tests are often helpful.

X-RAY
The plain x-ray appearance is normal; arthrography may reveal the tear.

Differential diagnosis

If the diagnosis is in doubt the first step is to start again, with a more detailed history and more careful examination. If doubt still persists it can be resolved by arthrography (especially useful for posterior tears), or by arthroscopy, or both. Disorders from which a torn medial meniscus must be differentiated include the following.

OTHER CAUSES OF TRUE LOCKING
Loose bodies The original history is different and the attacks are variable in character. A loose body may be palpable and is often visible on x-ray.

Recurrent dislocation of the patella The locking is more dramatic and may throw the patient to the ground. The apprehension test (page 279) is positive.

Fracture A fractured tibial spine (page 453) may be missed on x-ray. The joint cannot be fully extended but the history is different and tenderness is in front.

ATTACKS OF 'PSEUDOLOCKING'
Ligament injuries A partial tear of the medial ligament may lead to adhesions, with recurrent attacks of giving way, followed by pain and tenderness on the medial side. As with a meniscus injury, rotation is painful; but, unlike a meniscus injury, the grinding test gives less pain, and the distraction test more pain.

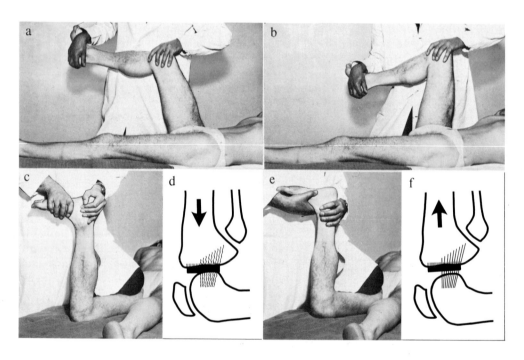

20.15 Torn medial meniscus – tests (a, b) McMurray's test is performed at varying angles of flexion. (c, d) The grinding test relaxes the ligaments but compresses the meniscus – it causes pain with meniscus lesions. (e, f) The distraction test releases the meniscus but stretches the ligaments and causes pain if these are injured.

Chondromalacia patellae Young adults complain that the knee gives way, especially on stairs. The friction test (page 279) causes pain.

Treatment

CONSERVATIVE
Conservative treatment is indicated in the following circumstances. (1) The patient is seen after the original injury and the joint is not locked. It is then justifiable to hope that the tear is peripheral and can repair. The knee is held straight in a plaster back slab for 4 weeks. Quadriceps exercises are practised. (2) Attacks are infrequent, not disabling, and the patient is willing to abandon those activities which provoke them.

MANIPULATIVE
Manipulation (if necessary, under anaesthesia) is indicated if a joint is locked but operation is inconvenient. The joint is rotated in varying degrees of flexion. Sometimes spurious unlocking is achieved because the torn fragment slips into the intercondylar fossa. Further symptoms are then inevitable.

OPERATIVE
Operation is indicated (1) if the joint cannot be unlocked, and (2) if symptoms are recurrent.

Closed partial meniscectomy (via the arthroscope) is feasible and postoperative recovery is rapid; but it is not easy and, except in experienced hands, open operation is wiser.

Technique of meniscectomy A thigh tourniquet is applied and the patient lies on his back with the knee bent to 90 degrees over the end of the table. The skin incision may be transverse (if the diagnosis is certain) or obliquely downwards and laterally (to avoid the infrapatellar branch of the saphenous nerve) if there is the slightest doubt. The capsule is incised, then the synovium, and the joint is inspected.

The anterior horn is separated from the tibia and the attachment to the tibia is cut off. A retractor is placed in the medial side of the joint and the front of the meniscus is pulled laterally. The remaining attachments to the tibia and to the medial ligament are carefully divided and the meniscus displaced into the centre of the joint. The attachment to the posterior tibial spine is then divided, taking care to avoid the cruciate ligaments, and the meniscus is removed. If the posterior horn is accidentally left behind it can be excised through a separate posteromedial incision. If the peripheral portion of the meniscus is intact, only the loose fragment need be excised.

For closure, the knee is first straightened; then the synovium and capsule are sutured separately. A pressure bandage is applied and the tourniquet removed. Quadriceps exercises are started next day.

Other meniscus lesions

Immobile meniscus

Degenerative fibrosis may limit the normal excursion of the medial meniscus on the tibia. The patient, usually aged 40–60 years, complains of aching and sometimes of swelling. The joint is tender over the meniscus and rotation is painful. The condition resembles an early osteoarthritic knee, but the x-ray appearance is normal. Heat, massage and deep frictions sometimes produce relief. Manipulation under anaesthesia accompanied by local hydrocortisone injection often helps. Meniscectomy cures the symptoms but is rarely necessary.

Torn lateral meniscus

The lateral meniscus is less likely to tear than the medial because its attachments permit freer mobility. An injury is followed by attacks of pain and giving way, but rarely locking. Tenderness is on the lateral side and rotation, especially medial, is painful. If the symptoms warrant, the meniscus should be excised.

Discoid lateral meniscus

In the fetus the meniscus is not semilunar but disc-like; if this shape persists, symptoms are likely. A young patient complains that, without any history of injury, the knee gives way and 'thuds' loudly. A characteristic clunk may be felt at 110 degrees as the knee is bent and at 10 degrees as it is being straightened. The meniscus should be excised.

Meniscal cysts

Cysts of the menisci are probably traumatic in origin; synovial cells become displaced into the vascular area between meniscus and capsule and

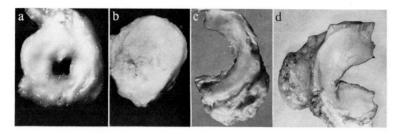

20.16 Other meniscus lesions   Whereas tears are much more common on the medial side, discoid meniscus and cysts are much more common on the lateral. (a) Partial and (b) complete discoid lateral meniscus; (c) cyst of lateral, and (d) of medial meniscus. These examples are all from left knees.

there multiply. The trauma is usually minor and often forgotten, but months or years later the patient complains of ache or a lump. The ache is localized and intermittent, often worse soon after going to bed and sometimes after activity. The lump also may appear to be intermittent, so that for months at a time there may be no symptoms.

The lateral meniscus is much more often cystic than the medial and the patient, usually an adult male, presents with a characteristic lump on the outer side of the knee. The lump is hard, almost bony, often just below the joint line, and most easily seen with the knee slightly flexed. Rotation may be painful and the grinding test positive. Medial meniscus cysts when they do occur are larger and softer.

If the symptoms warrant operation, the meniscus should be removed; excising the cyst alone is inadequate because recurrence is likely.

Extensor mechanism lesions

Strains, avulsions and ruptures

Resisted extension of the knee may tear the extensor mechanism. The patient stumbles on a stair, catches his foot while walking or running, or may only be kicking a muddy football. In all these incidents, active knee extension is prevented by an obstacle. The precise lesion varies with the patient's age. In the elderly, the injury is usually above the patella; in middle life, the patella fractures; in young adults the patellar ligament can rupture. In adolescents, the upper tibial apophysis is occasionally avulsed; much more often it is merely 'strained'.

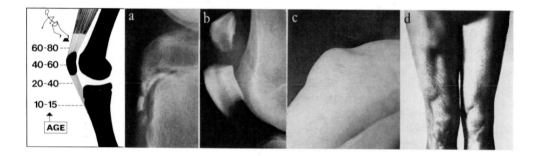

20.17 Extensor mechanism lesions   These follow resisted action of the quadriceps; they usually occur at a progressively higher level with increasing age (diagram). (a) Schlatter's disease – the only one which usually does not follow a definite accident; (b) gap fracture of patella; (c) ruptured quadriceps tendon (note the suprapatellar depression); (d) ruptured rectus femoris causing a lump with a hollow below.

Below the patella

OSGOOD–SCHLATTER'S DISEASE

This condition is common. Although often called osteochondritis, it is nothing more than a traction injury of the apophysis into which part of the patellar tendon is inserted (the remainder is inserted on each side of the apophysis and prevents complete separation).

There is no history of injury and sometimes the condition is bilateral. A young adolescent complains of pain after activity, and of a lump. The lump is tender and its situation over the tibial tuberosity is diagnostic. Sometimes active extension of the knee against resistance is painful and x-rays may show fragmentation of the apophysis.

Spontaneous recovery is usual, but takes time, and it is wise to restrict such activities as cycling and soccer. Occasionally symptoms persist and, if patience or wearing a back splint during the day are unavailing, a separated ossicle in the tendon is usually responsible; its removal is then worth while.

FRACTURE-SEPARATION OF UPPER TIBIAL EPIPHYSIS
(see page 454)

The displacement is reduced under anaesthesia and held in a plaster tube with the knee straight for 6 weeks.

JOHANSSON–LARSEN'S DISEASE

The patellar ligament is partially avulsed from the lower pole of the patella; a traction tendinitis develops, usually with calcification. The condition is comparable to Osgood–Schlatter's disease and usually recovers with rest.

Around the patella

Three lesions occur: transverse fracture of the patella; avulsion of the quadriceps tendon; and rupture of the patellar ligament. In all three the joint is swollen and held slightly flexed; a gap may be palpable and the patient is unable to lift his leg with the knee straight. The essential treatment is repair of the extensor mechanism.

TRANSVERSE FRACTURE OF PATELLA (see also page 455)

This, the commonest lesion, occurs in middle life. The fractured patella is repaired, but the essential is reconstitution of the extensor mechanism, including repair of the lateral expansions which are always torn. A plaster back slab is worn until active extension has been regained.

AVULSION OF QUADRICEPS TENDON

Avulsion from the upper border of the patella occurs in elderly people and is sometimes bilateral. Operative repair is essential

and the after-care is as for a fractured patella. Sometimes avulsion of the tendon is only partial and no operation is then needed.

RUPTURE OF PATELLAR LIGAMENT

This occurs in young adults. Sometimes the ligament is avulsed from the lower pole of the patella. Operative repair is necessary and the after-care is the same as for a fractured patella.

Above the patella

RUPTURE OF RECTUS FEMORIS

This lesion occurs in the belly of the rectus femoris muscle well above the knee. Usually the patient is elderly and, as the tissues are degenerate, suture is not feasible. The avulsed muscle fibres retract and form a characteristic lump, which becomes more obvious and harder when the muscle is put into action. Function is usually good, so that no treatment is required.

Occasionally a similar injury, but at the musculotendinous junction, occurs in young athletes. If it is diagnosed early, suture is probably advisable, or athletic prowess is likely to be reduced.

Recurrent dislocation of patella

Four varieties of patellar dislocation exist: (1) congenital, which is very rare, and in which the laterally displaced patella never returns to its correct position; (2) habitual, in which the patella dislocates every time the knee is bent, but reduces each time it is straightened; (3) traumatic dislocation (see page 461); and (4) recurrent dislocation, which is described below.

The causal factors in recurrent dislocation are as follows.

LAX LIGAMENTS

In generalized joint hypermobility (page 10) the knees hyperextend, and recurrent patellar dislocation is common.

WEAK MUSCLES

Following reduction of a traumatic patellar dislocation the muscles must be exercised vigorously; otherwise, weakness (especially of vastus medialis) facilitates recurrence.

ANATOMICAL ABNORMALITIES

With normal ligaments and muscles dislocation is prevented by a bony ridge on the lateral femoral

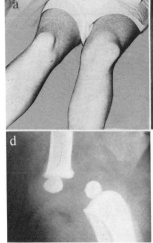
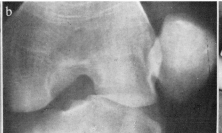
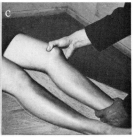

20.18 Dislocation of patella (a, b) The patella always dislocates laterally; the apprehension test (c) remains positive after even a single incident. Dislocation of the knee itself is almost always traumatic; but congenital dislocation (d) can occur.

condyle. This checking mechanism fails if the ridge is poorly developed, if the patella is too small or too high, or if the knee hyperextends. Genu valgum also favours dislocation because the line of quadriceps pull exerts a lateral force on the patella.

Pathology

Dislocation is always to the lateral side. The capsule on the medial side of the patella is torn and, if it fails to unite properly, lateral laxity persists. Repeated dislocation damages the contiguous surfaces of patella and femoral condyle; degenerative changes follow which may result in flattening of the condyle, so facilitating further dislocations.

Symptoms and signs

Sudden attacks occur without injury. The knee gets stuck (though often only momentarily) in a much more flexed position than with meniscus injuries, and the patient may be thrown to the ground. Although the patella always dislocates laterally, the patient may think it has displaced medially because the uncovered medial femoral condyle shows as a lump. Between attacks the patient has no symptoms.

Young adults, usually females, are affected, and the condition may be bilateral. If the knee is seen while the patella is dislocated, diagnosis is obvious.

Between attacks the patella may be too high (patella alta) or too small, and the knee may hyperextend, but one test is nearly always positive and is pathognomonic: if the patella is pushed laterally with the knee slightly flexed, the patient resists vigorously. (The term 'apprehension test' has been coined because the patient is apprehensive lest dislocation recur.) If the friction test also is positive, then chondromalacia has supervened.

Treatment

Only rarely is the patient seen during the first attack, when the ideal treatment would be operative repair of the torn medial structures. Usually the patella has been reduced and a back slab applied. Treatment then should concentrate on strengthening the quadriceps (especially vastus medialis). For recurrent dislocation, the only effective treatment is operation.

Two procedures give good results – realignment and patellectomy: with either, the capsule lateral to the patella should be incised ('released') and the medial capsule tightened by reefing. Realignment, which leaves a big scar, is indicated if the articular cartilage of the patella is normal; otherwise patellectomy, which leaves an almost invisible scar, is preferred. With manifest chondromalacia it is feasible to combine both procedures at the one operation.

REALIGNMENT The patellar ligament with the segment of bone into which it is inserted is freed and reattached further medially and further distally. Alternatively, the lateral half of the patellar ligament is detached, threaded through the medial half and reattached more medially and distally. Either procedure prevents dislocation, but if chondromalacia is already present it may progress and subsequent patellectomy will be required.

PATELLECTOMY The patella is excised and the resulting gap repaired. Chondromalacia is now impossible, but the repaired tendon itself occasionally dislocates, and then subsequent realignment as above is necessary. Either operation is therefore sometimes the precursor of the other.

Recurrent subluxation

Recurrent subluxation of the patella is probably more common than usually supposed. The apprehension test is usually positive and chondromalacia may supervene. Treatment is the same as for recurrent dislocation.

Chondromalacia patellae

Causes

The articular cartilage of the patella may be damaged by a single injury, by friction against a ridge on the medial femoral condyle or by recurrent displacement (subluxation or dislocation); even without displacement, if the path (or 'track') of the patella during flexion and extension is faulty, pressure on its articular cartilage may become excessive.

The causes of faulty patellar tracking include: (1) disorders above the knee (adduction deformity of the hip, excessive anteversion of the femoral neck, or medial displacement of the femoral shaft following fracture or osteotomy); (2) disorders at the knee (valgus deformity, a high patella or an irregular patella); and (3) disorders below the knee (abnormal tibial rotation, usually secondary to foot deformities). Whatever the cause, damage to the articular cartilage may lead to chondromalacia.

Pathology

Chondromalacia (cartilage softening) chiefly affects the central portion and both neighbouring facets of the articular cartilage; occasionally mirror-lesions are seen on the femur. The cartilage becomes soft, swollen and spongy; the surface loses lustre and may become fissured and fibrillated, looking like crab meat. Sometimes a 'blister' develops under the surface and may erupt. If the surface becomes eroded and the underlying bone exposed, this means that osteoarthritis has supervened.

The above description does not adequately explain the frequency of chondromalacia in teenage girls, nor the fact that most recover spontaneously. Goodfellow *et al.* (1976) postulate two kinds of cartilage degeneration: superficial, which is painless but does not heal; and deep, which hurts but usually heals. Aetiologically also there are two varieties: (1) secondary, from some known cause such as trauma, recurrent

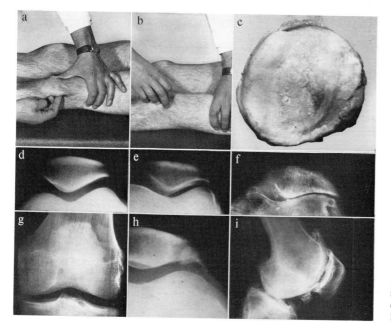

20.19 Chondromalacia patellae (a) Tenderness behind the patella; (b) pain on patellar friction; (c) well-marked chondromalacia.

Skyline views: (d) normal joint, (e) early degeneration, (f) late degeneration.

(g) Bipartite patella which may cause symptoms if (h) the small fragment is out of step; (i) gross osteoarthritis of patellofemoral joint.

displacement (dislocation or subluxation) or faulty patellar tracking; and (2) primary (idiopathic) in which no cause has so far been found.

Clinical features

The patient, usually a girl and often a teenager or young adult, may give a history of injury or of recurrent displacement. She complains of diffuse pain in front of the knee, chiefly after prolonged sitting or on stairs. The knee gives way and occasionally swells. Pseudolocking may occur, but not unlocking.

The knee usually looks normal, but sometimes the 'Q' angle (between the line of pull of the quadriceps muscle and the line of the patellar ligament) is increased; this is measured by drawing a line from the anterior superior iliac spine to the middle of the patella, and another from the mid-patella to the tibial tubercle.

Sometimes fluid is detectable. If the patella is pushed sideways, its posterior surface can be felt and is usually tender. Pressing the patella against the femur and then moving it (the friction test) causes pain. The tibiofemoral joint has full movement, though occasionally there is painful grating. X-rays are usually normal, but tomograms sometimes reveal patellar cysts.

Treatment

The patient is given analgesics and advised to avoid undue activity, but encouraged to practise non-weight-bearing exercises. Short-wave diathermy also appears to help some patients, but this may be coincidence because spontaneous recovery is not uncommon.

If symptoms are excessively prolonged, operation may need to be considered. Obvious deformity, such as genu valgum, should first be corrected. The patellar pull can be realigned by: (1) 'releasing' (incising) the lateral capsule; (2) combining lateral release with medial 'reefing' (tightening); (3) combining both with transfer of all or part of the patellar ligament further medially and distally; or (4) levering the tibial attachment of the ligament forwards – possibly combined with patellar realignment. Shaving or excising the damaged cartilage is unlikely to give permanent relief. If all else fails, patellectomy may be advisable.

Contracture of the quadriceps

The quadriceps muscle may become fibrosed and shortened because of congenital disorders, or as a result of repeated injections into the muscle. The vastus intermedius is most commonly involved and the child presents with progressive loss of knee flexion. If the vastus lateralis and iliotibial tract are involved, habitual dislocation of the patella is the usual sequel. Division of the affected muscle is necessary in either case.

The plica syndrome

A plica is the remnant of an embryonic synovial partition in the knee. It may well be present in 20 per cent of adults, but symptoms (ache, clicks or swelling) are rare. The plica is sometimes palpable and may be slightly tender; it is readily displayed by arthrography or arthroscopy. If symptoms persist and no other cause for them is found, the plica can be excised – via the arthroscope or at open operation.

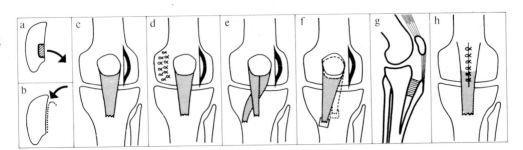

20.20 Chondromalacia patellae – treatment (a) Excision of diseased area; (b) 'shaving'; (c) incision of lateral capsule (release); (d) lateral release and medial reefing; (e) release and transfer of part of tendon (Goldthwait); (f) release and transfer of entire extensor insertion (Hauser); (g) tibial tubercle advancement; (h) patellectomy.

Bursae

Prepatellar bursitis (housemaid's knee)

An uninfected bursitis is due not to pressure but to constant friction between skin and patella. It occurs in carpet layers and miners but rarely in housemaids, who use vacuum cleaners. The swelling is circumscribed and fluctuant, but the joint itself is normal. Treatment consists of firm bandaging, and kneeling is avoided; occasionally aspiration is needed. In chronic cases the lump is best excised.

Infection (possibly due to foreign body implantation) results in a warm, tender swelling. Treatment is by rest, antibiotics and, if necessary, aspiration or incision.

Infrapatellar bursitis (clergyman's knee)

The swelling is superficial to the patellar ligament, being more distally placed than prepatellar bursitis because one who prays kneels more uprightly than one who scrubs. Treatment is similar to that for prepatellar bursitis. Occasionally the bursa is affected in gout or syphilis.

Semimembranosus bursa

The bursa between the semimembranosus and the medial head of gastrocnemius may become enlarged in children or adults. It presents usually as a painless lump behind the knee, more obvious with the knee straight. The lump is fluctuant but the fluid cannot be pushed into the joint, presumably because the muscles compress and obstruct the normal communication. The knee joint is normal. Occasionally the lump aches, and if so it may be excised through a transverse incision.

Two other swellings behind the knee may be confused with an enlarged semimembranosus bursa.

Popliteal cyst

This follows synovial rupture or herniation, so that the joint itself is abnormal; it may be osteoarthritic (the term Baker's cyst is then used) or, more commonly, rheumatoid. The lump is in the midline and fluctuates, but is not tender. It may diminish following aspiration and injection of hydrocortisone; excision is not advised, because recurrence is common unless the underlying condition also is treated (e.g. by synovectomy).

The cyst may leak or rupture; fluid then tracks down the calf, which becomes swollen and tender, mimicking a calf vein thrombosis.

POPLITEAL ANEURYSM
This is the commonest limb aneurysm and is sometimes bilateral. Pain and stiffness of the knee may precede the symptoms of peripheral arterial disease so that it is essential to examine any lump behind the knee for pulsation.

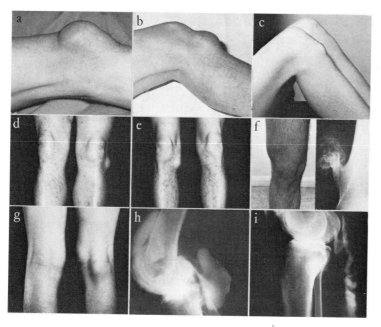

20.21 Lumps around the knee In front: (a) prepatellar bursa; (b) infrapatellar bursa; (c) Schlatter's disease.

On either side: (d) cyst of lateral meniscus; (e) cyst of medial meniscus; (f) cartilage-capped exostosis.

Behind: (g) semimembranosus bursa; (h) arthrogram of popliteal cyst; (i) leaking cyst.

Loose bodies

Cause and pathology

INJURY

A piece of bone and cartilage may be broken off by a single definite injury. Osteochondritis dissecans (see page 67) may be traumatic in origin.

DEGENERATION

In osteoarthritis small osteophytes may break off, and in Charcot's disease large loose bodies are common.

INFLAMMATION

Small fibrinous loose bodies may occur in chronic inflammatory conditions, but in these the underlying disorder is the dominant feature.

SYNOVIAL CHONDROMATOSIS

Cartilage metaplasia in an area of synovium may give rise to numerous cartilaginous loose bodies; these may ossify and are then visible on x-ray. Operative treatment is successful only if the area of metaplasia is identified and removed.

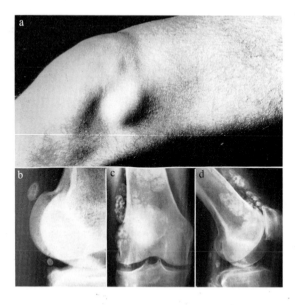

20.22 Loose bodies   (a) This loose body slipped away from the fingers when touched; the term 'joint mouse' seems appropriate. (b) Which is the loose body here? – not the large one (which is a fabella), but the small lower one opposite the joint line. (c, d) Synovial chondromatosis – the multiple loose bodies are characteristic.

Symptoms and signs

Loose bodies may be symptomless. The usual complaint is attacks of sudden locking without injury. The joint gets stuck in a position which varies from one attack to another. Sometimes the locking is only momentary and usually the patient can wriggle the knee until it suddenly unlocks.

In adolescents, a loose body is usually due to osteochondritis dissecans, rarely to injury. In adults, osteoarthritis is the most frequent cause.

Only rarely is the patient seen with the knee still locked. Sometimes, especially after the first attack, there is synovitis or there may be evidence of the underlying cause. A pedunculated loose body may be felt; one which is truly loose tends to slip away during palpation.

X-RAY   Most loose bodies are radio-opaque. The films also show any underlying joint abnormality.

Treatment

A loose body causing symptoms should be removed unless the joint is severely osteoarthritic. Operation should not be lightly undertaken, for the loose body may be difficult to find without wide exposure.

Osteochondritis dissecans
(see also page 67)

The likeliest cause is trauma, probably an osteochondral or subchondral fracture which remains un-united. It may be significant that, in full flexion, the patella makes contact with the classic site.

The lower or lateral part of the medial femoral condyle is usually affected, rarely the lateral condyle, and still more rarely the patella. An area of softened articular cartilage together with an underlying ovoid piece of bone becomes demarcated from the femoral condyle. Later, the segment becomes partly detached and finally broken off to form a loose body (sometimes two or three). A crater remains, at the periphery of which the cartilage is undermined.

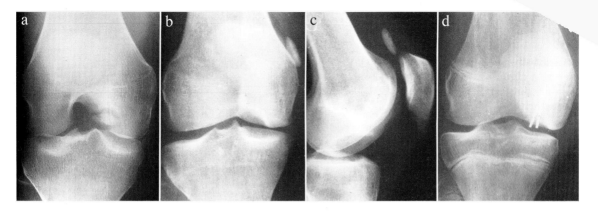

20.23 Osteochondritis dissecans (a) At first the affected area separates ('dissects') but still remains in position; the 'tunnel' view shown is often the most helpful. (b, c) Here the fragment is loose – the crater on the medial femoral condyle, from which it came, is clearly seen. (d) Pinning the fragment back is one method of treatment.

Symptoms and signs

The patient, usually aged 15–20 years, presents with intermittent ache or swelling. Later, there are attacks of giving way so that the knee feels unreliable, and locking may occur.

Soon after an attack, apart from swelling there are two signs which are almost diagnostic: (1) tenderness localized to one femoral condyle; and (2) Wilson's sign – if the knee is flexed to 90 degrees, rotated medially and then gradually straightened, pain is felt which is relieved by lateral rotation.

X-RAY At first, a fragment of bone is seen to be separated from the rest of the femur by a clear zone. Later, the fragment may be hinged on one side and project into the joint. Still later, there is a loose body, and its site of origin is visible.

Treatment

Before the fragment has separated spontaneous healing can probably occur, and the patient is merely taken off games for a few months; but healing is uncertain and, except in the very earliest cases, operation is probably wiser. If the fragment is partly detached, or even slightly loose, it is best removed (although pinning it back has been advocated); after removal, the crater is cleaned out and its base drilled to promote the formation of fibrocartilage.

Charcot's disease
(see also page 57)

Cause and pathology

Probably trauma to an insensitive joint is the immediate cause; the underlying cause is nearly always tabes. Destruction of bone is rapid and leads to instability. Loose pieces of bone break off into the joint. There is gross enlargement of the joint, with a thick but stretched capsule, ragged hypertrophy of the synovial membrane and increased fluid. Large calcified masses form in the capsule.

Clinical features

The patient chiefly complains of instability; pain (other than tabetic lightning pains) is unusual. The joint is swollen and often grossly deformed. It feels like a bag of bones and fluid, but is neither warm nor tender. Movements beyond the normal limits are a notable feature. Radiologically the joint is often subluxed, bone destruction is obvious and irregular calcified masses can be seen.

Treatment is difficult. A course of penicillin may alleviate lightning pains, but the joint instability is best treated with a caliper. Arthrodesis is feasible but demands a meticulous technique.

…eumatoid arthritis starts in the
…nic monarticular synovitis. Sooner
or … …ever, other joints become involved
and a… …us of the knee is only one aspect of a
widespread disease (page 35).

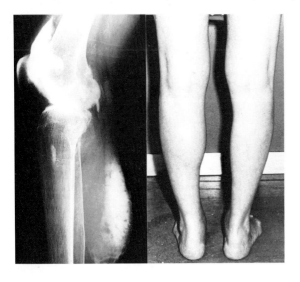

20.24 Rheumatoid arthritis This patient with early rheumatoid arthritis of her left knee had a considerable effusion which burst out of the back of the joint, causing the calf to become painful and swollen; she was sent to hospital with a mistaken diagnosis of calf-vein thrombosis.

Clinical features

During stage 1 (synovitis) the patient complains of pain and chronic swelling. There may be a large effusion and the thickened synovium is easily palpable. At this stage, while the joint is still stable and the muscles are reasonably strong, there is a danger of rupturing the posterior capsule; the joint contents are extruded into a large posterior bursa or between the muscle planes of the calf, causing sudden pain and swelling which closely mimic the features of calf vein thrombosis.

In stage 2 there is increasing instability of the joint and some loss of flexion and extension. X-rays may show loss of joint space and marginal erosions; the condition is easily distinguishable from osteoarthritis by the complete absence of osteophytes, but in the monarticular variety biopsy may be needed to exclude tuberculosis.

In stage 3 pain and disability are usually severe. In some patients stiffness is so marked that the patient has to be helped to stand and the joint has only a jog of painful movement. In others, cartilage and bone destruction predominate and the joint becomes increasingly unstable and deformed. The commonest deformities are fixed flexion and valgus; abnormal mobility (increased anteroposterior glide and lateral wobble) is present. X-rays show the bone destruction characteristic of advanced disease.

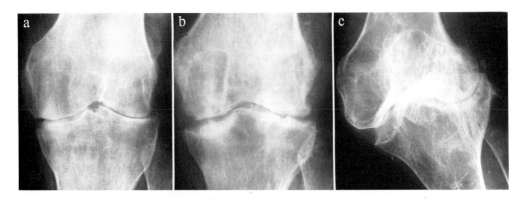

20.25 Rheumatoid arthritis (a) Early changes are cartilage erosion (giving a narrow joint space) and osteoporosis. (b) Later, joint destruction becomes more obvious, and (c) in severe cases gross deformity may result.

Treatment

In addition to general treatment, local splintage and injection of methylprednisolone and nitrogen mustard usually reduce the synovitis promptly; a more prolonged effect may be obtained by injecting radiocolloids such as yttrium-90 (^{90}Y). The majority of patients can be managed by conservative measures.

OPERATIVE TREATMENT

Synovectomy Only if other measures fail to control the synovitis (which nowadays is rare) is synovectomy indicated. Postoperatively any haematoma must be drained and movements are commenced as soon as pain has subsided.

Supracondylar osteotomy Marked valgus deformity in a reasonably stable knee is best dealt with by supracondylar osteotomy (an associated flexion deformity can be corrected at the same time). The bones are held by internal fixation and external plaster splintage for 4–6 weeks; thereafter movement is encouraged, but full weight-bearing is allowed only when union is secure.

Arthroplasty Total joint replacement is useful when joint destruction is advanced. However, it is less successful if the knee has been allowed to become very unstable or very stiff; consequently, timing of the operation is most important.

Osteoarthritis of the knee

Osteoarthritis of the knee does not often follow a single injury unless this has resulted in considerable incongruity. The oft-repeated injury of recurrent subluxation or dislocation, however, frequently gives rise to patellofemoral osteoarthritis. In the tibiofemoral joint, degeneration may result from the traumatic effects of a torn meniscus or a loose body; osteochondritis dissecans is liable to lead to osteoarthritis partly because the loose body inflicts articular damage and partly because the femoral condyle is irregular. Osteoarthritis may also follow chronic inflammation, especially rheumatoid arthritis.

Genu varum is often a precursor of osteoarthritis; moreover, if osteoarthritis develops in a previously straight knee, varus deformity may then follow. Valgus deformity and osteoarthritis are less often associated.

Pathology

The process appears to star cartilage. At the pressure area comes rough, fibrillated and thir flake off; beneath it the bone may the non-pressure areas the artic alage proliferates and calcifies, giving osteophytes which occasionally break off as loose bodies.

The synovial membrane often proliferates and excess fluid is formed.

Clinical features

Pain is the leading symptom, worse after use, or (if the patellofemoral joint is affected) on stairs. After rest, the joint feels stiff and it hurts to 'get going' after sitting for any length of time. Swelling is common, and giving way or locking may occur. With time, the pain and swelling tend to increase, though remissions may occur.

The patient is a fit adult, and the local signs are as follows.

- LOOK There may be swelling and slight wasting of the quadriceps muscle. Varus deformity is common, but occasionally the knee is valgus.

- FEEL Except during an exacerbation, there is little fluid and no warmth; nor is the synovial membrane thickened. The articular margins may be tender.

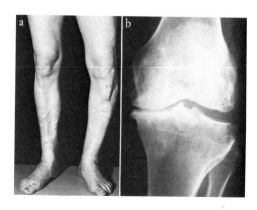

20.26 Osteoarthritis of the knee (a, b) Varus deformity and degeneration on the medial side.

Extremes of movement are usually slightly limited, and attempts to produce them are painful. If the patella is firmly pressed against the femur and then moved, pain is usually elicited.

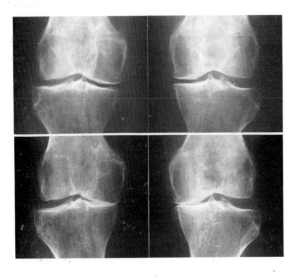

20.27 Osteoarthritis – x-rays The upper films, taken with the patient lying on the x-ray couch, show only slight narrowing of the medial joint space; but with weight-bearing, as in the lower films, it is clear that the changes are considerable.

- X-RAY The joint space is diminished at the patellofemoral joint or the tibiofemoral joint, or both. The true extent of tibiofemoral narrowing is best demonstrated by a weight-bearing film. Medial narrowing usually predominates, but occasionally lateral. Lipping and osteophytes are often seen and there may be loose bodies.

Treatment

CONSERVATIVE

If pain is not severe, conservative treatment is used. A useful first step, especially in early cases, is to manipulate the joint under anaesthesia (trying to restore full range) and to inject hydrocortisone; then to retain the increase and strengthen the knee by quadriceps exercises. Analgesics are prescribed, and warmth (e.g. radiant heat, short-wave diathermy or a bandage) is soothing. The patient is encouraged to use a stick, but will rarely tolerate a removable splint.

OPERATIVE

Three main operations are available: osteotomy, arthrodesis and arthroplasty. Osteotomy is particularly indicated when one compartment of the tibiofemoral joint is predominantly affected and the joint is stable; the results with a varus knee are particularly good. Arthrodesis is seldom performed because a stiff knee sticks out so awkwardly when sitting; it is, however, used to salvage a failed knee replacement. Arthroplasty (joint replacement) is indicated if degeneration is too advanced for osteotomy or if osteotomy has failed, and if the patient's activities are not likely to be excessive.

Knee operations

Osteotomy

When painful arthritis is associated with varus deformity, high tibial osteotomy is valuable. One method is to divide the upper end of the fibula, remove a laterally based wedge of tibia, fix the corrected position with staples and hold the leg in plaster till union has occurred.

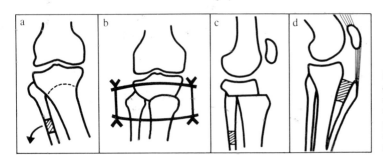

20.28 Osteoarthritis – treatment by osteotomy (a, b) Before and after 'barrel-stave' osteotomy for osteoarthritis with varus. This may be combined with (c) if patellofemoral osteoarthritis is also present. (d) Another method of treating patellofemoral osteoarthritis.

Maquet (1976) has devised a curved high tibial osteotomy in which no bone is excised and precise correction is controlled with transfixing pins; moving the lower fragment forward at the same time relieves patellofemoral pain. Low femoral osteotomy is used when the deformity is valgus, but the results are less satisfactory. Double osteotomy (low femur and upper tibia) has been advocated, especially when degeneration is secondary to rheumatoid arthritis (Benjamin, 1969).

Arthrodesis

A stiff knee is a considerable disability, and arthrodesis is not often performed. Nevertheless, it remains the only certain way of relieving pain permanently, and it may particularly be indicated for a failed knee replacement. A short period in plaster before operation enables the patient to decide if the inconvenience is tolerable.

Technique A vertical midline incision is used. If the operation is for tuberculosis the diseased synovium is excised, otherwise it is disregarded. The posterior vessels and nerves are protected and the ends of the tibia and femur removed by means of straight saw cuts. Thick Steinmann pins are inserted parallel to each other, through the tibia and femur. The bone ends are apposed and compressed by clamping the pins together (Charnley's method). For additional protection a padded plaster is applied. The clamps and pins are removed after 4–6 weeks and a new plaster cylinder is applied; this is worn for a further 6 weeks, after which, provided the x-rays show sufficient union, it is removed.

The optimum position for arthrodesis va. patient's needs; 15 degrees of flexion makes awkward, but standing and walking are easier with nearly straight.

Total knee replacement

Knee replacement is less satisfactory than hip replacement because: (1) stability is dependent on the integrity of ligaments and not, as in the hip, on the intrinsic shape; (2) complications are more frequent because the joint is so superficial; and (3) failure is more disastrous because the only salvage procedure is arthrodesis, a greater handicap than a Girdlestone hip arthroplasty.

The chief indication is pain, especially when combined with deformity and instability. Unilateral osteoarthritis is nearly always better treated by osteotomy; and rheumatoid arthritis (so often bilateral) is the commonest indication for replacement. The available prostheses are best grouped according to the needs of each individual patient.

(1) *Partial replacement* Unicompartmental replacement (e.g. Marmor) of the medial or lateral portion of the tibiofemoral joint can be used where the disease is appropriately localized; but the rest of the joint is rarely quite normal, and the results

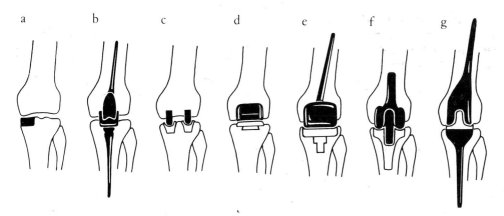

20.29 Osteoarthritis – treatment by joint replacement (a) MacIntosh, (b) Stanmore, (c) Gunston, (d) Freeman, (e) Denham, (f) Attenborough and (g) Sheehan; (a) is a hemiarthroplasty, (b) is a hinged prosthesis, (c), (d) and (e) are largely surface replacements, (f) and (g) are linked prostheses.

are seldom lasting. With MacIntosh's prosthesis a metal implant is fitted onto one or both tibial condyles; since the femur also is usually involved, the results are only moderate. Patellar resurfacing, a kind of partial replacement, is rarely performed alone; usually it is combined with surface replacement of the condyles.

(2) *Surface replacements* (e.g. Freeman, Denham, total condylar) constitute the largest group. Though variations are great (some have two components, others four) all have two important features in common: (*a*) they prevent contact between worn surfaces; and (*b*) they regain stability by 'jacking the joint apart', thereby restoring tension to the ligaments. Ligaments are rarely destroyed, even in rheumatoid arthritis; much more often they are lax because of bone and cartilage destruction.

(3) *Linked joints* (e.g. Attenborough, Sheehan) provide stability yet permit rotation. More bone is removed than with surface replacement, making salvage (if needed) more difficult. Their main indication at present is considerable deformity and instability.

(4) *Hinged joints* (e.g. Walldius, Guepar, Stanmore) are used when the joint is destroyed, stability lost and the patient fairly decrepit. The term 'hinge' implies constraint, and while hinges provide stability they lack rotation which the muscles impose; consequently they are liable to loosen, to break, or to erode the tibial or femoral shafts, unless inactivity severely limits their use.

Complications

Infection The methods for preventing and treating infection are similar to those used in hip replacement. If the prosthesis has to be removed, arthrodesis should be attempted; hence the advantage of non-bulky prostheses.

Loosening This results from faulty prosthetic design or inaccurate bone removal. It is important: (1) to overcome deformity (the knee should finally be 7 degrees valgus, no more and no less); (2) to promote stability (by tailoring the bone cuts so that the collateral ligaments are reasonably tight in full extension); (3) to permit rotation (otherwise cemented prostheses are liable to loosen). A loose prosthesis can be recemented, but unless the cause is dealt with loosening will recur.

Notes on applied anatomy

The knee joint combines two articulations – tibiofemoral and patellofemoral. The bones of the tibiofemoral joint have little or no inherent stability; this depends largely upon strong ligaments and muscles. The patellofemoral joint is so shaped that the patella moves in a shallow path (or track) between the femoral condyles; if this track is too shallow the patella readily dislocates, and if its line is faulty the patellar articular cartilage is subject to excessive wear. One important function of the patella is to increase the power of extension; it lifts the quadriceps forwards, thereby increasing its moment arm.

The shaft of the femur is inclined medially, while the tibia is vertical; thus the normal knee is slightly valgus (average 7 degrees). This amount is physiological and the term 'genu valgum' is used only when the angle exceeds 7 degrees; less than this amount is genu varum.

During walking, weight is necessarily taken alternately on each leg. The line of body weight falls medial to the knee and must be counterbalanced by muscle action lateral to the joint (chiefly the tensor fascia femoris). To calculate the force transmitted across the knee, that due to muscle action must be added to that imposed by gravity; moreover, since with each step the knee is braced by the quadriceps, the force which this imposes also must be added.

Clearly the stresses on the articular cartilage are (as they also are at the hip) much greater than consideration only of body weight would lead one to suppose. It is also obvious that a varus deformity can easily overload the medial compartment, leading to cartilage breakdown; similarly, a valgus deformity may overload the lateral compartment.

As the knee bends, the axis of the tibiofemoral 'hinge' moves further and further backwards, so that the rolling movement of the femoral condyles is accompanied by backward gliding of the tibia. As the knee straightens, these are reversed; in addition, during the final stages of extension the tibia rotates laterally (hence the differing shapes of the two femoral condyles). The complex combination of a rolling, gliding and rotating movement is difficult to analyse; it is even more difficult to reproduce in a prosthesis. This partly explains why, at the knee, joint replacement has been less successful than at the hip.

Situated as they are between these complexly moving surfaces, the fibrocartilaginous menisci are prone to injury, particularly during unguarded movements of extension and rotation on the weight-bearing leg. The medial meniscus is especially vulnerable because, in addition to its loose attachments via the coronary ligaments, it is firmly attached at three widely separated points: the anterior horn, the posterior horn and to the medial collateral ligament. The lateral meniscus more readily escapes damage because it is attached only at its anterior and posterior horns and these are close to each other.

The function of the menisci is not known for certain, but they certainly increase the contact area between femur and tibia. They play a significant part in weight transmission and this applies at all angles of flexion and extension: as the knee bends they glide backwards, and as it straightens they are pushed forwards.

The deep portion of the medial collateral ligament, to which the meniscus is attached, is fan-shaped and blends with the posteromedial capsule. It is, therefore, not surprising that medial ligament tears are often associated with tears of the medial meniscus and of the posteromedial capsule. The lateral collateral ligament is situated more posteriorly and does not blend with the capsule; nor is it attached to the meniscus, from which it is separated by the tendon of popliteus.

The two collateral ligaments resist sideways tilting of the extended knee. In addition, the medial ligament prevents the medial tibial condyle from subluxating forwards. Forward subluxation of the lateral tibial condyle, however, is prevented, not by the lateral collateral ligament, but by the anterior cruciate. Only when the medial ligament and the anterior cruciate are both torn can the whole tibia subluxate forwards (giving a marked positive anterior drawer sign). Backward subluxation of the tibia is prevented by the powerful posterior cruciate ligament in combination with the arcuate ligament on its lateral side and the posterior oblique ligament on its medial aside.

Further reading

Aichroth, P. (1971) Osteochondritis dissecans of the knee. *Journal of Bone and Joint Surgery* **53B**, 440–447; 448–454

Apley, A. Graham (1947) The diagnosis of meniscus injuries: some new clinical methods. *Journal of Bone and Joint Surgery* **29**, 78–84

Apley, A. Graham (1964) Editorial: Intelligent kneemanship. *Postgraduate Medical Journal* **40**, 519–520

Benjamin, A. (1969) Double osteotomy for the painful knee in rheumatoid arthritis and osteoarthritis. *Journal of Bone and Joint Surgery* **51B**, 694–699

Bentley, G. (1978) The surgical treatment of chondromalacia patellae. *Journal of Bone and Joint Surgery* **60B**, 74–81

Bose, K. and Chong, K. C. (1976) The clinical manifestations and pathomechanics of contracture of the extensor mechanism of the knee. *Journal of Bone and Joint Surgery* **58B**, 478–484

Goodfellow, J., Hungerford, D. S. and Zindel, M.; Goodfellow, J., Hungerford, D. S. and Woods, C. (1976) Patellofemoral joint mechanics and pathology. *Journal of Bone and Joint Surgery* **58B**, 287–290; 291–299

Hardaker, W. T., Whipple, T. L. and Bassett, F. H. (1980) Diagnosis and treatment of the plica syndrome of the knee. *Journal of Bone and Joint Surgery* **62A**, 221–225

Helfet, A. J. (1974) *Disorders of the Knee*. Philadelphia: Lippincott

Insall, J., Falvo, K. A. and Wise, D. W. (1976) Chondromalacia patellae. *Journal of Bone and Joint Surgery* **58A**, 1–8

Ireland, J., Trickey, E. L. and Stoker, D. J. (1980) Arthroscopy and arthrography of the knee. *Journal of Bone and Joint Surgery* **62B**, 3–6

Jackson, R. W. and Dandy, D. J. (1976) *Arthroscopy of the Knee*. New York, San Francisco, London: Grune & Stratton

Jackson, J. P. and Waugh, W. (1974) The technique and complications of upper tibial osteotomy. *Journal of Bone and Joint Surgery* **56B**, 236–245

Maquet, P. G. J. (1976) *Biomechanics of the Knee*. Berlin, Heidelberg, New York: Springer-Verlag

Milgram, J. W. (1977) Synovial osteochondromatosis. *Journal of Bone and Joint Surgery* **59A**, 792–801

Smillie, I. S. (1980) *Diseases of the Knee Joint*, 2nd edn. Edinburgh and London: Churchill Livingstone

Wilson, J. N. (1967) A diagnostic sign in osteochondritis dissecans of the knee. *Journal of Bone and Joint Surgery* **49A**, 477–480

The Ankle and Foot

21

Examination

Symptoms

The most common presenting symptoms are pain, deformity and swelling. It is important to know whether standing or walking provokes the symptoms and whether shoe pressure is a factor.

Signs with the patient standing and walking

The patient, whose lower limbs should be exposed from the knees downwards, stands first facing the surgeon, then with his back to the surgeon.

● LOOK   The legs, ankles, feet and toes are systematically inspected. Particular points to observe are the colour of the skin, and any swelling or deformity.

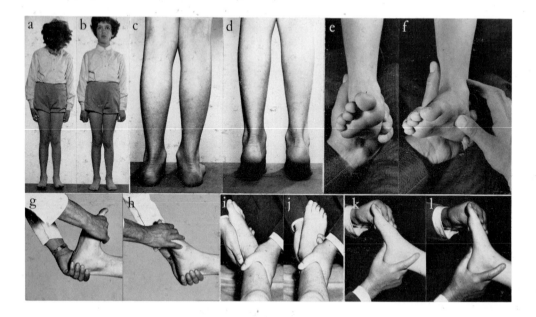

21.1 Examination   The patient examined standing, instinctively looks at her feet; this throws her off balance (a); she should look straight ahead (b). Next the feet are examined from behind (c) and on tiptoe (d); then held on the surgeon's lap with the heel square to see if the forefoot is varus (e), and to feel for tenderness (f). Ankle dorsiflexion (g) and plantarflexion (h) are examined; then subtalar inversion (i) and eversion (j). Finally, (k, l) midtarsal movements are tested.

FEEL   Palpation is postponed until the patient is sitting.

MOVE   The patient is asked to stand on tiptoes, then to walk normally and finally to walk on tiptoes.

Signs with the patient sitting or lying

The patient is next examined lying on a couch, or it may be more convenient if he sits opposite the surgeon and places his feet on the surgeon's lap.

LOOK   The heel is held square so that any foot deformity can be assessed. The sole and toes should be inspected for callosities.

FEEL   The skin temperature is assessed and the pulses are felt. If there is tenderness in the foot it must be correctly localized, for its site is often diagnostic. Any swelling, oedema or lumps must be examined. Sensation may be abnormal.

MOVE   The foot can be regarded as a series of joints which should be examined methodically.

Ankle joint   With the heel grasped in the left hand and the midfoot in the right, dorsiflexion and plantarflexion are tested.

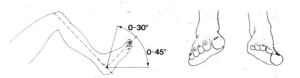

21.2 Normal range of movement All movements are measured from zero with the foot in the 'neutral' or 'anatomical' position: thus, dorsiflexion is 0–30 degrees and plantarflexion 0–45 degrees. Inversion is normally greater than eversion.

Subtalar joint   Grasping the heel alone, inversion and eversion are examined.

Midtarsal joint   The heel is held still with one hand while the other moves the tarsus up and down and from side to side.

Toes   Movement at the metatarsophalangeal and interphalangeal joints is tested.

SHOES   The shoe may be deformed or show uneven wear.

X-ray appearances

Anteroposterior and lateral views of the ankle and foot joints are examined in the routine way. Standing films, strain films and special views are sometimes needed.

Deformities of the foot

Most 'idiopathic' deformities are inherited, but muscle imbalance is clearly important since: (1) known neurological causes of imbalance give precisely the same deformities; and (2) electron microscopy and histochemical studies have shown motor unit abnormalities in some congenital deformities.

Congenital talipes equinovarus (club foot)

This relatively common deformity shows a polygenic pattern of inheritance. Boys are affected twice as often as girls and the condition is bilateral in one-third of cases. Identical deformities occur with myelomeningocele and in arthrogryposis.

Pathological anatomy

The talus points downwards (equinus) and slightly outwards in relation to the calcaneum, while the navicular and the entire forefoot are shifted medially and rotated into supination (the composite varus deformity). The soft tissues of the calf and the medial side of the foot may be short and underdeveloped. If the condition is not corrected early, secondary growth changes occur in the bones; these are permanent. Even with treatment the foot is liable to be short, and the calf may remain thin.

Clinical features

The ankle is in equinus, and the foot is supinated and adducted. The heel may be small and high, and the calf thin. The head of the talus may protrude on the dorsolateral surface of the foot.

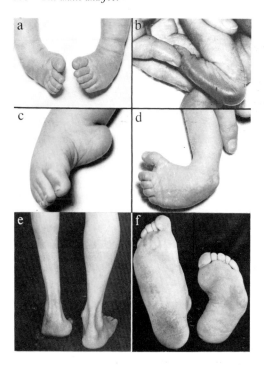

Gentle attempts at passive correction show the deformity to be fixed; in a normal baby with postural equinovarus (persistence of the intra-uterine position) the foot can be dorsiflexed and everted until the toes touch the front of the leg. The infant must always be examined for associated disorders such as spina bifida or arthrogryposis.

X-rays showing the shape and position of the tarsal ossific centres are helpful in assessing progress after treatment.

Treatment

The objectives are: (1) to correct the deformity early; (2) to correct it fully; and (3) to hold the corrected position until the foot stops growing. There seem to be two varieties of club foot: 'easy' and 'resistant' (Attenborough, 1966). Easy cases respond readily to stretching and splinting. Resistant cases respond poorly, relapse quickly and may tempt one to dangerously forceful manipulation; in them early operative correction is advisable so that manipulation and splintage can be gentle. Resistant cases are recognized by the thin calf and the small high heel; arthrogryotic club foot is notoriously resistant.

STRETCHING AND SPLINTING   Treatment begins within 2 or 3 days of birth. Each component of the deformity is corrected in turn, and always in the following order: first the forefoot adduction, then

21.3 Talipes equinovarus (club foot)   (a) True club foot is a fixed deformity, unlike (b) 'postural' talipes, which is easily correctible by gentle passive movement. (c) With true club foot the poorly developed heel is higher than the forefoot, which is also (d) varus. (e, f) The adult appearance when club foot has not been adequately corrected.

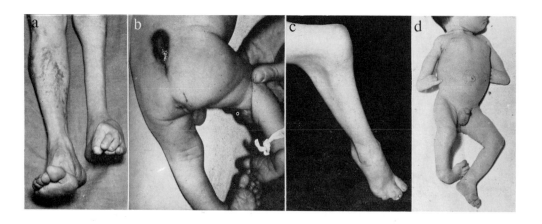

21.4 Other causes of club foot   (a) Old polio; (b) spina bifida; (c) arthrogryposis multiplex congenita; (d) multiple deformities in a thalidomide baby.

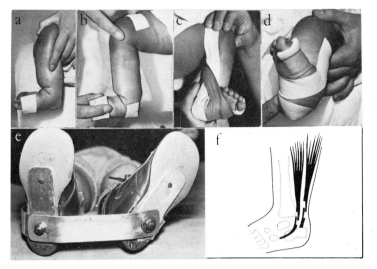

21.5 Treatment of congenital talipes
(a–d) Manipulation and strapping.

(e) Denis Browne night shoes. (f) Very early operation.

the supination and finally the equinus. Attempts to overcome equinus first may 'break' the foot in the mid-tarsal region, creating a highly refractory 'rocker-bottom' deformity.

Without anaesthesia the foot is gently moulded towards the desired position and held there by adhesive strapping with felt pads protecting the skin at points of pressure. (An alternative method is to apply a light plaster cast over a protective layer of strapping.) The process is repeated weekly; by 6 weeks it is usually apparent whether the case is 'easy' or 'resistant'. Final correction must be confirmed by x-ray: in the anteroposterior view the longitudinal axes of the talus and calcaneum should be separated by 20 degrees; in the lateral view the calcaneal axis should be at right angles (or less) to the tibia.

OPERATION   The resistant case is best operated on by 6 weeks. Through a medial incision the tendo Achillis is lengthened and tight tendons (usually the invertors and plantarflexors) are elongated or divided. The foot must be corrected fully and the corrected position held in plaster.

TREATMENT AFTER CORRECTION   Whether or not operation was needed, splintage continues; but now the moulding process need be repeated only at fortnightly or monthly intervals. This continues until the child starts walking; thereafter correction can be maintained by Denis Browne night splints and orthoses which permit walking in eversion. Splintage may need to be continued until puberty.

LATER OPERATIONS   If the previous methods have failed and the child is less than 5 years old, open division of the contracted soft tissues (including the posterior part of the medial talocalcaneal ligament and the posterior capsule of the ankle) is necessary for correction. Splintage is then continued.

Over the age of 5, correction of deformities is impossible without bone reshaping. This may take the form of a dorsolateral wedge-excision of the calcaneocuboid joint (Evans, 1961) or of osteotomy of the calcaneum to correct varus

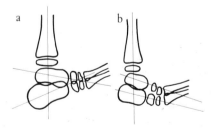

21.6 Treatment of congenital talipes (continued)   After a period of manipulation and splintage, correction is assessed both clinically and radiologically. (a) With the foot pushed up into maximum dorsiflexion the axis of the calcaneum should normally form an acute angle with that of the tibia and the talocalcaneal angle should be at least 20 degrees. (b) Dorsiflexion here has achieved only spurious correction; unless measurement of x-rays is satisfactory, the foot has not been adequately corrected.

(Dwyer, 1963). Over the age of 10 the best operation is probably a lateral wedge tarsectomy or, if the foot is mature, a triple arthrodesis.

Other varieties of 'talipes'

Sometimes the only deformity is an adducted forefoot, which is nearly always correctible by manipulation and splintage. Less than 10 per cent need operation: up to the age of 4 years, dividing the capsules and ligaments of all the tarsometatarsal joints seems to permit good realignment; for older children the possibilities are Evans' procedure (see above) or osteotomy of all five metatarsals. Neglected deformities in adults are treated by wedge-excision and arthrodesis of the tarsometatarsal joints.

Talipes calcaneus (the foot dorsiflexed) is common and often associated with valgus deformity. The deformity usually disappears spontaneously but, if it is severe or persistent, correction is easily and quickly obtained by manipulation and splintage. With calcaneovalgus deformity it is important to exclude congenital dislocation of the hip.

Flat foot

The medial arch of the foot may be normally low or normally high, but the term 'flat foot' implies that the apex of the arch has collapsed inwards.

Terminology in flat foot is confused. Thus, the terms 'pes planus', 'pes valgus' or 'pronated foot' are simply anatomical descriptions: as the arch collapses its apex drops and shifts medially; the heel becomes valgus and the foot pronates at the subtalar–midtarsal complex. The terms 'unstable', 'hypermobile' or 'postural' flat foot are descriptions of a common physiological predisposing factor; and terms such as 'foot strain' and 'rigid flat foot' describe sequels to the deformity.

Causes

ANATOMICAL   Five groups of anatomical peculiarities predispose to flat foot; their frequent inheritance explains the familial incidence.

Limb rotation   The entire limb may be externally rotated, or the leg only may be rotated from the knee downwards. In either case, the patient stands like Charlie Chaplin and the line of body weight, which should come between the first and second metatarsal bones, falls too far medially. As the body moves forwards its weight therefore tends to make the arch collapse.

Genu valgum   At the knee there may be genu valgum. In this, which is common in children, again the body weight is taken too far medially.

Equinus deformity   At the ankle there may be equinus deformity. If the tendo Achillis is short, the foot is unable to dorsiflex above the right angle in walking without the tendon taking a short cut. Consequently the arch collapses inwards.

Varus deformity   During walking, weight comes onto the forefoot; if this is varus, the medial border is forced downwards and medially, resulting in flat foot.

Congenital   This is rare, except with myelomeningocele. The foot is valgus and 'boat-shaped', being convex downwards (rocker foot) and very stiff. X-rays show the calcaneum in equinus; the talus is almost vertical and its head is dislocated. Forced manipulation of a club foot may produce a similar deformity.

PHYSIOLOGICAL   The bony arch of the foot is potentially unstable. It is bound together by ligaments, but these are capable of resisting short-term stress only; even an anatomically perfect foot will rapidly become flat unless there are muscles of good bulk and tone to support it (e.g. paralytic flat foot).

Infantile flat foot   Until an infant has learnt to control the balancing muscles, the foot collapses on weight-bearing. Sometimes the infantile lack of control persists long after walking, and consequently the foot remains flat for years.

Postural flat foot   The posture of some children is poor. They stand with a thoracic kyphosis, a lumbar lordosis and the pelvis tilted forwards. The gluteal, leg and foot muscles share in the generalized poor muscle tone and flat foot may result.

Middle-aged flat foot   In middle age muscles tend to become flabby. The housewife not only stands for long periods of time but is likely to put on weight. She gets less support just when she needs more. Flat foot is one of the results; subsequent joint degeneration may lead to stiffness.

Temporary flat foot   During prolonged illness in bed the muscles lose their bulk and tone, and on resumption of weight-bearing the feet may rapidly become flat; the ligament damage causes pain and tenderness ('acute foot strain').

Clinical features

Often there are no symptoms; but the school doctor may 'complain' that the feet look flat, or the mother that the shoes wear badly. Pain is not a feature except (1) with acute foot strain following prolonged recumbency, (2) if joint degeneration has supervened or (3) if secondary forefoot deformities (bunions or curly toes) have developed.

There are rarely any general signs, although with severe flat foot the back and the central nervous system should be examined. The local signs are as follows.

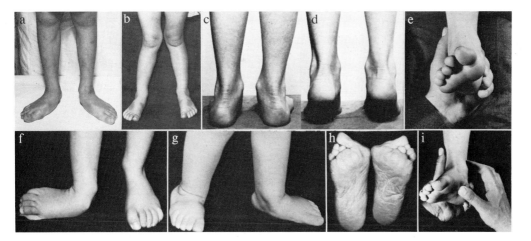

21.7 Flat foot – causal factors Flat foot may be associated with anatomical faults (upper row), or with physiological faults (lower row). (a) External rotation of the legs; (b) knock knees; (c) a tight tendo Achillis – note that standing on tiptoe (d) restores the arch; (e) a varus forefoot. (f) Paralytic flat foot from old polio; (g) infantile flat foot; (h) middle-aged splay foot; (i) tenderness in temporary flat foot (foot strain).

● LOOK   The legs are inspected for abnormal rotation and for knock knee. Then the feet themselves are examined; if the arch has collapsed the tuberosity of the navicular is unduly prominent. From behind, the heel is seen to be valgus (the tendo Achillis angulates laterally), but the deformity usually disappears when standing on tiptoe.

The patient now sits, and each foot is examined in turn while the surgeon holds it with the heel square. It is then possible to see if the forefoot is varus and to assess any associated toe disorders.

● FEEL   The foot is palpated for tenderness: first under the arch, then at the mid-tarsal region, and finally at the forefoot.

● MOVE   With the heel still held square and the knee straight, movements are tested. First the ankle: does it dorsiflex above a right angle? If there is a tight tendo Achillis, dorsiflexion does not occur without the heel moving into valgus. The subtalar, midtarsal and metatarsophalangeal joints are each examined in turn to determine their range of movement.

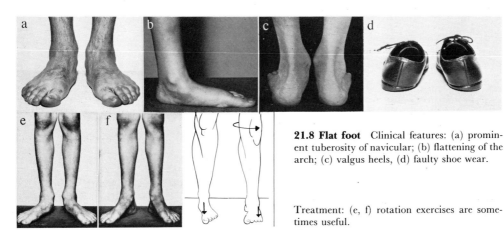

21.8 Flat foot Clinical features: (a) prominent tuberosity of navicular; (b) flattening of the arch; (c) valgus heels, (d) faulty shoe wear.

Treatment: (e, f) rotation exercises are sometimes useful.

Treatment

In the vast majority of cases flat foot is painless and no treatment is required. Exercises may strengthen the muscles, and supports may prop up the arch; the middle-aged patient with pain sometimes finds the combination comforting, but it does not restore the arch to normal. Children with painless flat foot are certainly best left untreated. The mother, who often demands treatment, should be told that the arch may develop during growth, but that treatment does not influence the outcome; supports or heel seats are justified only if their use cuts down wear on shoes.

Only two kinds of flat foot, both rare, need treatment: congenital flat foot and acute foot strain. Acute foot strain is painful, but the only treatment required is a period of rest combined with graduated exercises and a temporary support. With *congenital flat foot*, however, reduction of the talar dislocation is essential. It is probably best to operate through a posteromedial incision, first elongating the tendo Achillis and excising the navicular bone; the talus is then reduced, the tibialis anterior implanted into its neck and the reduction held with a Kirschner wire and plaster (Colton, 1973).

Spasmodic flat foot

The term is a misnomer: the foot is not flat, nor is the disorder spasmodic; but the foot is everted and the muscles are in spasm. The likeliest cause is an anatomical abnormality, for in many cases an abnormal bar of bone can be demonstrated joining the calcaneum to the talus or to the navicular; the term 'tarsal coalition' is used but the bar is not necessarily complete. The flaw presumably leads to a faulty pattern of movement at the remainder of the subtalar–midtarsal complex; hence the pain and spasm. Relatives of affected patients often show tarsal coalitions on x-ray, but in them symptoms are rare (Leonard, 1974).

Spasmodic flat foot may also occur in inflammatory disorders such as Reiter's disease.

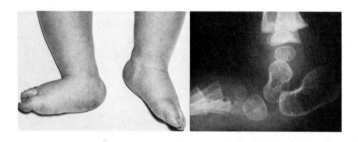

21.9 Flat foot – congenital   Note the 'rocker bottom' foot and the vertical talus.

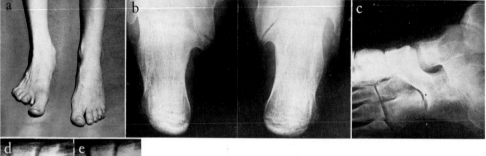

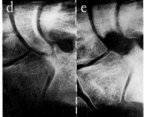

21.10 'Spasmodic' flat foot   (a) Evertor spasm, (b) Harris' axial view shows calcaneotalar coalition on the left; this is more difficult to see than (c) a calcaneonavicular bar; (d) before and (e) after excision of similar bar.

Symptoms and signs

Pain is the presenting symptom. The condition usually occurs between the ages of 12 and 16 years, is twice as common in boys and is often bilateral. The foot is held everted, and the peroneal and extensor tendons can be seen standing out in spasm under the skin. There may be diffuse tenderness around the tarsus. Ankle movements are normal. Subtalar joint movement is grossly restricted and often painful; even if no spasm was previously visible, attempted movement provokes it. Midtarsal movements also are restricted.

X-RAY   An abnormal bar of bone may be seen, although special views are sometimes needed to demonstrate it.

Treatment

CONSERVATIVE   A walking plaster is applied with the foot in its normal position (an anaesthetic may be necessary). The plaster is worn for at least 6 weeks. An outside iron and inside T-strap can then, if necessary, be worn for a further 3 months.

OPERATIVE   A calcaneonavicular bar can be excised and sometimes normal movement is restored. If this fails, or with a talocalcaneal bar, the pain can be relieved by a calcaneal osteotomy, taking out a medially based wedge (Cain and Hyman, 1978); or, if necessary, by a triple arthrodesis.

Pes cavus

Causes

MUSCLE IMBALANCE   The lumbrical and interosseous muscles normally flex the straight toes (i.e. they flex the metatarsophalangeal joints and extend the interphalangeal joints). If these short intrinsic muscles are weak, they are overpowered by the long toe muscles and claw foot and curly toes are produced. The muscle weakness may be due to neurological disease. Often, however, no cause is found and the condition is termed 'idiopathic'.

MUSCLE FIBROSIS   A similar deformity may occur if the intrinsic muscles shorten as a result of fibrosis (e.g. following Volkmann's ischaemia).

Pathological anatomy

The deformity resulting from muscle imbalance is complex. At the subtalar joint there is inversion of the heel. At the midtarsal joint there is plantaris deformity; that is, the forefoot is plantarflexed, bringing it below its normal level. The metatarsophalangeal joints are hyperextended, the interphalangeal joints flexed.

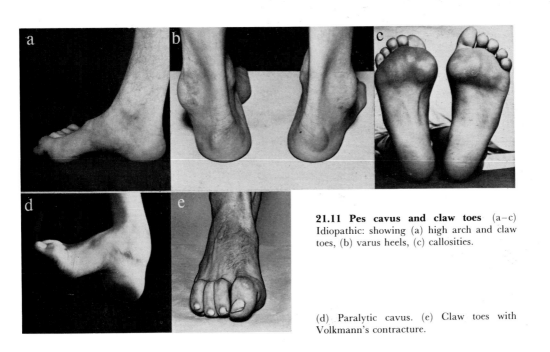

21.11 Pes cavus and claw toes (a–c) Idiopathic: showing (a) high arch and claw toes, (b) varus heels, (c) callosities.

(d) Paralytic cavus. (e) Claw toes with Volkmann's contracture.

After a time these deformities become fixed and the foot takes pressure over too small an area of the sole, where painful callosities develop under the metatarsal heads. There is not enough height in the shoe for the curly toes and callosities develop on their dorsum.

Clinical features

Deformity may be noticed by the mother or the school doctor before there is any pain. Usually, pain is felt at the site of callosities. Sometimes there is also a general aching of the foot and calf after exercise. The ankle may sprain easily because of the varus heel.

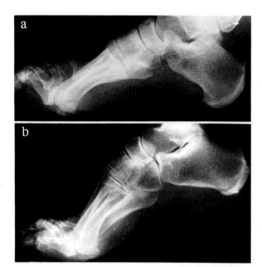

21.12 Pes cavus (a) In pes cavus there is a true elevation of the medial arch when the foot is placed on a flat surface; the x-ray in (b) looks similar, but this is due simply to plantar angulation of the metatarsals – the 'plantaris' deformity.

Idiopathic pes cavus is first noticed at the age of 8–10 years in an otherwise fit child. There is often a family history and as a rule both feet are affected. The deformities described are obvious: the extensor tendons stand out as tight bands under the skin. Callosities may be visible and are often tender. The ankle may move normally, but even when it is dorsiflexed the forefoot remains at a lower level than the heel (plantaris deformity). The subtalar joint is in fixed inversion. The midtarsal joint is in fixed plantaris and cannot be dorsiflexed. The metatarsophalangeal joints are fixed in hyperextension and are often subluxed or dislocated. The interphalangeal joints are fixed flexed.

Differential diagnosis

Before claw foot is labelled as idiopathic the following conditions must be excluded.

NEUROLOGICAL DISORDERS   These include Friedreich's ataxia and spina bifida, in both of which there is other evidence of the cause. In peroneal muscle atrophy the hands are usually affected as well.

VOLKMANN'S ISCHAEMIA   In Volkmann's ischaemia of the calf there is a history of injury; the claw foot results from contracture of the muscles.

Treatment

IN YOUNG CHILDREN   An attempt is made to strengthen the intrinsic muscles by exercises in which the straight toes are taught to flex at the metatarsophalangeal joints. Great care is necessary to see that the shoes are long enough and the heel low.

Operation may become necessary. Before the toe deformities become fixed the long flexor tendons of the outer four toes are transferred into the extensor tendons, and the interphalangeal joint of the hallux is arthrodesed. This straightens the toes, but if there is much cavus deformity Steindler's operation is performed at the same time: in this the tissues arising from the undersurface of the calcaneum are divided and the foot is wrenched until it flattens. The corrected position is held in plaster for at least 6 weeks.

IN ADOLESCENTS   If the toe deformities have become fixed it is best to arthrodese all the interphalangeal joints (so that the long flexors now flex the toes instead of bunching them up) and the long extensors are reinserted into the metatarsal necks (so that they elevate the forefoot). The outer four toes are held with wires and the hallux with a screw.

When varus deformity of the heel is a prominent feature a calcaneal osteotomy is valuable and can usefully be combined with Steindler's operation. If forefoot plantaris is severe the

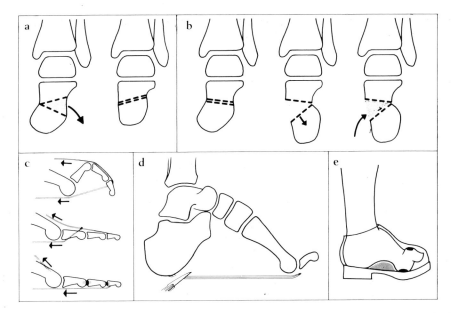

21.13 Treatment of pes cavus and claw toes   Correction of the varus heel by (a) excising a laterally based wedge of bone, or (b) inserting a medial wedge (Dwyer).
(c) Claw toes due to overaction of the long tendons may be dealt with by transferring flexor to extensor tendons or by arthrodesing the toe joints and reattaching the long extensors more proximally. (d) Division of the plantar fascia (Steindler). (e) Padding and special shoes for the late untreated case.

least mutilating operation is wedge-excision and arthrodesis of the tarsometatarsal joints (Jahss, 1980). This should only be done after bone maturity (14–16 years) and if there is no neurological disease.

IN ADULTS   Palliative treatment is usually all that is practicable in adults. A cork or sponge insole is fitted to distribute pressure evenly, and shoes are made specially. The shoe must be large enough to accommodate the foot, the claw toes and the insole, all without undue pressure. With care and chiropody, most patients can be made comfortable. Severe claw toes with painful callosities may need operation (page 319).

Hallux valgus

Hallux valgus is the commonest of the foot deformities (and probably of all musculoskeletal deformities). In the natural state (i.e. in people who have never worn shoes) the big toe is in line with the first metatarsal, retaining the slightly fan-shaped appearance of the forefoot. In people who wear shoes the hallux assumes a valgus position; but only if the angulation is excessive is it referred to as 'hallux valgus'.

Causal factors

VARUS FIRST METATARSAL   This, usually regarded as the basic deformity, may be congenital or acquired.

Congenital   The condition is often familial, and sometimes the first metatarsal is rotated (like a thumb), suggesting an atavistic abnormality.

Acquired   In middle age and with increasing weight, the intrinsic muscles weaken and the forefoot splays so that the first metatarsal becomes more varus.

SHOES   Shoes cannot produce metatarsus varus; but, when that deformity is present, they may force the hallux into valgus, because no modern shoe allows the toe to continue along the line of a varus first metatarsal. The importance of footwear in causing hallux valgus is disputed; its importance in causing the symptoms is undeniable.

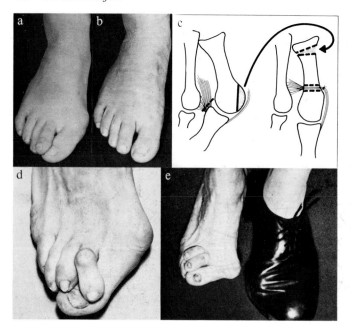

21.14 Hallux valgus (a, b) Adolescent, before and after operative correction; (c) principles of Simmonds' operation. (d) Severe deformity in middle age. (e) This patient was comfortable in wide shoes – the simplest treatment.

Pathological anatomy

The most obvious feature is prominence of the first metatarsal head. This is due to several factors: (1) increased width of the forefoot, with the first metatarsal shaft deviated medially away from the second; (2) the metatarsal head develops a protective bursa (bunion) where the shoe rubs; and (3) the proximal phalanx of the hallux is inclined laterally towards the second toe, which is crowded and may become deformed.

Into the gap between the first and second metatarsal heads, the long tendon of the hallux and the sesamoid bones are shifted laterally; once this shift has occurred, the 'bowstringing' effect tends to increase the toe deformity.

Clinical features

Often there are no symptoms apart from the deformity. Pain, if present, may be due to (1) an inflamed bunion, (2) a hammer toe, (3) an associated wide splay foot (with pain under the metatarsal heads) or (4) secondary osteoarthritis of the first metatarsophalangeal joint.

Hallux valgus is usually bilateral, and is commonest in the sixth decade and in females. There is a variety, strongly familial and by no means uncommon, which presents in adolescents.

● LOOK The forefoot is too wide and the first metatarsal head too prominent. There may be a painful and inflamed bursa over the metatarsal head. The proximal phalanx is valgus and often rotated. The extensor tendon can be seen standing out as a tight band. The second toe may overlap the first or underlap it, or be a hammer toe. There may be callosities under the metatarsal heads.

● FEEL The site of tenderness is important and must be accurately localized, for it may influence treatment. It may be (1) over the bunion, (2) in the joint or (3) between the metatarsals.

● MOVE The metatarsophalangeal joint, in spite of deformity, usually has a good range of movement.

● X-RAY The varus first metatarsal and the lateral shift of the sesamoid bones are clearly seen. The angle between first and second metatarsals can be measured.

Treatment

ADOLESCENTS Deformity is usually the only symptom, but the mother is anxious to prevent it

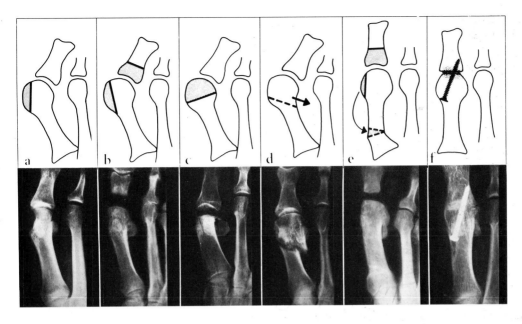

21.15 Hallux valgus – treatment Surgical procedures: (a) bevelling; (b) Keller's operation; (c) Mayo's operation; (d) Wilson's osteotomy; (e) Keller's operation combined with osteotomy; (f) arthrodesis.

becoming as severe as her own. Nothing short of operation can prevent the deformity from increasing.

It is possible to correct varus deformity of the first metatarsal by an osteotomy near its base, and to maintain correction by inserting into the osteotomy a wedge of bone removed from the prominent metatarsal head. A distal osteotomy of the metatarsal neck with lateral displacement of the head is equally effective, but care must be taken to prevent dorsal angulation of the distal fragment, as this can result in pain under the metatarsal. A simpler method is to osteotomize the first metatarsal obliquely through its distal third; the distal portion is displaced laterally and held in position by angulating the toe into varus (Wilson, 1963).

ADULTS All patients with hallux valgus can be made comfortable by careful attention to footwear. The shoe should be wide and the upper soft. Padding may be used to protect the bunion or a hammer toe. Foot exercises and an anterior platform type of support are useful when there is a splay foot with metatarsalgia.

In adults aged between 20 and 50 the big toe can be 'straightened out' by a varus osteotomy of the proximal phalanx. In elderly patients the simplest operation is an excision arthroplasty of the metatarsophalangeal joint. Two procedures are commonly performed.

Keller's operation The proximal third of the proximal phalanx is excised, and the prominent portion of the metatarsal head trimmed.

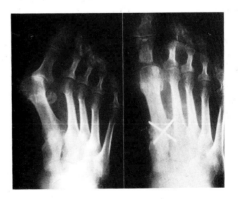

21.16 Hallux valgus – treatment (continued) If hallux valgus is accompanied by marked varus of the first metatarsal, both deformities may need correction. This patient has had an osteotomy of the base of the metatarsal (held by K-wires) and Keller's excision arthroplasty of the big toe.

Mayo's operation The metatarsal head is excised and the prominent portion of the proximal phalanx trimmed. In theory this weakens the foot more than Keller's operation but in practice results are the same.

With either Mayo's or Keller's operation it is often wise to elongate the extensor hallucis tendon and to shorten and straighten the second toe. If there is gross varus of the first metatarsal, Keller's operation may be combined with a metatarsal osteotomy.

Hallux rigidus

The 'rigidity' (joint stiffness) is due to degenerative arthritis, the result of local trauma, osteochondritis of the first metatarsal head, gout or pseudogout. In marked contrast to hallux valgus, males are more commonly affected.

Clinical features

Pain on walking, especially on slopes or rough ground, is the predominant symptom. The hallux is straight and the metatarsophalangeal joint is knobbly. Often there is a callosity under the medial side of the distal phalanx. The outer side of the sole of the shoe may be unduly worn – the result of rolling the foot outwards to avoid pressing on the big toe. The metatarsophalangeal joint feels enlarged and tender. Dorsiflexion is restricted and painful; plantarflexion also is limited, but less so. There may be compensatory hyperextension at the interphalangeal joint.

X-RAY The changes are those of osteoarthritis: the joint space is narrowed, there is bone sclerosis and, often, large osteophytes.

Treatment

A rocker-soled shoe may abolish pain by allowing the foot to 'roll' without the necessity for dorsiflexion at the metatarsophalangeal joint.

If walking is painful despite this adjustment, an operation is advised. Joint replacement, using a Silastic prosthesis, effectively relieves pain and may increase the range of dorsiflexion. Arthrodesis also abolishes pain but it is difficult to achieve a position which suits the requirements of the individual patient, and for women it may preclude the wearing of different-height heels.

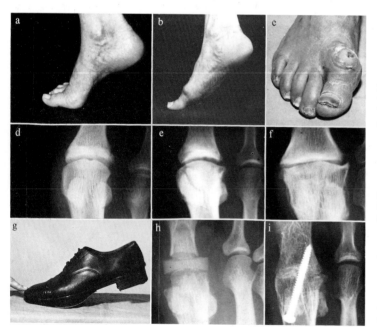

21.17 Hallux rigidus (a) In normal walking the hallux dorsiflexes considerably. With rigidus (b), dorsiflexion is limited; a dorsal callosity (c) may develop.

(d) Splitting osteochondritis or (e) a bipartite sesamoid may be precursors of (f) joint degeneration.

(g) A rocker sole relieves symptoms; operations include joint replacement with a Silastic spacer (h) and arthrodesis (i).

Claw toes

Flexion of the interphalangeal joints and hyperextension of the metatarsophalangeal joints constitute claw toes. This 'intrinsic-minus' deformity is seen in neurological disorders (e.g. poliomyelitis and peroneal muscular atrophy) and in rheumatoid arthritis. Usually, however, no cause is found and the condition may be associated with idiopathic pes cavus; in such cases there is often a positive family history.

Clinical features

The patient complains of pain in the forefoot (metatarsalgia) and under the metatarsal heads. Usually the condition is bilateral and walking may be severely restricted. At first the joints are mobile and can be passively corrected; later the deformities become fixed and the metatarsophalangeal joints dislocated. Painful callosities may develop on the dorsum of the toes and under the metatarsal heads. In the most severe cases the skin ulcerates at the pressure sites.

Treatment

So long as the toes can be passively straightened, 'dynamic' correction is possible by transferring the long toe flexors to the extensors. When the deformity is fixed it may either be accepted and accommodated by special footwear, or treated by one of the following operations.

Interphalangeal arthrodesis Even when the toe deformities are fixed, the metatarsophalangeal joints may remain mobile. In these cases (usually young adults) arthrodesis of the toe joints permits active flexion of the metatarsophalangeal joints by the long flexors; this is often combined with transfer of the extensor hallucis longus to the first metatarsal, partly in order to remove a deforming force and partly to provide dynamic 'lift' for the forefoot.

Joint excision If passive toe flexion is not possible, the metatarsal heads alone or the entire joints can be excised; the shortened toes fall into reasonable position even though the interphalangeal joints remain flexed, but occasionally they too must be excised and straightened.

Metatarsal osteotomy Oblique osteotomies of the outer four metatarsals (Helal, 1975), allowing the distal segments to slide proximally and dorsally, relax the dorsal structures and take pressure off the metatarsal heads.

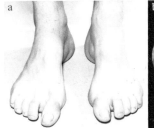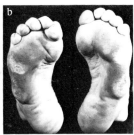

21.18 Claw toes Claw-toe deformity suggests muscle imbalance, with relative weakness of the intrinsics. Only occasionally, however (as in these examples of peroneal muscular atrophy), is definite neurological defect found.

Amputation Toes that are severely contracted, dislocated and ulcerated are worse than none. If the circulation is satisfactory and the patient is willing to accept the appearance, amputation of all ten toes (the 'pobble' procedure) is a useful palliative operation.

Hammer toe

The proximal toe joint is fixed in flexion, while the distal joint and the metatarsophalangeal joint are extended. The second toe of one or both feet is commonly affected, and hyperextension of the metatarsophalangeal joint may go on to dorsal dislocation. Shoe pressure may produce painful corns or callosities on the dorsum of the toe and under the prominent metatarsal head.

The cause is obscure: the similarity to boutonnière deformity of a finger suggests an extensor dysfunction, a view supported by the frequent association with a dropped metatarsal head, flat anterior arch and hallux valgus. A simpler explanation is that the toe was too long or the shoe too short.

Operative correction is indicated for pain or for difficulty with shoes. The toe is shortened and straightened by excising the joint. A large wedge of soft tissue and bone is removed (including the corn if present). When the wound edges are firmly sutured the toe straightens and the excised joint needs no internal fixation. The toe is splinted for 6 weeks using a collodion bandage.

Overlapping fifth toe

This is a common congenital anomaly. If symptoms warrant, the toe may be straightened by a V/Y-plasty, reinforced by transferring the flexor to the extensor tendon.

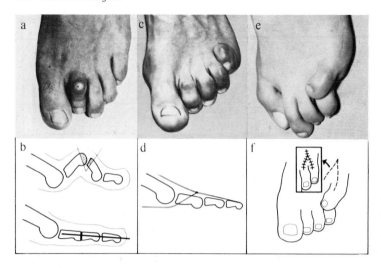

21.19 Toe disorders (a) Hammer toe, and (b) treatment by excision-arthrodesis. (c) Curly toes and (d) treatment by flexor-to-extensor transfer. (e) Overlapping fifth toe, and (f) treatment by V/Y-plasty.

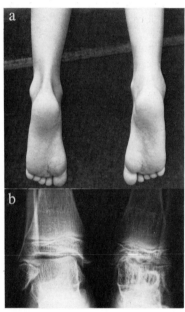

21.20 Tuberculous arthritis of the ankle (a) The swelling is best seen from behind; (b) shows rarefaction and joint destruction.

Tuberculous arthritis

This begins as a synovitis or as an osteomyelitis and, because walking is painful, may present before true arthritis supervenes. The ankle is swollen and the calf markedly wasted; the skin feels warm and movements are restricted. Sinus formation occurs early. X-rays show generalized rarefaction, sometimes a bone abscess and, with late disease, narrowing and irregularity of the joint space.

In addition to general treatment (Chapter 3) a removable splint is used to rest the foot in neutral position. If the disease is arrested early, the patient is allowed up non-weight-bearing in a caliper; gradually he takes more weight, then discards the caliper. Following arthritis, weight-bearing is harmless, but stiffness is inevitable and usually arthrodesis is the best treatment.

Rheumatoid arthritis

(see also page 35)

The ankle and foot are affected almost as often as the wrist and hand. During stage 1 there is synovitis of the metatarsophalangeal, intertarsal and ankle joints, as well as of the sheathed tendons (usually the peronei and tibialis posterior). In stage 2, joint erosion and tendon dysfunction prepare the ground for the progressive deformities of stage 3.

The ankle and hindfoot

The earliest symptoms are pain and swelling around the ankle. Walking becomes increasingly difficult and later deformities appear. On examination, swelling and tenderness are usually localized to the back of the medial malleolus (tenosynovitis of tibialis posterior) or the lateral malleolus (tenosynovitis of the peronei). Less often the ankle swells (joint synovitis) and its movements are restricted. Inversion and eversion may be painful and limited. In the late stages the tibialis posterior may rupture, or become ineffectual due to progressive erosion of the tarsal joints, and the foot gradually drifts into severe valgus deformity. X-rays show osteoporosis and, later, erosion of the tarsal and ankle joints. Soft-tissue swelling may be marked.

Treatment

In the stage of synovitis, splintage is essential (to allow inflammation to subside and to prevent deformity) while waiting for systemic treatment to control the disease. Initially tendon sheaths and joints may be injected with the 'anti-inflammatory cocktail' (methylprednisolone, nitrogen mustard and local anaesthetic), but this should not be repeated more than two or three times. A lightweight below-knee caliper with an inside supporting strap restores stability and may be worn almost indefinitely.

If the synovitis does not subside, operative synovectomy and (if necessary) tendon repair or

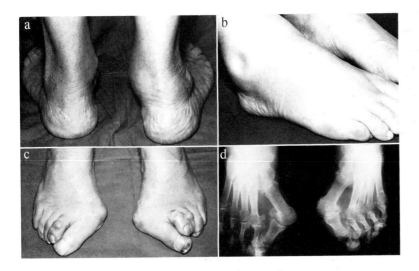

21.21 Rheumatoid arthritis Swelling of the hindfoot is more often due to tenosynovitis of tibialis posterior (a) or peronei (b), than to subtalar arthritis, though if tendon rupture occurs talar destruction and hindfoot deformity are inevitable. (c, d) Forefoot deformities are due primarily to progressive erosion of the metatarsophalangeal joints.

replacement are advisable. In the very late stage, arthrodesis of the ankle and tarsal joints can still restore modest function and abolish pain.

Arthrodesis of the ankle   is indicated for destructive arthritis (post-traumatic osteoarthritis, rheumatoid disease or tuberculosis) or for instability. The joint surfaces are rawed and held together by compression clamps, or by a tibial graft slotted into the talus, or by using the lower end of the fibula as an onlay graft. Plaster immobilization is maintained for 3 months and thereafter a supporting caliper is used for another 3 months. *Optimal position:* neutral for men; 10 degrees' plantarflexion for women who wear higher heels.

Tarsal arthrodesis (triple fusion)   is required for advanced arthritis (or to stabilize a paralysed foot). Three joints are involved: the talocalcaneal, talonavicular and calcaneocuboid. The joints are exposed from the outer side, dislocated, rawed and replaced in the plantigrade position. Depending on the existing deformity, this may require the removal of wedges in order to obtain a good fit.

The forefoot

Pain and swelling of the metatarsophalangeal joints are among the earliest features of rheumatoid arthritis. Shoes feel uncomfortable and the patient walks less and less. Tenderness is at first localized to the metatarsophalangeal joints; later the entire forefoot is painful on pressing or squeezing. With increasing weakness of the intrinsic muscles and joint destruction, the characteristic deformities appear: a flattened anterior arch, claw toes and hallux valgus. Subcutaneous nodules are common and may ulcerate. Dorsal corns and plantar callosities also may break down and become infected. In the worst cases the toes are dislocated, inflamed, ulcerated and useless.

X-rays show osteoporosis and periarticular erosions at the metatarsophalangeal joints. Curiously – in contrast to the hand – the smaller digits (fourth and fifth toes) are affected first.

Treatment

During the stage of synovitis, anti-inflammatory injections and attention to footwear may relieve symptoms. Once deformity is progressive, treatment is that of the claw toes and hallux valgus.

Degenerative disorders

Ruptured tendo Achillis

Probably rupture occurs only if the tendon is degenerate. Consequently most patients are aged over 40. While pushing off (running or jumping), the calf muscle contracts; but the contraction is resisted by body weight and the tendon ruptures. The patient feels as if he has been struck just above the heel, and he is unable to tiptoe. Soon after the tear occurs, a gap can be seen and felt 5 cm above the insertion of the tendon. Plantarflexion of the foot is weak and is not accompanied

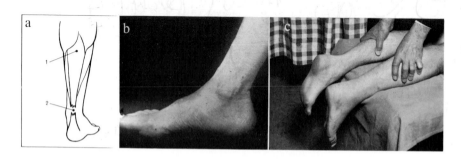

21.22 Tendo Achillis   (a) The soleus may tear at its musculotendinous junction (1) but the tendo Achillis itself ruptures 5 cm above its insertion (2). (b) The depression seen in this picture at the site of rupture later fills with blood. (c) Simmonds' test: both calves are being squeezed but only the left foot plantarflexes – the right tendon is ruptured.

by tautening of the tendon. Where doubt exists, Simmonds' test is helpful: with the patient prone, the calf is squeezed; if the tendon is intact, the foot is seen to plantarflex; if the tendon is ruptured the foot remains still.

Differential diagnosis

'INCOMPLETE' TEAR   This is uncommon, but is frequently diagnosed in error. The mistake arises because, if a complete rupture is not seen within 24 hours, the gap is difficult to feel; moreover, the patient may be able to stand on tiptoe (just), by using his long toe flexors. A correct diagnosis of incomplete tear is seldom possible without operation; if it can be made, probably a raised heel and reasonable caution are adequate.

TEAR OF SOLEUS MUSCLE   A tear at the musculotendinous junction causes pain and tenderness halfway up the calf. This recovers with the aid of physiotherapy and raising the heel of the shoe.

Treatment

If the patient is seen early, the ends of the tendon may approximate when the foot is passively plantarflexed. If so, plaster is applied with the foot in equinus and is worn for 8 weeks. A shoe with a raised heel is worn for a further 6 weeks. Operative repair is probably safer, but an equinus plaster for 8 weeks and a heel raise for a further 6 weeks are still needed.

Osteoarthritis

Osteoarthritis of the ankle may be the sequel to injury (a malunited fracture or recurrent instability), to osteochondritis dissecans of the talus or to

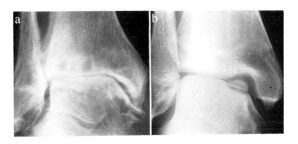

21.23 Osteoarthritis and osteochondritis   Osteoarthritis of the ankle (a) is always secondary to some recognizable disorder (usually trauma); note the loss of joint space and subchondral cysts. Osteochondritis dissecans of the talus (b) is an occasional cause of joint degeneration.

repeated bleeding with haemophilia. It does not necessarily cause symptoms, because extremes of range are not required with normal use. Only occasionally is operation (arthrodesis) required.

Gout

Swelling, redness, heat and exquisite tenderness of the metatarsophalangeal joint of the big toe ('podagra') is the epitome of gout. Other toes,

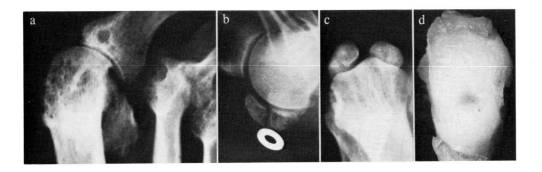

21.24 Other disorders of the hallux   Gout (a) is relatively uncommon. Sesamoid chondromalacia (b, c, d) is relatively common: (b) lateral view of bipartite sesamoid – the marker shows the tender spot; (c) skyline view of the same patient; (d) the sesamoid has been removed – cartilage degeneration was obvious and the symptoms were relieved.

however, and the tarsal joints also may be affected, and pain in the heel (fasciitis) is not uncommon.

Sesamoid chondromalacia

Softening of the articular cartilage on the medial sesamoid may cause pain on walking and localized tenderness. A local injection of methylprednisolone and local anaesthetic often helps; otherwise the sesamoid should be removed.

NOTE – OSTEOCHONDRITIS DISSECANS OF THE TALUS
Unexplained pain and slight limitation of movement in the ankle of a young person may be due to a small osteochondral fracture of the upper surface of the talus, though the injury may have been forgotten. X-rays taken at appropriate angles to produce tangential views of the talar surface show the small bony separation (no more than a few millimetres in diameter) at either the anteromedial or the posterolateral part of the superior surface of the talus. If symptoms cannot be tolerated, the fragment may be excised.

The paralysed foot

Weakness or paralysis of the foot may be symptomless, or may present in one of three characteristic ways: the patient may complain of difficulty in walking; he may 'catch his toe' on climbing stairs (due to weak dorsiflexion); or he may stumble and fall (due to instability).

Clinical features

UPPER MOTOR NEURON LESIONS   Spastic paralysis may occur in children with cerebral palsy or in adults following a stroke. Muscle imbalance usually leads to equinus or equinovarus deformity. The reflexes are brisk but sensation is normal. The entire limb (or both lower limbs) is usually abnormal.

LOWER MOTOR NEURON LESIONS   Poliomyelitis was (and in some parts of the world still is) a common cause of foot paralysis. If all muscle groups are affected, the foot is flail and dangles from the ankle; if knee extension also is weak, the patient cannot walk without a caliper. With unbalanced weakness, the foot develops fixed deformity; it may also be smaller and colder than normal, but sensation is normal. Other lower motor neuron disorders such as spinal cord tumours, peroneal muscular atrophy and severe nerve root compression are rare causes of foot weakness or deformity.

PERIPHERAL NERVE INJURIES   The sciatic, lateral popliteal or peroneal nerve may be affected. The commonest abnormalities are drop foot and weakness of peroneal action. Post-operative or post-immobilization drop foot is due to pressure

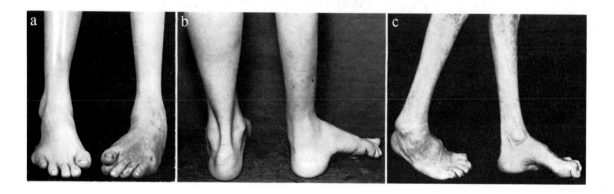

21.25 The paralysed foot   (a) In spina bifida – the small ulcer is an indication of insensitive skin. (b) Poliomyelitis, and (c) peroneal muscular atrophy, in both of which sensation is normal.

on the lateral popliteal or on the peroneal nerve as the leg rolls into external rotation. In addition to motor weakness there is an area of sensory loss. Unless the nerve is divided, recovery is possible but may take many months.

Treatment

The weakness may need no treatment at all, or only a splint.

The drop foot following nerve palsy can be treated by transferring the tibialis posterior through the interosseous membrane to the mid-tarsal region.

Spastic paralysis can be treated by tendon release and transfer, but great care is needed to prevent overaction in the new direction. Thus, a spastic equinovarus deformity may be converted to a severe valgus deformity by transferring tibialis anterior to the lateral side; this is avoided if only half the tendon is transferred.

Fixed deformities must be corrected first before doing tendon transfers. If no adequate tendon is available to permit dynamic correction, the joint may be reshaped and arthrodesed; at the same time muscle rebalancing (even of weak muscles) is necessary, otherwise the deformity will recur.

The painful foot

Painful heel

The causes of pain in the region of the heel may conveniently be classified according to the age group in which they commonly occur.

Children

Sever's disease (apophysitis) usually occurs in boys of about 10. It is not a 'disease' but a mild traction injury. Pain and tenderness are localized to the tendo Achillis insertion. The x-ray report usually refers to increased density and fragmentation of the apophysis, but often the painless heel looks similar. The heel of the shoe should be raised a little and strenuous activities restricted for a few weeks.

Adolescents

In girls aged 15–20, a calcaneal knob (often bilateral) is common. The posterolateral portion of the calcaneum is too prominent and the shoe rubs on it, causing pain. If attention to footwear does not help, the knob is removed.

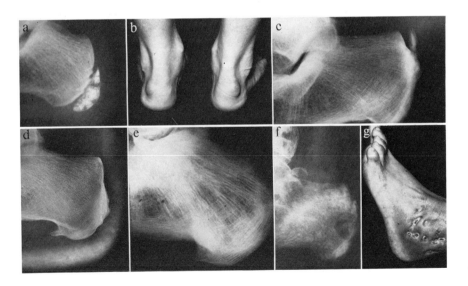

21.26 Heel disorders   (a) Sever's disease – the apophysis is dense and fragmented. (b) Bilateral heel knobs. (c) Achillis bursitis, in this case with calcification. (d) 'Policeman's heel' – both heels had spurs but only one side was painful. (e) Paget's disease. (f, g) Tuberculosis of the calcaneum.

Young adults

Bursitis just above the insertion of the tendo Achillis may result from ill-fitting footwear, especially in young women and army recruits. Localized pain and tenderness occur. Pain is relieved by removing the stiffener from the heel of the shoe.

Peritendinitis of the tendo Achillis occurs in athletes. The acute form may be relieved by rest, ice-packs, strapping or a hydrocortisone injection (not into the tendon!). The chronic form may need operation. Dividing the crural fascia and freeing adhesions may be adequate (Kvist and Kvist, 1980), but if there is a necrotic area of the tendon itself, this may need excision.

Acute plantar fasciitis occurs as a 'reactive' disorder associated with gonorrhoea, Reiter's disease and ankylosing spondylitis. Pain and tenderness are localized to the undersurface of the front of the calcaneum. The underlying cause should be treated and the painful area protected from pressure, if necessary with a padded plaster cast.

Older adults

'Policeman's heel' affects patients aged 40–60. It is sometimes called plantar fasciitis, but neither cause nor pathology is known. The only abnormal physical sign is localized tenderness beneath the calcaneum. A pad is made to transfer pressure away from the tender area. An injection of hydrocortisone occasionally helps. The pain slowly subsides in 6–12 months, and only rarely is division of the plantar fascia indicated. A bony spur projecting forwards from the undersurface of the calcaneal tuberosity is sometimes seen on x-ray.

Paget's disease may affect the calcaneum; it causes a deep-seated ache which is resistant to treatment.

Chronic bone infection

At any age, the calcaneum may be the site of chronic bone infection. A Brodie's abscess has a well-defined margin with surrounding bone sclerosis, whereas a tuberculous infection shows widespread rarefaction and the abscess margin is ill-defined.

Painful tarsus

In children, pain in the midtarsal region is rare; one cause is Köhler's disease (osteochondritis of the navicular). The bony nucleus of the navicular becomes dense and fragmented. The child, under the age of 5, has a painful limp, and a tender warm thickening over the navicular. If the foot is strapped, and activity restricted for a few weeks, symptoms disappear. The foot eventually becomes normal clinically and radiologically. A comparable condition occasionally affects middle-aged women (Brailsford's disease); the navicular becomes

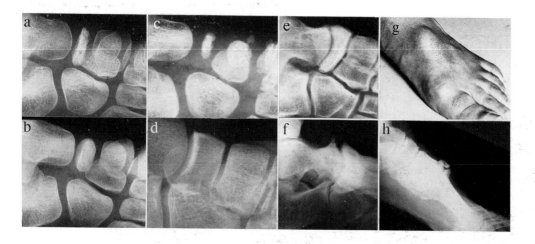

21.27 Painful tarsus   (a) Köhler's disease compared with (b) the normal foot. (c) Another example of Köhler's disease, and (d) the same foot fully grown – it has become normal. (e) Brailsford's disease, the adult equivalent of Köhler's disease. (f) Degeneration of the talonavicular joint. (g, h) The 'over-bone' at the first cuneiform-metatarsal joint.

dense, then altered in shape, and later the midtarsal joint may degenerate.

In adults, especially if the arch is high, a ridge of bone sometimes develops on the adjacent dorsal surfaces of the medial cuneiform and the first metatarsal ('the overbone'). A lump can be seen which feels bony and may become bigger and tender if the shoe presses on it. If shoe adjustment fails to provide relief the lump may be bevelled off.

Painful forefoot (metatarsalgia)

Any foot abnormality which results in faulty weight distribution may produce metatarsalgia. The causes are therefore numerous.

THE FOOT AS A WHOLE   A splay foot is wide and often associated with hallux valgus and curly toes. It is commonly seen in middle-aged women who have put on weight. A cavus foot with claw toes causes pain under the metatarsal heads because weight is taken over too limited an area.

INDIVIDUAL TOES   Hallux disorders, including failed operations, are the commonest causes of pain in the metatarsal region, because of faulty weight distribution (Scranton, 1980). If any of the other toes is painful or deformed so that it does not take its proper share of weight, pain under its metatarsal head is liable to occur. Thus, hammer toe, claw toes and curly toes may all produce metatarsalgia.

Special varieties

Freiberg's disease This is a 'crushing' type of osteochondritis of the second metatarsal head (rarely the third). It affects young adults, usually women. A bony lump (the enlarged head) is palpable and tender; the joint is irritable. X-rays show the head to be wide and flat, the neck thick and the joint space increased.

Stress fracture Stress fracture, usually of the second or third metatarsal, occurs in young adults after unaccustomed activity. The affected shaft feels thick and tender. The x-ray appearance is at first normal, but later shows fusiform callus around a fine transverse fracture.

Morton's metatarsalgia This condition is associated with a painful neuroma on a digital nerve. The neuroma occurs at the level of the metatarsal necks just proximal to the division of the digital nerves of the third or fourth clefts. Women aged 40–50 are mainly affected. Sharp intermittent pain shoots into the toes, but is felt only when shoes are worn, possibly because the metatarsal bones are then squeezed together ('compression metatarsalgia'). Tenderness is localized to the neuroma and sensation may be diminished in the affected cleft. An enlarged intermetatarsal bursa may press on a normal digital nerve, producing similar symptoms.

Clinical features

The patient, his feet and his shoes need to be methodically examined. The age may suggest the diagnosis. In young adolescents one thinks of idiopathic pes cavus or acute hallux rigidus; in young adults of Freiberg's disease or a stress fracture; and in older people of splay foot, hallux disorders, curly toes or Morton's metatarsalgia.

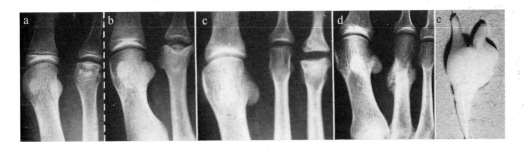

21,28 Metatarsalgia   (a, b) Stages in the development of Freiberg's disease; (c) the comparable disorder in the third metatarsal (Köhler's second disease); (d) stress fracture; (e) neuroma excised from patient with Morton's metatarsalgia.

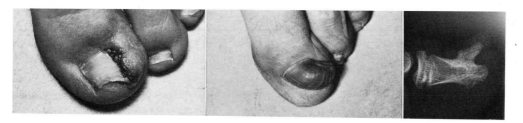

21.29 Toenail disorders   From left to right: ingrown toenail, overgrown toenail (onychogryphosis), and undergrown toenail (by a subungual exostosis).

Treatment

This largely depends upon the cause.

CONSERVATIVE   Pads or insoles can divert pressure from tender areas. Adequate footwear is important. Exercises are given to strengthen the foot muscles.

OPERATIVE   It may be advisable to operate on the hallux or other toes. If Morton's metatarsalgia does not respond to protective padding, the neuroma is excised through a plantar incision. If Freiberg's disease remains painful, the metatarsal head is excised through a dorsal incision. If one (or more) of the middle three metatarsal heads is unduly prominent with a painful callosity, symptoms can be relieved by an oblique osteotomy of the metatarsal shaft (Helal, 1975).

Tarsal tunnel syndrome

Pain in the medial part of the forefoot, unrelated to weight-bearing, may be due to compression of the posterior tibial nerve behind and below the medial malleolus. The pain is often worse at night and the patient may seek relief by walking around or stamping his foot. Sometimes there is paraesthesia or sensory loss. The diagnosis is difficult to establish, but nerve conduction studies may show slowing of conduction.

To decompress the nerve it is exposed behind the medial malleolus and followed into the sole of the foot; sometimes it is trapped by the belly of adductor hallucis arising more proximally than usual.

Toenail disorders

The toenail of the hallux may be ingrown, overgrown or undergrown.

INGROWN   The nail burrows into the nail groove; this ulcerates and its wall grows over the nail, so that the term 'embedded toenail' would be better. The patient is taught to cut the nail square, to insert pledgets of wool under the ingrowing edges and always to keep the feet clean and dry. If these measures fail, the 'gutter' treatment is worth trying. A small wedge of soft tissue (where the nail digs in) is excised; a fine polythene tube is cut vertically in half and a segment inserted between nail and soft tissue (Wallace *et al.*, 1979). More radical measures include partial or complete removal of the nail, taking care to remove the germinal matrix.

OVERGROWN (ONYCHOGRYPHOSIS)   The nail is hard, thick and curved. A chiropodist can usually make the patient comfortable, but occasionally the nail may need excision.

UNDERGROWN   A subungual exostosis grows on the dorsum of the terminal phalanx and pushes the nail upwards. The exostosis should be removed.

Notes on applied anatomy

The ankle and foot function as an integrated unit, and together provide stable support, proprioception, balance and mobility.

THE ANKLE   The ankle fits together like a tenon and mortise; the tibial and fibular parts of the mortise are bound together by the inferior tibiofibular ligament, and stability is augmented by the collateral ligaments. The medial ligament fans out from the tibial malleolus to the talus, the superficial fibres forming the deltoid ligament. The lateral ligament has three thickened bands: the anterior and posterior talofibular ligaments and, between them, the calcaneofibular ligament. Tears of these ligaments may cause tilting of the talus in its mortise. Forced abduction or adduction may disrupt the mortise altogether by (1) forcing the tibia and fibula apart (diastasis of the tibiofibular joint), (2) tearing the collateral ligaments or (3) fracturing the malleoli.

THE FOOT   The footprint gives some idea of the arched structure of the foot. This derives from the tripodial bony framework between the calcaneum posteriorly, and the first and fifth metatarsal heads. The medial arch is high, with the

if either is forced at the ankle, the mortise fractures. Pronation and supination occur at the intertarsal and tarsometatarsal joints; the foot rotates about an axis running through the second metatarsal, the sole turning laterally (pronation) or medially (supination) – movements analogous to those of the forearm. The combination of plantarflexion, adduction and supination is called inversion; the opposite movement of dorsiflexion, abduction and pronation is eversion.

FOOT POSITIONS AND DEFORMITIES   A downward-pointing foot is said to be in equinus; the opposite is calcaneus. If only the forefoot points downwards the term 'plantaris' is used. Supination with adduction produces a varus deformity; pronation with abduction causes pes valgus. An unusually high arch is called pes cavus. Many of these terms are used as if they were definitive diagnoses when, in fact, they are nothing more than Latin translations of descriptive anatomy.

21.30 Footprints   (a) The normal foot, (b) flat foot (the medial arch touches the ground), and (c) cavus foot (even the lateral arch barely makes contact).

Further reading

Attenborough, C. G. (1966) Severe congenital talipes equinovarus. *Journal of Bone and Joint Surgery* **48B**, 31–39

Cain, T. J. and Hyman, S. (1978) Peroneal spastic flat foot. *Journal of Bone and Joint Surgery* **60B**, 527–529

Colton, C. L. (1973) The surgical management of congenital vertical talus. *Journal of Bone and Joint Surgery* **55B**, 566–574

Dwyer, F. C. (1963) The treatment of relapsed club foot by the insertion of a wedge into the calcaneum. *Journal of Bone and Joint Surgery* **45B**, 67–75

Evans, D. (1961) Relapsed club foot. *Journal of Bone and Joint Surgery* **43B**, 722–733

Helal, B. (1975) Metatarsal osteotomy for metatarsalgia. *Journal of Bone and Joint Surgery* **57B**, 187–192

Jahss, M. H. (1980) Tarsometatarsal truncated-wedge arthrodesis for pes cavus and equinovarus deformity of the fore part of the foot. *Journal of Bone and Joint Surgery* **62A**, 713–722

Kvist, H. and Kvist, M. (1980) The operative treatment of chronic calcaneal paratenonitis. *Journal of Bone and Joint Surgery* **62B**, 353–357

Leonard, M. A. (1974) The inheritance of tarsal coalition and its relationship to spastic flat foot. *Journal of Bone and Joint Surgery* **56B**, 520–526

Perkins, G. (1961) *Orthopaedics*. London: Athlone Press

Scranton, P. E. (1980) Metatarsalgia: diagnosis and treatment. *Journal of Bone and Joint Surgery* **62A**, 723–732

Wallace, W. A., Milne, D. D. and Andrew, T. (1979) Gutter treatment for ingrowing toenails. *British Medical Journal* **2**, 168–171

Wilson, J. N. (1963) Oblique displacement osteotomy for hallux valgus. *Journal of Bone and Joint Surgery* **45B**, 552–556

navicular as its keystone; the lateral arch is flatter. The anterior arch, formed by the metatarsal bones, thrusts maximally upon the first and fifth metatarsal heads and flattens out (spreading the foot) during weight-bearing; it can be pulled up by contraction of the intrinsic muscles, which flex the metatarsophalangeal joints.

MOVEMENTS   The ankle allows movement in the sagittal plane only – plantarflexion and dorsiflexion. Adduction and abduction (turning the toes towards or away from the midline) are produced by rotation of the entire leg below the knee;

Part 3 — Fractures and Joint Injuries

Principles of Fractures **22**

How fractures happen

The patient who breaks a bone has been subjected to physical force. With normal bone the amount of force determines whether the fracture is complete or not; in children the bones are still springy, and incomplete (greenstick) fractures are common. If the force was insufficient to break normal bone, the fracture is 'pathological' and further investigation is essential.

With a direct force the bone breaks at the point of impact; the soft tissues also must be damaged. With an indirect force the bone breaks at a distance from where the force is applied; soft-tissue damage at the fracture site is not inevitable.

An indirect force may be: (1) twisting, which causes a spiral fracture; (2) bending, which causes a transverse fracture; (3) bending and compressing, which results in a fracture that is partly transverse but with a separate triangular 'butterfly' fragment; or (4) a combination of twisting, bending and compressing, which causes a short oblique fracture.

A direct force may be: (1) tapping, which causes a transverse fracture and some skin damage; or (2) crushing, which causes a comminuted fracture often with extensive soft-tissue damage.

The above description applies mainly to the long bones. A cancellous bone, such as a vertebra or the calcaneum, when subjected to sufficient force, sustains a comminuted crush fracture. At the knee or elbow resisted extension may cause an avulsion fracture of the patella or olecranon; and in a number of situations resisted muscle action may pull off the bony attachment of the muscle.

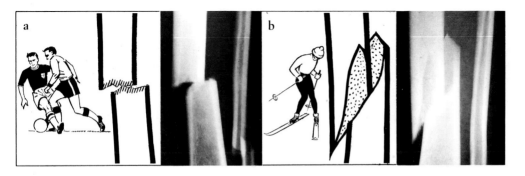

22.1 Mechanisms of injury (1) (a) A direct blow causes a transverse fracture. (b) A twisting force causes a spiral fracture.

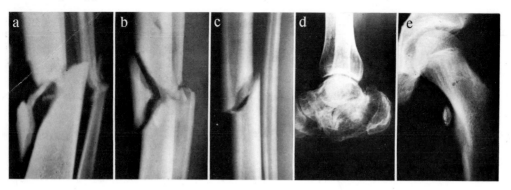

22.2 Mechanisms of injury (2) (a) A direct crushing force causes a comminuted fracture with considerable soft-tissue damage. (b) Angulation + axial compression causes a 'butterfly' fracture. (c) Angulation + axial compression + rotation causes a short oblique fracture. (d) Cancellous crushing of calcaneum. (e) Avulsion of lesser trochanter apophysis.

How fractures heal

It is commonly supposed that, in order to unite, a fracture must be immobilized. This cannot be so since, with few exceptions, fractures unite whether they are splinted or not; indeed, without a built-in mechanism for union, land animals could scarcely have evolved. It is, however, naive to suppose that union would occur if a fracture were kept moving indefinitely; the bone ends must, at some stage, be brought to rest relative to one another. But it is not mandatory for the surgeon to impose this immobility artificially – Nature can do it, with callus; and callus forms in response to movement, not to splintage. *We splint most fractures, not to ensure union but (1) to alleviate pain, and (2) to ensure that union takes place in good position.*

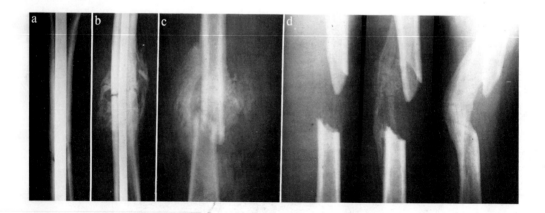

22.3 Callus and movement Four patients with femoral shaft fractures. (a) and (b) are both 6 weeks after fixation – in (a) the K-nail fitted tightly, preventing any movement, and there is no callus; in (b) the nail fitted loosely, permitting movement, so there is callus. (c) This patient had cerebral irritation and thrashed around wildly – at 3 weeks callus is already excessive. (d) This man, who left part of his femur in the road, was treated on traction without a splint – the fracture was never 'immobilized'.

a DIRECT

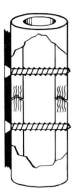

b INDIRECT

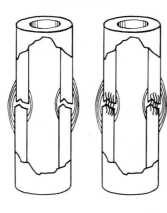

22.4 The healing process (a) Rigid fixation may permit direct union, but it inhibits callus. (b) When a fracture heals 'naturally' (without rigid fixation) callus forms first; then bone grows across the fracture – the process may be less direct but it has distinct advantages.

Union begins with resorption of the fracture haematoma and infiltration of the area by a fibrinous inflammatory exudate. New blood vessels and bone-forming cells begin to appear within a day or two of the fracture; they give rise to cartilage, bone and fibrous tissue, so that a bridge of callus forms around the fractured bone ends. Over the succeeding weeks this callus provides a measure of stability and allows direct bridging of the gap by both membranous bone formation and endochondral ossification. The callus is replaced by a network of woven bone and gradually this changes to strong mature bone as the trabeculae arrange themselves along the lines of stress (re-modelling).

Clinical and experimental studies (McKibbin, 1978) have shown that callus is the response to movement at the fracture site. If a fracture is fixed rigidly with metal, healing still occurs but, the surgeon having implanted a metal bridge, the natural bridge of callus is not needed and does not form; osteoclasts followed by osteoblasts grow directly across the fracture gap. This process has been called primary union, but the implication of superiority is misleading and the term 'direct' union is better.

Healing by callus ('indirect' union) has distinct advantages: it ensures mechanical strength while the bone ends heal; and, with increasing stress, the callus grows stronger and stronger (an example of Wolff's law). With rigid metal fixation, on the other hand, the absence of callus means that there is a long period during which the bone depends upon the metal implant for its integrity. Moreover, the implant diverts stress away from the bone, which becomes osteoporotic and cannot recover fully until the metal is removed. Flexible implants are now being tried in the hope of overcoming these drawbacks.

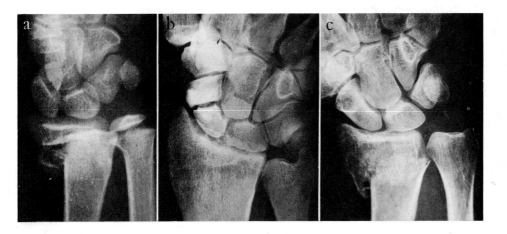

22.5 The patient's age Many fractures have a limited age distribution: each of these patients fell on the outstretched hand. (a) Aged 8 – fracture-separation of lower radial epiphysis; (b) aged 30 – fractured scaphoid; (c) aged 60 – Colles' fracture.

Clinical features

A fracture is usually followed by pain and loss of function. A pathological fracture may, in addition, have been preceded by pain or by symptoms of an underlying cause (such as a tumour).

General signs

A broken bone is part of a patient. It is important to look for evidence of: (1) shock or haemorrhage; (2) associated damage to brain, spinal cord or viscera; and (3) a predisposing cause (such as Paget's disease).

Local signs

A possible fracture must be handled gently. To elicit crepitus or abnormal movement is unnecessarily painful; x-ray diagnosis is more reliable.

Nevertheless the familiar headings of clinical examination should always be considered, or damage to arteries and nerves may be overlooked.

● LOOK
Swelling, bruising and deformity may be obvious, but the important point is whether the skin is intact; if the skin is broken, whether from within or without, the fracture is open (compound).

● FEEL
There is localized tenderness, but it is necessary also to examine distal to the fracture in order to feel the pulse, and to detect loss of sensation.

● MOVE
Crepitus and abnormal movement may be present, but it is more important to ask if the patient can move the joints distal to the injury.

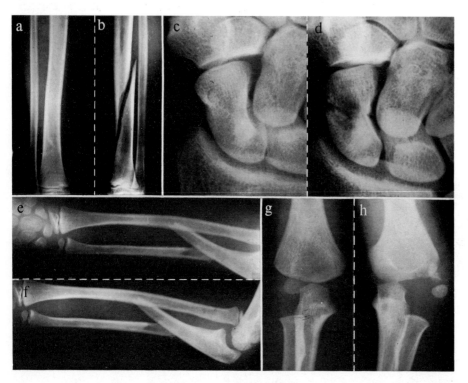

22.6 X-ray examination must be 'adequate'   (a, b) Two films of the same tibia: the AP fails to show the fracture. (c) Fractured scaphoid not visible on the day of injury, but clearly seen (d) 2 weeks later. (e, f) Monteggia fracture-dislocation: failure to include both joints in forearm fractures (e) may result in a radioulnar dislocation (f) being missed. (g, h) Fractured lateral condyle (h) – in a child comparison with the uninjured side (g) is useful.

● X-RAY

X-ray examination enables a fracture to be accurately described and is essential for medicolegal purposes. Certain pitfalls must be avoided, as follows.

Two views A fracture or a dislocation may not be seen on a single x-ray film, and at least two views (anteroposterior and lateral) must be taken.

Two occasions Soon after injury, a fracture (e.g. of the carpal scaphoid) may be difficult to see. If doubt exists, further examinations must be carried out 10 days later, by which time bone resorption at the fracture site makes diagnosis easier.

Two joints In the forearm or leg, one bone may be fractured and angulated. Angulation, however, is impossible unless the other bone also is broken, or a joint dislocated. The joints above and below the fracture must both be included on the x-ray films.

Two limbs In x-rays of a child's elbow, normal epiphyses may confuse the diagnosis of a fracture, and films of the uninjured elbow are then helpful.

Description

Diagnosing a fracture is not enough; the surgeon should picture it (and describe it) in all its complexity. (1) Is it open or closed? (2) Which bone is broken, and where? (3) Has it involved a joint surface? (4) What is the shape of the break? A transverse fracture is slow to join because the area of contact is small; if the broken surfaces are accurately apposed, however, the fracture is stable on compression. A spiral fracture joins more rapidly (because the contact area is large) but is not stable on compression. Short oblique fractures, those with a separate 'butterfly' fragment and comminuted fractures are all slow to join and unstable on compression.

DISPLACEMENT

Displacement can be resolved into three components.

(1) *Shift* (backwards, forwards, sideways, or longitudinally with impaction or overlap).

(2) *Tilt* (sideways, backwards or forwards).

(3) *Twist* (rotation in any direction).

Treatment of closed fractures

General treatment is the first consideration: to treat the patient, not simply the part. The sequence is: (1) first aid; (2) transport; and (3) the treatment of shock, haemorrhage and associated injuries. These are discussed in the next chapter.

Treatment of the fracture itself is based upon three injunctions.

(1) REDUCE – only, of course, if the fracture is displaced.

(2) HOLD – though not necessarily with total rigidity.

(3) EXERCISE – until maximum function is regained.

The problem is how to hold a fracture adequately and yet use the limb sufficiently: this is a conflict ('*Hold* v *Move*') which the surgeon seeks to resolve as rapidly as possible (e.g. by internal fixation); but he also wants to avoid unnecessary risks – here is a second conflict ('*Speed* v *Safety*'). This dual conflict epitomizes the four factors that dominate fracture management (the term 'fracture quartet' seems appropriate).

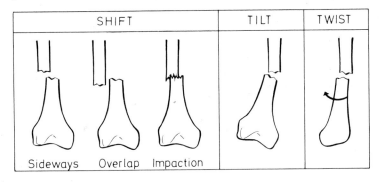

22.7 Fracture displacements

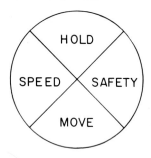

The fracture
quartet

Reduce

Closed reduction

Accurate reduction by closed manipulation demands a methodical approach. The doctor should
first study the x-ray films (thereby deducing the
causal force if possible); then, if inexperienced, he
should rehearse the manoeuvres needed for reduction. Next, the patient should be appropriately anaesthetized and muscle relaxation assured.
The first step in reduction is usually traction
along the line of the bone, which is sometimes
sufficient to achieve reduction. A force, the re-

verse of that which caused the fracture, is then
applied (e.g. with an external rotation ankle
fracture the foot is twisted inwards). Reduction
must be confirmed by x-ray.

With shaft fractures the periosteum on one side
is usually intact; this acts as a soft tissue hinge
which can be used to facilitate reduction.

Open reduction

Operative reduction is indicated if closed reduction is impossible or insufficiently accurate.

CLOSED REDUCTION IMPOSSIBLE
Closed reduction may fail because (1) a small
fragment is unmanageable, (2) a fragment is
trapped in a joint or (3) soft tissues are interposed.

CLOSED REDUCTION INACCURATE
With any fracture, accuracy of reduction is desirable; in some it is imperative because (1) fractures
involving a joint surface, unless perfectly reduced,
are likely to be followed by joint degeneration,
and (2) fractures of the radius and ulna in adults,
unless perfectly reduced, result in limited rotation.

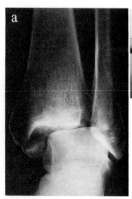

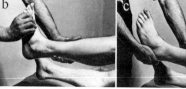

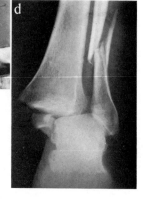

22.8 Closed reduction   These two ankle fractures look somewhat similar but are caused by
different forces (see page 469). The causal force
must be reversed to achieve reduction: (a)
requires internal rotation (b); an adduction
force (c) is needed for (d).

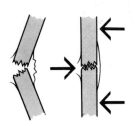

22.9 Reduction   Intact periosteum facilitates reduction.

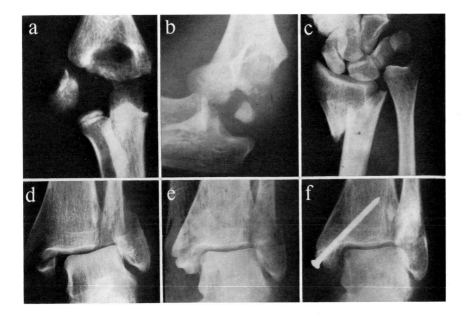

22.10 Indications for open reduction (a) The elbow was grossly swollen and this fractured lateral condyle could not be reduced by closed manipulation. (b) Similarly this medial epicondyle could be extricated from the joint only by open operation. (c) The sharp fragment of radius had impaled muscle and could not be freed without operation. (d, e, f) This ankle fracture (d) was manipulated closed and the position (e) looks reasonable; but it lacks the accuracy desirable at a joint surface, so open reduction (f) was performed.

Hold reduction

The word 'immobilization' has been deliberately avoided since the objective is seldom immobility; usually it is the prevention of displacement. The available methods are: (1) continuous traction, often followed by functional bracing; (2) plaster splintage of conventional type, sometimes used only temporarily and followed by functional bracing; and (3) metal fixation, internal or external.

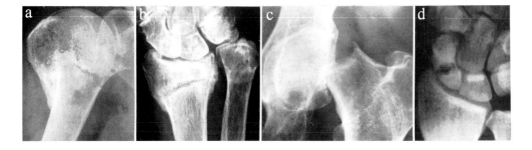

22.11 Two reasons for splintage Most fractures, such as (a) and (b), always unite, and the object of splinting them is simply to prevent re-displacement after reduction; only a few, such as (c) and (d) need to be held still in order to prevent non-union.

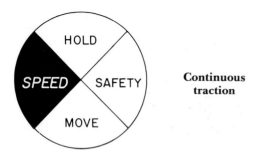

Continuous traction

Technique

TRACTION BY GRAVITY ALONE

This applies only to upper limb injuries. Thus, with a wrist sling, the weight of the arm provides continuous traction to the humerus; for comfort and stability, especially with a transverse fracture, a U-slab of plaster may be bandaged on or, better, a removable plastic sleeve from the axilla to just above the elbow is held on with Velcro.

SKIN TRACTION

Skin (or Buck's) traction will sustain a pull of no more than 4 or 5 kg. Holland strapping or one-way-stretch Elastoplast is stuck to the shaved skin and held on with a bandage. The malleoli are protected by Gamgee tissue, and cords or tapes are used for traction.

SKELETAL TRACTION

A Kirschner wire, Steinmann pin or Denham pin is inserted, usually behind the tibial tubercle for hip, thigh and knee injuries, lower in the tibia or through the calcaneum for tibial fractures. If a pin is used, hooks which can swivel freely are attached, and cords tied to them for applying traction.

Mechanics   Traction must always be opposed by countertraction; that is, the pull must be exerted against something, or it merely drags the patient down the bed.

Fixed traction   The pull is exerted against a fixed point; for example, the tapes are tied to the cross-piece of a Thomas' splint and pull the leg down until the root of the limb abuts against the ring of the splint.

Continuous traction

Continuous traction is used (1) for shaft fractures involving the femur, humerus and sometimes the tibia; and (2) for articular fractures, especially of the hip, knee and shoulder.

Traction cannot hold a fracture still, but it can pull a long bone straight and hold it out to length. The aim is to hold the reduced position while making the patient comfortable enough to exercise his muscles and to move his joints.

Traction is safe enough, provided it is not excessive and care is taken when inserting the traction pin. The problem is 'speed': not because the fracture unites slowly (it does not), but because lower limb traction keeps the patient in hospital. Consequently, as soon as the fracture is 'sticky' (deformable but not displaceable), traction should be replaced by functional bracing, if this method is feasible.

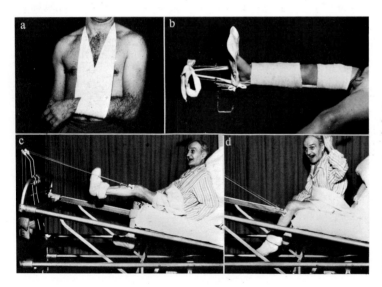

22.12 Continuous traction   (a) By means of gravity. (b) Skin traction fixed to the cross-piece of a Thomas' splint.

(c, d) Balanced skeletal traction – the patient can move his joints while traction holds position; people imagine that without a splint the patient must be uncomfortable – but look at his face!

Balanced traction The pull is exerted against an opposing force provided by the weight of the body when the foot of the bed is raised. The cords may be tied to the foot of the bed, or run over pulleys and have weights attached.

Combined traction A Thomas' splint is used. The tapes are tied to the end of the splint and the splint is suspended, or is tied to the end of the bed, which is raised.

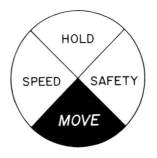

Plaster

Plaster

As a splint for holding the reduced fracture, plaster is widely used; for distal limb fractures and for most children's fractures it is often the method of choice.

Plaster is safe enough, so long as a limb which may swell is not encased in an unsplit cast, and provided pressure sores are avoided. The speed of union is neither greater nor less than with trac-

tion, but the patient can go home sooner. Holding reduction is usually no problem. Immobilized joints, however, are liable to stiffen; and stiffness (the 'fracture disease') is the problem with conventional plasters. If the haematoma of a fractured shaft is not milked away by exercises, adhesions form which bind muscle fibres to each other and to the bone; with articular fractures, plaster perpetuates surface irregularities (closed

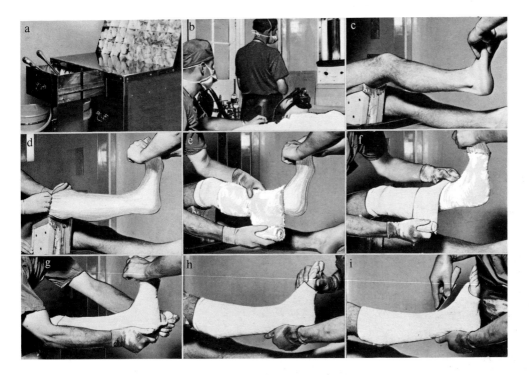

22.13 Plaster technique Applying a well-fitting and effective plaster needs experience and attention to detail. (a) A well-equipped plaster trolley is invaluable. (b) Adequate anaesthesia and careful study of the x-ray films are both indispensable. (c) For a below-knee plaster the thigh is best supported on a padded block. (d) Stockinette is threaded smoothly onto the leg. (e) For a padded plaster the wool is rolled on and it must be even. (f) Plaster is next applied smoothly, taking a tuck with each turn, and (g) smoothing each layer firmly onto the one beneath. (h) While still wet the cast is moulded away from the bony points. (i) With a recent injury the plaster is then split.

reduction is seldom perfect) and lack of movement inhibits the healing of cartilage defects.

Stiffness can be minimized by: (1) delayed splintage – that is, by using traction until movement has been regained, and only then applying plaster; or (2) starting with a conventional cast but, after a few days, when the limb can be handled without too much discomfort, replacing the cast by a functional brace which permits joint movement.

Technique

After the fracture has been reduced, stockinette is threaded over the limb and the bony points are protected with wool. Plaster is then applied. While it is setting the surgeon moulds it away from bony prominences; with shaft fractures three-point pressure can be applied to keep the intact periosteal hinge under tension and thereby maintain reduction.

If the fracture is recent, further swelling is likely; the plaster and stockinette are therefore split from top to bottom, exposing the skin.* Check x-rays are essential and the plaster may need to be wedged.

With fractures of the shafts of long bones, rotation is controlled only if the plaster includes the joints above and below the fracture. In the lower limb, the knee is usually held slightly flexed, the ankle at a right angle and the tarsus and forefoot neutral (this 'plantigrade' position is essential for normal walking). In the upper limb the position of the splinted joints varies with the fracture. Splintage must not be discontinued (though a functional brace may be substituted) until the fracture is consolidated; if plaster changes are needed, check x-rays are essential.

Functional bracing

The term 'bracing' implies the use of an external splint; if this is made of plaster, the term 'cast-bracing' is used. The splints are 'functional' in that joint movements are much less restricted than with conventional casts. Bracing can be employed for most limb fractures, and is being used increasingly. Functional bracing does not 'immobilize' fractures, but immobility is not needed for fracture healing. The method is effective because: (1) activity stimulates bone formation; and (2) even with weight-bearing, little shortening occurs, because a snugly fitting splint prevents the increase in girth which shortening would cause.

Functional bracing comes out well on all four of the basic requirements. The fracture can be *held* reasonably well; the joints can be *moved*; the fracture joins at normal *speed* (or perhaps slightly quicker) without keeping the patient in hospital; and the method is *safe*.

Technique

Considerable skill is needed to apply an effective brace. First the fracture is 'stabilized': by a few days on traction or in a conventional plaster for tibial fractures; and by a few weeks on traction for femoral fractures (till the fracture is sticky – i.e. deformable but not displaceable). Then a hinged cast or splint is applied which holds the fracture snugly but permits joint movement; functional activity, including weight-bearing, is encouraged.

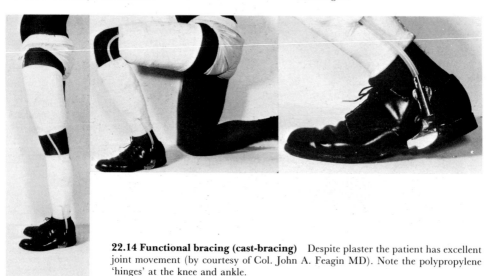

22.14 Functional bracing (cast-bracing)   Despite plaster the patient has excellent joint movement (by courtesy of Col. John A. Feagin MD). Note the polypropylene 'hinges' at the knee and ankle.

*'Down to – but not including – skin', is the slogan.

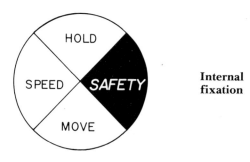

Internal fixation

movement) may be lost. The risk of infection depends upon: (1) the patient – devitalized tissues, a dirty wound and an unfit patient are all dangerous; (2) the surgeon – thorough training, a high degree of surgical dexterity and adequate assistance are all essential; and (3) the facilities – a guaranteed aseptic routine, a full range of implants and a staff familiar with their use are all indispensable.

Internal fixation

Properly applied, internal fixation holds a fracture so securely that movements can begin at once; and with early movement the 'fracture disease' (stiffness and oedema) is abolished. As far as speed is concerned, the patient can leave hospital as soon as the wound is healed, but he must remember that, even though the bone moves in one piece, the fracture is not united – it is merely held by a metal bridge; weight-bearing is unsafe until the bone itself has united and this takes a considerable length of time. The greatest danger, however, is sepsis; if infection supervenes, all the manifest advantages of internal fixation (precise reduction, immediate stability and early

Indications

Internal fixation is never essential; but in adults it is often desirable. The chief indications are as follows.

DIFFICULT FRACTURES
(1) Those prone to non-union, especially the femoral neck; (2) those prone to malunion, especially fracture-subluxations of the ankle and wrist, which are often unstable, and mid-shaft fractures of the forearm; (3) those prone to be pulled apart by muscle action, especially transverse fractures of the patella and olecranon.

PATHOLOGICAL FRACTURES
Those through malignant deposits, in which the malignancy may prevent healing; femoral shaft

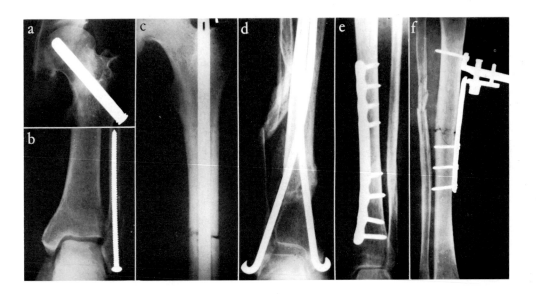

22.15 Examples of internal fixation Inlay techniques: (a) trifin nail; (b) intramedullary screw; (c) Küntscher nail; (d) Rush nails.
Onlay techniques: (e) plate and screws; (f) compression being applied before plating is completed – thus enhancing the fixation.

fractures through osteoporotic bone come into this category.

MULTIPLE FRACTURES

With two major fractures in one limb, fixation of one facilitates closed treatment of the other. With fractures of more than one limb the indication for fixation is still greater.

NURSING DIFFICULTIES

(1) Unless elderly patients lying in bed are skilfully nursed, a dangerous chain of complications may ensue – poor pulmonary ventilation, oedema, pressure sores and mental deterioration; (2) patients with traumatic paraplegia and those with multiple injuries also are difficult to nurse. In such instances internal fixation may simplify the management.

Note Internal fixation is often used to get the patient out of hospital quickly – either for personal reasons or because the surgeon needs the bed. These are not surgical indications; moreover, any gain in time may be more than offset if complications develop.

Technique

If a plate is used it must be strong and it must be fixed securely with at least two screws penetrating both cortices on each side of the fracture; to avoid undue compressive strain, plates should be applied to the tensile surface, which is usually the convex side of the bone. For the femoral shaft an intramedullary nail is preferred; for the femoral neck multiple pins or a compression screw and plate are used; for small bones or small fragments transfixing wires may suffice.

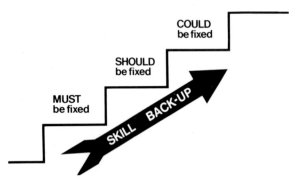

22.16 The indications staircase   The indications for fixation are not immutable; thus, if the surgical skill or back-up facilities (staff, sterility and equipment) are of a low order, internal fixation is indicated only when the alternative is unacceptable (e.g. with femoral neck fractures). With average skill and facilities, fixation is indicated when alternative methods are possible but very difficult (e.g. multiple injuries). With the highest levels of skill and facilities, fixation is reasonable if it saves time, money or beds.

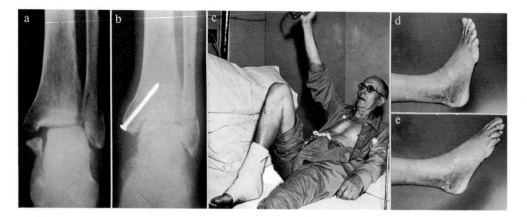

22.17 Delayed splintage   This patient's fractured ankle (a) was screwed (b). For the next few days he exercised it actively (c) but took no weight on the leg. When the wound was healed he walked in a below-knee plaster. After 6 weeks the plaster was removed: (d, e) show the ankle range 10 minutes later. Function was rapidly regained – of course it was! The patient was Professor George Perkins, the pioneer of delayed splintage.

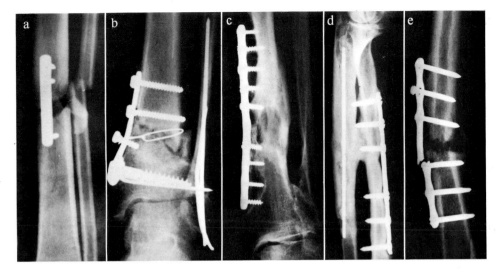

22.18 Bad fixation (how not to do it) (a) Timidity. (b) Over-exuberance. (c) The screws are too short and the bone is infected. (d) Unorthodoxy has resulted in cross-union. (e) Any plate is liable to break unless protected from stress until the fracture has joined.

Internal fixation alone is inadequate to withstand much stress. Thus, a patient with a recently plated tibia needs two crutches for the first 3 months; he should go through the motions of walking but take almost no weight ('shadow walking'). After that time, if union is proceeding satisfactorily, he can progress to two sticks or one crutch. An alternative is 'delayed splintage'. The leg is unsplinted and weight-bearing forbidden but exercises are encouraged; once movement has been regained, a full plaster or a functional brace is applied and weight-bearing can begin. Pain at the fracture site is a danger signal and must be investigated.

It is important not to remove metal implants too soon, or the bone may refracture. A year is the minimum and 18 or 24 months safer; for several weeks after screw removal the bone is weak, and care or protection is needed.

Complications*

Infection Iatrogenic infection is now the commonest cause of chronic osteitis; the metal does not predispose to infection, but the operation does.

Mechanical failure Until some union of the fracture has occurred metal implants are precarious; unless stress is avoided or the limb is protected by a splint the implant may break.

Non-union Totally rigid fixation prevents callus formation, so that union is slow – but it still occurs. If, however, the bones have been fixed rigidly but with the ends still apart, then non-union may well occur.

External fixation

External fixation is used chiefly for fractures of the tibia, but also to a lesser extent for those of the femur, humerus and pelvis; it has even been applied to hand fractures. The main indication is where the treatment of severe soft-tissue injuries, especially of blood vessels and skin, demands immediate stability but internal fixation is unsafe.

*Most complications are due to poor technique, poor equipment or poor operating conditions.

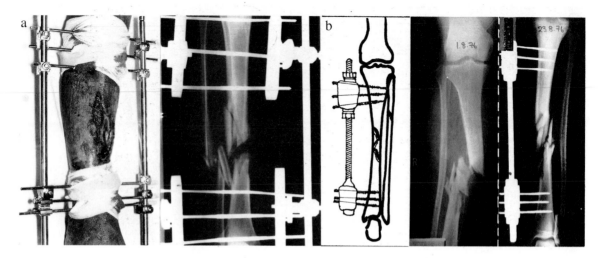

22.19 External fixation   (a) Through-and-through fixation holds the fracture rigidly and is sometimes used for a severe compound injury; (b) one-sided fixation is slightly less rigid but easier to apply and may form callus more quickly; the method illustrated (the 'Portsmouth method') was devised by R. A. Denham, whose patient this was.

Technique

Two main types of fixation are used.

(1) *Through-and-through*   Strong pins are driven completely through healthy bone above and below the fracture. The fracture is reduced and strong rods are attached to the pins on each side of the limb, so that a rigid system is set up.

(2) *One-sided*   Threaded pins are screwed into but not through the bone; their protruding ends are connected by a single rod.

With either system adjustments permit accurate reduction and long-axis compression enhances stability.

The time factor

Repair of a fracture is a continuous process; any stages into which it is divided are necessarily arbitrary. In this book the terms 'union' and 'consolidation' are used, and they are defined as follows.

UNION
Union is incomplete repair; the ensheathing callus is calcified. Clinically the fracture site is still a little tender and, though the bone moves in one piece (and in that sense is united), attempted angulation is painful. X-rays show the fracture line still clearly visible, with fluffy callus around it. Repair is incomplete and it is not safe to subject the unprotected bone to stress.

CONSOLIDATION
Consolidation is complete repair; the calcified callus is ossified. Clinically the fracture site is not tender, no movement can be obtained and attempted angulation is painless. X-rays show the fracture line to be almost obliterated and crossed by bone trabeculae, with well-defined callus around it. Repair is complete and further protection is unnecessary.

TIMETABLE
How long does a fracture take to unite and to consolidate? No precise answer is possible because age, constitution, blood supply, type of fracture and other factors all influence the time taken.

Approximate prediction is possible and Perkins' timetable is delightfully simple. A spiral fracture in the upper limb unites in 3 weeks; for consolidation multiply by 2; for the lower limb multiply by 2 again; for transverse fractures multiply again by 2. A more sophisticated formula is as follows. A

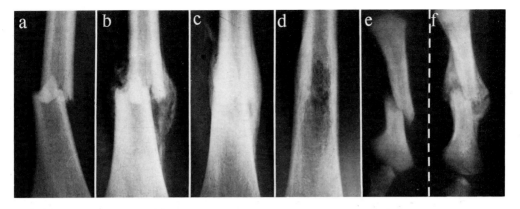

22.20 The processes of repair (a) Fracture; (b) union; (c) consolidation; (d) bone remodelling. The fracture must be protected until consolidated; the time required can be roughly forecast from Perkins' timetable. In children the process is much more rapid: this birth fracture (e) has a mass of callus (f) in only 19 days.

spiral fracture in the upper limb takes 6–8 weeks to consolidate; the lower limb needs twice as long. Add 25 per cent if the fracture is not spiral or if it involves the femur. Children's fractures, of course, join more quickly. These figures are only a rough guide; there must be clinical and radiological evidence of consolidation before full stress is permitted without splintage.

Treatment of the soft tissues

If a broken bone is badly treated malunion or non-union may result, but salvage is still possible. If the soft tissues around a fracture are badly treated (and neglect is bad treatment), then prolonged disability is likely and it may be permanent. The objectives of soft-tissue treatment are: to pump away oedema fluid and restore a healthy circulation; to prevent muscle fibres sticking to each other or to bone; and to encourage the healing of articular cartilage by keeping damaged joints moving. The essence of soft-tissue treatment may be summed up thus: *elevate and exercise; never dangle; never force.*

Elevation

An injured limb usually needs to be elevated; after reduction of a leg fracture, the foot of the bed is raised and exercises are begun. If the leg is in plaster the patient is not allowed up until swelling subsides. Then the limb must, at first, be dependent for only short periods; between these periods, the leg is elevated on a chair. The patient is allowed, and encouraged, to exercise the limb actively, but not to let it dangle. When plaster is finally removed, the leg is bandaged and a similar routine of activity punctuated by elevation is practised until circulatory control is fully restored.

Injuries of the upper limb also need elevation. A sling must not be a permanent passive arm-holder; the limb must be elevated intermittently or, if need be, continuously.

Exercises

All unsplinted joints must be used actively from the very start. A patient with a Colles' fracture, for example, must use the fingers, elbow and shoulder as soon as possible and as normally as possible.

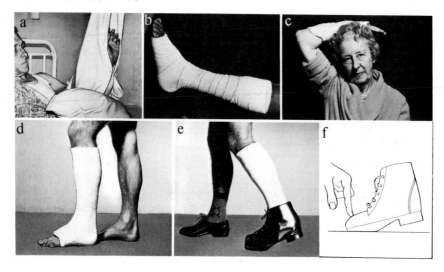

22.21 Some aspects of soft-tissue treatment   Swelling is minimized by (a) elevation and (b) firm support. Stiffness is minimized by exercises: this patient (c) with a Colles' fracture is in no danger of a stiff shoulder. To exercise muscles under a plaster is less easy – a walking plaster should be plantigrade (d); an over-boot with rocker action (e, f) facilitates normal walking and muscle activity.

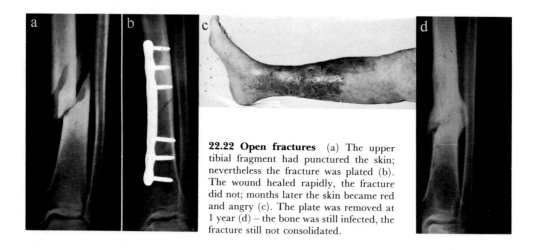

22.22 Open fractures   (a) The upper tibial fragment had punctured the skin; nevertheless the fracture was plated (b). The wound healed rapidly, the fracture did not; months later the skin became red and angry (c). The plate was removed at 1 year (d) – the bone was still infected, the fracture still not consolidated.

Joints encased in plaster cannot, of course, be moved, but the muscles passing over them can and must be exercised. A patient with a fractured leg, for example, is fitted with a special boot over the plaster; this has a rockered sole to compensate for lack of ankle movement. The patient is then taught to walk, using the normal heel–toe gait so that the long toe muscles are actively exercised. Even if weight-bearing is unsafe and crutches must be used, the patient should still go through the motions of correct walking ('shadow walking').

Forced movements are never permitted, and even gentle passive movements are usually considered unwise, especially at the elbow. Recently, however, machines have been devised to move injured limbs passively and continuously from the time of operation; the method is still experimental, but surprisingly good results are being reported.

Aphorisms of fracture management

Think before you start Are you treating the patient? Or merely the x-ray?

Think before you reduce Have you worked out how to do it? And how to hold your reduction?

Think before you hold Is your splint necessary? Is it harmful?

Think before you operate Are your facilities good enough? Are you good enough?

Treatment of open fractures

An open, or compound, fracture is one in which skin damage permits bacteria to enter and contaminate the fracture haematoma. The skin may be perforated, or cut, or there may be actual skin loss; no matter which, and no matter whether the fracture is open from within or without, contamination must be assumed and operation is needed urgently.

Treatment begins at the scene of the accident, where the primary objectives are to save life and minimize shock; the essentials are morphine, splintage and a dressing. In hospital, anti-shock measures are begun. Further treatment is based on the following considerations: (1) bacteria have entered the wound (therefore prophylactic antibiotics and anti-tetanus precautions); (2) bacteria may multiply in the wound (therefore wound toilet); and (3) tension may build up (therefore leave the wound open).

Wound toilet (débridement*)

The operation aims to leave the wound devoid of dead tissue and of foreign material, with a good blood supply throughout. Under general anaesthesia the patient's clothing is removed, while an assistant maintains traction on the limb and holds it still. A sterile pad is placed over the wound and the surrounding skin is cleaned and shaved. The wound itself is then gently cleaned with a harmless detergent. A tourniquet is not used; it would endanger the circulation still further and make it difficult to recognize which structures are devitalized. The tissues are then dealt with as follows.

SKIN
Only the merest sliver of skin is excised from the wound edges; as much skin as possible is spared. The wound often needs to be extended by planned incisions to obtain adequate exposure; once it is enlarged, clothing and other foreign material may be picked out.

FASCIA
Fascia is divided extensively, so that the circulation is not impeded.

MUSCLE
Dead muscle is dangerous; it provides food for bacteria. All dead and doubtfully viable muscle is excised.

BLOOD VESSELS
Large bleeding vessels are tied meticulously but, to minimize the amount of catgut left in the wound, small vessels are clamped with artery forceps and twisted.

NERVES
It is usually best to leave a cut nerve undisturbed. If, however, the wound is clean and the nerve ends present without dissection, the sheath is sutured using non-absorbable material for ease of later identification.

TENDONS
As a rule, cut tendons are also left alone. As with nerves, suture is permissible only if the wound is clean and dissection unnecessary.

BONE
The fractured surfaces are gently cleaned and replaced in correct position. Bone, like skin, should be spared, and fragments removed only if they are small and totally detached. Immediate screwing or plating of severe open fractures is dangerous; with small skin wounds, however, internal fixation is permissible if strongly indicated.

JOINTS
Open joint injuries are best treated by wound toilet, closure of synovium and capsule, and systemic antibiotics; drainage or suction irrigation are used only if contamination is severe.

*Débridement (from *débrider*, to unbridle) literally means to relieve tension by an incision; it has also come to imply the removal of débris and dead tissue.

Wound closure

Immediate closure is dangerous because, as tension rises within the wound, tissues may become avascular, providing food for bacteria, especially anaerobes. The wound is best left open, covered with tulle gras. Closure is postponed until the dangers of tension and infection have passed (delayed primary suture). A well-padded plaster is applied; both plaster and wool must be widely split so that skin is visible. Alternatively, external fixation is used, especially if soft-tissue injury is severe.

After-care

In the ward, the limb is elevated and its circulation carefully watched. Shock may still require treatment. Chemotherapy is continued; the organism is cultured and, if necessary, a different antibiotic is substituted.

If the wound has been left open it is inspected at 5–7 days. Delayed primary suture is then often safe, or, if there has been much skin loss, split-skin grafts are applied. If toxaemia or septicaemia persists in spite of chemotherapy, the wound is drained (the only safe treatment if an infected fracture is not seen until 24 hours after injury).

When all reasonable danger of infection has been overcome, definitive treatment of the fracture is carried out.

Sequels to open fractures

SKIN
If there has been skin loss or contracture, grafting may be necessary. When reparative or reconstructive surgery to deeper tissues is required, a full-thickness skin graft is highly desirable.

BONE
Infection may lead to sequestra and to sinuses. Small sequestra should be removed early, but large pieces of bone should not be excised.

Delayed union is inevitable after an infected fracture, but union will occur if infection is controlled and treatment continued for sufficient time.

JOINTS
When an infected fracture communicates with a joint, the principles of treatment are the same as with bone infection; namely, drugs, drainage and splintage. The joint should be splinted in the optimum position for ankylosis, lest this occur.

With any open fracture, even if not communicating with a joint, some stiffness is almost inevitable. It can be minimized by slowly increasing active exercises once it is certain that infection has been overcome.

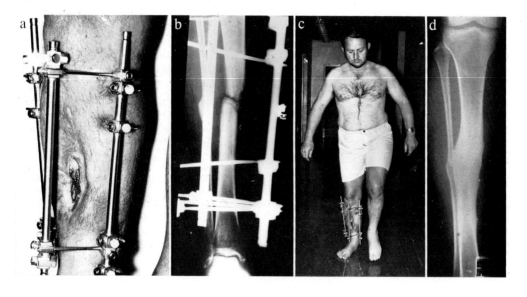

22.23 Infected fractures   (a) Infected fracture of the tibia treated by wound excision and external fixation; (b) the x-ray after 6 weeks; (c) he was able to walk around with his apparatus, and gradually the wound healed; at 1 year (d) the fracture was completely solid.

General complications of fractures

Shock

For a discussion of shock, see page 372.

Crush syndrome

The crush syndrome may occur if a large bulk of muscle is crushed, as by fallen masonry, or if a tourniquet has been left on too long. When compression is released, acid myohaematin, from muscle breakdown, is carried in the circulation to the kidney and blocks the tubules. An alternative explanation is that renal artery spasm occurs and the anoxic tubule cells necrose.

Shock is profound. The released limb is pulseless and later becomes red, swollen and blistered; sensation and muscle power may be lost. Renal secretion diminishes and a low-output uraemia with acidosis develops. If renal secretion returns within a week the patient survives; most patients become increasingly drowsy and die within 14 days.

To avert disaster, a limb crushed severely and for several hours should be amputated. Thus, if a tourniquet has been left on for more than 6 hours the limb must be sacrificed. Amputation is carried out above the site of compression and before compression is released.

Once the compression force has been released, amputation is valueless. The limb must be kept cool and the patient's shock treated. If oliguria develops, fluid and protein intake are reduced, carbohydrates given (by mouth or into a large vein), protein catabolism is reduced (by giving neomycin and an anabolic steroid) and the serum electrolyte balance maintained. Renal dialysis may be life-saving.

Venous thrombosis and pulmonary embolism

The veins most liable to thrombose are those of the pelvis and lower limbs. The primary cause is hypercoagulability of the blood, due mainly to activation of factor X by thromboplastins released from damaged tissues. Once thrombosis has been initiated, secondary factors become important: stasis may result from a tourniquet or tight bandage, pressure against the operating table or mattress, and prolonged immobility; endothelial damage and an increase in the number and stickiness of platelets may result from trauma or operation.

Diagnosis

With calf-vein thrombosis there may be pain and tenderness in the midline of the calf, increased warmth, swelling, pain on passive dorsiflexion of the foot (Homan's sign), slight pyrexia and tachycardia. Unfortunately, clinical features are unreliable and often negative. Diagnostic aids include ultrasonic demonstration of obstruction to the venous outflow, increased uptake of ^{125}I-labelled fibrinogen, and more rapid clearance of the isotope. Most reliable of all is phlebography, which also demonstrates the exact position of the thrombus – an important factor in gauging the risk of embolization.

With thrombosis of the thigh veins, clinical features are more reliable; pain and tenderness may extend up to the groin and the whole limb becomes swollen. Ultrasound flow detection is most useful here.

A pulmonary embolus, if small, causes few symptoms but is a warning that larger emboli may follow. Signs also are few: specific tests include perfusion scanning, ventilation scanning and selective pulmonary angiography. Large emboli (which almost always originate in the pelvis or thigh) cause pain, haemoptysis and dyspnoea; there is a pleural rub and evidence of lung consolidation. The occasional patient is seized with sudden chest pain, turns pale and falls dead.

Chronic lower limb oedema and leg ulcers (the post-phlebitic syndrome) occur in almost all patients with iliofemoral thrombosis and in 10 per cent of those with calf thrombosis.

Prophylactic treatment

To await pulmonary embolism and then treat it is dangerous; prophylaxis is far better. This is achieved by (1) reducing the hypercoagulable

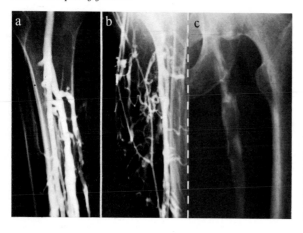

22.24 Deep vein thrombosis – phlebograms This patient's right calf (a) is normal, but his left calf (b) shows thrombosis; his left femoral vein (c) also is thrombosed; the filling defect is surrounded by contrast on all sides so the thrombosis is potentially mobile, but it does not look recent so the danger is not great. (By courtesy of Dr N. W. T. Grieve).

state, and (2) preventing stasis and platelet aggregation.

Low-dose heparin, which enhances the effect of anti-thrombin III, is the best available prophy- lactic, but is much less effective with hip opera- tions than with abdominal operations. An accepted programme is to give 5000 units sub- cutaneously 2 hours before operation and 8- hourly for 1 week after. This should not be used in elderly patients unless the plasma heparin levels can be monitored. Aspirin and hydroxychloro- quine, which only affect platelet aggregation, are inadequate on their own. Recently, smaller doses of heparin have been combined with dihydro- ergotamine, which diminishes venous stasis.

Prophylactic drugs are indicated for *high-risk patients* (those with a history of previous thrombo- sis, patients who are obese or who have just spent several days in bed, those with malignant disease and those taking contraceptive pills); and under *high-risk circumstances* (following pelvic and hip fractures, or before hip operations).

Pressure can be reduced by the use of Sorbo heel pads, and stasis minimized by electrical stimulation of the calf muscles, elastic stockings, pneumatic calf cuffs, and by getting the patient up, or at least moving about in bed, as early as possible.

Treatment of established thromboembolism

ANTICOAGULANTS
These are strongly indicated if pulmonary embol- ism has already occurred, and with a definite diagnosis of pelvic or thigh-vein thrombosis. Calf-

vein thrombosis is a less definite indication, but the absence of more proximal thrombosis needs to be demonstrated. A tendency to bleed and peptic ulcer are contraindications.

Heparin given intravenously acts as an anticoagulant with- in minutes (dose 10000 units 6-hourly, with protamine as the antidote should bleeding occur). Warfarin (loading dose 30–40 mg) is given orally at the same time and takes 48 hours to act. The heparin is then discontinued and the prothrombin time estimated; this is used to control the subsequent dosage of warfarin (usually given twice daily).

OTHER MEASURES
Vein ligation (to prevent emboli migrating) is not often practised, because emboli do not necessarily come from the obviously affected veins, or even from the clinically abnormal limb; but recurrent pulmonary emboli with x-ray evidence of a loose thrombus is an indication for thrombectomy.

When venous thrombosis has occurred the limb should be supported by a crêpe bandage, elastic bandage or elastic stocking until symptoms have subsided and the limb no longer swells. Streptokinase has been used in the attempt to dissolve the thrombus, but its administration is not without risk of haemorrhage and of anaphylaxis.

If pulmonary embolism has occurred antibiotics are given to prevent lung infection, but it should be remembered that broad-spectrum antibiotics potentiate the action of phenin- dione (aspirin and phenylbutazone have a similar action).

Tetanus

The tetanus organism flourishes only in dead tissue. It produces an exotoxin which passes to the central nervous system via the blood and the perineural lymphatics from the infected region. The toxin is fixed in the anterior horn cells and thereafter cannot be neutralized by antitoxin.

Established tetanus is characterized by tonic, and later clonic, contractions, especially of the muscles of the jaw and face (trismus, risus sardonicus), those near the wound itself, and later of the neck and trunk. Ultimately, the diaphragm and intercostal muscles may be fixed in spasm and the patient dies of asphyxia.

PROPHYLAXIS

Active immunization of the whole population by tetanus toxoid is an attainable ideal. To the patient so immunized booster doses of toxoid are given after all but trivial skin wounding. In non-immunized patients prompt and thorough wound toilet together with antibiotics may be adequate, but if the wound is contaminated, and particularly with delay before operation, then antitoxin is advisable. Horse serum carries a considerable risk of anaphylaxis, and human antitoxin (ATG) should be used. The opportunity is taken to initiate active immunization with toxoid at the same time.

TREATMENT

With established tetanus, intravenous antitoxin (again human for choice) is advisable. Heavy sedation and relaxant drugs may help; endotracheal intubation and controlled respiration are employed for the patient with respiratory and swallowing embarrassment.

Fat embolism

Circulating fat globules larger than 10 μm in diameter, and histological traces of fat emboli in the lungs, occur in most adults after closed fractures of long bones; fortunately only a small percentage of such patients develop respiratory insufficiency or systemic emboli.

The patient with symptoms is usually a young adult with a lower limb fracture. Early warning signs (within 72 hours of injury) are a slight rise of temperature and pulse rate. In more pronounced cases there is breathlessness and mild mental confusion or restlessness; petechiae should be sought on the front and back of the chest and in the conjunctival folds. In the most severe cases there may be marked respiratory distress and coma, due partly to hypoxia and partly to cerebral emboli.

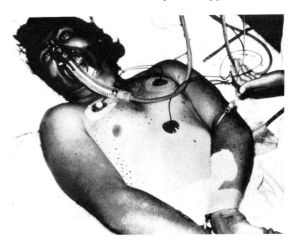

22.25 Fat embolism This man with bilateral femoral shaft fractures (closed) sustained fat embolism. When this photograph was taken he was unconscious, his face was congested and he was on continuous oxygen with cardiac monitoring. The petechiae were smaller and fainter than shown here; they have been accentuated for clarity and to show their distribution.

Hypoxaemia can be diagnosed in the absence of clinical signs by measuring the blood gases in all young patients with long bone fractures; a fall in Po_2 to below 60 mmHg (8 kPa) is highly suggestive. However, fat embolism is only one aspect of the post-traumatic pulmonary insufficiency syndrome, and inappropriate fluid replacement or the advent of sepsis may turn a serious situation into a disaster (Alho, 1980).

TREATMENT

In mild cases no treatment is required, but accurate monitoring of blood Po_2 and fluid balance is essential. If there are signs of hypoxia, oxygen should be given; patients with severe respiratory distress require intensive care, with sedation, assisted ventilation, and Swan–Ganz catheterization for monitoring cardiac function.

Fluid balance must be maintained, and other supportive measures have their advocates; e.g. heparin to counteract thromboembolism, steroids to help reduce pulmonary oedema, or aprotinin (Trasylol) which may prevent the aggregation of chylomicrons.

Other general complications

'FRACTURE FEVER'

This is a doubtful entity, though it is true that the absorption of a haematoma often causes slight pyrexia. If fever persists for more than 72 hours it is wise to presume the presence of infection.

DELIRIUM TREMENS

This may follow injury in a chronic alcoholic, and lead to alarming but characteristic symptoms. Chlormethiazole is useful.

ACCIDENT NEUROSIS

This condition, which can follow even minor injury, is closely associated with compensation. The patient is not a malingerer, but resolutely denies that he is fit for work or that any treatment is helping him. Prophylaxis is largely a social problem; treatment includes legal settlement of the case.

Local complications of limb fractures

Skin complications

The most important local complication is skin damage. The treatment of open fractures has already been described (page 349).

FRACTURE BLISTERS

These are due to elevation of the superficial layers of skin by oedema, and can sometimes be prevented by firm bandaging. They should be covered with a sterile dry dressing.

PLASTER SORES

Plaster sores occur where skin presses directly onto bone. They should be prevented by padding the bony points and by moulding the wet plaster so that pressure is distributed to the soft tissues around the bony points. While a plaster sore is developing the patient feels localized burning pain. A window must immediately be cut in the plaster, or warning pain quickly abates and skin necrosis proceeds unnoticed.

BED SORES

Bed sores occur in elderly or paralysed patients. The skin over the sacrum and heels is especially vulnerable. Careful nursing and early activity can usually prevent bed sores; once they have developed treatment is difficult, and it may be necessary to excise the necrotic tissue and apply skin grafts.

Muscle complications

TORN MUSCLE FIBRES

Torn muscle fibres are common with any fracture. Unless the muscle is actively exercised the torn fibres may become adherent to untorn fibres, capsule or bone; if adhesions have been allowed to develop, lengthy rehabilitation will be necessary after the fracture has consolidated. The fracture and the torn muscles both need treatment: it is better to serve two sentences concurrently than consecutively.

DISUSE ATROPHY

Like adhesions, disuse atrophy is largely the result of neglect in treatment, and is usually preventable by repeated active muscle exercises.

Tendon complications

TORN TENDON

A torn tendon is rare in association with a closed fracture, except in transverse fractures of the patella or olecranon process; in these fractures, the loss of continuity of the extensor mechanism of the joint is the essential feature.

AVULSION FRACTURES

Avulsion fractures, in which the tendon remains intact but pulls off a small flake of bone, occur at the shoulder (supraspinatus tendon), the fingers (mallet finger), the knee (patellar tendon), the pelvis and the lesser trochanter (psoas tendon).

LATE RUPTURE

Late rupture of the extensor pollicis longus tendon may occur 6–12 weeks after a fracture of the lower radius, and late rupture of the long head of biceps after a fractured neck of humerus.

TENDINITIS

Tendinitis may affect the tibialis posterior tendon following medial malleolar fractures. It should be prevented by accurate reduction, if necessary at open operation.

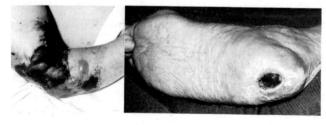

22.26 Skin complications Blisters may be difficult to avoid, but pressure sores usually can be prevented – and every effort should be made to prevent them, since they are painful and very slow to heal.

Nerve complications

NERVE INJURY

Nerve injury (Chapter 11) is not uncommon in association with a fracture. Usually the lesion is a neurapraxia which quickly recovers. Axonotmesis is liable to occur when the injury (fracture or dislocation) imposes severe traction on the nerve. Neurotmesis is rare with closed fractures.

Nerve damage should be diagnosed during the initial examination of the patient. In closed fractures recovery is usual and should be awaited. If recovery has not occurred by the expected time, the nerve should be explored as soon as the fracture has consolidated; but preliminary electromyography is a useful safeguard against unnecessary exploration.

COMPRESSION

Nerve compression may damage the lateral popliteal nerve if an elderly or emaciated patient lies with the leg in full external rotation. Radial palsy may follow the faulty use of crutches. Both conditions are due to lack of supervision.

LATE ULNAR NEURITIS

This condition results from a valgus elbow following an un-united lateral condyle fracture (see page 391).

Arterial complications

In this section, ischaemia of soft tissues is discussed; avascular necrosis of bone is considered on page 357.

Arteries may be cut, compressed or contused; and even with a closed injury the intima may be torn, sealing off the entrance to collaterals, or promoting thrombus formation. Pulsation proximal to the injury and an empty vessel distal to it may suggest spasm; but this appearance is spurious, for spasm is rare (and treatment based on the possibility dangerously time-wasting). If sufficiently severe, arterial ischaemia leads to gangrene, or to a compartment syndrome followed by contracture.

Gangrene

All the tissues are ischaemic, the most distal (fingers or toes) being the most severely affected.

The distal limb becomes cold and pulseless and, unless the ischaemia is relieved without delay, the tissues die, become discoloured and a line of

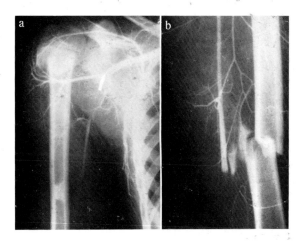

22.27 Gangrene In both these patients the peripheral part of the limb was cold and pulseless; arteriography shows a cut-off of a major artery in association with (a) a fractured neck of humerus, and (b) a fractured shaft of femur.

demarcation develops; amputation is then inevitable. Before this stage is reached, prompt reduction of a fracture or dislocation may restore pulsation; if not, exploration (preceded by arteriography) is imperative with a view to arterial repair or grafting.

Compartment syndromes (Volkmann's ischaemia)

PATHOLOGY

Unlike gangrene, a compartment syndrome does not involve all the tissues; moreover, the fingers and toes are usually not ischaemic, though they may be numb and paralysed. What happens is that, within a confined space (an osteofascial compartment) oedema leads to an increase of pressure; this reduces the capillary flow, which leads to still more oedema. A vicious circle develops, resulting in ischaemia of the tissues within the compartment; this is Volkmann's ischaemia.

The tissues are not all affected equally by ischaemia. Nerve, though it is the most sensitive and can survive only 2–4 hours, is theoretically capable of regeneration; but muscle, though it can

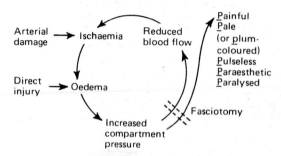

22.28 The vicious circle of Volkmann's ischaemia (Modified from the *Journal of Bone and Joint Surgery*, 1979, **61B**, 298 by kind permission of Mr C. E. Holden and the Editor).

survive longer (probably 6–8 hours), once infarcted can never recover – it is replaced by fibrous tissue which contracts (Volkmann's contracture).

Two varieties of compartment syndrome are described: (1) where the main artery proximal to the compartment is damaged; and (2) where direct injury occurs within the compartment itself. Both lead to rising pressure within the compartment and, unless relieved promptly by fasciotomy, to ischaemic necrosis and contracture. The most important compartments are in the forearm (back or front) and in the leg (anterior tibial, peroneal and deep posterior compartments). The injuries most likely to result in compartment syndromes are: (1) supracondylar fractures of the humerus in children; (2) fractures of the proximal third of the tibia; (3) fractures of the femur in infants treated on overhead (Bryant's or gallows) traction; and (4) lying or squatting awkwardly on a hard surface while in a drug-induced coma.

CLINICAL FEATURES

Ischaemia of the flexor compartment of the forearm is described here, but comparable features apply at other sites.

Pain is the dominant symptom – severe, unremitting, often agonizing pain – made still worse by passive extension of the fingers. This is the key feature; others must be sought, but their absence does not exclude an acute compartment syndrome.

The skin of the hand often looks pale or slightly cyanosed; the pulse is usually absent and sensation in the fingers blunted or absent; and the belly of the forearm feels tense and tender. Pain plus any one of these signs is sufficient for a diagnosis.*

On rare occasions, if nerve damage is extensive, pain may be only slight. Diagnosis is then difficult, but it can be established by measuring the intracompartmental pressure with a cannula attached to a pressure transducer; 30 mmHg or above is the signal for urgent action.

TREATMENT

(1) The front half of any encircling splints or bandages must at once be removed so that the skin of the entire front of the limb is exposed.
(2) The elbow, if acutely flexed, is straightened a little to ensure that the artery is not unduly kinked.
(3) The fracture is x-rayed and, if the position of the bones suggests that the artery is being compressed or kinked, prompt reduction is necessary.
(4) The limb is kept cool to reduce its metabolic requirements.
(5) Preparations are made for emergency operation.

One hour later the patient is re-examined. Unless the signs of ischaemia have abated, immediate operation is necessary. Extensive fasciotomy is the essential feature. Then the artery is exposed. A bleeding vessel may need ligation, or the damaged segment may need to be excised and bypassed or grafted. Arterial surgery is facilitated if the fracture is first fixed internally. The wound is left open and delayed primary suture performed a few days later.

A hyperbaric chamber has been used to reduce the effects of ischaemia.

AFTER-CARE

Prolonged physiotherapy (wax baths, exercises and prolonged stretching on a special splint) may minimize the contracture.

Volkmann's contracture

Ischaemic muscles fibrose and contract, though ischaemic nerves sometimes recover, at least partially. Thus the patient presents with deformity and stiffness, but numbness is inconstant.

If the flexor compartment of the forearm was affected, the forearm is thin and the hand clawed;

*If the fracture site is painful, or the skin is coloured plum;
If the radial pulse is absent, or the fingers feeling numb;
If the flexors don't like stretching, or the forearm feels too tense;
You must take off all the splints, and ring the Medical Defence.
(*With apologies to Rudyard Kipling*)

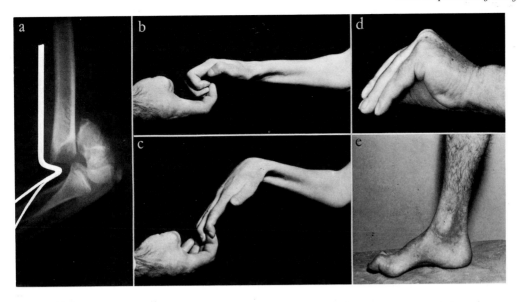

22.29 Volkmann's ischaemia (a) Kinking of the main artery is an important cause. (b, c) Volkmann's contracture of the forearm; the fingers can be straightened only when the wrist is palmarflexed (the constant-length phenomenon). (d) Ischaemic contracture of the small muscles of the hand (Bunnell). (e) Ischaemic contracture of the calf muscles with clawing of the toes.

all the fingers are flexed at the proximal and distal interphalangeal joints. Because the flexor muscles are contracted the patient can extend his fingers only by flexing the wrist; and he can grip (often feebly) only by extending the wrist. Sensation may be diminished or absent.

TREATMENT
Two methods of treating Volkmann's contracture of the forearm flexors are available. (1) The origin of the flexor muscles is moved distally; deformity is reduced, but function may be little improved. (2) The necrotic muscles are excised and contracted tendons divided; the wrist dorsiflexors or other functioning tendons are then transferred to the cut distal end of the finger flexors. Considerable improvement in function may follow and, if necessary, the procedure may be supplemented by grafting the median nerve.

Ischaemia at other sites

Ischaemia of the hand may follow forearm injuries, or swelling of the fingers associated with a tight forearm bandage or plaster. The intrinsic hand muscles fibrose and shorten, pulling the fingers into flexion at the metacarpophalangeal joints, but the interphalangeal joints remain straight. The thumb is adducted across the palm (Bunnell's 'intrinsic-plus' position).

Ischaemia of the calf muscles may follow injuries or operations involving the popliteal artery or its divisions. This is commoner than is usually supposed. The symptoms, signs and subsequent contracture are similar to those following ischaemia of the forearm. Occasionally, ischaemia may affect the intrinsic muscles of the foot.

Wherever ischaemia occurs, the principles of treatment are those outlined above.

Bone complications

Avascular necrosis

Bone dies when deprived of its blood supply. The bones affected are as follows.

Femoral head Avascular necrosis of the femoral head may follow cervical fracture or traumatic dislocation. Segmental necrosis may follow nailing a cervical fracture.

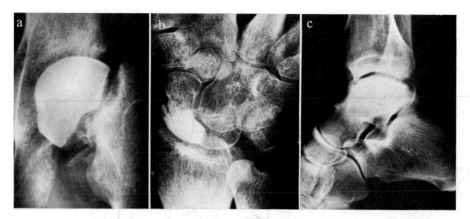

22.30 Avascular necrosis   If the fracture cuts off the blood supply to part of the bone the avascular part becomes dense on x-ray. Three common sites are: (a) head of femur, (b) proximal portion of scaphoid, (c) posterior half of talus.

Carpal bones   The proximal portion of the carpal scaphoid and the lunate may become avascular following carpal fracture or dislocation (pages 408 and 410).

Other sites   Part of the talus may become avascular after a fracture, or the whole bone after a dislocation. The head of the humerus rarely becomes avascular. Following fractures into joints, small fragments of bone not infrequently become avascular.

Avascular necrosis is not exclusively a complication of fractures and dislocations. Thus, the femoral head may become avascular after forcible reduction of a congenital hip dislocation or a slipped epiphysis, and 'spontaneously' in Perthes' disease. Other sites of avascular necrosis are described in Chapter 6.

EFFECTS
At first there are no radiological changes, but within a few weeks the avascular bone may look dense if the area has been immobilized; this is a relative change because the affected bone cannot share in the rarefaction of the surrounding bones which follows immobilization. Still later, absolute increase of density occurs as new bone is laid down on top of dead trabeculae.

Delayed union is inevitable in the presence of avascular necrosis, but union follows if the bones can be held together until revascularization has taken place; otherwise non-union is likely.

Osteoarthritis is liable to follow avascular necrosis if the dead bone is allowed to crush with stress.

Delayed union

The timetable on page 346 is no more than a rough guide to the period in which a fracture may be expected to unite and consolidate. It must never be relied upon in deciding when treatment may be discontinued. If the time is unduly prolonged, the term 'delayed union' is used.

CAUSES
Inadequate blood supply   Whenever a fracture occurs through bone which is bare of muscle fibres there is the risk of delayed union. The vulnerable bones include those which are liable to avascular necrosis, and also the lower tibia (especially a double fracture).

Infection   An open fracture is slow to join, probably because there is little fracture haematoma in which ensheathing callus can form; infection delays union still further.

Incorrect splintage   This includes (1) insufficient splintage; thus, a standard below-knee plaster does not hold a fractured shaft of tibia adequately; and (2) excessive traction, which pulls the bones apart.

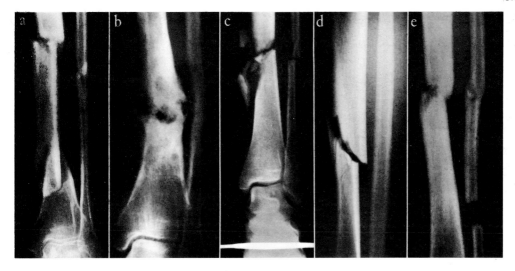

22.31 Delayed union Causes of delay include (a) a double fracture, (b) infection, (c) excessive traction, and (d) an intact fibula. In (e) both bones were fractured but the fibula joined first and splinted the tibia apart; the delayed union is obvious – 2.5 cm of fibula was therefore excised.

Internal fixation Open reduction with internal fixation of a fracture delays union, partly because the fracture haematoma escapes.

Intact fellow bone If one bone in the forearm or leg is unbroken, the fractured ends of the other may be held apart, and some delay then follows.

SIGNS
The fracture site is usually tender. The bone may appear to move in one piece; if, however, it is subjected to stress, pain is immediately felt and the bone may angulate; the fracture is not consolidated.

X-ray The fracture site is still clearly visible, but the bone ends are not sclerosed.

TREATMENT
Conservative Delayed union is the signal to continue treatment of the fracture, and to continue it efficiently until consolidation is complete. If plaster is being used, it must be sufficiently extensive and must fit accurately. If traction is being used it must not be excessive; it is sometimes better replaced by plaster splintage. Functional bracing is an effective method of promoting bony union.

Operative If a fractured tibia is being held apart by a fibula which was not fractured or which has united quickly, it is worth while excising 2.5 cm of fibula and reapplying plaster.

Non-union

CAUSES
Unless delayed union is recognized, and the fracture adequately treated, non-union is liable to result. Other causes include too large a gap and interposition of tissues.

Too large a gap If the fracture surfaces are too widely separated, union takes a very long time or may never occur. The gap may be due to a gunshot fracture which destroys a large section of bone, to muscle retraction in which the patient's own muscles pull the fragments apart (as in a fractured patella), or to treatment with excessive traction.

Interposition Non-union may develop when any one of the following tissues is interposed between the bone ends: periosteum (e.g. a flap of periosteum in association with a fractured medial malleolus); muscle (e.g. a fractured femur may spike through the quadriceps muscle); cartilage (e.g. a fractured lateral condyle of humerus may be so rotated that its cartilaginous articular surface faces the shaft).

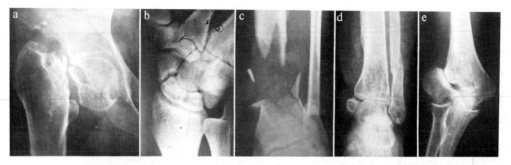

22.32 Non-union (1)   The femoral neck (a) and the carpal scaphoid (b) are two common sites of non-union. This tibia (c) could hardly be expected to unite – so much bone had been left at the scene of the accident. (d) This medial malleolus failed to unite, presumably because a flap of periosteum was interposed. (e) This lateral condyle had rotated so that articular cartilage prevented union.

CAUSES OF NON-UNION

THE INJURY	THE BONE	THE SURGEON	THE PATIENT
1. Soft tissue loss	1. Poor blood supply	1. Distraction	1. Immense
2. Bone loss	2. Poor haematoma	2. Poor splintage	2. Immoderate
3. Intact fellow bone	3. Infection	3. Poor fixation	3. Immovable
4. Soft tissue interposition	4. Pathological lesion	4. Impatience	4. Impossible

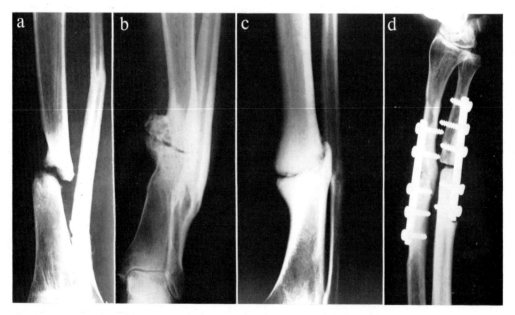

22.33 Non-union (2)   (a) Atrophic non-union – bone grafting is needed. (b) Hypertrophic non-union – rigid fixation would probably suffice. (c) The so-called elephant's foot appearance – although partly hypertrophic, fixation plus grafting would be wise. (d) This patient had atrophic non-union of both forearm bones – both were plated, but grafts were added only to the radius and (predictably) it alone has united.

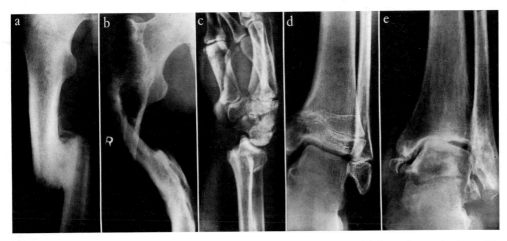

22.34 Malunion Primary malunion (a) with overlap, (b) with angulation. (c) Secondary malunion – this Colles' fracture was reduced satisfactorily, but displaced in plaster. (d) Secondary malunion following damage to the lower tibial epiphysis. (e) Osteoarthritis, the sequel to malunion.

SIGNS
Movement can be elicited at the fracture site, and this movement (unless excessive) is painless; such painless movement is diagnostic of non-union as distinct from delayed union.

X-ray The fracture is visible and the bone on each side of it may be sclerosed. Two varieties of non-union can be distinguished: (1) hypertrophic, with bulbous bone ends, indicating osteogenic activity (as if in the attempt to form bridging callus); and (2) atrophic, with no calcification around the bone ends.

TREATMENT
Conservative Non-union is occasionally symptomless, needing no treatment or, at most, a removable splint. Even if symptoms are present, operation is not the only answer; with hypertrophic non-union, functional bracing may be sufficient to induce union, but treatment often needs to be prolonged. Electrical stimulation promotes osteogenesis and also is sometimes successful; an induced current can be applied through a plaster cast, or electrodes may be implanted.

Operative With hypertrophic non-union and in the absence of deformity, very rigid internal fixation alone may lead to union. With atrophic non-union, fixation alone is not enough and bone grafts should be added; it is wise first to excise any fibrous tissue interposed between the bone ends, and it is important also to correct any deformity.

Malunion
CAUSES
Primary The fracture was never reduced and has united in a deformed position. Shortening is, of course, one type of deformity.

Secondary The fracture was reduced but reduction was not held. Redisplacement may occur during the first week, and a check x-ray at 1 week is advisable.

SIGNS
The deformity is usually obvious. There may be painful limitation of joint movement (e.g. osteoarthritis of the ankle years after a malunited Pott's fracture). At the elbow, valgus deformity may present with delayed ulnar palsy.

TREATMENT
Conservative If shortening is the main feature a raised shoe is usually sufficient. Often no treatment is required, either because a bone may grow straight,* or because a neighbouring ball-and-socket joint compensates for the deformity.

Operative Osteotomy may be necessary if deformity is unsightly or to prevent the development of osteoarthritis.

*Malunion in a child will remodel – provided the fracture is near a bone end and not malrotated.

Growth disturbance

Provided it is accurately reduced, fracture-separation of an epiphysis does not disturb growth: the epiphysis and growth disc are displaced together; the line of fracture is immediately next to the growth disc on its metaphyseal side, and the growth disc is consequently undamaged. A crushing injury to the growth disc, or a vertical fracture through it, however, may well disturb growth and lead to malunion.

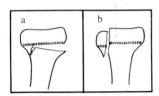

22.35 Ephiphyseal injuries (a) Fracture-separation – much the commonest epiphyseal injury: the epiphysis, the growth disc and a triangle of metaphysis all move together and, following reduction, growth is undisturbed. Other varieties of epiphyseal injury, such as (b), can, and do, influence future growth.

Joint complications

Instability

Following injury a joint may give way. Causes include the following.

Ligamentous laxity, especially at the knee (page 458), the ankle (page 467) and the metacarpophalangeal joint of the thumb (page 415).

Muscle weakness, especially if splintage has been excessive or prolonged, and exercises have been inadequate (again the knee and ankle are most often affected).

Bone loss, especially after a gunshot fracture or severe compound injury.

Injury may also lead to another form of instability; namely, *recurrent dislocation*. The commonest sites are: (1) the shoulder – if the glenoid labrum has been detached (page 382); and (2) the patella – if, after traumatic dislocation, the capsule heals poorly (page 294).

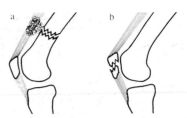

22.36 Two causes of stiffness (a) Fibrosis limiting muscle excursion; (b) malunion at an articular surface.

Stiffness

Limited movement at a joint, one of the commonest complications of a fracture, has a variety of causes.

INACTIVITY
This, the most important cause, is largely preventable. Active exercises are an essential part of the treatment of any fracture. Inactivity leads to adhesions, particularly after prolonged splintage or with persistent oedema. If stiffness has developed, the joint can be manipulated under anaesthesia once the fracture is consolidated; at the knee, quadriceps-plasty should be considered.

INFECTION
Infection following a compound fracture nearly always causes considerable stiffness of long duration.

MALUNION
Malunion may restrict movement; for example, malunion of the radius and ulna limits forearm rotation; cross-union, which is rare, prevents all rotation.

MYOSITIS OSSIFICANS
In traumatic myositis ossificans, heterotopic bone forms in the fleshy part of the muscle over the fracture; movement of the nearby joint becomes restricted. The cause is unknown but it is thought to be related to muscle damage or too early and too vigorous joint movement.

The commonest site is the elbow. A few weeks after injury, movement, instead of increasing, is found to be getting less. The elbow may be painful and almost totally stiff. X-rays show a fluffy mass of calcification in front.

At the first hint that movement is decreasing, the elbow should be rested in a plaster gutter. Months later, the fluffy mass of callus appears smaller and more discrete; its removal then is sometimes followed by increased movement.

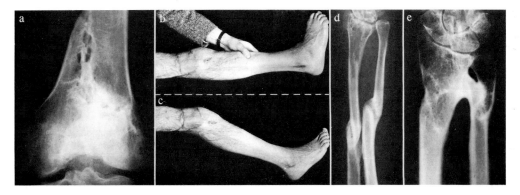

22.37 Joint stiffness (1) (a) This heavily compound fracture inevitably caused gross knee stiffness (b, c), which was eventually treated by quadriceps-plasty. (d) Malunion caused limited rotation of this forearm. (e) Cross-union here abolished rotation.

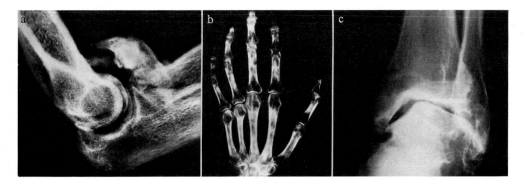

22.38 Joint stiffness (2) (a) Myositis ossificans following a fractured head of radius. (b) Sudeck's atrophy following a relatively minor injury of the wrist. (c) Osteoarthritis following malunion.

Myositis ossificans may occur without bony injury, as after a kick on the front of the thigh. A large haematoma of the thigh should if possible be aspirated; ice-packs and ultrasound may reduce the risk of myositis ossificans in such injuries.

SUDECK'S ATROPHY

Sudeck's atrophy occasionally affects the foot, but more usually the hand, often after relatively trivial wrist or forearm injuries. Pain and stiffness of fingers come on a few weeks after injury. The fingers are puffy, patchily discoloured, unduly moist, hyperaesthetic and stiff. X-rays show patchy rarefaction of the bones.

With prolonged physiotherapy (heat, elevation and graduated exercises) recovery is slow but steady over many months. Recovery can be accelerated by: (1) serial injections of long-lasting local anaesthetics into the stellate ganglion (or other appropriate site); (2) the use of guanethidine injections

as described in the treatment of causalgia (see page 138); or (3) a short course of steroids in fairly high dosage.

OSTEOARTHRITIS

Osteoarthritis is liable to follow malunion when the joint surfaces remain incongruous, or when the direction of stress transmission is abnormal. Avascular necrosis is another potent precursor of joint degeneration.

UNREDUCED DISLOCATIONS

With every day that passes, reduction of a dislocation becomes more difficult and more dangerous. After a few days or weeks (varying with the joint and the patient's age) closed reduction is unwise; open reduction may still be feasible. Still later, neither should be attempted, but function can sometimes be improved by osteotomy, or by a 'sham reduction' (see page 397).

Pathological fractures

Pathological fractures are of two kinds: those occurring in apparently normal bone (stress fractures), and those occurring in bone which is clearly abnormal.

Stress fractures

A stress or fatigue fracture is one occurring in the normal bone of a healthy patient. It is caused, not by a specific traumatic incident, but by frequently repeated forces, which are of two main kinds – bending and compression.

Bending forces, which breach one cortex; healing begins, but with repeated stress the breach may extend across the bone. This variety affects young adults and is probably due to muscular action, which tends to deform bone; the athlete in training or the military recruit builds up muscle power quickly but bone strength only slowly and a stress fracture may result.

Compression forces, which act on soft cancellous bone; with frequent repetition an impacted fracture may follow.

NOTE   It has been suggested that a stress fracture is the initial lesion in some of the osteochondritides; e.g. Freiberg's disease.

SITES AFFECTED
Least rare are the following: shaft of humerus (adolescent cricketers); pars interarticularis of fifth lumbar vertebra (causing spondylolysis); pubic rami (inferior in children, both in adults); femoral neck (at any age); femoral shaft (chiefly lower third); patella (children and young adults); tibial shaft (proximal third in children, middle third in athletes, distal third in the elderly); distal shaft of fibula (the 'runner's fracture'); calcaneum (adults); metatarsals (especially the second – see page 327).

Clinical features

There may be a history of unaccustomed and repeated activity. A common sequence of events is: pain after exercise – pain during exercise – pain without exercise. Occasionally the patient presents only after the fracture has healed; he may then complain of a lump (the callus).

The patient is usually healthy. The affected site may be swollen or red. It is sometimes warm and usually tender; the callus may be palpable. 'Springing' the bone (attempting to bend it) is often painful.

X-RAY
The fracture is difficult to see; several views, tomograms or a technetium scan may be helpful. A small cortical breach, or a faint line like a vessel marking, may reveal the fracture. Compression stress fractures (especially of the femoral neck and upper tibia) may show as a hazy transverse band of sclerosis with (in the tibia) peripheral callus.

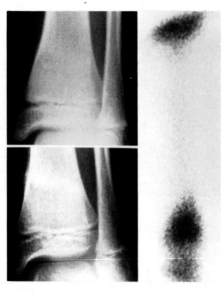

22.39   Stress   fracture –   diagnosis
Because of pain after activity the upper x-ray was taken, and reported as normal. But a stress fracture was suspected, so a scan was done immediately and shows a hot spot just above the ankle. The lower film was taken 17 days later and now at last the stress fracture is clearly seen.

Diagnosis

Many disorders, including osteomyelitis, scurvy and the battered baby syndrome, may be confused with stress fractures. The great danger, however, is a mistaken diagnosis of osteosarcoma. Scanning shows increased uptake in both conditions and even biopsy may be misleading (see

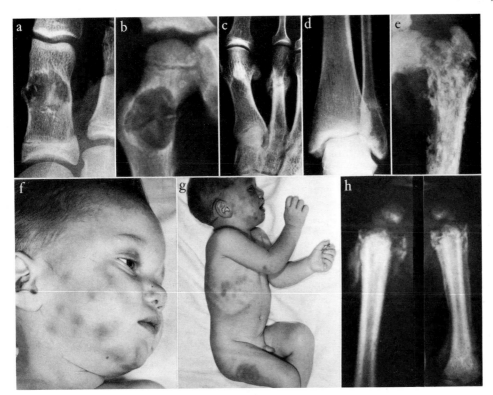

22.40 Pathological fractures – in the young (a) Through a chondroma of the hallux; (b) through a cyst of the femoral neck; (c) stress fracture of second metatarsal; (d) stress fracture of the fibula – a less common site; (e) fracture through bone weakened by acute osteomyelitis.
(f, g, h) The battered baby syndrome. The fractures are not pathological but the family is; the metaphyseal lesions in each humerus (h) are characteristic.

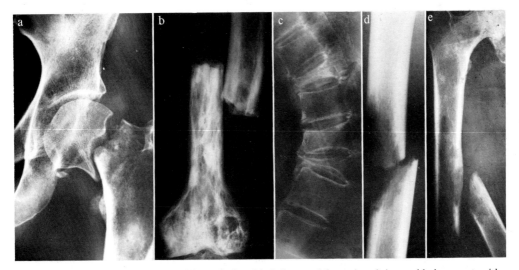

22.41 Pathological fractures – in older people (a) A fractured femoral neck in an elderly woman with osteoporosis is probably the commonest. Fractures through Paget bone (b) also are usually in old people. Fractures through secondary deposits (c and d) and through myelomatosis (e) may occur somewhat earlier.

page 104); but if the clinician alerts the pathologist to the possibility of a stress fracture, this
disastrous mistake can be avoided.

Treatment

Most stress fractures need no treatment other
than an elastic bandage and avoidance of the
painful activity. An important exception is femoral neck fractures which (after reduction if necessary) need to be held; in children two threaded
pins suffice, in adults more sturdy fixation is
needed.

Other pathological fractures

A great variety of disorders may weaken bone and
predispose to pathological fracture. Most of the
causal conditions are described elsewhere; they
can be classified into easily remembered groups
as follows:

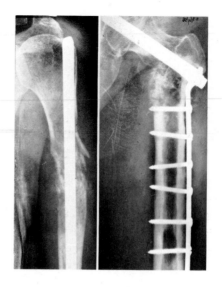

**22.42 Pathological fractures – treat-
ment** Fractures such as these, through
secondary deposits, are nearly always
treated by internal fixation.

Defective bone (congenital)	Disused bone (or faulty use)	Diseased bone	Displaced bone (i.e. replaced)	Disordered bone (faulty metabolism)
Brittle bones	Post-traumatic disuse	Paget's disease	Solitary cyst	Osteoporosis
Marble bones	Paralysed limbs	Acute osteomyelitis	Fibrous dysplasia	Osteomalacia
Congenital pseudarthrosis	Rheumatoid arthritis	Syphilitic osteitis	Deposits	Hyperpara-thyroidism

Investigations

General symptoms

A history of many previous fractures may suggest
a diagnosis of brittle bones.

An operation, no matter how long ago, may
have been performed for the removal of a tumour;
the present fracture may be the first evidence of
metastasis.

Symptoms such as loss of weight, pain, a lump,
cough or haematuria suggest that the fracture
may be through a secondary deposit.

Local symptoms

Three questions are important. Was the force
insufficient to break normal bone? Was the fracture preceded by pain (for example, of a tumour,
or Paget's disease)? Was the bone bent before it
fractured (as in Paget's disease)?

General signs

AGE
Under the age of 20 the common causes are
chondroma (in a finger or toe), cyst (in the
metaphysis of a long bone) and stress fracture.

Over the age of 40 the common causes are Paget's disease (especially of the upper femur), osteoporosis (in the spine or femoral neck), myelomatosis and secondary carcinoma (in the spine, pelvis, humerus or femur).

GENERAL APPEARANCE

The underlying cause may be suggested by cachexia (malignant disease) or by multiple gross deformities (brittle bones, generalized Paget's disease or von Recklinghausen's disease).

GENERAL EXAMINATION

A thorough general examination is necessary and it is useful to proceed systematically, in the following manner.

Head There may be evidence of Paget's disease or rickets.

Neck Cervical lymph nodes or the thyroid gland may be enlarged.

Chest Lumps may be palpable in a breast or axilla, and examination of the lung may suggest a tumour.

Abdomen The abdominal viscera, kidneys and groins must be palpated.

Pelvis Examination of the pelvis is incomplete without rectal and vaginal examination.

Central nervous system There may be evidence of a brain, spinal cord or root tumour, or of neurosyphilis.

Local signs

SITE

The site of the fracture often suggests the cause.

Spine Osteoporosis, secondary deposit and myelomatosis.

Femoral neck Osteoporosis, secondary deposit and irradiation.

Femoral shaft Paget's disease and secondary deposit.

Near end of a long bone Solitary cyst, giant-cell tumour and sarcoma.

Fingers Chondroma and cyst.

Feet March (stress) fracture and chondroma.

X-RAY OF THE BONE AS A WHOLE

Shape A bent bone suggests brittle bones, Paget's disease or old rickets.

Density Generalized decreased density is seen in disuse atrophy and in metabolic bone disease.

Architecture The bone architecture is abnormal in Paget's disease, haemangioma and fibrous dysplasia.

X-RAY OF THE FRACTURE

The appearance of the bone around the fracture may reveal the underlying cause.

Periosteum The periosteum may show callus with a stress fracture or sun-ray spicules and Codman's triangle with a sarcoma.

Cortex The cortex may be thinned or eroded by a tumour, or thickened in Paget's disease.

Medulla The medulla may contain a rarefied area with well-defined borders (solitary cyst, giant-cell tumour, chondroma), a rarefied area with an ill-defined border (malignant tumour), an area of altered architecture (fibrous dysplasia, Paget's disease) or an area of increased density (bone infarct, prostatic deposit).

NOTE ON VERTEBRAE An ordinary crush fracture is nearly always of the upper border. With a fracture through malignant disease the anterior border may be eroded; with osteoporotic fractures the discs are ballooned.

Additional investigations

X-RAY EXAMINATION X-ray of other bones, the lungs and the urogenital tract may be necessary to exclude malignant disease.

BLOOD INVESTIGATION Investigations should always include a full blood count, sedimentation rate, protein electrophoresis, and tests for syphilis and metabolic bone disorders.

URINE EXAMINATION Urine examination may reveal blood from a tumour, or Bence Jones protein in myelomatosis.

SCANNING Local radionuclide imaging may help elucidate the diagnosis, and scanning elsewhere (or, better, whole-body scanning) may reveal other deposits.

Treatment

The treatment of stress fractures has already been described. With other pathological fractures the underlying disease should, if possible, be treated.

Nearly all pathological fractures unite, and many at normal speed; most can be treated in the same way as fractures through normal bone. Fractures through Paget's disease, however, are prone to delayed union or non-union; internal fixation, though difficult, is often preferred. Fracture through a benign tumour is best treated by curetting or excising the tumour; bone grafting is then often necessary. Fracture through a sarcoma is often an indication for amputation.

Fractures through secondary deposits may unite with conservative treatment, especially with radiotherapy and control of the hormone environment (by drugs or operation). Internal fixation is, however, often preferred; it enables the patient to enjoy activity during his remaining months of life. With internal fixation for fractures through malignant deposits (or with osteoporosis), the bone may be too weak for the metal to hold securely; one answer is to pack the bone interior with acrylic cement before plating.

A pathological compression fracture of the spine may lead to paraplegia; if a metastasis or myeloma is suspected, the smallest sign of neurological disturbance (e.g. difficulty with micturition) signals an emergency, and local radiotherapy should be commenced even before investigations and diagnosis are complete. If this fails to halt deterioration, surgical decompression (laminectomy) may still succeed.

Further reading

Alho, A. (1980) Fat embolism syndrome. Etiology, pathogenesis and treatment. *Acta Chirurgica Scandinavica* Suppl. 499, 75–85

Bassett, C. A. L., Mitchell, S. N. and Gaston, S. R. (1981) Treatment of ununited tibial diaphyseal fractures with pulsing electromagnetic fields. *Journal of Bone and Joint Surgery* **63A,** 511–523

Charnley, J. (1961) *The Closed Treatment of Common Fractures,* 3rd edn. Edinburgh: Livingstone

Devas, M. (1975) *Stress Fractures.* Edinburgh, London, New York: Churchill Livingstone

Holden, C. E. A. (1979) The pathology and prevention of Volkmann's ischaemic contracture. *Journal of Bone and Joint Surgery* **61B,** 296–300

Lowe, L. W. (1981) Venous thrombosis and embolism. *Journal of Bone and Joint Surgery* **63B,** 155–167

McKibbin, B. (1978) The biology of fracture healing in long bones. *Journal of Bone and Joint Surgery* **60B,** 150–162

Müller, M. E., Allgöwer, M., Schneider, R. and Willeneger, H. (1979) *Manual of Internal Fixation,* 2nd edn. Trans. by J. Schatzker. Berlin, Heidelberg, New York: Springer-Verlag

Perkins, G. (1958) *Fractures and Dislocations.* London: Athlone Press

Roper, B. (1981) Editorial: Functional bracing of femoral fractures. *Journal of Bone and Joint Surgery* **63B,** 1–2 (see also 2 succeeding articles)

Sarmiento, A. and Latta, L. L. (1981) *Closed Functional Treatment of Fractures.* Berlin, Heidelberg, New York: Springer-Verlag

Watson-Jones, R. (1976) *Fractures and Joint Injuries,* 5th edn. Ed. by J. N. Wilson. Edinburgh: Churchill Livingstone

The Management of Major Accidents

The scene of the accident

Multiple accidents

The first duty of a doctor arriving at the scene of a major accident is to introduce calm and order into the prevailing chaos. His actions should be swift yet unhurried, cautious yet purposeful. Until the police or other authorities arrive he should assume control and, after rapidly assessing the situation, decide on priorities. If unskilled help is at hand messages are sent to the emergency services (ambulance, police and fire); the nearest accident centre is alerted and, where mobile operating theatres and surgical teams are available, they may need to be summoned.

The individual patient

Treatment of the individual patient begins as soon as possible. A useful sequence (modified to suit the circumstances) is: obtain access; ensure airway; examine; extricate; arrest haemorrhage; combat shock; splint fractures; and transport.

ACCESS
When a patient is trapped or buried, the objects covering him should be moved, rather than pulling him out from beneath them. Priority is given to freeing the head and trunk. If the patient is conscious he will need immediate reassurance.

AIRWAY
If the unconscious patient is breathing stertorously the angle of the jaw is pulled forwards and the head hyperextended; should the difficulty persist a finger is inserted into the mouth to ensure that breathing is not being obstructed by the tongue,

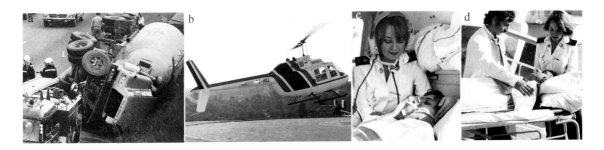

23.1 The major accident   (a) Major accidents call for (b) a rapid response, (c) expert care during transport and (d) a 24-hour medical service in the Accident Centre.

false teeth or any other foreign body. If, despite clearing the upper airway, the patient still cannot breathe freely, he may have a sucking wound of the chest wall, which should be covered with a dressing strapped firmly in position.

EXAMINATION

A detailed examination is neither practicable nor essential, but the pulse is felt, the respirations are observed, and the head, chest, abdomen and limbs, if accessible, are quickly palpated.

EXTRICATION

A patient with fractures should not be dragged forcibly from overlying impedimenta. When obstructions have been lifted he can be gently moved. Twisting and flexion must be avoided if there is the possibility of spinal injury.

HAEMORRHAGE

External bleeding can usually be stopped by pressure with a finger, forceps or a firm pad. Tourniquets are rarely necessary; if one must be used, a label stating the time of its application is attached to the patient in a prominent position.

SHOCK

Morphine is invaluable and, for a severely injured adult, it is probably best to give both 10 mg intravenously and 10 mg intramuscularly; again, adequate labelling is essential. Morphine should not be given to patients with abdominal or head injuries. Where facilities are available, intravenous fluids may be given (see later). *No food or fluids should be given by mouth*: if the patient is unconscious these may enter the trachea, and even if he is conscious their presence in the stomach increases the hazards of anaesthesia during the next few hours.

SPLINTAGE

A broken limb should be gently straightened by traction. A fractured arm is easily splinted by bandaging it to the trunk, and a leg by tying it to the other leg if this is intact. Ambulances should carry inflatable splints, and only occasionally are improvised splints needed; an umbrella, walking-stick, piece of wood or tubular steel is nearly always available. Open wounds are covered with a clean dressing.

TRANSPORT

To move a severely injured patient onto a stretcher at least two, but preferably three, people are required, so that he is transferred 'in one piece' without serious disturbance; this is particularly important with spinal fractures. The unconscious patient is best transported in the semi-prone position. The airway and pulse should be checked once more before the patient leaves in the ambulance.

Ambulances should be equipped with splints, dressings, airways, oxygen and transfusion apparatus. They should be in two-way radio communication with the accident unit. In difficult terrain helicopter ambulances are almost essential. Ambulance attendants are usually highly trained, but every effort should be made by the staff of the accident unit to keep them continually informed, up to date and interested in their work. Their observations on the patient's state of consciousness and general condition are invaluable.

Accident centres

Peripheral casualty services (cottage hospitals, health centres and first-aid posts) should deal only with minor injuries. Accident centres are quite different; they must be able to deal with any emergency – medical or surgical. Each centre should therefore be part of a general hospital; but it also needs the support of a central unit with

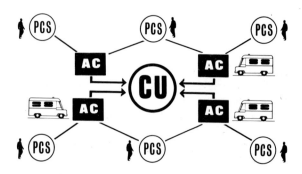

23.2 The organization A three-tier structure is needed: peripheral casualty services (PCS) are for minor injuries and the 'walking wounded'; accident centres (AC) must be able to cope with any emergency, but may need the support of a specialized central unit (CU).

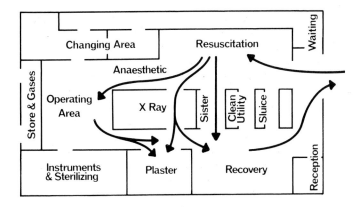

23.3 Plan of an accident centre Note (1) central positon of x-ray department; (2) open planning to permit a variety of flow patterns; (3) operating theatres, although not essential here, must be close by.

highly specialized services such as neurosurgery, thoracic surgery and dialysis. It is best designed on an open plan system permitting flexibility of use, and needs to be generously supplied with equipment for communications, patient transport and all forms of emergency care. Of particular importance is equipment for resuscitation, airway management, electrolyte investigations and radiology (portable equipment is inadequate and heavy duty equipment within the centre essential). Staffing also must be generous, but the leader need not be a surgeon. He must be expert in the diagnosis and management of emergencies, a born organizer, a natural diplomat and a dedicated enthusiast. Such individuals are rare; they deserve the status of bishops and the pay of pop singers.

The severely injured patient

The management of the severely injured patient is an urgent and complex task. The greatest problem is to decide on a sequence of procedures and to allot priorities. No rigid rules can apply to every patient and the account which follows aims at providing guidance for those with limited experience. The three essential phases of management, for ease of memory, may be expressed as revive, review and repair.

Revive

The term 'revive' implies rapid appraisal and urgent resuscitation. There are two causes of early death following an accident: (1) circulatory failure from bleeding and shock; (2) respiratory failure from airway obstruction, from paralysis of the respiratory centre (with head injuries), or from insufficient lung ventilation (with major chest injuries). The most urgent necessities are a clear airway, blood transfusion, the closure of a sucking chest wound and the immobilization of a flail segment of the chest wall.

Review

'Review' is a slightly more deliberate procedure. An attempt is made to find out if the patient is a diabetic, or is taking such drugs as steroids or anticoagulants. Then he is stripped, external bleeding arrested and a brief but orderly examination carried out. The head, chest, abdomen, spine and limbs are carefully but rapidly examined in turn. X-ray examination is frequently necessary for injuries of the chest, abdomen and pelvis; with head injuries x-rays are rarely helpful at this early stage, and with limb injuries major fractures are clinically apparent. Throughout the phase of review blood replacement is continuing, and, unless head or abdominal injuries contraindicate it, morphine is now given.

Repair

'Repair' is the term for the emergency operative procedures which resuscitation has made possible. The patient is anaesthetized and transfusion is continued. An orderly sequence is important. (1) Continued bleeding must be stopped; in order of importance are intracranial, intrathoracic and intra-abdominal bleeding. (2) Major chest injuries must be dealt with and this may necessitate tracheostomy. (3) Ruptured abdominal viscera must be repaired. (4) Open wounds are excised and dressed. (5) Fractures are splinted; where fractures are multiple, internal fixation may be necessary, but the temptation to surgical virtuosity should be resisted.

During and after these operations blood replacement is continued as necessary, with the patient's general condition and the central venous pressure as important guides. A fluid-balance chart is kept, and electrolyte balance maintained.

Shock

NEUROGENIC SHOCK
This occurs with painful injuries, emotional disturbances, or both. The blood volume is unchanged but its distribution is faulty, with excess in the non-essential circulation (splanchnic vessels and skeletal muscles) and insufficient in the essential circulation (cerebral and cardiac vessels).

OLIGAEMIC SHOCK
This is the result of bleeding, whether internal or external. The blood volume is reduced, but the harmful effects of this reduction are mitigated, again by redistribution: the peripheral and splanchnic vessels contract, so that a higher proportion of the reduced volume becomes available for the heart and brain. This compensatory mechanism may fail if the blood loss is great or rapid; the peripheral vessels then become dilated, the cardiac output and blood pressure drop and the circulation fails. This dangerous condition of peripheral vasodilatation is sometimes induced or hastened by heating the patient or giving him alcohol.

The bystander who faints at the sight of an accident is suffering from transient neurogenic shock. The injured person also is suffering from neurogenic shock but, because of blood loss, oligaemic shock may supervene. He becomes ill, apathetic and thirsty, his breathing shallow and rapid; the lips and skin are pale and the extremities feel cold and clammy. As compensation fails, the pulse becomes rapid and feeble while the blood pressure drops. Shock must not be diagnosed as purely neurogenic unless careful examination has failed to reveal any serious injury.

Treatment

Neurogenic shock is treated by elevating the legs, relieving pain and dispelling fear. If rapid recovery does not occur, the patient is suffering from oligaemic shock.

The treatment of oligaemic shock is urgent: the essentials are to arrest bleeding and to replace lost blood. Morphine (preferably given intravenously)

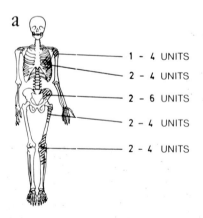

a

1 – 4 UNITS	
2 – 4 UNITS	
2 – 6 UNITS	
2 – 4 UNITS	
2 – 4 UNITS	

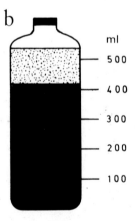

b

ml
500
400
300
200
100

23.4 Severe injuries – danger point (1)   (a) Range of probable blood loss in closed fractures. (b) From a 540 ml container the patient gets only 400–420 ml of actual blood – the rest is anticoagulant and space. *Moral* – The severely injured patient may lose more blood than you think, and get less; do not be afraid of overtransfusion.

is of great value, but must be withheld if there are head injuries or undiagnosed abdominal injuries. Giving oxygen and the early reduction and splintage of fractures are valuable. The intravenous injection of 100 mg of hydrocortisone sodium succinate may relieve a desperate situation, but vasopressor drugs are of doubtful value.

The essential feature of treatment, however, is early and adequate transfusion to restore the volume of circulating blood. Accurate blood grouping takes time, and group O Rh-negative blood may be used in emergency until cross-matched blood is available. Plasma and plasma-substitutes are of much less value; they should be used only as a stopgap and a specimen of blood for cross-matching must be taken first. (With burns, on the contrary, the shock is associated with an initial haemoconcentration, and plasma is the ideal transfusion fluid.)

It is important not only to give blood, but to give enough blood. Even with closed injuries there is far more bleeding into the tissues than is commonly appreciated. Two or three units may be lost with a single major limb fracture and up to 6 units with three major fractures; in trunk fractures with visceral damage, as much as half the blood volume may be lost. Rapid transfusion may be important, for which purpose a Martin pump is valuable. In the previously healthy patient 100 ml/min may be given until the blood pressure reaches 100 mm. With large transfusions the danger of introducing too much sodium citrate must be borne in mind, and countered by injecting the patient with a solution of calcium gluconate (1 g for each 500 ml of blood). If shock is not abating despite transfusion, concealed haemorrhage into the chest or abdomen is probable and must be treated.

Head injuries

The commonest head injury is concussion. It requires no special treatment beyond rest, but careful observation is necessary because compression (from intracranial haemorrhage or oedema) may supervene.

Examination

(1) The degree of impairment of consciousness is important. A history, usually obtained from the ambulance attendants, of a lucid interval between unconsciousness at the scene of the accident and unconsciousness on arrival at the hospital indicates rising intracranial pressure; so also does increasing depth of unconsciousness.

(2) The head is inspected for external wounds, depressed fracture and escaping cerebrospinal fluid. Gentle handling is vital; the patient with a head injury should be assumed also to have injured his cervical spine until the contrary is proved.

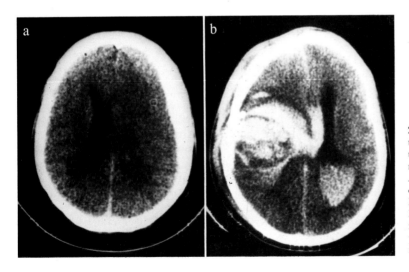

23.5 Head injuries – computerized tomography   'Cross-sections' through the skull obtained by CT scanning give invaluable information. (a) An extradural haematoma (right side of picture) has caused collapse of the lateral ventricle on that side. (b) A large intracerebral clot and surrounding oedema (left side of picture) has pushed the right lateral ventricle away from the midline.

(3) With generalized increase of intracranial pressure the breathing becomes stertorous, the pulse slow and bounding, and the pupils dilated. If the pupils become widely dilated and fixed, or flaccid limb paralysis becomes spastic, a dangerous level of intracranial pressure has been reached and its treatment is urgent.

(4) With a depressed fracture, or localized brain damage, the pupils may become unequal in size or the limbs on the two sides of the body unequal in tone. These signs also are a signal for urgent action, but it must be remembered that enlargement of one pupil may be the result of purely local damage to the eye or orbit.

(5) *Special investigations.* Carotid angiography, though valuable, is being supplanted by computerized tomography (CT scanning), which is safe and non-invasive. Lesions such as intra- or extracerebral haematomata, contusions and oedema can be diagnosed with precision, thus simplifying management.

Emergency treatment

(1) A clear airway is essential and the administration of oxygen is useful to lessen hypoxia, which increases cerebral congestion.

(2) Bleeding from the scalp can be arrested with artery forceps or a stitch. A depressed fracture with localizing signs needs to be elevated.

(3) Restlessness is difficult to control, because sedatives mask the important sign of deepening unconsciousness. A full bladder increases restlessness and should be emptied by catheterization.

(4) Generalized increase of intracranial pressure can sometimes be relieved by intravenous injection of hypertonic solutions, such as triple-strength plasma.

(5) A dangerous rise of intracranial pressure which is not relieved by the above measures may require craniotomy.

(6) The patient with a basal fracture and leaking cerebrospinal fluid is given antibiotics and instructed not to blow his nose.

(7) In all cases careful and regular observation is essential.

Respiratory obstruction

The injured and unconscious patient is in danger of suffocation. Respiratory obstruction, probably the commonest single cause of death soon after injury, is preventable. The respiratory passages may be obstructed by the tongue, dentures, blood, mucus or vomit. Breathing becomes laboured and stertorous, and the patient cyanosed.

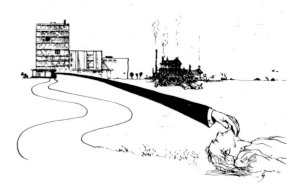

23.6 Severe injuries – danger point (2) This drawing (reproduced by kind permission of Mr R.S. Garden and the Editor of *Injury*) emphasizes the vital (literally) importance of a clear airway, and how it can usually be achieved.

Treatment

The obstruction must be removed immediately. If pulling the angle of the jaw forwards proves inadequate, a finger in the mouth is used to pull the tongue forwards or to dislodge and remove any other solid obstacle. Fluid is wiped out or aspirated with a sucker. Often these measures prove adequate and the insertion of a simple airway ensures comfortable breathing. If they fail, laryngoscopy or bronchoscopy may be necessary, but when the obstruction cannot be cleared by way of the mouth there should be no hesitation in performing immediate tracheostomy.

Chest injuries

Chest injuries may damage the rib cage, the lungs, the heart or the great vessels; precise diagnosis may be vital (literally). Clinical assessment must establish which (if any) of the following is present: (1) a simple fracture of one or two ribs; (2) multiple fractures with a flail segment or stove-in chest; (3) a pneumothorax – open or closed; (4) a haemothorax; (5) cardiac tamponade. Three warnings are important: (1) unconscious patients often have serious chest injuries; (2) small wounds may hide serious complications; and (3) pneumothorax can take many hours to develop, so repeated examination is necessary.

Examination

(1) The skin is inspected for open wounds (small ones are the most dangerous) and for bruising (which suggests a crushing injury). The shape of the chest also is noted; a stove-in chest may show obvious asymmetry.

(2) Fractured ribs or a stove-in segment can sometimes be palpated.

(3) Respiration is observed. Is the patient fighting for breath? During inspiration, if one side of the chest remains still, the lung on that side is probably collapsed; but if one side is sucked in, this paradoxical respiration is diagnostic of a flail segment.

(4) Percussion and auscultation may reveal signs of pulmonary collapse, fluid in the chest and mediastinal shift.

(5) X-rays are essential; they may show fractures, or a pleural effusion, or lung collapse and mediastinal displacement.

Emergency treatment

(1) With all severe chest injuries three measures are important: blood replacement (but not with crystalloid fluids, which aggravate pulmonary congestion); the administration of oxygen; and adequate analgesics (but not respiratory depressants).

(2) Open wounds that communicate with the pleural cavity cause a sucking pneumothorax and lung collapse. A moist swab strapped over the hole may suffice temporarily, but the wound should be securely stitched as soon as possible; an intercostal tube connected to an underwater seal allows the lung to expand.

(3) A tension pneumothorax occurs when there is no open wound but the injured lung leaks air into the pleural cavity. Increasing respiratory distress follows, with poor chest movements and absent breath sounds. If this lethal condition is even suspected, a needle should be inserted into the second interspace anteriorly, about 6 cm from the midline. This immediately relieves the tension. It can later be replaced by an intercostal catheter connected to an underwater seal, which is retained until the lung re-expands.

(4) Haemothorax (from a torn lung or blood vessel) can be diagnosed by withdrawing blood through a needle. The blood is drained by an intercostal catheter through a low intercostal space. Breathing exercises are encouraged.

(5) A stove-in chest with only moderate respiratory difficulty can be treated by strapping a large pack over the mobile segment and administering oxygen. More severe cases need endotracheal intubation and positive pressure ventilation; a chest drain connected to an underwater seal is essential in case there is an associated lung leak. (If ventilation is to be continued for several days a tracheostomy is needed.) The flail segment can be stabilized by rib traction (using wires or towel clips) or by internal fixation.

(6) Uncomplicated rib fractures need no treatment other than analgesics. The patient with multiple fractures and extensive bruising should, however, be kept in hospital until complications have been positively excluded.

Abdominal injuries

The most important abdominal injuries are ruptures of viscera and of blood vessels. There is a real danger that abdominal injuries may be overlooked, either because an unconscious patient can give no history, or because a conscious but shocked patient may not complain even with serious injury.

Examination

(1) The abdomen is inspected for perforating wounds, for bruising and to observe respiratory movements.

(2) Palpation may reveal localized tenderness, the boggy fullness of extensive bleeding, or board-like rigidity over a ruptured viscus. It must be remembered that considerable bleeding, especially if retroperitoneal, may not be detected on palpation, and rigidity may not develop despite a ruptured viscus if the patient is severely shocked.

(3) Auscultation tends to be forgotten but the complete absence of bowel sounds is an important sign of intra-abdominal damage.

(4) Percussion may disclose the presence of fluid, or of a decreased area of liver dullness due to gas from a ruptured viscus.

(5) Rectal and pelvic examination must not be omitted and, with lower abdominal injuries, the bladder, urethra and urine must be examined. An emergency urethrogram or intravenous pyelogram may be indicated.

(6) Intubation of the stomach is often wise; apart from the advantage of aspirating gastric contents prior to anaesthesia, the withdrawing of blood may suggest gastric injury.

(7) Peritoneal lavage is sometimes helpful, particularly in diagnosing bleeding from a ruptured spleen or liver.

Emergency treatment

(1) An open wound needs to be closed. A temporary dressing is sufficient and formal closure must not be performed if the integrity of the abdominal viscera is in doubt, for laparoscopy or laparotomy is then essential.

(2) Continued abdominal bleeding demands emergency transfusion and laparotomy. The patient with oligaemic shock who is not responding to transfusion is probably bleeding into his abdomen and, even if the signs are equivocal, exploration is justified.

(3) A ruptured viscus must be repaired when the patient has been resuscitated.

Burns

The patient with extensive burns suffers from neurogenic shock because of pain, and from oligaemic shock because (1) fluid exudes copiously from the burnt area, (2) fluid is lost into the tissues, and (3) red cells have been damaged. The amount of fluid loss varies with the area of the burn and can be assessed by a special formula (the rule of 9) or from pyrogram charts. Often the depth of the burn cannot be determined until superficial sloughs separate.

Emergency treatment

(1) Treatment of the shock is urgent. Morphine is given and fluid replacement begun. Every moment of delay in starting the transfusion makes the prognosis worse. For deep burns, whole blood is given; for superficial burns, plasma is used first, though blood usually becomes necessary later.

(2) With burns of the face or neck, immediate intubation or tracheostomy may be necessary.

(3) With chemical burns, the surface is gently washed. In all other cases the burnt area is not disturbed or treated with topical applications. If the environment is suitable the burn is left exposed, otherwise it is covered with sterile towels.

(4) If transfer to a special burns centre is unavoidably delayed, further measures become necessary. Fluid losses must continually be made good with blood, plasma, or plasma and saline solution as required. Antibiotics are started and sedation is continued. Metabolic requirements are met by oral feeding or, in children, intravenously. At least every 4 hours the patient is examined; the skin colour, pulse, blood pressure and urine output are noted. An indwelling catheter is useful in assessing the all-important fluid balance. In severe cases the blood haemoglobin, electrolytes and urea are examined 4-hourly and used as a guide to further treatment.

Further reading

Cole, W. H. and Puestow, C. B. (1972) *Emergency Care*, 7th edn. London: Butterworths

Ellis, M. (1970). *The Casualty Officer's Handbook*, 3rd edn. London: Butterworths

Keen, G. (1974) Chest injuries. *Annals of the Royal College of Surgeons of England* **54,** 124–131

Odling-Smee, W. and Crockard, A. (Ed.) (1981) *Trauma Care*. London, Toronto, Sydney: Academic Press; New York, San Francisco: Grune & Stratton

Tubbs, N. and London, P. S. (Ed.) (1980) *Topical Reviews in Accident Surgery*, vol. 1. Bristol: John Wright

I *Injuries of the shoulder and upper arm*

The great bugbear of upper limb injuries is stiffness – particularly of the shoulder, but sometimes of the elbow and hand as well. Two points should be constantly borne in mind: (1) in elderly patients it is often best to disregard the fracture and to concentrate on regaining movement; (2) whatever the injury, and however it is treated, the fingers should be exercised from the start.

Fractured clavicle

A fall on the outstretched hand breaks the clavicle; the outer fragment is pulled down by the weight of the arm and the inner half is held up by the sternomastoid muscle.

Special features

A subcutaneous lump is usually obvious and occasionally a sharp fragment threatens the skin. Though vascular complications are rare, it is prudent to feel the pulse and gently to palpate the root of the neck.

X-RAY
The fracture is usually in the middle third of the shaft, and is at right angles to the length of the bone. The outer fragment lies below the inner; often there is a separate central fragment.

Treatment

● REDUCE
Accurate reduction is neither possible nor essential. If displacement is considerable, pulling the patient's shoulders firmly backwards (without anaesthetic) may improve the position.

● HOLD
Axillary loops, linked posteriorly, or a figure-of-eight bandage, is customary though not always essential. But a sling must be worn, and is needed for about 3 weeks.

● EXERCISE
The elbow, wrist and fingers must be exercised from the start. Active shoulder movements should also be begun early; the patient feels reassured if the fracture is 'protected' by the physiotherapist's hand.

When the sling is discarded, full shoulder movements are quickly regained.

Complications

EARLY
Damage to vessels or nerves is very rare.

LATE
Non-union rarely occurs unless a surgeon has been unwise enough to operate on the fracture.

Malunion is invariable and leaves a lump; in a child the lump always disappears in time, and in an adult it usually does. A girl anxious to obtain a good cosmetic result quickly may be willing to undergo more drastic treatment: the fracture is manually reduced under anaesthesia and held reduced by a plaster cuirasse. The patient must remain in bed for 3 weeks.

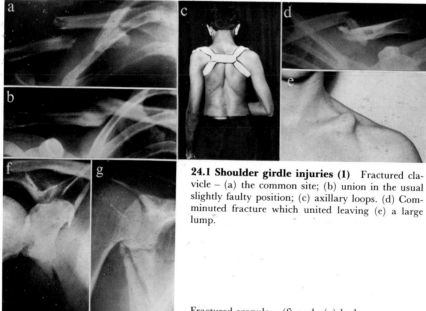

24.1 Shoulder girdle injuries (1) Fractured clavicle – (a) the common site; (b) union in the usual slightly faulty position; (c) axillary loops. (d) Comminuted fracture which united leaving (e) a large lump.

Fractured scapula – (f) neck; (g) body.

Stiffness of the shoulder is common but temporary; it results from fear of moving a fracture. Unless the fingers are exercised, they also may become stiff and take months to regain movement.

Fracture at either end

Occasionally the clavicle fractures near one or other end. The injury resembles a subluxation or dislocation of the nearby joint and is treated like such an injury.

Fractured scapula

The body of the scapula is fractured by a crushing force, which usually also fractures ribs and may dislocate the sternoclavicular joint. The neck of the scapula may be fractured by a blow or by a fall on the shoulder. The coracoid process may fracture across its base or be avulsed at the tip.

Special features

Shoulder movements are painful but possible. If breathing also is painful, then thoracic injury must be excluded.

X-RAY
The films may show a comminuted fracture of the body of the scapula, or a fractured scapular neck with the outer fragment pulled downwards by the weight of the arm. Occasionally a crack is seen in the acromion or the coracoid process.

Treatment

Reduction is impossible and unnecessary. The patient wears a sling for comfort, and from the start practises active exercises to the shoulder, elbow and fingers.

Acromioclavicular joint injuries

A fall on the shoulder tears the acromioclavicular ligaments, and upward subluxation of the clavicle may occur; more severe injury also tears the conoid and trapezoid ligaments, permitting dislocation.

Special features

The patient can usually point to the site of injury, where, unless obscured by swelling, an unduly high 'step' is visible; it is also palpable, but tender. Shoulder movements are limited.

X-RAY
The films show either a subluxation with only slight elevation of the clavicle, or dislocation with considerable elevation. Stress films (with the patient carrying a weight) are helpful.

Treatment

● REDUCE
Pressure on the outer end of the clavicle effects reduction.

● HOLD
Maintaining reduction by closed methods (felt pads over the olecranon and outer clavicle, held approximated with encircling strapping) is rarely effective and may cause skin necrosis. It is better to leave a subluxation untreated (wearing a sling for comfort) and to treat a dislocation (in a young patient) by internal fixation using threaded pins or a screw.

● EXERCISE
The fingers and elbow are exercised from the start, and the shoulder as soon as possible.

Complications

An unreduced subluxation causes no disability. An unreduced dislocation is ugly and sometimes affects function. If necessary, the outer 2.5 cm of the clavicle may be excised, or the clavicle anchored down to the coracoid process. Alternatively, the coracoid process may be detached and, with its muscles, fixed to the clavicle, thus stabilizing the joint.

Sternoclavicular dislocations

(a) Anterior

This rare injury is caused by a fall on the shoulder which forces the inner end of the clavicle forwards and upwards.

Special features

The dislocated medial end of the clavicle forms a prominent lump, which is tender. Shoulder movements may be painful.

X-RAY
The films are difficult to interpret, but enable dislocation to be distinguished from a fractured medial end of clavicle.

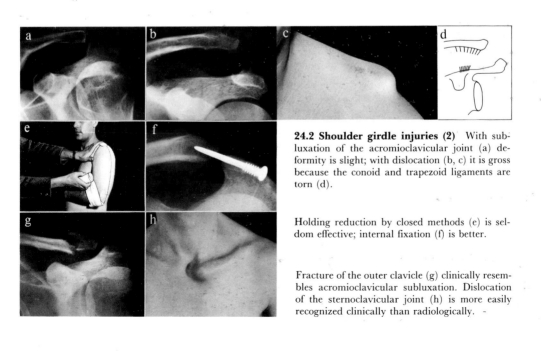

24.2 Shoulder girdle injuries (2) With subluxation of the acromioclavicular joint (a) deformity is slight; with dislocation (b, c) it is gross because the conoid and trapezoid ligaments are torn (d).

Holding reduction by closed methods (e) is seldom effective; internal fixation (f) is better.

Fracture of the outer clavicle (g) clinically resembles acromioclavicular subluxation. Dislocation of the sternoclavicular joint (h) is more easily recognized clinically than radiologically. -

Treatment

● REDUCE
With the patient anaesthetized, the medial end of the clavicle can be pushed into position.

● HOLD
Strapping, or a firm pad and bandage, is worth trying and, if effective (which is unlikely), is retained for 6 weeks; a sling is worn.

If the patient is prepared to accept a lump, a sling worn for a few days is the only treatment necessary. Full function will be regained, though not for several months. Internal fixation is unnecessary and can be dangerous (because of the large vessels behind the sternum).

● EXERCISE
Elbow and fingers are exercised from the start, and the shoulder as soon as possible.

Complications

An unreduced dislocation or a *recurrent dislocation*, if troublesome, may be held down using subclavius as a tenodesis (Burrows, 1951).

(b) Posterior

Backward subluxation of the inner end of the clavicle is very rare; it results from a direct blow. Ribs are broken, shock is profound, and dangerous pressure on the trachea or innominate vein may develop quickly. Reduction is urgent; the medial end of the clavicle is grasped with bone forceps and pulled forwards.

Anterior dislocation of the shoulder

This common injury is caused by a fall on the hand. The humerus is driven forward, tearing the capsule or avulsing the glenoid labrum. Occasionally the posterolateral part of the head is crushed. Rarely, the acromion process levers the head downwards and luxatio erecta (with the hand pointing upwards) results; nearly always the arm then drops, bringing the head to its subcoracoid position.

Special features

The patient supports his arm, which is held abducted and appears too long. The contour is angular, because of the unduly prominent acromion process and the flat deltoid muscle. The humeral head is difficult to feel unless the axilla is palpated. Shoulder movements are impossible.

Note   The limb must always be tested for nerve and vessel injury.

X-RAY
Even if the dislocation is obvious, x-rays are taken to see if a fracture coexists.

Treatment

● REDUCE
Under anaesthesia with full relaxation, reduction is generally easy; an assistant pulls on the arm in abduction while the surgeon thumbs the head into place.

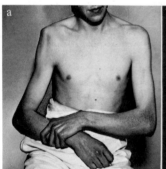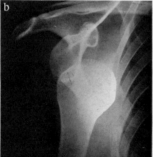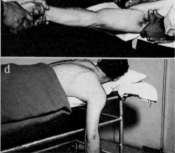

24.3 Shoulder dislocations – anterior (1)   (a, b) Anterior dislocation of the shoulder. (c, d) Two methods of reduction.

Even without anaesthesia, however, reduction is often possible, and three methods are available. (1) The patient lies prone on a couch with his injured arm hanging vertically for a few minutes; reduction may occur spontaneously, or then be easily achieved. (2) Hippocrates' method: the surgeon places his stockinged foot in the patient's axilla, pulls on the arm, and levers the head of the humerus into position. It is easier if an assistant pulls on the arm while the surgeon thumbs the head back into place. (3) Kocher's method: the surgeon pulls on the flexed elbow, rotates the humerus laterally, then adducts it while rotating it medially.

An x-ray picture is taken to confirm reduction and exclude a fracture.

● HOLD
When the patient is fully awake, active abduction is gently tested; if abduction is impossible, there may be a circumflex nerve palsy or supraspinatus tendon avulsion. The complication is noted, but the treatment in any event is a sling for 2 or 3 weeks.

● EXERCISE
Elbow and finger movements are started at once. Shoulder movements are encouraged, but for 3 weeks lateral rotation should not be combined with abduction.

Complications

EARLY
A torn supraspinatus tendon should be recognized early, although treatment (surgical reattachment) is rarely advisable.

Nerve injury is common and usually affects the circumflex nerve. It should be recognized before reduction by demonstrating a small patch of anaesthesia over the deltoid muscle, or soon after

reduction by the patient's inability to contract the muscle. The lesion is usually a neurapraxia which recovers spontaneously, though this may take many months.

Fractures are sometimes associated. (1) The greater tuberosity may be sheared off during dislocation. It usually falls into place during reduction, and no special treatment is then required. If it remains displaced, surgical reattachment is feasible but rarely needed. (2) The neck of the humerus may fracture with the initial injury or during unskilled reduction. The combined lesion is known as a fracture-dislocation. The detached head remains dislocated and capsized; it may undergo avascular necrosis. Closed reduction is attempted, using the same method as for an uncomplicated dislocation, and if it succeeds, treatment is similar. If closed reduction fails, open reduction should be attempted only in the young, for it is difficult and dangerous; in the elderly, it is better to leave the dislocation and to try to regain some movement.

LATE
Following dislocation, the joint may remain unduly stiff, or unstable (recurrent dislocation). These complications are considered separately.

Joint stiffness after dislocation

There are two reasons why, after dislocation, a shoulder may fail to regain full movement.

Immobilization in the sling position

After a shoulder injury the arm is usually rested in a sling, which necessarily holds the shoulder in medial rotation. Damaged capsule or muscle, if splinted in this position, soon loses the ability to stretch, especially in patients over the age of 40 years. There is consequent loss of lateral rotation, which automatically limits abduction.

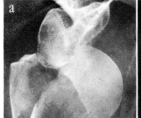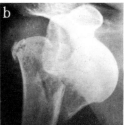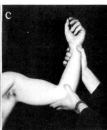

24.4 Shoulder dislocations – anterior (2) complications Associated fractures of (a) greater tuberosity; (b) neck of humerus. (c) The 'apprehension test' for recurrent dislocation.

Treatment   Active exercises can usually cure stiffness if immobilization has not been prolonged. They are practised vigorously, bearing in mind that full abduction is not possible until lateral rotation has been regained. Manipulation under anaesthesia is advised only if progress has halted and at least 6 months have elapsed since injury. Lateral rotation should be restored before abduction, and the manipulations should be gentle and repeated rather than forceful.

Unreduced dislocation

Surprisingly, a dislocation of the shoulder sometimes remains undiagnosed.

Treatment   Closed reduction is worth attempting up to 6 weeks after injury; manipulation later may fracture the bone or tear vessels or nerves.

Operative reduction is indicated after 6 weeks only in the young, because it is difficult, dangerous and followed by prolonged stiffness. An anterior approach is used, and the vessels and nerves are carefully identified before the dislocation is reduced. 'Active neglect' summarizes the treatment of unreduced dislocation in the elderly. The dislocation is disregarded and gentle active movements are encouraged. Moderately good function is often regained.

Recurrent dislocation

If an anterior dislocation tears the shoulder capsule, repair occurs spontaneously and the dislocation does not recur; but if, instead, the glenoid labrum is detached, repair is less likely and recurrence common. Bandaging the arm to the side after reducing the acute dislocation does not seem to influence the outcome. Detachment of the labrum occurs particularly in young patients, and if at injury a bony defect has been gouged out of the posterolateral aspect of the humeral head, then recurrence is even more likely.

The history is diagnostic. The patient complains that the shoulder dislocates with relatively trivial everyday actions. Often he can reduce the dislocation himself. Any doubt as to diagnosis is quickly resolved by one simple test: if the patient's arm is passively placed behind the coronal plane in a position of abduction and lateral rotation, his immediate resistance and apprehension are pathognomonic.

Treatment

Conservative treatment is useless. An operation which uses an anterior approach to the shoulder is almost uniformly successful. *Bristow's, Bankart's* and the *Putti–Platt* operation are described.

OPERATIONS
A vertical incision along the deltopectoral groove is the easiest but may leave an unsightly scar; an axillary approach is feasible though more difficult. The deltoid and pectoralis major muscles are separated, exposing the coracoid process; this is divided near its base and reflected downwards with its attached muscles. A vertical incision is made through subscapularis and the joint capsule; through this the front of the scapular neck is rawed and the coracoid process screwed to the raw area (Bristow's operation). Movements can safely begin within a few days, but a sling for 5 weeks is wise.

Many other operations using the same approach are described, the best known being Bankart's (the labrum and capsule are reattached via drill holes through the anterior edge of the glenoid), and the Putti–Platt (the capsule and subscapularis are each sutured with 2 cm of overlap). After either procedure the coracoid process is replaced and the arm bandaged to the side for 4 weeks.

Recurrent subluxation

This is fairly common and often not diagnosed. Following an initial acute dislocation, the patient complains of recurrent episodes of sudden pain and 'paralysis' of the shoulder. Disability may be considerable and require operation as for dislocation.

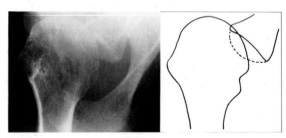

24.5 Recurrent subluxation   X-ray showing anterior subluxation; the humeral head is riding on the lip of the glenoid.

Voluntary dislocation

Occasionally someone discovers that the trick of habitually dislocating a lax shoulder (in any direction) can win friends and influence people. A strong admonition is better than a strong operation.

Posterior dislocation of the shoulder

This commonly missed injury is not a complete dislocation but a fracture-subluxation. It is usually caused by forced internal rotation of the abducted arm or by a direct blow on the front of the shoulder. It should always be suspected after an epileptic fit or an electric shock.*

Special features

The diagnosis is frequently missed because, in the anteroposterior film, the humeral head may seem to be in contact with the glenoid. But clinically the condition is unmistakable because the arm is held in medial rotation and is locked in that position. The front of the shoulder looks flat with a prominent coracoid, but swelling may obscure this deformity; seen from above, however, the posterior displacement is usually apparent.

X-RAY
In the anteroposterior film the humeral head, because it is medially rotated, looks abnormal in shape (like an electric light bulb). A lateral film is essential; it shows posterior subluxation and sometimes a piece gouged out of the humeral head.

Treatment

● REDUCE   The arm is pulled and rotated laterally, while the head of the humerus is pushed forwards.

● HOLD   If reduction feels stable a sling is enough; otherwise the shoulder is held widely abducted and laterally rotated in a plaster spica for 3 weeks.

● EXERCISE   Shoulder movement is regained by active exercises.

Complications

UNREDUCED DISLOCATION
Up to about 8 weeks from dislocation open reduction is worth while; the posterior approach has the advantage of permitting capsular repair and reefing in the hope of preventing recurrence. Late dislocations, especially in the elderly, are best left, but movement is encouraged.

RECURRENT DISLOCATION
The posterior capsule can be repaired with overlap; if this is combined with a posterior bone block and the shoulder is held abducted and laterally rotated for 6 weeks, then further recurrence is less likely. An alternative operation is to approach the shoulder from in front, detach the subscapularis at its insertion and fix this tendon securely in the defect on the humeral head; muscle action draws the humerus forwards and keeps it reduced.

Fractured neck of humerus

The patient falls on the outstretched hand, fracturing the surgical neck; the upthrust may shear off the greater tuberosity. The injury is common in the elderly, not uncommon in adolescents, but rare between these ages.

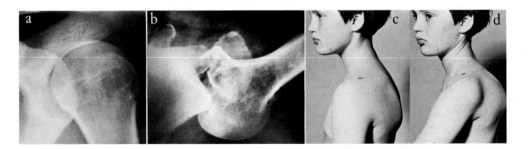

24.6 Shoulder dislocations – posterior   (a) The anteroposterior view may look almost normal, but (b) the lateral view shows obvious subluxation. (c, d) Habitual (voluntary) dislocation: the clue is the unconcerned expression.

*Electric shock/Epileptic fit + Painful shoulder = Posterior dislocation.

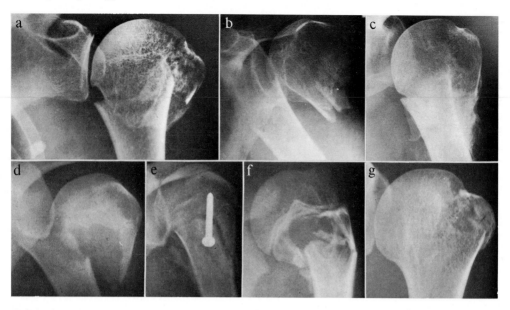

24.7 Fractures of the upper humerus   (a) The common impacted fracture of the neck. (b) A severely displaced fracture which, treated only with a sling, has united (c) in good position. (d) Fracture-separation of the upper humeral epiphysis with gross displacement which, very unusually, needed (e) open reduction. (f) In a young child, fracture is rare except through a cyst. (g) Fractured greater tuberosity, usually associated with a dislocation.

Special features

Because the fragments are often impacted, a large tell-tale bruise may be the first sign of the fracture – swelling and painful movement having previously been regarded as a 'sprain' (though shoulder sprains are rare).

X-RAY

In the elderly, a transverse fracture extends across the surgical neck, and often the greater tuberosity also is fractured. The shaft is usually impacted into the head in an abducted position. Occasionally no impaction occurs and the shaft may shift medially.

In adolescents, fracture-separation of the upper humeral epiphysis occurs; the shaft shifts upwards and forwards; the head, with a large triangular piece of the metaphysis attached, remains in position.

In young children, fracture through the upper humerus is rare except through a solitary cyst.

Treatment

● REDUCE

Usually reduction is unnecessary, and with impaction in the elderly it is unwise. But with considerable displacement in the adolescent approaching skeletal maturity, or in the young adult, reduction is worth while, either by manipulation or, very occasionally, by open operation.

● HOLD

Only a sling is necessary, whether or not reduction has been attempted. The weight of the arm tends to correct displacement. Union occurs in 3 weeks and consolidation in 6 weeks.

● EXERCISE

Pendulum exercises of the shoulder are begun at once, and the patient is encouraged to abduct the arm actively as soon as possible. In the elderly it is especially important to concentrate on regaining shoulder movements.

NOTE   Neer (1970) describes two-part, three-part and four-part proximal humeral fractures: two-part fractures are treated closed; three-part fractures may need open reduction; four-part fractures may suffer avascular necrosis and prosthetic replacement is advocated.

Complications

Stiffness of the shoulder is common and important, but is minimized by early and persistent exercises. Unlike a frozen shoulder, the stiffness is maximal at the outset.

Malunion is not uncommon. In the elderly it causes little disability; in the young adolescent the bone grows straight.

Fractured greater tuberosity

The greater tuberosity may sustain a 'direct' injury when the patient falls on the abducted arm, and the tuberosity impinges against the acromion process; the fracture is common in association with a dislocated shoulder. Occasionally an 'indirect' or avulsion fracture occurs in a young adult who is trying to save himself from falling, when the action of the supraspinatus muscle is resisted by an obstacle; the tuberosity is then pulled off.

Special features

The only notable feature, apart from swelling and local tenderness, is that abduction is severely limited and the attempt painful.

X-RAY
The tuberosity is usually undisplaced; it is demarcated from the shaft by a fracture line, or is comminuted. Occasionally the tuberosity is avulsed by the supraspinatus tendon; it is pulled upwards and appears as a thin slice of bone just under the acromion process.

Treatment

In the absence of displacement, reduction is unnecessary; a sling is worn for a week or two. The rare displaced avulsion fracture is best reduced operatively and the fragment fixed back with a screw; a sling for 3 weeks is advisable. In all cases stiffness must be avoided; it is best to begin gentle pendulum exercises as soon as possible.

Fractured shaft of humerus

A fall on the hand may twist the humerus, causing a spiral fracture. A fall on the elbow with the arm abducted may hinge the bone, causing a slightly oblique or transverse fracture. A heavy blow on the arm causes a fracture which is either transverse or grossly comminuted.

Special features

Active extension of the fingers should be examined, since the radial nerve is occasionally damaged. The usual features of a fracture – swelling, bruising, tenderness and abnormal movement – are, of course, also present.

X-RAY
The site of the fracture, its line (transverse, spiral or comminuted) and any displacement are readily seen. The possibility that the fracture may be pathological should be remembered.

Treatment

● REDUCE
Provided it is supported in a wrist sling, the weight of the arm is usually sufficient to effect reduction.

● HOLD
The continuous pull of gravity is also capable of holding reduction while union proceeds; but it is difficult to keep the arm vertical when sitting or lying, and the fracture tends to angulate. Consequently support is advisable. A U-slab of plaster can be bandaged onto the arm (with the loop of the U over the shoulder for high fractures and under the elbow for low ones). This can be worn continuously until the fracture is united; but the patient is more comfortable and uses the limb better if, after only 1 week, the plaster is replaced by a functional brace, such as a removable prefabricated 'sleeve' of polypropylene held together with Velcro straps.

Spiral fractures unite in about 6 weeks; the other varieties take 4 or 6 weeks longer. Once united, only a sling is needed until the fracture is consolidated.

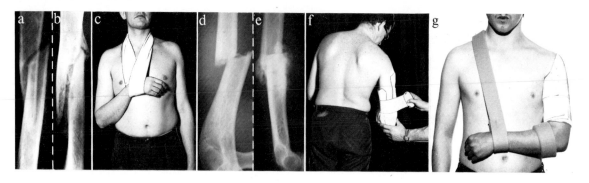

24.8 Fractured shaft of humerus – closed treatment   (a) This spiral fracture united in 6 weeks (b); the only 'splint' was (c) a wrist sling.
A transverse fracture, such as (d), takes a little longer to unite (e); it is less stable and the patient is more comfortable with (f) a U-slab of plaster or (g) a functional brace made of polypropylene.

Internal fixation   is indicated if closed treatment is impracticable because of associated soft-tissue damage or injuries elsewhere. The fracture can be fixed by plating (the radial nerve must be found and protected), or by intramedullary nailing.

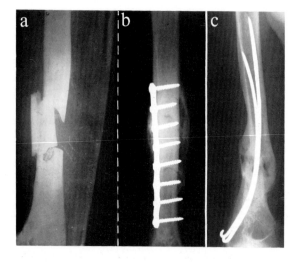

24.9 Fractured shaft of humerus – open treatment   (a) This segmental fracture was treated by (b) plating. Rush nails (c) are easier but the fixation is less stable. Neither method is recommended except in special circumstances.

● EXERCISE
The wrist and fingers are exercised from the start. The patient is taught to contract the elbow flexors and extensors actively. Pendulum exercises of the shoulder are begun within a week, but active abduction of the shoulder is postponed until the fracture is clinically and radiologically consolidated.

Complications

EARLY
Radial nerve palsy   is usually temporary. A 'lively' splint is used to support the wrist and hand while recovery is awaited. If recovery does not occur by 6 weeks, the nerve should be explored; if divided, it can be repaired, but tendon transfers may ultimately be required.

LATE
Delayed union   may occur in transverse fractures, especially if excessive traction has been used (e.g. a hanging cast) or if the patient has not actively exercised the elbow flexors and extensors.

Non-union   may follow. The dangerous combination is incomplete union and a stiff joint. If elbow or shoulder movements are forced before consolidation, the humerus refractures, and non-union may occur.

The treatment of established non-union is operative. The bone ends are freshened, bone chips packed around them and an intramedullary nail is inserted or a plate screwed on.

Joint stiffness   may be minimized by early activity, but transverse fractures (in which shoulder abduction is dangerous) may limit shoulder movement for several months.

II *Injuries of the elbow and forearm*

Elbow fractures in children differ from those in adults. Beneath the heading of each fracture is indicated whether it occurs in childhood or in adult life.

Supracondylar fracture

(a) With posterior displacement (children)

This common injury is caused by a fall on the hand with the elbow bent. The humerus breaks just above the condyles. The distal fragment, with the forearm, is pushed backwards and (because the forearm is usually in full pronation) twisted inwards.

Special features

The child holds the forearm with his other hand; unless obscured by swelling the deformity is usually apparent. An x-ray is mandatory, so that it is unnecessary (and cruel) to feel or move the fracture. It is, however, essential to feel the pulse, and wise to examine the hand for evidence of nerve injury.

X-RAY
The lateral film shows the fracture line proximal to the growth plate and running obliquely downwards and forwards; usually the distal fragment is shifted backwards and tilted backwards. The anteroposterior view often shows that the fragment is also shifted and tilted sideways and is twisted, usually medially. (The anteroposterior film may be unobtainable without causing pain; if so, it is postponed until the child is anaesthetized prior to reduction.)

Treatment

● REDUCE
Reduction must be carried out methodically with the child relaxed under anaesthesia. The uninjured arm should first be examined to assess the carrying angle, and to decide how far the arm and forearm together rotate at the shoulder.
(1) With one hand the surgeon then pulls on the injured forearm with the elbow 20 degrees flexed; he maintains traction for 1 minute. (2) Without releasing traction he grasps the distal fragment with his other hand and corrects sideways shift, tilt and twist. (3) He then flexes the elbow while pushing the lower humerus forwards with his thumb. The intact triceps prevents overreduction. (4) The radial pulse is then palpated. If it cannot be felt, the elbow must be extended a few degrees until the pulse returns, then a further 10 degrees for safety. (5) Anteroposterior and lateral films are taken to confirm reduction. The elbow must not be straightened; the anteroposterior film is taken through the flexed upper forearm. Slight shift may be accepted, but tilt or twist should be fully corrected. If necessary, the manipulations are repeated.

Open reduction (held by two Kirschner wires) has been advocated but is difficult and hazardous. If an acceptable position cannot be obtained by manipulation, or if, with the

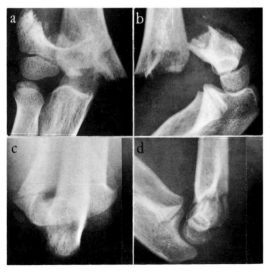

24.10 Supracondylar fractures (1) (a, b) This considerably displaced fracture was reduced (c, d) by the method shown in Fig. 24.11. Note that the anteroposterior view in (c) is taken with the elbow flexed.

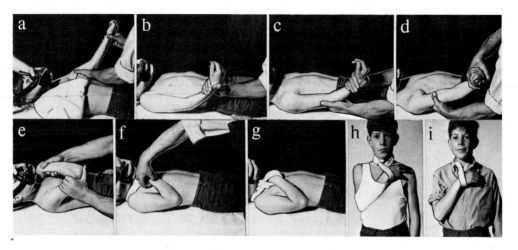

24.11 Supracondylar fractures (2) – treatment of displaced fracture   (a) The uninjured arm is examined first; (b) traction on the fractured arm; (c) correcting lateral shift and tilt; (d) correcting rotation; (e) correcting backward shift and tilt; (f) feeling the pulse; (g) the elbow is kept well flexed while x-ray films are taken; (h) for the first 3 weeks the arm is kept under the vest; after this (i) it is outside the vest.

elbow flexed as little as 90 degrees, the pulse is obliterated, then Dunlop traction can be used: the child lies supine with the shoulder abducted and the elbow nearly straight; a sling and weights hold the lower humerus; skin traction is applied to the forearm via a metal frame fixed to the bed.

● HOLD

A collar and cuff is applied to hold the elbow flexed. The more the elbow is flexed, the more stable is reduction, and during the next few days, as swelling subsides, the link between the collar and the cuff is tightened, provided the pulse remains palpable.

Occasionally the elbow cannot be sufficiently flexed without obliterating the pulse. A less flexed position, at which the pulse is palpable, must be accepted, and a posterior plaster slab is used in addition to the collar and cuff. The slab extends two-thirds of the way round the limb, from below the shoulder to above the wrist, and is held on with a crêpe bandage. A few days later the plaster is removed, the elbow flexed further and x-rays are taken; occasionally remanipulation proves necessary.

Union takes 3 weeks; during this time the hand must not be taken out of the cuff and the limb is kept beneath the shirt. For the succeeding 3 weeks (until consolidation) the limb is supported outside the clothing.

● EXERCISE

For the first 3 weeks, only finger and wrist movements are practised. After that time the child may take his hand out of the cuff during supervised activities, such as washing, dressing and writing. Elbow flexion is encouraged, but not extension, which returns gradually with use. Passive movements are prohibited at all times; the elbow must never be pulled, pushed or passively stretched by carrying weights.

Note   Occasionally a supracondylar fracture occurs with little or no displacement. Reduction is unnecessary and the child only needs a sling for 3 weeks.

Complications

EARLY

Volkmann's ischaemia   is the danger. Undue pain, plus any one positive sign (absent pulse, tense tender forearm, pain on passive extension of the fingers, or blunted sensation) demands urgent action (page 356).

Nerve injuries   are common, but usually recover spontaneously.

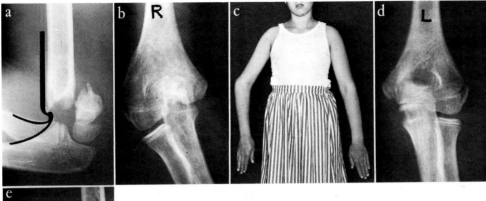

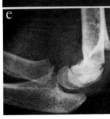

24.12 Supracondylar fractures (3) · The most serious complication is arterial damage (a) leading to Volkmann's ischaemia. (b, c, d) Varus deformity of right elbow following poor reduction (rotation was never corrected). (e) Supracondylar fracture with anterior displacement is uncommon (compare the position with (a) above).

LATE

Myositis ossificans is a possibility. If, at 3 or 4 weeks, movement is decreasing instead of increasing, the elbow should immediately be rested in a plaster gutter.

Elbow stiffness, even without myositis, is common, and extension in particular may take months to return. It must not be hurried. Passive movements (which include carrying weights) or forced movements are prohibited.

Malunion is common. With backward or sideways shift, the humerus gradually grows straight. Forward or backward tilt may limit flexion or extension, but consequent disability is slight.

Uncorrected sideways tilt or rotation is more important. It may lead to a varus deformity, which is ugly and sometimes requires osteotomy; or rarely to a valgus deformity, which may cause late ulnar palsy. Epiphyseal damage is often blamed for these deformities, but usually faulty reduction is responsible.

Note Very occasionally, in babies (especially battered babies) or young children the entire distal humerus is displaced posteromedially. It should be reduced by closed manipulation under anaesthesia and held for 3 weeks in an above-elbow plaster with the elbow at 90 degrees and the forearm pronated.

(b) With anterior displacement (children)

This rare injury is caused by a fall on the hand with the elbow straight. The humerus breaks just above the growth disc and the fragment is tilted forwards.

Special features

Bruising and swelling may be considerable. It is important to test for neurovascular complications.

X-RAY

The fracture line is oblique and is lower posteriorly. To assess the forward tilt a line may be drawn down the front of the humeral shaft; normally its projection bisects the epiphysis.

Treatment

● REDUCE   The arm is pulled, the elbow fully straightened and the carrying angle restored.

● HOLD   A posterior slab is bandaged on, holding the elbow straight. After 3 weeks the slab is removed.

● EXERCISE   The child is allowed to regain elbow flexion gradually.

Complications

If the fracture has not been reduced, extension remains limited but the disability is rarely severe.

T-shaped and Y-shaped fractures (adults)

A fall on the point of the elbow drives the olecranon process upwards, splitting the condyles apart.

Special features

Swelling is often considerable and the arm is held immobile.

X-RAY

The fracture extends from the lower humerus into the elbow joint; it may be T-shaped, Y-shaped or comminuted. Often the condyles are separated, and either may be tilted in any direction.

Treatment

ORTHODOX TREATMENT

The forearm is pulled in the straight position and the bones are moulded into shape. A posterior plaster slab, bandaged on with the elbow a little straighter than a right angle, is retained for 3 weeks. The shoulder, wrist and fingers are exercised from the start. When the plaster is removed the patient tries to regain elbow flexion.

TREATMENT BY ACTIVITY

The orthodox treatment usually leaves a permanently stiffish elbow, and if flexion is much limited, the disability is considerable. If comminution has occurred, it is probably better to disregard the fracture and to concentrate on the joint. The arm is held above a right angle in a collar and cuff. Active movements are encouraged, and often mould the fragments into reasonable position. The final range is usually better than expected.

OPERATIVE TREATMENT

A high degree of skill is needed and may be rewarding, but considerable stiffness is not uncommon. Through a posterior approach the ulnar nerve is identified, the trochlea fixed in position, then the remainder of the jig-saw is pieced together and held with Kirschner wires or screws.

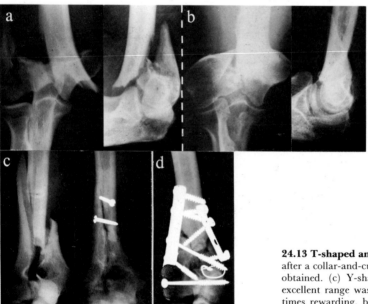

24.13 T-shaped and Y-shaped fractures (a) Before and (b) after a collar-and-cuff plus activity – reasonable movement was obtained. (c) Y-shaped fracture fixed with two screws – an excellent range was obtained; (d) surgical virtuosity is sometimes rewarding, but not always – this ended up with a stiff elbow.

Fracture-separation of lateral condylar epiphysis (children)

The child falls on the hand. A large fragment, which includes the lateral condyle, breaks off and is pulled upon by the attached wrist extensors. In severe injuries probably the elbow dislocates posterolaterally; the condyle is 'capsized' by muscle pull and remains capsized while the elbow reduces spontaneously.

Special features

Because the dorsiflexors arise from the lateral condyle, active wrist dorsiflexion is painful (as, of course, are elbow movements). Tenderness may be confined to the lateral side.

X-RAY
With so-called incomplete fractures displacement is slight; comparison with films of the normal elbow is useful. The commoner complete fracture is often grossly displaced and may carry with it a triangular piece of the metaphysis.

Treatment

● REDUCE
Accurate reduction is important. Under anaesthesia the forearm is pushed posterolaterally, as if

to reproduce the dislocation, and then pulled forwards again. This manoeuvre feels unconvincing but is often successful.

If closed reduction fails, a complete fracture should be reduced open. The fragment is exposed, replaced in position and held with catgut sutures, a small screw or pins.

● HOLD
A posterior plaster slab is applied, extending from below the shoulder to just short of the knuckles, with the elbow just above a right angle and the wrist dorsiflexed (to relax the extensor muscles). After 3 weeks, the plaster is removed but a collar and cuff is worn for a further 3 weeks.

● EXERCISE
The fingers and shoulder are exercised from the start. Elbow and wrist movements are regained later.

Complications

Non-union and malunion　If the condyle is left capsized non-union is inevitable; with growth the elbow becomes increasingly valgus, and ulnar nerve palsy is then likely to develop, requiring

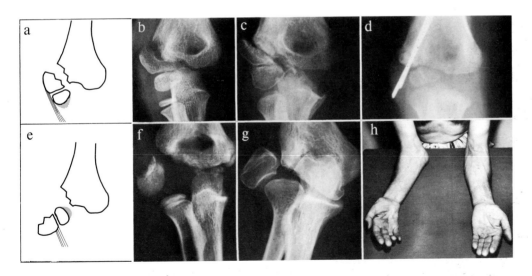

24.14 Fractured lateral condyle (a, b) A large fragment of bone and cartilage is avulsed; even with reasonable reduction, union is not inevitable (c), and open reduction with fixation (d) is often wise. (e, f) Sometimes the condyle is capsized; if left unreduced non-union is inevitable (g) and a valgus elbow with delayed ulnar palsy (h) the likely sequel.

anterior transposition. Even minor displacements sometimes lead to non-union, and even slight malunion may lead to ulnar palsy; it is for these reasons that open reduction (and internal fixation) is often preferred.

Recurrent dislocation   Occasionally condylar displacement results in posterolateral dislocation of the elbow. The only effective treatment is reconstruction of the bony and soft tissues on the lateral side.

Fractured capitulum (adults)

The patient falls on the hand, usually with the elbow straight. The anterior half of the capitulum and the trochlea are broken off and displaced proximally.

Special features

Fullness in front of the elbow is the most notable feature. Flexion is grossly restricted.

X-RAY
In the lateral view the capitulum is seen in front of the lower humerus, and the radial head no longer points directly towards it.

Treatment

● REDUCE
While the arm is being pulled straight an attempt is made to thumb the fragment back into position.

If closed reduction fails operation is essential, or flexion will remain permanently limited. The elbow is approached from the outer side and the

capitulum sutured in position with catgut; but if there is difficulty the fragment can be removed.

● HOLD
A collar and cuff is sufficient.

● EXERCISE
The shoulder, wrist and fingers must be exercised from the start. Elbow movements are regained when active movement is comfortable.

Separation of medial epicondylar epiphysis (adolescents)

The medial epicondylar epiphysis begins to ossify at the age of about 5 and fuses to the shaft at about 16; between these ages it may be avulsed by a fall on the hand. The epiphysis is pulled distally by the attached wrist flexors. With more severe injuries the joint dislocates laterally and the epiphysis is pulled into the joint. The elbow may remain dislocated, or may reduce spontaneously and trap the epicondyle.

Special features

If the elbow is still dislocated, deformity is of course obvious. But even without dislocation the diagnosis should be suspected if injury is followed by pain on the medial side. Sensation in the ulnar fingers should be tested to exclude nerve damage.

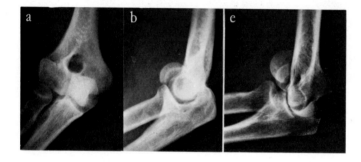

24.15 Fractured capitulum (a, b) Anteroposterior and lateral views showing proximal displacement and tilting; in (c) the capitulum has been sheared off vertically.

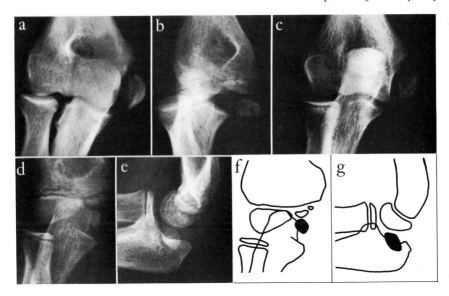

24.16 Fractured medial epicondyle   (a) Avulsion of the medial epicondyle following valgus strain. (b) Avulsion associated with dislocation of the elbow – (c) after reduction. Sometimes the epicondylar fragment is trapped in the joint (d, e); the serious nature of the injury is then liable to be missed unless the surgeon specifically looks for the trapped fragment, which is emphasized in the tracings (f, g).

X-RAY

In the anteroposterior view, the medial epicondylar epiphysis may be tilted or shifted downwards; if the joint is dislocated the epiphysis lies distal to the lower humerus. A lateral view may show the epicondyle looking like a loose body in the joint.

● HOLD

A collar and cuff is worn for 3 weeks.

● EXERCISE

The shoulder is exercised from the start and elbow range is regained when the collar and cuff has been removed.

Treatment

● REDUCE

Minor displacement may be disregarded; but an epicondyle trapped in the joint must be freed. Manipulation with the elbow pulled into valgus is sometimes successful. Another possible manoeuvre is to hold the fingers extended and apply a faradic current to the forearm flexors, which may then pull the fragment out of the joint. If closed methods fail, operation is essential. An incision is made on the medial aspect of the elbow, and the ulnar nerve, which may be kinked into the joint, is carefully exposed. The epicondyle is replaced in position or excised and the ulnar nerve transposed to the front of the elbow.

Complications

EARLY

Ulnar nerve damage   is not uncommon, but recovery is usual unless the nerve is left kinked in the joint.

LATE

Stiffness   of the elbow is common and extension often limited for months; but provided movement is not forced, it will eventually return.

Late ulnar nerve palsy   may follow friction in the roughened bony groove.

Fractured neck of radius
(children)

The child falls on the outstretched hand while the elbow is slightly valgus.

Special features

Painful forearm rotation and tenderness on the lateral side are the only notable features.

X-RAY

The fracture line is transverse. It is either situated immediately distal to the growth disc, or there is true separation of the epiphysis with a triangular fragment of shaft. The proximal fragment is tilted distally, forwards and outwards. Sometimes the upper end of the ulna is also fractured.

Treatment

● REDUCE

Up to about 15 degrees of tilt is acceptable. Beyond that reduction is needed. The arm is pulled into extension and slight varus. With his thumb the surgeon pushes the displaced radial fragment proximally, medially and backwards. If

necessary the manoeuvre is repeated in varying positions of pronation and supination.

If this fails, open reduction is performed. The head of the radius must never be excised in children or the ulna will outgrow the radius; the inferior radioulnar joint then subluxates and rotation becomes limited.

● HOLD

A posterior plaster slab extending two-thirds of the way round the limb is bandaged on. It is usual for the elbow to be held in 90 degrees of flexion, but the angle at which reduction seems stable should be maintained.

The slab is worn for 3 weeks, and a collar and cuff for a further 3 weeks.

● EXERCISE

The elbow is allowed to regain movement spontaneously after the collar and cuff has been removed.

Fractured head of radius (adults)

A fall on the outstretched hand forces the elbow into valgus and pushes the radial head against the

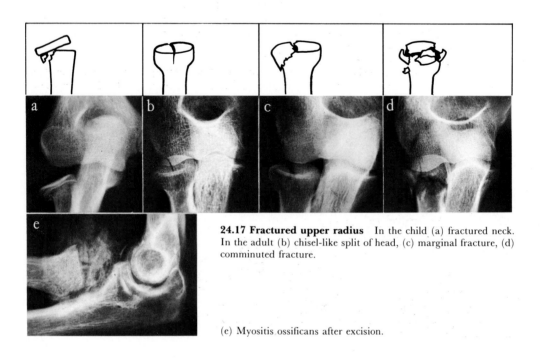

24.17 Fractured upper radius   In the child (a) fractured neck. In the adult (b) chisel-like split of head, (c) marginal fracture, (d) comminuted fracture.

(e) Myositis ossificans after excision.

capitulum. The radial head may be split or broken. In addition, the articular cartilage of the capitulum may be bruised or chipped; this cannot be seen on x-ray but is an important complication.

Special features

This fracture is sometimes missed, but painful rotation of the forearm and tenderness on the lateral side of the elbow should suggest the diagnosis.

X-RAY
The films may show (1) a vertical split in the radial head; or (2) a single fragment of the lateral portion of the head broken off and usually displaced distally; or (3) the head broken into several fragments.

Treatment

With an undisplaced split the arm is held in a collar and cuff for 3 weeks; active flexion and extension may be encouraged, but rotation should be left to return by itself.

A single large fragment may be pinned back with a Kirschner wire.

A severe fracture is best treated by excising the radial head; Silastic replacements are available, but simple excision is probably adequate.

Technique A tourniquet is applied, the elbow is flexed and an incision 5 cm long is made extending from the lateral epicondyle towards the thumb. The capsule is incised and the radial head removed. The excised portions should be fitted together to ensure that no fragment has been left behind. The capsule

and the skin are sutured. After-care is the same as that following closed treatment.

Complications

Joint stiffness is common and may involve both the elbow and the radioulnar joints. Occasionally myositis ossificans develops. Stiffness may occur whether the radial head has been excised or not. Probably, however, the prognosis with a comminuted fracture is better after operation.

Fractured olecranon (adults)

(a) Comminuted

A direct blow or fall on the point of the elbow causes a comminuted fracture of the olecranon process with little displacement.

Special features

A graze or bruise over the point of the elbow is the tell-tale feature. The triceps is intact and the elbow can be extended against resistance.

X-RAY
The olecranon process may be broken into several fragments, but usually there is little displacement.

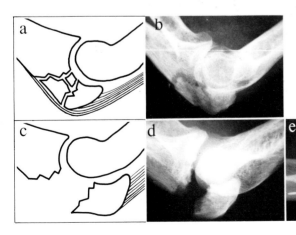
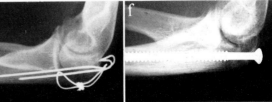

24.18 Fractured olecranon (a, b) Comminuted fracture – best treated by activity. (c, d) Gap fracture – the extensor mechanism is not intact: treatment by tension-band wiring (e), or by a long screw (f).

Treatment

The injury should be treated as a bruise and the fracture disregarded. A sling is worn for comfort and active movements are encouraged.

(b) Transverse

The patient falls onto the hand while the triceps muscle is in action. The olecranon process fractures transversely and its proximal portion is pulled upwards by the triceps muscle.

Special features

There is no skin damage over the point of the elbow, but often swelling and sometimes a visible or palpable gap. The patient cannot extend the elbow against resistance.

X-RAY
The fracture is transverse and the avulsed fragment is pulled proximally.

Treatment

Closed treatment is useless; although reduction is easy, it can be held only by splinting the arm straight – and stiffness in that position would be disastrous.

The extensor mechanism should be repaired operatively. The fracture is reduced and held with a screw or by tension band wiring. If the fragment is very small it may be excised and the triceps reattached to the ulna. A sling is worn for 3 weeks.

Elbow dislocation (children or adults)

A fall on the hand may dislocate the elbow. The forearm is pushed backwards. Once posterior dislocation has taken place, lateral shift may also occur.

Special features

The patient supports his forearm with the other hand. Deformity is usually very obvious and the elbow is held immobile. It is important to exclude damage to vessels or nerves.

X-RAY
Even though the dislocation is clinically obvious, x-ray films must be taken to exclude an associated fracture.

Treatment

- REDUCE
  The patient should be fully relaxed under anaesthesia. The surgeon pulls on the forearm while the elbow is slightly flexed. With one hand, sideways displacement is corrected, then the elbow is further flexed while the olecranon process is pushed forward with the thumbs. Unless almost full flexion can be obtained, the olecranon is not in the trochlear groove.

- HOLD
  The arm is held in a collar and cuff with the elbow flexed above 90 degrees. After 1 week the patient gently exercises his elbow; at 3 weeks he discards the collar and cuff.

- EXERCISE
  Shoulder and finger exercises are begun at once. Elbow movements are allowed to return spontaneously and are never forced.

Complications

EARLY
Nerve injuries　nearly always recover spontaneously.

Associated fractures　are common. Small flakes off the coronoid need no special treatment, and epicondylar fractures with lateral dislocation have already been described (page 392). Other associated fractures are:

(1) Head of radius. Combined with a dislocation, this is a serious injury. The dislocation should first be reduced; 3 weeks later, unless the fragments are in satisfactory position, the radial head is probably best excised.
(2) Olecranon process. This fractures with the rare forward dislocation of the elbow; 2 cm of the olecranon is left behind as a separate fragment. Open reduction with internal fixation is the best treatment.

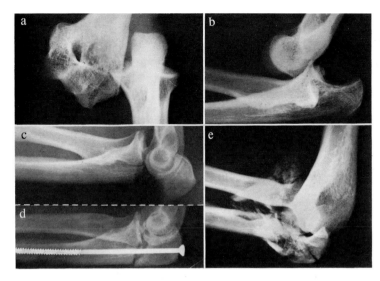

24.19 Elbow dislocations (a, b) The usual uncomplicated dislocation.

(c) Forward dislocation with fractured olecranon; this needs (d) reduction, with stabilization of the olecranon. (e) Side-swipe fracture-dislocation.

(3) Side-swipe fracture-dislocation. Typically, this occurs when a car-driver's elbow, protruding through the window, is struck by another car.* The result is forward dislocation with fractures of any or all of the bones. It is best to reduce the dislocation first, then hold it reduced in a split plaster, and treat the fractures when the joint becomes stable.

LATE

Myositis ossificans To minimize the risk of this complication, passive movements must be prohibited. If movement is diminishing, or if x-rays show calcification, the elbow should be rested in a plaster gutter.

Unreduced dislocation A dislocation may not have been diagnosed; or only the backward displacement corrected, leaving the olecranon process still displaced sideways. Up to 6 weeks from injury, manipulative reduction is worth attempting. After that a 'sham reduction' can be tried: under anaesthesia the elbow is manipulated to a more flexed position, held in a sling and activity encouraged. Often a useful range of movement is regained, but if the elbow remains stiff and painful, arthroplasty may be considered.

Recurrent dislocation If this occurs, any loose bodies in the elbow should first be removed; then the lateral ligament and capsule are repaired or reattached to the lateral condyle. A plaster with the elbow at 90 degrees is worn for 4 weeks.

Fractured radius and ulna

A twisting force (commonly a fall on the hand) causes a spiral fracture with the bones broken at different levels. A direct blow or an angulating force causes a transverse fracture of both bones at the same level. Additional rotation deformity may be produced by the pull of muscles attached to the radius: they are the biceps and supinator muscles to the upper third, the pronator teres to the middle third, and the pronator quadratus to the lower third.

Special features

The fracture is usually quite obvious, but the pulse must be felt and the hand examined for circulatory or neural deficit.

X-RAY

Both bones are broken, either transversely and at the same level, or obliquely with the radial fracture usually at a higher level. In children, the fracture is often incomplete (greenstick) and only angulated. In adults, displacement may occur in any direction – shift, overlap, tilt or twist.

Closed treatment

● REDUCE

A greenstick fracture is easily straightened by firm pressure. A complete fracture, whether spiral or transverse, is reduced by traction and rotation. The elbow is bent so that the forearm is vertical. Traction is applied to the fingers (either directly or via Chinese finger-traps) while an assistant resists the pull by holding the upper arm. The

* 'Don't stick your elbow out too far – it may go home in another car.'

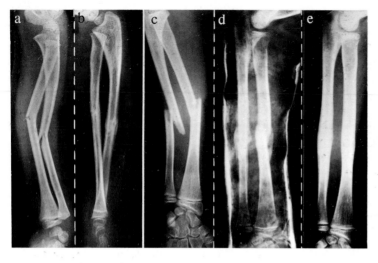

24.20 Fractured radius and ulna in children Green-stick fractures (a) only need correction of angulation (b), and plaster.

Complete fractures (c) are harder to reduce: but provided alignment is corrected and held in plaster (d) slight lateral shift remodels with growth (e).

hand is then rotated until the fragments are aligned; the forearm usually needs to be supinated when the radial fracture is high, pronated when it is low, and neutral between the two.

In adults, perfect reduction is essential; in children slight overlap is unimportant, provided no angulation or rotation deformity persists.

● HOLD

While traction is maintained, plaster is applied from just below the axilla to just above the

knuckles. The elbow is held at 90 degrees, the wrist dorsiflexed and the forearm in that degree of rotation at which reduction was obtained. X-ray films are taken to confirm reduction.

As soon as the plaster has set it is split from top to bottom to expose the skin. The patient is returned to the ward, and his arm elevated. When swelling has subsided, the plaster is completed or renewed.

In adults a spiral fracture consolidates in about 6 weeks, and a transverse fracture in 10–12

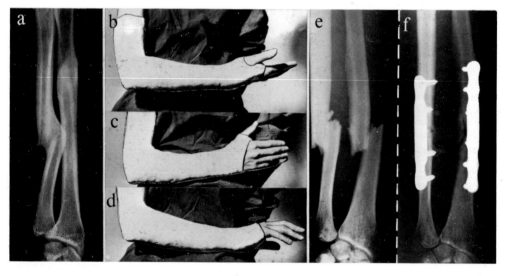

24.21 Fractured radius and ulna in adults Adult fractures also can be treated in plaster, but the danger is malunion (a). The radius is the difficult bone: with high fractures the forearm usually needs to be supinated (b); in the middle third usually in mid-rotation (c), and in the lower third pronated (d). If closed reduction is imperfect, open reduction and plating (e, f) is the answer; many surgeons, indeed, regard it as the standard method, although longer plates with six screws are usually preferred.

weeks; in children, these times are considerably shorter. When consolidation may be expected to have occurred, the plaster is removed and the fracture assessed clinically and radiologically. Unless consolidation has occurred a complete plaster must be reapplied.

● EXERCISE
Shoulder and finger movements are practised from the start. When the plaster is removed the patient wears a sling and regains elbow and radioulnar movements by graduated activity.

Sarmiento has shown that functional bracing can be used for forearm fractures. The brace permits movements at the elbow and wrist but controls rotation.

Operative treatment

With closed fractures in adults, perfect function cannot be ensured unless perfect reduction has been achieved. If closed reduction fails or redisplacement occurs in plaster, then operation is advisable; it is probably best performed 2 weeks after injury.

In open fractures wound toilet is, of course, necessary. The fracture is reduced under direct vision; if reduction is stable the fracture is treated in plaster; if reduction is unstable, the patient an adult and the wound not heavily contaminated, then the fractures are plated.

● REDUCE
The fractures are exposed by two separate incisions, one for each bone (if one incision only is used, there is danger of cross-union). An assistant pulls on the arm and rotates it, while the surgeon reduces the fracture under direct vision.

● HOLD
The fracture in each bone is held by means of a plate and screws. A plaster slab is bandaged on if the patient cannot be trusted to take reasonable care.

Consolidation takes at least as long as if the fractures had not been plated, and the usual practice, once the wounds have healed, is to replace the plaster slab by a complete plaster for at least 8 weeks.

● EXERCISE
Plated forearm fractures are eminently suited to the 'delayed splintage' technique: the day after operation a physiotherapist shows the patient how to exercise all the joints of the injured limb. This is repeated twice daily until the wounds have healed. A complete plaster is then applied and, when it is removed, full movement is rapidly regained. Alternatively, a removable functional brace is used.

Very occasionally open reduction may be desirable in a child, but plating is never essential.

Complications

EARLY
Ischaemia must be suspected if there is undue pain; passive extension of the fingers should always be tested.

LATE
Non-union may occur if the plaster has been removed before consolidation. It is particularly liable to follow plating of comminuted fractures. Non-union is treated by freshening the bone ends and screwing on a cortical bone graft, or by applying cancellous bone strips around the fracture; plaster splintage is, of course, also necessary.

Malunion is usually due to redisplacement within a loose plaster. The arm looks ugly and rotation is limited. Operative correction and plating may be necessary.

Temporary stiffness of the elbow and radioulnar joints may be unavoidable but, unless there is malunion, full movement will be regained with activity. Shoulder and finger stiffness result from neglect.

Fractures of one forearm bone only

Fracture of the radius alone or of the ulna alone is uncommon and usually caused by a direct blow. It is important for two reasons. (1) An associated dislocation may be undiagnosed; if only one forearm bone is broken and there is displacement, one or other radioulnar joint must be dislocated; as a precaution the entire forearm must always be x-rayed. (2) Non-union is liable to occur unless it is realized that one bone takes just as long to consolidate as two.

Special features

Ulnar fractures are easily missed – even on x-ray. If there is local tenderness, a further x-ray a few days later is wise.

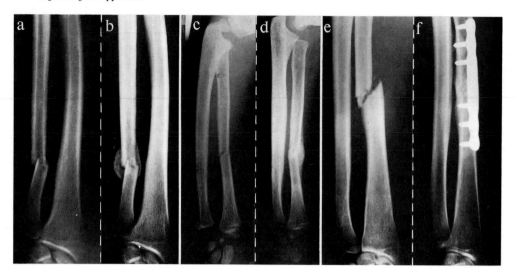

24.22 Fractured radius or ulna   A fracture of the ulna alone (a) usually joins satisfactorily (b) with treatment in plaster. This fracture of the radius alone in a child (c) also joined (d) in plaster; but in adults a fractured radius (e) is sometimes better treated by plating (f); delayed splintage is then used.

X-RAY
The fracture may be anywhere in the radius or ulna. The fracture line is transverse and displacement is slight (or else there must be a fracture-dislocation – see below).

Treatment

● REDUCE
Ulnar fractures are rarely displaced. With radial fractures there may be rotary displacement; to achieve reduction the forearm usually needs to be supinated for upper third fractures, neutral for middle third fractures, and pronated for lower third fractures.

● HOLD
A complete plaster is applied, to include the elbow and wrist joints, exactly as though both forearm bones were broken. The fracture is transverse; therefore it may be 12 weeks before consolidation is complete.

● EXERCISE
Exercises, as for fractures of both bones, are carried out.

NOTE   Because one bone is intact the ends of the broken bone cannot impinge upon one another;

union is liable to be delayed and many surgeons therefore advise internal fixation by a plate and screws. A plated ulna probably needs no plaster, but a plated radius in a manual worker must be protected by a plaster which includes the elbow and wrist.

Fracture-dislocation: (a) upper (Monteggia)

Usually the cause is a fall on the hand; if at the moment of impact the body is twisting, its momentum may forcibly pronate the forearm. The radial head dislocates forwards and the upper third of the ulna fractures and bows forwards. Sometimes the causal force is hyperextension.

Special features

The ulnar deformity is usually obvious but the dislocated head of radius is masked by swelling.

X-RAY
The head of the radius, which normally points directly to the capitulum, is dislocated forwards; and there is a fracture of the upper third of the ulna with forward bowing.

Closed treatment

- REDUCE
An assistant holds the arm while the surgeon pulls on the forearm, supinates it fully, and tries to thumb the radial head back into place. The manoeuvre rarely succeeds except in children.

- HOLD
If reduction is successful plaster is applied, from the axilla to the knuckles, with the elbow at a right angle and the forearm fully supinated.

   Consolidation of the ulnar fracture takes about 12 weeks, and the plaster must be retained until it occurs.

- EXERCISE
The shoulder and fingers are exercised from the start. Elbow and radioulnar movements take many months to return; they must not be forced.

Operative treatment

In children, if closed reduction fails, operation is wise. In adults, although closed reduction can sometimes be achieved, it tends to be unstable; open reduction with internal fixation is usually preferred.

Technique The ulna is exposed and reduced under direct vision. It is held reduced by a plate and screws or by an intramedullary nail. With perfect reduction of the ulna, the dislocation of the radial head is reduced automatically; but if the ulna cannot be perfectly reduced, the radial head should be exposed; it may need to be levered back through the orbicular ligament. Then the ulna is plated. After operation, the delayed splintage method is employed, the application of a complete plaster being postponed until movements have been regained.

Complications

Malunion of the ulna causes little disability but, unless the ulna has been perfectly reduced, the radial head remains dislocated and limits elbow flexion. In children no treatment is advised. In adults excision of the head of the radius may be needed.

Non-union of the ulna should be treated by bone grafting. If the radial head is dislocated it should be excised.

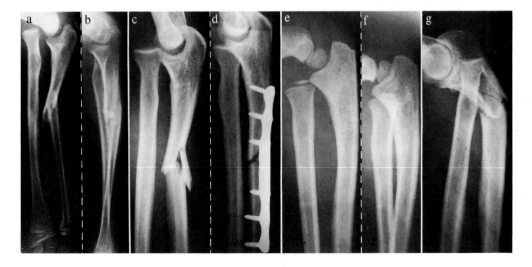

24.23 Fracture-dislocation – Monteggia (a) The ulna is fractured and the head of the radius no longer points to the capitulum; in the child closed reduction and plaster (b) is usually satisfactory. (c) In the adult open reduction and plating (d) is preferred.
(e) Forward dislocation of the radial head without an ulnar fracture also can follow pronation injury; (f) shows the dislocation reduced by supination. (g) The rare backward type of Monteggia injury with posterior dislocation of the radial head.

Backward Monteggia

In this variety the head of the radius dislocates backwards and the ulnar fracture bows backwards. Although manipulative reduction is relatively easy, it can only be held in plaster with the elbow extended, and disabling stiffness is likely. Operative treatment with internal fixation of the ulna is therefore better.

Dislocation of the radial head

This may follow a pronation injury without fracture of the ulna. The dislocation is reduced by supination and direct pressure, and the arm held supine in plaster for 6 weeks.

Dislocation of the radial head may be congenital and if the patient injures his elbow, the unwary surgeon may attempt an impossible reduction. Congenital dislocation may be forwards or backwards, and is usually bilateral; but in all cases the radial head is dome-shaped, distinguishing it from traumatic dislocation (page 171).

Pulled elbow

A child aged 3 or 4 is brought with a painful elbow which he supports with the other hand. The probable cause is distal subluxation of the radial head which becomes impacted in the orbicular ligament, preventing rotation. Spontaneous recovery occurs if the arm is rested in a sling for a few days; dramatic improvement may follow forcible supination in the course of examination.

Fracture-dislocation: (b) lower (Galeazzi)

The usual cause is a fall on the hand; probably a rotation force is superimposed. The radius fractures in its lower third and the inferior radio-ulnar joint dislocates. The injury is an almost exact counterpart of the Monteggia fracture-dislocation.

Special features

The prominent lower end of the ulna is the striking feature. It is important also to test for an ulnar nerve lesion, which is common.

X-RAY
A transverse or short oblique fracture is seen in the lower third of the radius, with angulation or overlap. The inferior radioulnar joint is dislocated.

Treatment

Closed reduction is sometimes successful and can be held by a full above-elbow plaster, which must be maintained for at least 3 months. It is probably better, however, to reduce and plate the radius at open operation. Accurate reduction of the radius ensures replacement of the radioulnar dislocation.

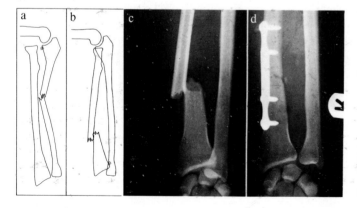

24.24 Fracture-dislocation – Galeazzi The diagrams show the contrast between (a) Monteggia and (b) Galeazzi fracture-dislocations. (c, d) Galeazzi type before and after reduction and plating.

III   *Injuries of the wrist and hand*

Colles' fracture

The patient is usually an elderly woman, often osteoporotic. She falls on the dorsiflexed hand, breaking the radius transversely just above the wrist. Probably the momentum of the body imposes a supination force and the lower radius, with the hand, is twisted and tilted backwards and radially.

Special features

We can recognize this fracture (as Abraham Colles did long before radiography was invented) by the 'dinner-fork' deformity, with prominence on the back of the wrist and a depression in front. In patients with less deformity there may only be local tenderness and pain on wrist movements.

X-RAY

There is a transverse fracture of the radius less than 2.5 cm from the wrist, and often the ulnar styloid process is broken off. The radial fragment is (1) shifted and tilted backwards, (2) shifted and tilted radially, and (3) impacted.

Treatment

● REDUCE

Under anaesthesia the fracture is reduced in three stages.

(1) *Disimpaction*   Disimpaction may be achieved by pulling on the hand. If this fails, the backward tilt should be temporarily increased and then traction resumed.

(2) *Pronation*   The patient's wrist is palmarflexed and the forearm strongly pronated.

(3) *Pressure*   To ensure that reduction is complete, the surgeon presses the lower radius firmly forwards and towards the ulna.

● HOLD

While the forearm is still held pronated and the wrist slightly palmarflexed and ulnar deviated, a plaster slab is applied. It extends from just below the elbow to the metacarpal necks and two-thirds of the way round the circumference of the wrist. It is held in position by a crêpe bandage. While the plaster slab is setting the surgeon holds the reduction by firm pressure with his thenar eminences. Post-reduction x-rays are taken.

Next day, if the fingers are swollen, cyanosed or painful, there should be no hesitation in splitting the bandage. At 7–10 days fresh x-rays are taken; redisplacement is not uncommon and requires re-reduction.

The fracture unites in 6 weeks and, even in the absence of radiological proof of union, the slab may safely be discarded and replaced by a temporary crêpe bandage.

● EXERCISE

The patient should not be allowed to go home until she can comb her hair and move her fingers fully. Regular active exercises of the shoulder and fingers must be insisted upon – they are more important than treatment of the broken bone.

When the plaster has been removed, return of wrist and radioulnar movements is encouraged by the regular practice of such normal activities as washing up.

Complications

EARLY

The circulation   in the fingers must be checked; the bandage holding the slab may need to be split or loosened.

Nerve injury   is rare, and even compression of the median nerve in the carpal tunnel is surprisingly uncommon.

LATE

Malunion   is common, either because reduction was not complete or because displacement within the plaster was overlooked. The appearance is ugly, and weakness and loss of rotation may persist. In most cases treatment is not necessary. Where the disability is severe and the patient relatively young, the lower 2.5 cm of the ulna may be excised to restore rotation and the radial deformity corrected by osteotomy.

Delayed union and non-union   of the radius do not occur, but the ulnar styloid process often joins by fibrous tissue only and remains painful and tender for several months.

Stiffness   of the shoulder, from neglect, is probably the commonest complication. Stiffness of the wrist may follow persisting with splintage despite poor position in plaster – the patient has the worst of both worlds. Finger stiffness can nearly always be avoided by active use but, rarely, Sudeck's atrophy (page 363) develops and stiffness then persists for months.

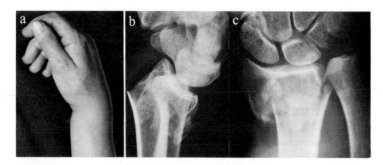

24.25 Colles' fracture (1) (a) Dinner-fork deformity. (b,c) The fracture is not into the wrist joint: the chief displacements are backwards and radially.

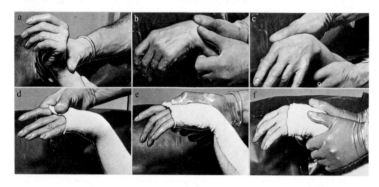

24.26 Colles' fracture (2) Reduction: (a) disimpaction (not always necessary), (b) pronation and forward shift, (c) ulnar deviation.

Splintage: (d) stockinette, (e) wet plaster slab, (f) slab bandaged on and reduction held till plaster set.

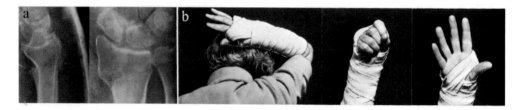

24.27 Colles' fracture (3) (a) Post-reduction films are satisfactory (Fig. 24.25 were the pre-reduction films of this patient); (b) before going home she is taught these movements and persuaded to practise them regularly.

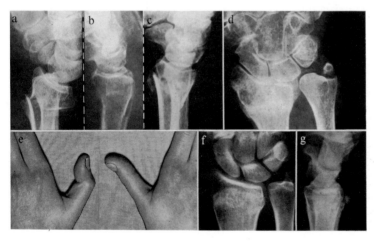

24.28 Colles' fracture (4) Malunion: backward shift (a) was reduced (b), but recurred (c). Slight malunion of radius with non-union of ulna (d). Delayed rupture of extensor pollicis longus (e) is not a complication of a true Colles' fracture, but of this apparently trivial fracture (f, g).

Rupture of the extensor pollicis longus tendon occasionally occurs a few weeks after an apparently trivial undisplaced fracture of the lower radius. The patient should be warned of the possibility and told that operative treatment is available (page 191).

Helal believes rupture follows swelling within the tight compartment between bone and ligament; with displaced fractures the ligament ruptures and consequently there is no tension so that tendon rupture does not occur.

Other fractures of lower radius

Juvenile Colles' fracture

The force which in an older person causes a Colles' fracture may, in a child, cause a fracture-separation of the lower radial epiphysis. The epiphysis is shifted and tilted backwards and may also be shifted and tilted radially. As it displaces, it carries with it a triangular fragment of the radial metaphysis. The fracture is reduced and held in the same way as a Colles' fracture.

Fracture-separation of the lower radial epiphysis does not interfere with growth of the bone; but a minor crush of the radial epiphysis without displacement may do so, and premature epiphyseal fusion then occurs. The ulna outgrows

the radius and the ulnar head dislocates. It may subsequently be necessary to excise the lower 2.5 cm of the ulna.

Fractured radial styloid

This injury is caused by forced radial deviation of the wrist and may occur after a fall, or when a starting handle 'kicks back'. The fracture line is transverse, extending laterally from the articular surface of the radius; the fragment, much more than the radial styloid, is often undisplaced.

If there is displacement it is reduced, and the wrist is held in ulnar deviation by a plaster slab round the outer forearm extending from below the elbow to the metacarpal necks. Imperfect reduction may lead to osteoarthritis; therefore if closed reduction is imperfect the fragment should be screwed back, or held with Kirschner wires.

Comminuted fractures

Instead of the lower radius breaking transversely above the wrist as in a true Colles' fracture, there may be a T-shaped fracture into the joint, or the lower radius may be comminuted. Accurate reduction can sometimes be achieved by manual traction, and possibly held in an above-elbow plaster for 6 weeks. If the patient is young and reduction is inaccurate, an external fixation device connecting the second metacarpal to the

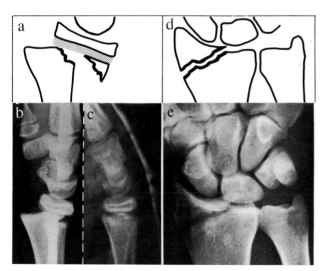

24.29 Other fractures of the lower radius (a, b) Juvenile Colles' fracture – lateral view. Note that displacement is not through the growth disc but just proximal to it; (c) after reduction. (d, e) Radial styloid.

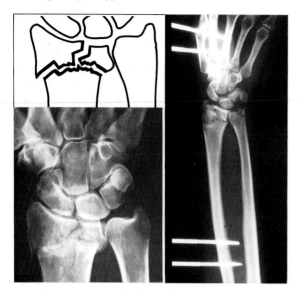

24.30 Comminuted fractures of the lower radius A severely comminuted fracture of the lower radius can be held in position by external fixation; pins passed through the second metacarpal and the proximal radius are connected by an external rod.

radius can be used. Usually the patient is elderly and it is then best to apply a plaster slab (purely for comfort), removing it after a few days for active exercises; the carpal bones mould the radial fragments into reasonable position and quite good function is regained.

Fractures with forward displacement

The terms reversed Colles' and Smith's fracture are used misleadingly. In 1847 Smith described a transverse fracture just above the wrist – a true reversed Colles' fracture. The injury to which his name is usually applied is a fracture-dislocation, and was described in 1839 by Barton.

A true *reversed Colles' fracture* (a transverse fracture of the lower radius with forward shift and tilt) is rare, and occurs mainly in elderly women. It is reduced by disimpaction and held dorsiflexed, preferably in supination and in an above-elbow plaster, for 6 weeks.

Fracture-dislocation (Barton's fracture) is commoner. The radial fracture is oblique, extending upwards and forwards from the wrist joint; the separated anterior fragment of radius shifts proximally, carrying the hand with it. Reduction can usually be achieved by strong traction and supination but is unstable; open reduction with internal fixation (using a small anterior plate) is preferable. A forearm plaster is applied for 6 weeks, after which wrist movements are encouraged.

Note A comparable fracture-dislocation with a dorsal fragment occasionally occurs; treatment is similar, but the plate should be posterior.

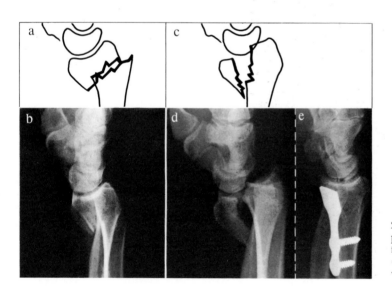

24.31 Fractures with forward displacement (a, b) True reversed Colles' fracture. (c, d) Fracture–dislocation (Barton's fracture), reduced and held (e) with a small anterior plate.

Fractured carpal scaphoid

A fall on the dorsiflexed hand may fracture the scaphoid. Probably the force is a combination of dorsiflexion and radial deviation. The deviation occurs between the two rows of carpal bones; the scaphoid, lying partly in each row, fractures across its waist. The injury is rare in children and in the elderly.

Special features

The appearance may be deceptively normal, but the astute observer can usually detect fullness in the anatomical snuffbox; precisely localized tenderness in the same situation is an important diagnostic feature.

X-RAY
Anteroposterior, lateral and oblique views are all essential; often a recent fracture shows only in the oblique view. Usually the fracture line is transverse, and through the narrowest part of the bone (waist), but it may be more proximally situated (proximal pole fracture). Sometimes only the tubercle of the scaphoid is fractured. There is rarely much displacement.

Diagnosis

Sprains of the wrist are rare and must not be diagnosed unless repeated x-rays have excluded a fracture. Immediately after injury a fracture of the scaphoid may be almost invisible; where there is the slightest doubt, further x-rays must be taken 2–3 weeks after the injury, when the fracture can be clearly seen.

Wrist sprains may remain uncomfortable for many weeks, but splintage is not helpful. A crêpe bandage for a few days is comforting, but activity should be encouraged. Sometimes a lateral x-ray shows a flake fracture off the back of the triquetrum; this injury also should be regarded as a sprain and treated by active use.

Treatment

Fracture of the scaphoid tubercle needs no splintage and should be treated as a wrist sprain (see above). All other scaphoid fractures are treated as follows.

● REDUCE
Displacement is not common, but when it is present an attempt should be made to reduce it by manipulation under anaesthesia. Rarely, manipulation fails, and if displacement is substantial, open reduction is worth considering; it can usefully be followed by inserting a screw across the fracture (Maudsley and Chen, 1972).

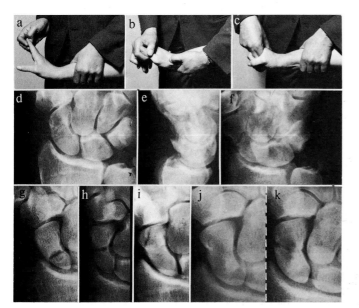

24.32 Scaphoid fractures – diagnosis Clinical signs: (a) pain on dorsiflexion, (b) localized tenderness, (c) pain on gripping.

X-ray signs: the AP view (d) and the lateral (e) often fail to show the fracture; even in an oblique view (f) it may be difficult to see.

Fracture may be through (g) the proximal pole, (h) the waist, or (i) the tubercle. Even when no fracture is seen at first (j), a repeat film at 2 weeks (k) shows it clearly.

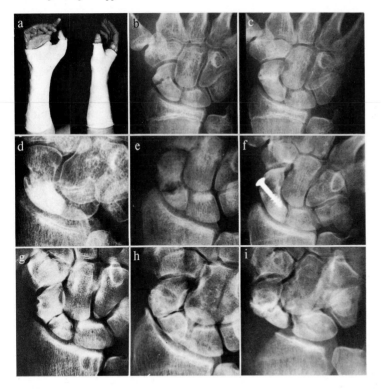

24.33 Scaphoid fractures – treatment and complications (a) Scaphoid plaster – position and extent. (b, c) Before and after treatment: in this case radiological union was visible at 10 weeks.

(d) Avascular necrosis of proximal half; (e) early non-union, treated successfully by (f) inserting a screw.

(g) Established non-union with sclerosis; (h) non-union with localized osteoarthritic changes; (i) osteoarthritis treated by excising the radial styloid.

● HOLD

A complete plaster is applied from the upper forearm to just short of the metacarpophalangeal joints of the fingers, but incorporating the proximal phalanx of the thumb. The wrist is held dorsiflexed and the thumb forwards in the 'glass-holding' position. The plaster must be carefully moulded into the hollow of the hand, and is not split. It is retained (and if necessary repaired or renewed) for 6 weeks.

After 6 weeks the plaster is removed and the wrist examined clinically. A further plaster for 4 weeks is applied only if the wrist is tender and uncomfortable, or with a proximal pole fracture. Otherwise the wrist is left free; often radiological union becomes obvious only after several months. It is possible that too short a time in plaster occasionally leads to non-union; but the risk of painful non-union is smaller than the risk of painful stiffness after prolonged splintage.

● EXERCISE

Shoulder movements are practised from the start, and the plaster is so designed that function of the hand is limited as little as possible. Wrist movements are regained when the plaster is removed.

Complications

● *Avascular necrosis* The proximal fragment may die, especially with proximal pole fractures, and then at 2–3 months it appears dense on x-ray. Although revascularization and union are theoretically possible, they take years. If pain is present, the dead fragment and the radial styloid should be excised.

● *Early non-union* It may be apparent in 3–6 months that the bone ends at the fracture are becoming sclerosed. The fracture may be fixed in compression with a screw, or a bone graft inserted. Plaster is worn for 3 months.

● *Established non-union* A patient may be seen because of a recent injury, but x-rays show an old, un-united fracture with sclerosed edges. He may recall a previous 'sprain' which was in reality an undiagnosed scaphoid fracture. The wrist soon became painless, fortifying both patient and doctor in their error. Provided avascular necrosis has not occurred, non-union of the scaphoid does not necessarily cause symptoms, but there is an increased likelihood of pain following overuse or further injury.

The patient who presents with a wrist sprain and established non-union is put in plaster for 2–4 weeks; often the wrist becomes painless and strong again. If symptoms persist, or repeated sprains occur, the radial styloid process should be excised.

Osteoarthritis   Osteoarthritis of the wrist may be a sequel to non-union of the scaphoid, especially when there has been avascular necrosis. The patient may complain of repeated sprains and later of weakness, stiffness and pain. If a wrist strap or polythene splint fails to relieve symptoms, the wrist may need to be arthrodesed.

Scaphoid subluxation

Persistent, unexplained tenderness over the scaphoid may be due to subluxation. The x-ray appearance is pathognomonic: a gap between scaphoid and lunate. If closed manipulation fails, the bone may be repositioned by open operation and held in place with a Kirschner wire for 3 weeks.

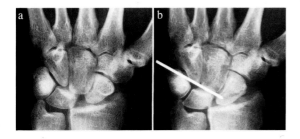

24.34 Subluxation of the scaphoid   After a fall this patient had pain and tenderness in the anatomical snuff-box. The scaphoid is intact but (a) there is an obvious gap between the lunate and scaphoid. After open reduction the scaphoid was held in position with a K-wire (b) until capsular healing was complete.

Carpal dislocations

A fall on the dorsiflexed hand may displace the hand and most of the carpus backwards, leaving only the lunate in contact with the radius (*perilunar dislocation*); this may be associated with fractures of the radial styloid or any carpal bone. Usually the hand immediately snaps forwards again but, as it does so, the lunate is levered forwards out of position (*lunate dislocation*). A lunate dislocation can possibly occur without preceding perilunar dislocation; during forced dorsiflexion the bone might conceivably be ejected like an orange pip.

If the dorsiflexion injury has also fractured the scaphoid, its proximal half remains alongside the lunate in whatever position that bone lies.

Special features

Swelling is considerable and obscures the dislocation. But the wrist is almost immobile, and there are two features which strongly suggest insufficient room in the carpal tunnel: (1) blunting of sensation in the median nerve territory, and (2) difficulty in flexing the fingers actively.

X-RAY
In the anteroposterior view, the lunate has lost its normal somewhat quadrilateral shape; instead it comes to a point distally. The scaphoid may also have fractured.

In the lateral view it is easy to distinguish a perilunar from a lunate dislocation. The dislocated lunate is grossly tilted forwards and is displaced in front of the radius, while the os magnum and metacarpal bones are in line with the radius. With a perilunar dislocation the lunate is tilted forwards only slightly, and is not displaced forwards; and the os magnum and metacarpals lie behind the line of the radius.

Treatment

● REDUCE
The surgeon pulls strongly on the dorsiflexed hand. While maintaining traction he slowly palmarflexes the wrist, at the same time squeezing the lunate backwards with his other thumb. These manoeuvres usually effect reduction; they also prevent conversion of perilunar to lunate dislocation.

Reduction is imperative, and if closed reduction fails, the bone is exposed by an anterior approach which has the advantage of decompressing the carpal tunnel. While an assistant pulls on the hand, the lunate is levered into place. If at operation the bone is seen to be totally detached, some surgeons advise its immediate excision, because avascular necrosis is inevitable; but excision leaves some weakness and Silastic replacement is worth considering.

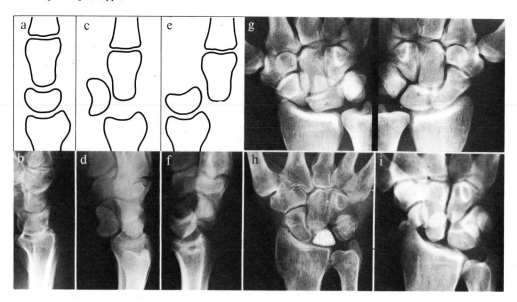

24.35 Lunate and perilunar dislocations   (a, b) Lateral view of normal wrist; (c, d) lunate dislocation; (e, f) perilunar dislocation. (g) AP of both wrists with dislocated left lunate – note the triangular appearance. (h) Avascular necrosis following reduction. (i) Associated fracture of scaphoid.

- HOLD
Reduction is stable, but a plaster slab holding the wrist neutral is comforting, and is worn for 3 weeks.

- EXERCISE
Finger movements are begun at once.

Complications

Nerve injury   Median nerve compression in the carpal tunnel occurs almost invariably, but recovers after reduction.

Unreduced dislocation   This presents as a painful stiffish wrist, with median paraesthesia. The lunate should be excised through an anterior incision; it is worth seeing if a Silastic replacement can be fitted into the gap.

Fractured scaphoid   It is important always to exclude a scaphoid fracture by x-ray after reduction of the dislocation (which will automatically have reduced the fractured scaphoid). Following reduction, an anterior plaster slab is applied which, after 1 week, is replaced by a full scaphoid plaster; the injury is then treated as a fractured scaphoid.

Avascular necrosis   The lunate and the proximal half of the scaphoid may become avascular. Osteoarthritis of the radiocarpal joint is likely to ensue.

Fractures of the hand

Management

In the hand, even more than elsewhere, function is a vital consideration. Fingers stiffen easily and a stiff finger is often worse than no finger. Fractures in the hand almost invariably unite and even if angulation persists, malunion is less disabling than stiffness.

The guiding principles of treatment are as follows.

SWELLING
Swelling must be controlled by elevating the hand and by early and repeated active exercises.

SPLINTAGE
Splintage must be kept to a minimum. If it is essential, it is best to attach the injured finger to its neighbour (by strapping or by a double Tubigrip), so that both move as one. Apart from this, only the injured finger should be splinted and then only in the correct position – with the knuckle joint flexed 90 degrees and the finger joints straight (page 203). Sometimes an external splint, to be effective, would need to immobilize other fingers; if so, it is preferable to use internal splintage with Kirschner wires. The wires can conveniently be cut short enough to close the skin and are subsequently removed under local anaesthesia.

SKIN DAMAGE
Skin damage demands wound toilet followed by suture or skin grafting. Treatment of the skin takes precedence over treatment of the fracture. (Open injuries of the hand are discussed in full on page 200.)

Fractured base of thumb

An unskilled boxer may, while punching, sustain a fracture of the first metacarpal base. Localized swelling and tenderness are found, and x-ray shows a transverse fracture about 6 mm distal to the carpometacarpal joint, with outward bowing and usually impaction.

Treatment

To reduce the fracture, the surgeon pulls on the abducted thumb and, by levering the metacarpal outwards against his own thumb, corrects the bowing. A firm crêpe bandage usually suffices to prevent redisplacement, but if the fracture feels unstable a plaster slab is applied, extending from the forearm to just short of the interphalangeal thumb joint; the thumb is in the position of function where the index finger can make pulp-to-pulp contact with it. The slab is removed after 3 weeks and movement usually recovers rapidly.

Bennett's fracture-dislocation

This fracture, too, occurs at the base of the first metacarpal bone and is commonly due to punching; but the fracture is oblique, extends into the carpometacarpal joint and is unstable. The thumb looks short and the carpometacarpal region swollen. X-rays show that a small triangular fragment has remained in contact with the medial half of the trapezium, while the remainder of the thumb has subluxated proximally.

Treatment

REDUCTION AND SPLINTAGE
The fracture is easily reduced by pulling on the thumb, abducting it and extending it. To hold reduction is difficult and three methods are available.

24.36 Fractures of the first metacarpal base A transverse fracture (a) can be reduced and held in plaster (b).

A Bennett's fracture-dislocation can often be reduced and held in plaster (c, d); alternative methods are internal fixation (e, f), or treatment by activity (g, h).

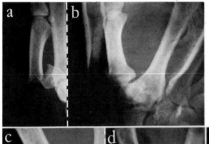
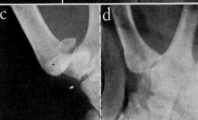
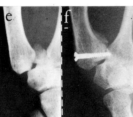
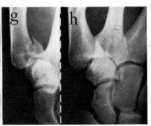

Plaster may be applied with a felt pad over the fracture, and the first metacarpal held abducted and extended (usually best achieved by *flexing* the metacarpophalangeal joint). If x-ray shows that perfect reduction is being held, the plaster is worn for 3 weeks; otherwise the method is abandoned.

Continuous skin traction can be employed using a strong wire splint incorporated in plaster. Again 3 weeks' treatment is needed and the method is abandoned if reduction is not successful.

Internal fixation is usually the method of choice; it can be achieved by inserting a small screw, or by driving short lengths of Kirschner wire through the metacarpal base (bypassing the fracture) into the carpus; the protruding ends are incorporated in a small plaster slab. After 3 weeks the slab is removed and the wires are pulled out.

FUNCTIONAL TREATMENT
If the fracture is disregarded and active use encouraged, painless function is quickly regained. The fracture unites but in faulty position. It is widely supposed (with little evidence) that osteoarthritis is the inevitable sequel.

Fractured metacarpal shafts

A direct blow may fracture one or several metacarpal shafts transversely, often with associated skin damage. A twisting or punching force may cause a spiral fracture of one or more shafts. There is local pain and swelling, sometimes deformity, and one knuckle may have receded.

Treatment

Spiral fractures or transverse fractures with slight displacement require no reduction. Splintage also is unnecessary, but a crêpe bandage worn for a few days may be comforting; this should not be allowed to discourage the patient from active movements of the fingers, which should be practised assiduously.

Transverse fractures with considerable displacement are reduced by traction and pressure. Reduction can be held by a plaster slab extending from the forearm over the fingers (only the damaged ones). The slab is maintained for 3 weeks and the undamaged fingers are exercised. A more elegant method is to insert a short length of Kirschner wire across the fracture through a dorsal incision; alternatively the distal fragment, after reduction, may be transfixed to the neighbouring undamaged metacarpal by transverse wires. In either case no external splint is necessary and early movements are encouraged.

Complications

It sometimes happens that an undetected rotational deformity becomes apparent as movement returns; the patient cannot properly close the fist and osteotomy may be needed.

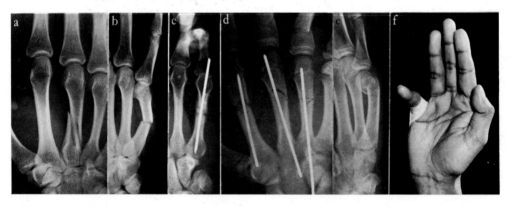

24.37 Other metacarpal fractures (a) A spiral fracture of a single metacarpal (especially an 'inboard' one) is adequately held by neighbouring bones and muscles; (b) a displaced fracture (especially an 'outboard' one) is often best held by a wire (c). With several adjacent metacarpals fractured (d), internal fixation may be the only safe way to avoid stiffness. With a fractured neck of the fifth metacarpal (e), if reduction feels stable, strapping in this position (f) is useful.

Fractured metacarpal necks

A blow may fracture the metacarpal neck of the fifth finger or occasionally of the index finger. A lump is visible and x-rays show a transverse fracture with backward angulation.

Treatment

Slight displacement may be disregarded and the patient is encouraged to use his hand; a small lump may remain, but full function is rapidly regained.

If displacement is considerable it is reduced by direct pressure between the surgeon's finger on the front of the metacarpal head and his thumb on the dorsum of the fracture. The reduction can be held by a plaster slab which extends from the wrist to the proximal finger joint, but no further; if the reduction feels stable, plaster is unnecessary, and strapping may suffice. If, however, the plaster is ineffective, the small distal fragment can (after reduction) be transfixed by a small piece of Kirschner wire anchoring it to the neighbouring metacarpal head.

Fractured phalanges

Fractures of the proximal or middle phalanx result from direct violence, and may be open. The phalanx fractures transversely, often with forward angulation which may damage the flexor tendon sheath.

The fracture is reduced by pulling on the bent finger and thumbing the phalanx straight. A flexed position must be maintained to hold the reduction, and is most simply achieved by placing a rolled bandage in the palm and holding the flexed finger over it with a crêpe bandage. To prevent rotation deformity, the flexed finger must point towards the scaphoid bone. It is unwise to keep finger joints flexed for long, and after 10 days the bandage should be removed. A removable posterior plaster slab is substituted; it is taken off several times a day and the patient exercises the finger while he protects the fracture with his other hand.

The terminal phalanx may be struck by a hammer, or caught in a door, and the bone shattered. The fracture is disregarded and treatment is focused on controlling swelling and regaining movement.

Fractures into joints

Any finger joint may be injured by a direct blow (often the overlying skin is damaged), or by an angulation force, or by the straight finger being forcibly stubbed. The affected joint is swollen, tender and too painful to move. X-rays may show that a fragment of bone has been sheared off or avulsed.

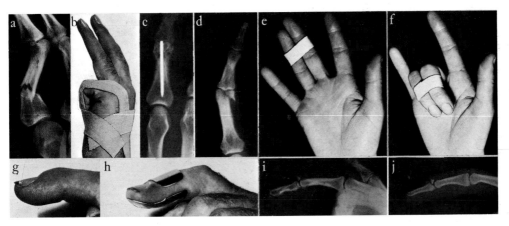

24.38 Phalangeal fractures   Fractured proximal phalanx (a) held reduced by strapping in flexion (b), or with a wire (c). A fracture into a joint (d) can either be treated by internal fixation, or by movement with the finger strapped to its neighbour (e, f).
Mallet finger (g) treated by a splint (h); this is adequate when the bony fragment (if any) is small (i), but a large fragment (j) needs fixation.

It is usually best to disregard the fracture, to strap the finger to its neighbour with a garter, and to concentrate on regaining movement. If a bone fragment is grossly displaced, recovery of function may be hastened by fixing it back in position with a Kirschner wire, or by removing the fragment and repairing the soft tissue defect.

With *mallet finger* (see also page 191) the extensor tendon may avulse a fragment from the base of the terminal phalanx; but there are two distinct varieties. With the bed-making type of injury only a tiny flake is avulsed and treatment in a splint for 6 weeks is satisfactory. With a stubbing injury, such as mis-catching a cricket ball, the avulsed fragment is much larger; unless it reduces accurately with hyperextension, the fragment should be fixed back with a small piece of Kirschner wire, otherwise painful stiffness is likely to develop.

Dislocations

Carpometacarpal

The thumb is most frequently affected and clinically the injury then resembles a Bennett's fracture-dislocation; but x-rays show proximal subluxation of the first metacarpal bone without a fracture. The dislocation is easily reduced by traction, but reduction is unstable and can be held only by one of the methods used for a Bennett's fracture-dislocation; namely, plaster, skin traction, a wire splint, or Kirschner wires driven through the metacarpus into the carpus. Splintage is discontinued after 3 weeks.

Dislocations at the other carpometacarpal joints occur typically when a motorcyclist holding the handlebars, strikes an object; one hand is driven backwards, leaving the carpus, thumb and forearm projecting forwards. Closed manipulation is usually successful and a protective slab for 6 weeks restores stability.

Metacarpophalangeal

Usually the thumb is affected, sometimes the fifth finger, and rarely the other fingers. A hyperextension force may dislocate the phalanx backwards, and the capsule and muscle insertions in front of the joint may be torn. If the metacarpal head has been forced like a button through the hole, closed reduction may be impossible.

Closed reduction is first attempted by pulling on the thumb and levering the phalanx forwards. If this fails, the joint is exposed from behind and, while strong traction is applied, the metacarpal head is levered into place. The joint is then strapped in the flexed position for 1 week.

Interphalangeal

Backward dislocation at the distal joint is common and is easily reduced by pulling. The joint may be strapped flexed for a few days.

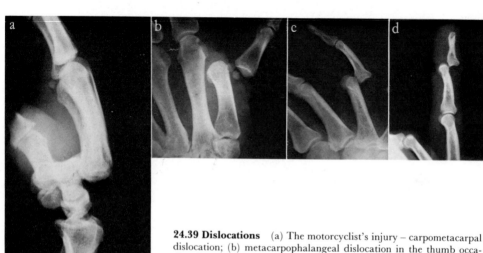

24.39 Dislocations   (a) The motorcyclist's injury – carpometacarpal dislocation; (b) metacarpophalangeal dislocation in the thumb occasionally buttonholes and needs open reduction; (c, d) interphalangeal dislocations are easily reduced and easily missed if not x-rayed.

Sprains

Sprains of the finger joints are common, and usually due to an angulation force. Sometimes a small bony fragment is avulsed.

The injured finger should be strapped to its neighbour by means of a garter and active movements encouraged. The patient must be warned that, following a sprain, the joint is likely to remain swollen, slightly painful and stiffish for 6–12 months.

Sprain of the metacarpophalangeal joint of the thumb ('gamekeeper's thumb') is more serious. If the ulnar collateral ligament ruptures completely (usually at its proximal attachment), it may not repair even with several weeks in plaster. Injury to this joint merits careful examination; if instability is demonstrable, immediate operative repair is advised. The neglected injury leads to weakness of pinch, which is probably best treated by arthrodesis, although in early cases without articular damage, stability may be preserved by advancing the insertion of adductor pollicis to the base of the phalanx or by reinforcing the ligament with the tendon of extensor pollicis brevis.

Further reading

Barton, N. (1977) Fractures of the phalanges of the hand. *The Hand* **9,** 1–10

Burrows, H. J. (1951) Tenodesis of subclavius in the treatment of recurrent dislocation of the sterno-clavicular joint. *Journal of Bone and Joint Surgery* **33B,** 240–243

Fisk, G. R. (1980) An overview of injuries of the wrist. *Clinical Orthopaedics and Related Research,* **149,** 137–144

Maudsley, R. H. and Chen, S. C. (1972) Screw fixation in the management of the fractured carpal scaphoid. *Journal of Bone and Joint Surgery* **54B,** 432–441

Mikić, Z. (1975) Galeazzi fracture-dislocation. *Journal of Bone and Joint Surgery* **57A,** 1071–1080

Neer, C. S. (1970) Displaced proximal humeral fractures. *Journal of Bone and Joint Surgery* **52A,** 1077–1089; 1090–1103

Protzman, R. R. (1980) Anterior instability of the shoulder. *Journal of Bone and Joint Surgery* **62A,** 909–918

Rowe, C. R., Pierce, D. S. and Clark, J. G. (1973) Voluntary dislocation of the shoulder. *Journal of Bone and Joint Surgery* **55A,** 445–460

Sarmiento, A., Kinman, P. B., Galvin, E. G., Schmitt, R. H. and Phillips, J. G. (1977) Functional bracing of fractures of the shaft of the humerus. *Journal of Bone and Joint Surgery* **59A,** 596–601

Smith, R. J. (1977) Post-traumatic instability of the metacarpophalangeal joint of the thumb. *Journal of Bone and Joint Surgery* **59A,** 14–21

Because the question of cord damage is dominant, spine fractures are best classified as stable or unstable. In *stable fractures* the cord is rarely damaged and movement of the spine is safe. In *unstable fractures* the cord may have been damaged but, if it has escaped, it may be injured by subsequent movement.

Stability depends, not on the fracture itself, but on the integrity of the ligaments and in particular the posterior ligament complex; this complex consists of the supraspinous ligament, the interspinous ligaments, the capsules of the facet joints and possibly also the ligamentum flavum. Fortunately, only 10 per cent of spinal injuries are unstable.

Mechanism of injury

In order to understand which fractures are stable it is necessary to consider the forces which produce injury. Their study is simplified if we exclude avulsion injuries of the transverse or spinous processes; these should not be regarded as fractures of the spinal column, for essentially they are muscle injuries.

In the lumbar spine resisted muscle effort may avulse transverse processes; in the cervical spine usually the seventh spinous process is avulsed ('clay-shoveller's fracture'). Avulsion fractures should alert the doctor to inspect the x-ray films with even more than usual care so as to exclude

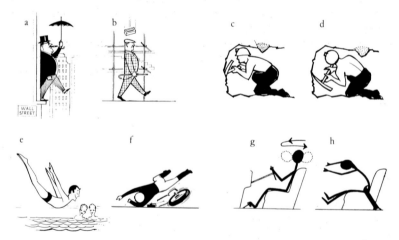

25.1 Mechanisms of spinal injuries Examples of the forces producing spine fractures: (a) and (b) may cause 'burst' fractures; (c) a fall of roof in this position might cause an anterior wedge fracture; (d) the trunk is twisted and a fracture-dislocation may result; (e) might cause an extension hinging injury to the neck; (f) with rotation a fracture-dislocation is likely to occur; (g) whiplash injury and (h) a seat-belt fracture – both involve forward shearing forces.

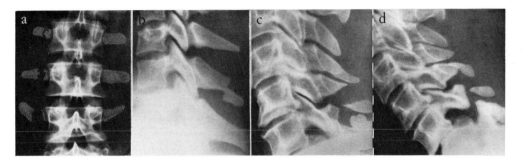

25.2 Avulsions   (a) Fractured lumbar transverse processes; (b) clay-shoveller's fracture. (c) This patient was at first thought to have a simple avulsion, but a subsequent flexion film (d) showed the serious nature of the injury – a severe fracture–dislocation.

other and more important injuries; but in themselves these 'muscle injuries' require no splintage and are best treated by activity.

The important damaging forces are: (1) compression; (2) hinging; and (3) shearing (especially rotation).

Compression forces

Compression can be applied only to a straight portion of the spine. The thoracic spine is always kyphosed and cannot suffer compression, but the cervical and lumbar spines may sometimes be straight. The lumbar spine may be compressed by a fall from a height, and the cervical spine when a weight falls on the head. The nucleus pulposus splits the vertebral end plate and fractures the vertebra vertically; with greater force, disc material is forced into the vertebral body, causing a 'burst' fracture.

Hinging forces

EXTENSION
A backward hinging force may damage the neural arch but does not tear the posterior ligaments. In the neck a hyperextension force (caused, for example, by diving into shallow water) may fracture the arch of the atlas or of the axis. Usually this injury is stable, but fracture of the pedicle of C2 ('hangman's fracture') is unstable. In the lordotic cervical spine further extension may also crush the vertebral body, forcing bone backwards into the cord (the 'teardrop' fracture). Occasionally, instead of the bone breaking, the anterior longitudinal ligament tears; this injury also (unlike a tear of the posterior ligaments) is stable.

Lumbar extension injuries are less common than cervical. Backward hinging can, however, occur and may result in a fracture of the pars interarticularis.

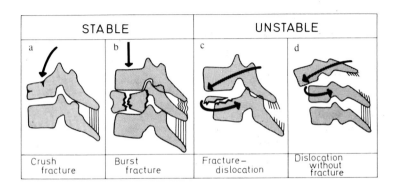

STABLE		UNSTABLE	
a	b	c	d
Crush fracture	Burst fracture	Fracture–dislocation	Dislocation without fracture

25.3 Stability   If the posterior ligaments are intact, the spine is stable; if they are torn it is unstable.

FLEXION

Forward hinging (flexion) injuries are most common in the lumbar spine following a fall in the bent position or a weight falling on the bent back. The posterior ligaments remain intact, so that the injury is stable, but the front of the vertebral body crumples. Forward hinging less often damages the cervical spine because the chin abuts against the sternum, and rarely involves the thoracic spine which is secured by the ribs.

Shearing forces

Shearing forces tear ligaments and cause instability. Rotation is a particularly important cause of ligamentous damage. Usually the rotation is associated with flexion. In the lumbar spine likely causes are a weight falling asymmetrically onto the back, or a fall from a height with the body twisted; most of these injuries are between T10 and L1. The posterior ligament complex tears as the spine rotates and shears forward. Bony injury is liable to occur at the same time; a slice of bone may be sheared off the top of one vertebra and the posterior facets may be fractured. In the neck a comparable injury can follow a fall from a motorcycle or horse.

It may well be that a similarly unstable injury can result, not from rotation, but from the combination of a flexion force with purely forward shearing. A whiplash injury of the neck, for example, may tear the posterior ligaments and permit forward dislocation; it should be noted that the facets are relatively horizontal in the neck, so that forward dislocation can readily occur without facet fracture. In the lumbar spine a comparable mechanism occurs in the seat-belt fracture; the pelvis is anchored by the lap strap and, following a collision, the body is thrown forwards and jack-knifed. The posterior ligaments are torn but there may be no bony fracture. The spine, however, is angulated and the upper facet may leap-frog over the lower.

Cervical spine injuries

Diagnosis

The most important diagnostic aid is clinical awareness. Pain and stiffness should never be regarded lightly; nor should weakness or sensory loss. The force producing a serious head injury (e.g. a road traffic accident or a fall from a height onto the head) may also injure the neck. Consequently it should be a rule that in every patient unconscious from a head injury, a fractured cervical spine should be suspected.

An abnormal position of the neck may be suggestive, but palpation is rarely helpful and

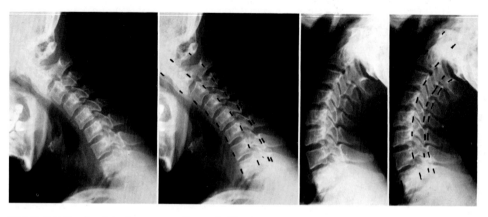

25.4 Cervical spine injuries – x-ray diagnosis (1)   In lateral films taken in both flexion and extension, four parallel lines can be traced unbroken from C1 to C7. They are formed by: (1) the anterior surfaces of the vertebral bodies; (2) the posterior surfaces of the bodies; (3) the posterior borders of the lateral masses; and (4) the bases of the spinous processes.

movement is dangerous; x-ray examination is mandatory. With the conscious patient the neck can be examined, but the gap where the posterior ligament has been torn is much less easy to detect than in the lumbar spine. Movements should be extremely gentle and, if painful, are best postponed until the neck has been x-rayed. Pain or paraesthesia in the limbs is significant, and the limbs should always be examined for evidence of cord or root damage. X-ray films must be of high quality and should be inspected methodically. Note the following points.

(1) In the anteroposterior view the lateral outlines should be intact, and the spinous processes and tracheal shadow in the midline. An open-mouth view is necessary to show C1 and C2 (odontoid and lateral mass fractures).

(2) The lateral view must include all seven cervical vertebrae and T1, otherwise a low injury will be missed. Count the vertebrae; if necessary re-x-ray while applying downward traction to the arms. The smooth lordotic curve should be followed, tracing the four parallel lines formed by the front of the vertebral bodies, the back of the bodies, the lateral masses and the bases of the spinous processes; any irregularity suggests a fracture or displacement. An unduly wide interspinous space suggests anterior luxation. The trachea may be displaced by a soft-tissue haematoma.

(3) The distance between the odontoid peg and the back of the anterior arch of the atlas should be no more than 4.5 mm in children or 3 mm in adults and does not vary with flexion.

(4) To avoid missing a dislocation without fracture, lateral films in flexion and extension are occasionally necessary. Flexion should be guided by the doctor himself and must stop immediately if the patient experiences any arm or leg symptoms.

(5) Forward shift of a vertebral body on the one below is important. Displacement of less than half the vertebral body width suggests unilateral facet dislocation and oblique views are needed to show the involved side; greater displacement suggests bilateral displacement.

(6) Unclear or doubtful lesions require tomography.

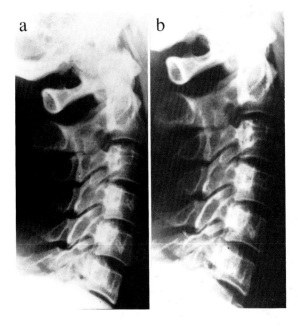

25.5 Cervical spine injuries – x-ray diagnosis (2) (a) Following a traffic accident this patient had a painful neck and consulted her doctor three times; on each occasion she was told 'the x-rays are normal'. But count the vertebrae! There are only six in this film. (b) When a strenuous effort was made to show the entire cervical spine a dislocation of C6 on C7 could be seen at the very bottom of the film.

Management of fractures of C1 and C2

Neural arches

Hyperextension is the likely cause of neural arch fractures, which are probably stable; but the appearance and situation are sufficiently alarming to justify wearing a polythene collar for 3 months.

A similar force may fracture the pedicles of the axis ('hangman's fracture'). This sinister term is applied to two different injuries. In one, hyperextension is associated with distraction and is lethal. The other, caused by hyperextension and compression, frequently has no neurological damage; a collar should, however, be worn for 3 months.

The ring of the atlas may, under load, fracture at its weakest point, where the posterior arch and the lateral masses join (the bursting fracture of Jefferson). Again the survivors often escape neurological damage and need only a collar. But if x-ray shows sideways spreading of the lateral masses, then the transverse ligament has ruptured; this injury is unstable and should be treated by 6 weeks' skull traction followed by a further 6 weeks in a collar. Alternative methods are early fixation in a halo-body cast and fusion of C2 to the skull.

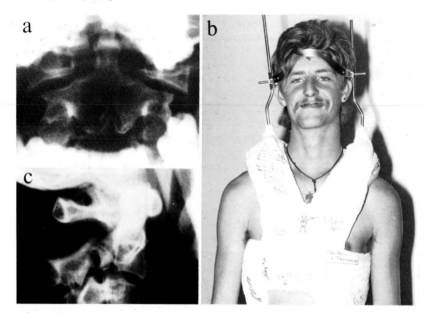

25.6 Fractures of C1 and C2 – neural arches   (a) Fracture of C1 with disruption of the arch (Jefferson fracture). The open-mouth view shows spreading of the lateral masses; the spine is unstable, and a halo-body cast (b) may be indicated. (c) Fracture of the pedicle or lateral pillar of C2 is usually due to a flexion injury ('hangman's fracture').

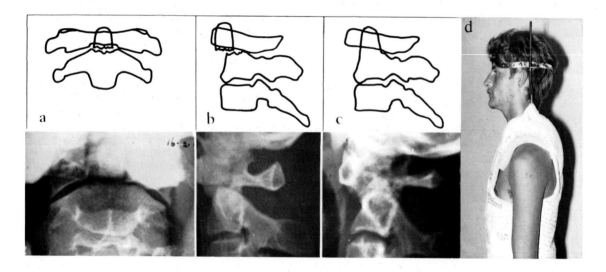

25.7 Odontoid fractures   (a, b) Fractured base of odontoid peg, permitting forward shift of the atlas and skull. (c) Similar forward shift follows rupture of the transverse ligament. The safest treatment is (d) immobilization in a halo-body cast.

Odontoid fractures

These result from high-velocity accidents or severe falls; the precise mechanism is unknown but rotation or shearing forces may be involved. Diagnosis usually requires open-mouth views and possibly tomograms. The odontoid peg ossifies from a separate epiphysis; fracture-separation can occur, but the normal growth disc should not be mistaken for a fracture. Clinicians find that cord damage is suprisingly uncommon, because only the fortunate patients present to them; those with major cord damage rarely survive.

Provided the fracture is treated early, is reduced accurately and is held securely, firm union occurs in about 12 weeks and no late displacement follows. Reduction is best achieved by fitting a metal halo and applying traction with the skull in extension; the halo is attached to a body cast and the patient allowed up. If union has not occurred by 12 weeks (as shown by flexion and extension x-rays) posterior fusion of C1 to C2 is advisable.

Management of fractures and dislocations of C3–7

Anterior wedge fracture

This uncommon injury is stable. A collar may be worn for comfort but can safely be removed to allow washing.

Burst fractures

These also are stable, but they are painful and the bony fragments are close to the cord; it is therefore prudent to restrict movement. A plaster collar is the safest; after 6 weeks it can be replaced by a polythene collar which is worn until interbody fusion is seen on x-ray.

Some burst fractures are severely comminuted (the 'teardrop' fracture), causing cord damage and, often, quadriplegia. These severe injuries need skull traction for 6 weeks, after which a polythene collar is worn until interbody fusion is seen on x-ray (usually another 6–12 weeks).

NOTE ON TRACTION   All unstable cervical fractures should be treated on traction. Halter traction becomes uncomfortable within a few hours and skeletal skull traction is better; techniques include the halo device, Crutchfield's tongs, Cone's or Blackburn's caliper. X-ray control is needed; an excessive pull may exacerbate the neurological signs.

Hyperextension injuries

The bone is undamaged, but the anterior longitudinal ligament may be torn. The history and facial bruising or lacerations often suggest the mechanism. Neurological damage is variable and probably due to compression between the disc and the ligamentum flavum; oedema and haematomyelia may cause the acute central spinal cord syndrome (page 428). X-rays show no fracture, but an extension film shows a gap between the front of two vertebral bodies. These injuries are stable in the neutral position, in which they should be held by a collar for 6 weeks.

Sometimes no gap is seen, even in extension; instead the films show old spondylosis. Again there may be cord or root damage. The neck should be held in a collar in the neutral position for 6 weeks.

Dislocation without fracture

Subluxation   The mildest flexion injury is a subluxation. There is vertebral tilting and opening up of the interspinous space at one level. There may be associated disc rupture. A collar for 3–6 weeks is adequate.

Bilateral facet dislocation   The posterior ligaments are ruptured and the spine is unstable. Skull traction is applied, starting with 10 kg and increasing to 20 kg over 2–3 hours. Progress is checked by frequent x-rays. Usually reduction is

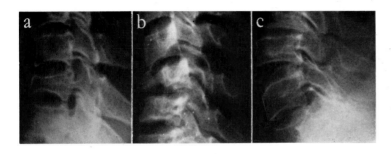

25.8 Uncommon neck injuries (a) Anterior wedge fracture (posterior ligament intact, therefore stable). (b) Comminuted fracture with 'teardrop' anteriorly and posterior fragment displaced backward (posterior ligament torn, therefore unstable). (c) Extension injury (anterior ligament torn, but stable in flexion).

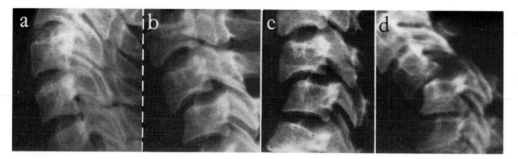

25.9 Unstable neck injuries   In (a) the cervical spine looks normal, but the film in flexion (b) shows forward subluxation – the posterior ligaments are torn. (c) Fracture-dislocation with moderate forward shift signifying a unilateral facet dislocation; (d) another fracture-dislocation with severe forward shift.

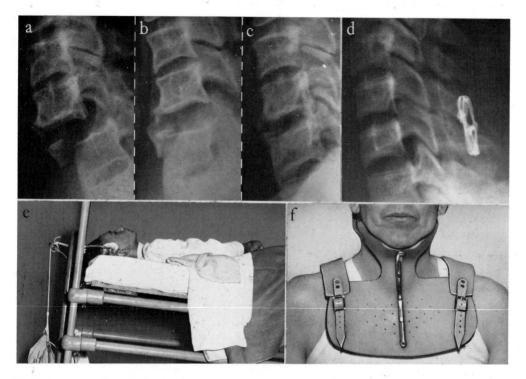

25.10 Treatment of cervical spine fractures   (a, b, c) Stages in the reduction of a fracture-dislocation by skull traction; (d) subsequent wiring to ensure stability. (e) The patient was kept on skull traction until the wound was healed. A polythene collar as in (f) was then applied.

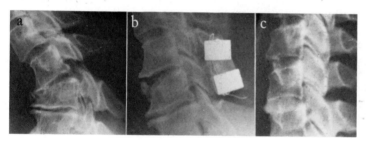

25.11 Treatment of cervical spine fractures (continued)   (a) Late redisplacement some months after treatment by external splintage alone; (b) stability has been restored by posterior fixation. Sometimes an anterior bone graft, as in (c), is preferred.

achieved; if not, gentle manipulation under anaesthesia is permissible. If the dislocation is reduced, traction is kept on for 6 weeks; some prefer a halo-body cast while awaiting spontaneous fusion – which may take 3–4 months. If this does not occur, posterior operative fusion is indicated; a collar is retained until the graft is incorporated. If skull traction fails to reduce the dislocation, operative reduction and posterior fusion are carried out within the first 2 days.

Unilateral facet dislocation The treatment is essentially the same as for bilateral dislocation, but the lesion is more stable and, once reduced, does not require either prolonged immobilization or spinal fusion. Three weeks' skull traction and 6 weeks in a collar are adequate.

Fracture-dislocations

These are extremely unstable and often associated with cord damage. They are most satisfactorily reduced by skull traction. The method advocated by Evans (1966) is to anaesthetize the patient, pass an endotracheal tube, and then to x-ray the neck and see if the fracture is reduced. If not, gentle manual traction associated with rotation may achieve reduction; but, whether or not the fracture is reduced, skull traction is then applied.

Many surgeons prefer to apply skull traction as the first manoeuvre. The next step depends upon the precise nature of the injury: with unilateral facet dislocation traction is maintained while the neck is rotated and tilted away from the dislocated side, then twisted back to neutral and, finally, extended; with fractured facets or bilateral facet dislocation a straight pull may be sufficient to obtain reduction. By adjusting the angle and the amount of traction, and judging the results on lateral films, reduction can usually be achieved within a few hours. Once reduction is satisfactory, the neck is held slightly extended with only light traction (5 kg).

Whichever method of reduction is used the patient remains on traction for 3 weeks and then a lateral x-ray is taken. If this shows that callus is forming (and therefore that spontaneous interbody fusion will follow) the traction is retained unchanged for a further 3 weeks, after which it is removed and a collar applied. If the film taken at 3 weeks shows no callus then interbody fusion is not likely to occur; the injury is mainly ligamentous and a bone grafting operation is performed as for a pure dislocation. Again the traction is maintained during the operation and afterwards until the wound is healed. Following grafting a polythene collar is sufficient until the graft is incorporated.

Thoracic spine injuries

Between T1 and T8 the rib cage imparts great stability to the spinal column. Only two varieties of injury occur.

ANTERIOR WEDGE FRACTURES These of course are stable and can safely be treated by activity. It should be borne in mind, however, that a considerable proportion of anterior wedge fractures in the thoracic spine are pathological in nature, occurring as a result of osteoporosis or malignant deposits.

A TRUE FRACTURE-DISLOCATION Almost invariably, paraplegia results and, in any event, the displacement is quite irreducible. Consequently it is the paraplegia which should be treated rather than the fracture itself.

Thoracolumbar injuries

Management clearly depends upon precise diagnosis, but in one respect it must precede diagnosis. *When the patient is seen at the site of the accident it is essential that he is handled in such a way that, even if he has an unstable fracture, displacement will not be increased.* He must be moved onto the stretcher 'in one piece': traction is applied to the head and legs and the spine is kept straight.

Diagnosis

Usually the patient is first seen lying supine on a stretcher or trolley. The opportunity should be taken to examine the chest and abdomen first for associated injuries. It must be remembered that, while abdominal pain and tenderness are suggestive of intra-abdominal damage, they can occur with a purely spinal injury. Next, the lower limbs are examined for evidence of neurological damage.

To examine the back, the patient is carefully turned (at least two and preferably three people are needed) onto one side. First, the skin is inspected for abrasions or bruising; either indicates the probable level of injury. Next, the spinous processes are palpated systematically. With unstable injuries a gap can be felt where the ligament has been torn; this important physical sign is surprisingly easy to elicit. Spinal movements should not be examined; the attempt may imperil the cord.

Finally, x-rays are taken. As they must be of high quality, portable apparatus is quite inadequate. The minimum requirements are anteroposterior and lateral views, but two laterals are better – one centred over the vertebral bodies and the other over the spinous processes; oblique views and tomograms also may be helpful. Interpreting films is not always easy and it is important in both the anteroposterior and lateral views to inspect carefully: (1) the alignment of the vertebrae – is there any angulation or shift at any one point? (2) the shape of the individual vertebral bodies – is there any loss of the normal box-like appearance? (3) the neural arches – is there any evidence of fracture or of dislocation?

Management of stable fractures

Anterior wedge fractures

These result from forward hinging and are stable. The best treatment is by activity. For the first few days, while the back is painful and the muscles are in spasm, the patient is turned onto his face several times each day, radiant heat is applied and he is taught to use his spinal muscles. Analgesics may be necessary for the first week. As soon as he is comfortable he is got up and encouraged to use his back fully and actively.

If loss of vertebral height is greater than 50 per cent, progressive collapse may occur. A well-fitting brace or plaster jacket is indicated; if painful kyphosis seems inevitable, spinal fusion may be necessary.

Burst fractures

Burst fractures also are stable because the posterior ligament complex is undamaged. They are, however, associated with considerable pain and the posterior portion of the vertebral body is perilously close to the dura and nerve roots. Consequently, these fractures are usually treated in a plaster jacket despite their stability. The jacket should be applied, not with the spine hyperextended, but in the neutral position. After 6 weeks it can safely be replaced by a polythene jacket which is taken off for washing and sleeping; and at 12 weeks from the time of injury it can be discarded altogether.

A burst fracture may cause paraplegia. Treatment of the spine is essentially the same, but a plaster jacket is not used.

Laminar fractures

These probably result from hinging the back into extension and are frequently missed. It has been shown that some patients thought to have sustained disc prolapse have, in fact, sustained lami-

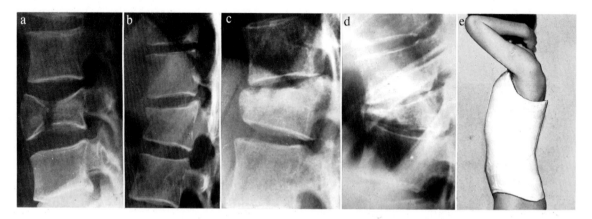

25.12 Stable thoracolumbar fractures (a) Burst fracture. (b) Trivial anterior wedge fracture. (c) Wedge fracture with a little less than 50 per cent loss of height in front. (d) Severe wedge fracture with more than 50 per cent loss of height. (e) Plaster jacket such as would be used in treating (a) and (d).

nar fractures which can best be demonstrated on oblique radiographs. If these fractures are untreated, non-union is likely and, at L4 or L5, forward displacement may subsequently occur which results in spondylolisthesis. Consequently these injuries, too, are best treated in a plaster jacket; after 6 weeks this can be replaced by a polythene jacket, which should not be discarded until x-rays demonstrate union.

Management of unstable fractures

In these the problem of paraplegia dominates management.

Fractures with paraplegia

In the presence of anaesthetic skin, treatment in plaster is not safe, because pressure sores are likely to develop rapidly. Two methods of management are available.

Conservative The patient is turned every 2 hours onto his side; three assistants are needed so that he is moved in one piece. While on his side his skin is carefully cleaned and the sheets are meticulously smoothed. In this way pressure sores can be avoided and, after a few days or weeks, the patient can be moved more easily and without discomfort.

Operative The spine is fixed without delay; plates are attached on each side of the spinous processes and fix two processes above and two below the torn ligament; alternatively two small Harrington rods may be used. Fixation facilitates nursing and turning is made comfortable; moreover, further damage to nerve roots is prevented.

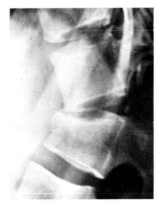

25.13 Thoracolumbar injuries Whereas forward flexion usually crushes bone but leaves the posterior ligaments intact, this injury has done the reverse – the posterior ligaments are completely torn, the bone only slightly crushed. The patient had a seatbelt injury as in Fig. 25.1 (h).

The advocates of closed treatment point out that fixation often fails; the plates or rods break out of the bony processes, the fracture redisplaces, the implants press on the skin, and sepsis follows. It may well be that poorly applied plates break out but, in the hands of a skilled spinal surgeon, fixation is safe and on the whole is the more satisfactory method.

Unstable fractures without paraplegia

The spine must be held because movement may damage the cord. Stability can be achieved by plating as already described; but, in the absence of paraplegia, closed treatment in plaster is safe.

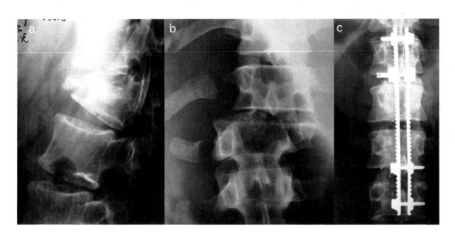

25.14 Thoracolumbar unstable fractures (a) Fracture-dislocation with considerable forward shift; (b) AP view of another patient with gross displacement and paraplegia; such fractures are well treated by (c) open reduction and internal fixation.

A reasonable routine is as follows. The patient is placed prone on an operating table and in that position re-x-rayed. Provided reduction has been achieved (and it often has) plaster is applied to the back half of the trunk and legs, as the first step towards making a plaster bed. When this is complete the patient lies in the back half, but for cleaning purposes he is turned over into the front half at least once a week. After 6 weeks the fracture is less unstable and a plaster jacket is applied with the spine in neutral position. The patient is then allowed up. He wears the jacket for a further 6–12 weeks, the precise time being determined by x-ray; the plaster is not discarded until bony fusion is seen between the fractured vertebra and its neighbour.

Sometimes the prone position fails to achieve reduction. This usually indicates locked facets and it is worth while to hinge the operating table at the level of the fracture. If the facets are still locked the patient is anaesthetized. Gentle manipulation combined with traction may achieve reduction but, if not, there should be no hesitation in exposing the fracture operatively and reducing it under direct vision. Facetectomy is not often necessary and laminectomy hardly ever indicated. Following open reduction, internal fixation is used. Where there is considerable bony (as distinct from ligamentous) damage, plates and bolts are sufficient because spontaneous interbody fusion will occur before the bolts become loose. But if the injury is mainly ligamentous (as in seat-belt fractures) it is wise to apply bone grafts as well because spontaneous ligament repair cannot be relied upon to prevent late displacement.

Injuries with neural damage

In spinal injuries the displaced structures may damage the cord, or nerve roots, or both; cervical lesions may cause *quadriplegia*, thoracolumbar lesions *paraplegia*. The damage may be temporary or permanent. Three varieties of lesion occur.

CORD CONCUSSION
Motor paralysis (flaccid), sensory loss and visceral paralysis occur below the level of the cord lesion. The disturbance is one of function without a demonstrable anatomical lesion. Recovery begins within 8 hours and eventually becomes complete.

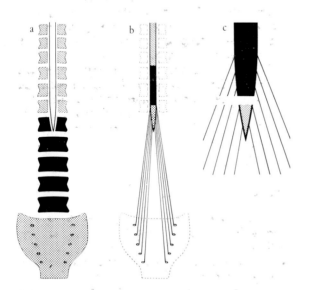

Thoracic segments (bony and neural)

Lumbar segments (bony and neural)

Sacral segments (bony and neural)

25.15 Traumatic paraplegia   (a) In the adult the cord ends at the lower border of L1. (b) Shows the disposition of the nerve roots. In (c) an injury to the 12th thoracic vertebra has transected the cord between the lumbar and sacral segments; on one side the roots also are transected, on the other there has been root escape.

CORD TRANSECTION

Motor paralysis, sensory loss and visceral paralysis occur below the level of the cord lesion; as with cord concussion the motor paralysis is at first flaccid. This is a temporary condition known as cord shock, but the injury is anatomical and irreparable.

After a time, however, the cord below the level of transection recovers from the shock and acts as an independent structure; that is, it manifests reflex activity. In a few hours the anal and penile reflexes return, and the plantar responses become extensor. In a few days or weeks the flaccid paralysis becomes spastic, with increased tone, increased tendon reflexes and clonus; flexor spasms and contractures may develop but sensation never returns. The presence of anal and penile reflexes in the absence of sensation in the legs is diagnostic of cord transection.

ROOT TRANSECTION

Motor paralysis, sensory loss and visceral paralysis occur in the distribution of the damaged roots. Root transection, however, differs from cord transection in two ways: (1) regeneration is theoretically possible; and (2) residual motor paralysis remains permanently flaccid.

Anatomical levels

CERVICAL SPINE

With cervical spine injuries, the segmental level of cord transection nearly corresponds to the level of bony damage. Not more than one or two additional roots are likely to be transected. High cervical cord transection is fatal because all the respiratory muscles are paralysed. At the level of the fifth cervical vertebra cord transection isolates the lower cervical cord (with paralysis of the upper limbs), the thoracic cord (with paralysis of the trunk) and the lumbar and sacral cord (with paralysis of the lower limbs and viscera). With injury below the fifth cervical vertebra, the upper limbs are partially spared and characteristic deformities result.

BETWEEN FIRST AND TENTH THORACIC VERTEBRAE

The first lumbar cord segment in the adult is at the level of the tenth thoracic vertebra. Consequently, cord transection at that level spares the thoracic cord but isolates the entire lumbar and sacral cord, with paralysis of the lower limbs and viscera. The lower thoracic roots may also be transected but are of relatively little importance.

BELOW TENTH THORACIC VERTEBRA

The cord forms a slight bulge (the conus medullaris) between the tenth thoracic and first lumbar vertebrae, and tapers to an end at the interspace between the first and second lumbar vertebrae. The second lumbar to fourth sacral nerve roots arise from the conus medullaris and stream downwards in a bunch (the cauda equina) to emerge at successive levels of the lumbosacral spine. Therefore, spinal injuries above the tenth thoracic vertebra cause cord transection, those between the tenth thoracic and first lumbar vertebrae cause cord and nerve root lesions, and those below the first lumbar vertebra only root lesions.

The sacral roots innervate (1) sensation in the 'saddle' area, a strip down the back of the thigh and leg, and the outer two-thirds of the sole; (2) motor power to the muscles controlling the ankle and foot; (3) the anal and penile reflexes, plantar responses and ankle jerks; (4) control of micturition.

The lumbar roots innervate (1) sensation to the entire lower limb other than that portion supplied by the sacral segment; (2) motor power to the muscles controlling the hip and knee; and (3) the cremasteric reflexes and knee jerks.

It is essential, when the bony injury is at the thoracolumbar junction, to distinguish between *cord transection with root escape* and *cord transection with root transection*. A patient with root escape is much better off than one with cord and root transection.

Signs

Clinical examination of the back nearly always shows the signs of an unstable fracture; however, a 'burst' fracture with paraplegia is stable. The nature and level of the bone lesion are demonstrated by x-ray.

Neurological examination should be painstaking. Without detailed information, accurate diagnosis and prognosis are impossible; rectal examination is mandatory.

COMPLETE CORD LESIONS

Complete paralysis and anaesthesia below the level of injury suggest cord transection. During the stage of *spinal shock* when the anal reflex is absent (seldom longer than the first 24 hours) the diagnosis cannot be absolutely certain; if the anal reflex returns and the neural deficit persists, the cord lesion is complete.

INCOMPLETE CORD LESIONS

Persistence of any sensation distal to the injury (perianal pinprick is most important) suggests an incomplete lesion and therefore a favourable prognosis. The commonest is the *central cord syndrome* where the initial flaccid weakness is followed by lower motor neuron paralysis of the upper limbs with upper motor neuron (spastic) paralysis of the lower limbs, and preservation of bladder control and perianal sensation (sacral sparing). With the less common *anterior cord syndrome* there is complete paralysis and anaesthesia but deep pressure and position sense are retained in the lower limbs (dorsal column sparing). The *posterior cord syndrome* is rare (only deep pressure and proprioception are lost), and the *Brown-Séquard syndrome* (cord hemisection, with ipsilateral paralysis and contralateral loss of pain sensation) is usually associated with thoracic injuries. Below the tenth thoracic vertebra discrepancies between neurological and skeletal levels are due to *transection of roots* descending from segments higher than the cord lesion.

Management of traumatic paraplegia and quadriplegia

Decompression of the cord seems a tempting possibility, but laminectomy alone has proved a failure; its only effect is to make an already unstable spine even more so. Anterior decompression has been used with some success (Riska, 1973), but the procedure is still not widely accepted. Operation simply to fix an unstable injury may facilitate nursing and speed rehabilitation.

No matter whether the paraplegia is complete or partial, temporary or permanent, it is the overall management which is important, and especially the management in the first 24 hours. The patient must be transported with great care to avoid further damage, and preferably taken to a spinal centre. The strategy is outlined below.

SKIN

Within a few hours anaesthetic skin may develop enormous pressure sores; these must be prevented by meticulous nursing. Immediate fixation of the spine (page 425) enables these essential nursing procedures to be carried out much more easily and without discomfort to the patient. Creases in the sheets and crumbs in the bed are not permitted. Every 2 hours the patient is gently rolled onto his side and his back is carefully washed (without rubbing), dried and powdered. After a few weeks the skin becomes a little more tolerant and the patient can turn himself. Later he should be taught how to relieve skin pressure intermittently during periods of sitting. If sores have been allowed to develop, they may never heal without excision and skin grafting.

BLADDER AND BOWEL

For the first 24 hours the bladder distends only slowly, but, if the distension is allowed to progress, overflow incontinence occurs and infection is probable. In special centres it is usual to manage the patient from the outset by intermittent catheterization under sterile conditions. If early transfer to a paraplegia centre is not possible, continuous drainage through a fine Silastic catheter is advised. The catheter drains in a closed manner into a disposable bag, and is changed twice weekly to avoid blockage. When infection supervenes, antibiotics are given.

Bladder training is begun at 1 week if possible. Although retention is complete to begin with, partial recovery may lead to (1) an automatic bladder which works reflexly, or (2) an expressible bladder which is emptied by manual suprapubic pressure.

A few patients are left with a high residual urine after emptying the bladder. They need special investigations, including cystography and cystometry; transurethral resection of the bladder neck or sphincterotomy may be indicated but should not be performed until at least 3 months of bladder training have been completed.

The bowel is more easily trained, with the help of enemas, aperients and abdominal exercises.

MUSCLES AND JOINTS

The paralysed muscles, if not treated, may develop severe flexion contractures. These are usually preventable by moving the joints passively through their full range twice daily. Later, splints become necessary.

With lesions below the cervical cord, the patient should be up within 3 months; standing and walking are valuable in preventing contractures. Calipers are usually necessary to keep the knees straight and the feet plantigrade. The calipers are removed at intervals during the day while the patient lies prone, and while he is having physiotherapy. The upper limbs must be trained until they develop sufficient power to enable the patient to use crutches and a wheelchair.

If flexion contractures have been allowed to develop, tenotomies may be necessary. Painful flexor spasms are rare unless skin or bladder infection occurs. They can sometimes be relieved by tenotomies, neurectomies, rhizotomies or the intrathecal injection of alcohol.

Heterotopic ossification may restrict or abolish movement, especially at the hip. It is doubtful whether ossification can be prevented, but once the new bone is mature it can safely be excised.

MORALE

The morale of a paraplegic patient is liable to reach a low ebb, and the restoration of his self-confidence is an important part of treatment. Constant enthusiasm and encouragement by doctors, physiotherapists and nurses is essential. Their scrupulous attention to his comfort and toilet are of primary importance; the unpleasant smells associated with skin or urinary infection must be avoided. The earlier the patient gets up the better, and he must be trained for a new job as quickly as possible.

Further reading

Anderson, L. D. and D'Alonzo, R. T. (1974) Fractures of the odontoid process of the axis. *Journal of Bone and Joint Surgery* **56A,** 1663–1674

Evans, D. K. (1966) Fractures and dislocations of the spine. In *Clinical Surgery,* vol. 12, *Fractures and Dislocations.* Ed. by R. Furlong. London: Butterworths

Hardy, A. G. and Rossier, A. B. (1975) *Spinal Cord Injuries.* Stuttgart: Georg Thieme

Harris, J. H. (1978) *The Radiology of Acute Cervical Spine Trauma.* Baltimore: Williams & Wilkins

Holdsworth, Sir F. W. (1970) Fractures, dislocations and fracture-dislocations of the spine. *Journal of Bone and Joint Surgery* **52A,** 1534–1551

Lewis, J. and McKibbin, B. (1974) The treatment of unstable fracture-dislocation of the thoraco-lumbar spine accompanied by paraplegia. *Journal of Bone and Joint Surgery* **56B,** 603–612

Riska, E. B. (1973) Antero-lateral decompression as a treatment of fresh paraplegia following vertebral fractures. *Acta Orthopaedica Scandinavica* **44,** 89–91

Injuries of the Pelvis

The symmetrical halves of the pelvis articulate anteriorly at the pubic symphysis to form part of a bony ring which is completed posteriorly by the sacrococcygeal segments of the spine and the sacroiliac joints. The pelvic basin contains the lower intestinal tract, the urogenital structures and many large vessels and nerves; in pelvic fractures, injuries of these soft tissues are more serious than the bony lesions.

A fracture of the pelvis should be suspected and excluded by x-ray in every patient with serious abdominal or lower limb injuries. Local bruising or abrasions may be obvious; ecchymoses may extend into the thigh, labia or scrotum. Pain may be elicited if the pelvic ring is sprung by gentle but firm pressure – first from side to side on the iliac crests, then outwards on the anterior superior iliac spines, and then directly on the symphysis pubis. During a rectal examination the coccyx and sacrum can be felt; more important, the position of the prostate may indicate a urethral injury.

Haemorrhage and shock may be severe, and resuscitation should be started even before x-ray examination. Ideally, four views should be obtained: a standard anteroposterior view, an inlet view with the tube tilted 20–30 degrees caudad, and two oblique 45-degree views taken with the patient rolled gently first onto one buttock and then onto the other.

If the patient cannot pass urine he *must not be catheterized*; gentle retrograde urethrography is harmless and may show a urethral tear.

Pelvic fractures fall into four groups. (1) Isolated fractures with an intact ring. (2) Fractures with a broken ring; these may be stable or unstable. (3) Fractures of the acetabulum; although these are ring fractures, involvement of the joint raises special problems and therefore they are considered separately. (4) Sacrococcygeal fractures.

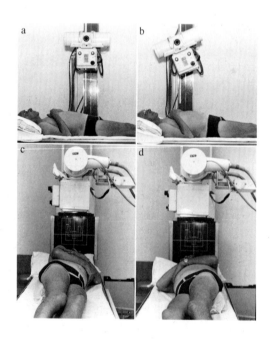

26.1 Pelvic fractures – x-ray diagnosis Four views are essential: (a) anteroposterior; (b) inlet view with tube tilted 20–30 degrees; (c) and (d) right and left oblique views.

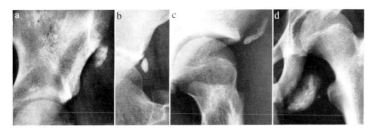

26.2 Avulsion injuries These all result from powerful muscle action. (a) Avulsion of sartorius attachment; this should not be confused with (b) an os acetabuli, which is well-defined on all sides. (c) Avulsion of rectus origin. (d) Avulsion of hamstring origin – the clinical condition is much less alarming than the x-ray.

Isolated fractures with an intact ring

AVULSION FRACTURES are due to violent muscle action in athletes. The sartorius may pull off the anterior superior iliac spine, the rectus femoris the anterior inferior iliac spine, the adductor longus a piece of the pubis, and the hamstrings part of the ischium. All are essentially muscle injuries, needing only rest for a few days and reassurance. Pain may take months to disappear and, because there is often no history of injury, biopsy of the callus may lead to an erroneous diagnosis of a tumour.

DIRECT FRACTURES of the ischium or of the iliac blade may follow a fall. Bed rest until pain subsides is adequate.

STRESS FRACTURES of the pubic rami are fairly common (and often quite painless) in severely osteoporotic patients.

Fractures with a broken ring

It has been cogently argued that, because of the rigidity of the pelvis, a break at one point in the ring must be accompanied by disruption at a

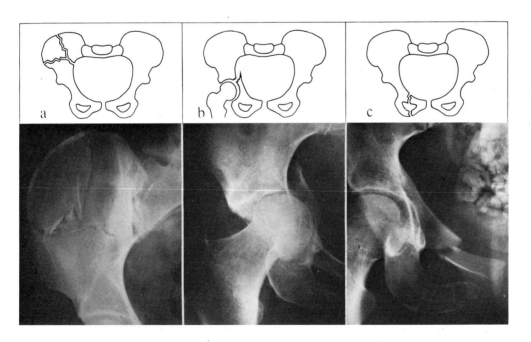

26.3 Stable pelvic ring fractures The ring is broken in only one place. (a) The blade of the ilium; (b) the floor of the acetabulum; (c) the ischiopubic ramus.

second point; exceptions are fractures due to direct blows (including fractures of the acetabular floor), or ring fractures in children, whose symphysis and sacroiliac joints are springy. Often, however, the second break is not visible – either because it is reduced immediately, or because the sacroiliac joints are only partially disrupted; in these circumstances the visible fracture is not displaced and the ring is stable. A fracture or joint disruption that is markedly displaced, and all obvious double ring fractures, are unstable. This distinction has more practical value than a pedantic classification into 'single' and 'double' ring fractures.

Stable ring fractures

Undisplaced fractures of one or both ipsilateral pubic rami may be due to direct violence or to a fall on the side of the pelvis. If the inferior ramus alone is fractured, oblique views almost invariably show a second fracture into the floor of the acetabulum. These lesions are stable and pelvic viscera are seldom damaged; but the patient has pain on attempting to walk. Treatment is symptomatic: bed rest until discomfort subsides, then up, with a stick or crutches for a few weeks.

Undisplaced fractures of the posterior part of the ring (usually close to the sacroiliac joint) are uncommon and most often due to direct violence posteriorly. There is bruising over the buttock and often tenderness over the pubic symphysis, suggesting a strain or partial disruption. The injury is severe and the patient should be kept in bed for 4–6 weeks; if there is displacement, this period should be doubled.

Unstable ring fractures

The ring is clearly disrupted by a displaced fracture or by separation of the pubic symphysis or sacroiliac joint. The main causes are crushing injuries, falls from heights and road accidents. Perkins distinguished three mechanisms: (1) anteroposterior compression, which fractures the pubic rami on both sides; (2) a hinge force, which is applied to one blade of the ilium and 'opens' the pelvis (e.g. when a patient is run over); and (3) a vertical force due to a fall onto one leg, causing vertical displacement of the pubis and ilium on the same side.

These are all extremely serious injuries, with a high incidence of visceral damage and a significant mortality rate. The patient is in pain, cannot stand and may be unable to pass urine. Haemorrhage is often considerable and shock severe.

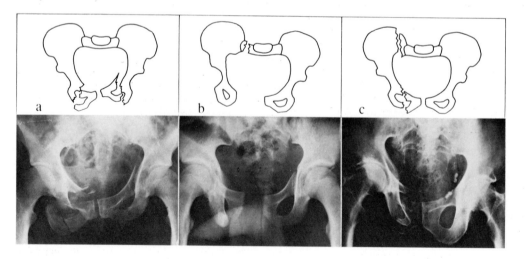

26.4 Unstable pelvic ring disruptions   The ring is broken in more than one place. (a) Anteroposterior crush; (b) hinge type of injury; (c) vertical force fracture.

Urogenital damage may be indicated by the presence of blood at the external meatus.

There may be a graze or perineal bruising and swelling. A gap at the symphysis is occasionally felt. Tenderness may be too great or too diffuse to be of diagnostic value. One leg may be partly anaesthetic because of sciatic nerve damage. About one-third of these patients have urethral injuries.

X-RAY
There may be fractures of the pubic rami bilaterally, symphyseal separation, ipsilateral fractures of anterior and posterior elements, or contralateral injuries (e.g. pubic rami on one side and the sacroiliac joint on the other).

Treatment of ring fractures

EMERGENCY TREATMENT
Shock For the treatment of shock, see page 372.

Urogenital damage Compression fractures are the usual cause of urogenital tract damage; but with all pelvic ring disruptions, damage must be excluded. However, all that needs to be provided urgently in a seriously ill patient is adequate urinary drainage, which is accomplished by suprapubic cystostomy. Definitive repair may well be delayed whilst the patient's general condition improves and expert urological advice is sought.

The patient is asked to pass urine; provided he can, and if the urine is clear, all is well. If he cannot, or if there is blood at the external meatus, the temptation to pass a catheter in the less-than-ideal surroundings of the casualty reception room should be resisted for fear of converting a partial to a complete rupture of the urethra. Gentle retrograde urethrography using dilute aqueous medium will establish the presence and site of a urethral leak. If the urethra is intact, the bladder will be outlined. The uncommon condition of gross upward dislocation of the prostate may be safely demonstrated by intravenous urography, as will ruptures of the bladder.

Intrapelvic rupture of the urethra is treated by suprapubic cystostomy for urinary drainage, a retropubic corrugated or suction drain, and an indwelling fenestrated urethral catheter to provide alignment of the urethra as well as drainage of blood and secretions from its lumen. If the bladder is floating high it is repositioned and held down by a sling-suture passed through the apex of the prostate, through the perineum lateral to the urethra, and anchored to the thighs by elastic bands.

Rupture of the bladder is treated by suprapubic cystostomy with, in addition, suture of the tear if it is intraperitoneal or drainage of the retropubic space if extraperitoneal.

TREATMENT OF THE FRACTURE
Compression type Reduction is neither possible nor necessary; consequently splintage is not required. The patient lies free in bed for 3 weeks; active movements of the hip and spine are encouraged. He is then allowed to walk normally; weight-bearing is quite safe because the line of weight transmission does not pass through the fracture area.

Hinge type Under anaesthesia the patient is rolled onto his unaffected side. The surgeon leans on the upper half of the pelvis and by this means 'closes' the pelvis. Reduction is usually stable, and a firm binder or lumbosacral corset is sufficient protection. If reduction fails (or if urogenital surgery is being done), metal fixation may be used: the vertical rami of the pubis are plated together; an alternative is external fixation with rods.

For the first 4–6 weeks the patient remains in bed, but is encouraged to move his limbs. The external fixation device can be removed after 4 weeks. He is then allowed up, using crutches at first, and within 12 weeks should have regained full activity. The corset is discarded after 3 months.

Vertical force type Under anaesthesia, the leg on the side of the pelvis which has shifted upwards is forcibly pulled down. Skeletal traction is applied and the patient remains on traction for 6 weeks. He is then allowed up with crutches but should not take weight for 3 months from the injury.

Complications

Persistent sacroiliac pain is fairly common after hinge fractures and may occasionally necessitate arthrodesis of the sacroiliac joint. Sciatic nerve injury usually recovers but sometimes exploration later proves necessary. Severe urethral injuries may result in impotence.

Fractures of the acetabulum

Fractures of the acetabulum combine the complexities of pelvic fractures (notably the frequency of associated soft-tissue injury) with those of joint

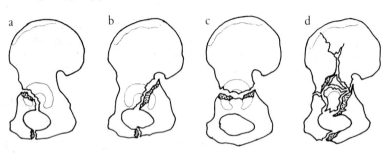

26.5 Acetabular fractures The four types of injury: (a) simple fracture of the anterior pillar; (b) fracture of the posterior pillar; (c) transverse fracture, which usually lies just above the cotyloid notch; and (d) a composite fracture. The transverse fractures (occasionally) and the composite fractures (almost always) damage the weight-bearing surface and may cause post-traumatic osteoarthritis.

disruption (namely, the attendant risks of stiffness and secondary osteoarthritis).

There are four major types of acetabular fracture; though they are distinguished on anatomical grounds, it is important to recognize that they also differ in their ease of reduction, their stability after reduction and their long-term prognosis.

(1) ANTERIOR FRACTURE   The fracture runs through the thin anterior part of the acetabulum separating a segment between the anterior inferior iliac spine and the obturator foramen. It is uncommon, does not involve the weight-bearing area and has a good prognosis.

(2) POSTERIOR FRACTURE   This fracture runs upwards from the obturator foramen into the sciatic notch, separating the posterior ischiopubic column of bone and breaking the weight-bearing part of the acetabulum. It is usually associated with a posterior dislocation of the hip and may injure the sciatic nerve. Treatment is more urgent and usually involves internal fixation to obtain a stable joint.

(3) TRANSVERSE FRACTURE   This is an uncomminuted fracture running transversely through the acetabulum and separating the iliac portion above from the pubic and ischial portions below. It is usually fairly easy to reduce and to hold reduced.

(4) COMPLEX FRACTURES   Most acetabular fractures are complex injuries which damage either the anterior or the posterior segments (or both) as well as the roof of the acetabulum. There is no value in precise subdivision, since the differences between the various types are much less important than their similarities. They all share the following features: (a) the injury is severe; (b) the joint surface is disrupted; (c) they are difficult to reduce; (d) they always need expert treatment, often operative; and (e) the end result is likely to be less than perfect.

Clinical features

There has usually been a severe injury – either a traffic accident or a fall from a height. Associated fractures are not uncommon and, because they may be more obvious, are liable to divert attention from the more urgent pelvic injuries. Whenever a fractured femur, a severe knee injury or a fractured calcaneum is diagnosed, the hips also should be x-rayed.

The patient may be severely shocked, and the complications associated with all pelvic fractures should be sought. There may be bruising around the hip and the limb may lie in internal rotation (if the hip is dislocated). No attempt should be made to move the hip.

X-RAY
At least four views should be taken in every case: a standard anteroposterior view, the pelvic inlet view and two 45-degree oblique views (to show the anterior and posterior columns separately). The type of fracture, degree of comminution and the amount of displacement are noted.

Treatment

Emergency treatment should consist only of counteracting shock and reducing a dislocation. Traction is then applied to the limb (10 kg will suffice) and during the next 3 or 4 days the patient's general condition is brought under control. Definitive treatment of the fracture is delayed until he is fit and operation facilities are optimal; but the delay should not exceed 7 days.

With simple anterior or posterior fractures closed reduction under general anaesthesia is attempted. If this is successful, traction is maintained for a further 6 weeks. If closed reduction fails and adequate surgical expertise is available, operative reduction and internal fixation with lag screws or a compression plate are advisable; for anterior fractures a modified Smith-Peterson approach is used, and for posterior fractures a 'southern' approach.

Complex fractures are difficult to reduce, and in elderly patients operative intervention is not advised unless a persistent posterior dislocation needs to be stabilized. In younger patients, however, the likelihood of osteoarthritis is so great that operative reduction and fixation is justified. This sometimes requires a wide lateral approach, exposing both the anterior and the posterior columns; it should not be attempted in the absence of ideal operating facilities, ample blood for transfusion and adequate surgical expertise.

If comminution is so severe that the architecture cannot be restored, again operation should not be attempted. Traction is continued and exercises started as soon as possible. If necessary, arthroplasty of the hip can be carried out years later when union is complete and function has stabilized.

Injuries to the sacrum and coccyx

A blow from behind, or a fall onto the 'tail' may fracture the sacrum or coccyx, or sprain the joint between them. Women seem to be affected more commonly than men.

Bruising is considerable and tenderness is elicited when the sacrum or coccyx is palpated from behind or per rectum. Sensation may be lost over the distribution of sacral nerves.

X-rays may show (1) a transverse fracture of the sacrum, in rare cases with the lower fragment pushed forwards; (2) a fractured coccyx, sometimes with the lower fragment angulated forwards; or (3) a normal appearance if the injury was a sprain of the sacrococcygeal joint.

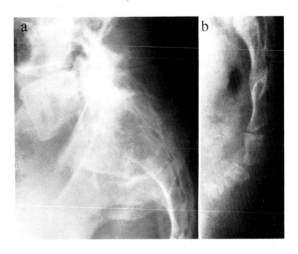

26.6 Sacrococcygeal fractures (a) Fractured sacrum; (b) fractured coccyx.

If the fracture is displaced, reduction is worth attempting. The lower fragment may be pushed backwards per rectum. The reduction is stable, which is fortunate. The patient is allowed to resume normal activity, but is advised to use a rubber ring or Sorbo cushion when sitting.

Persistent pain, especially on sitting, is common after coccygeal injuries. If the pain is not relieved by the use of a Sorbo cushion or by the injection of local anaesthetic into the tender area, excision of the coccyx may be considered.

Further reading

Perkins, G. (1966) Fractures of the pelvis. In *Clinical Surgery*, vol. 12, *Fractures and Dislocations*. Ed. by R. Furlong. London: Butterworths

Senegas, J., Liorzou, G. and Yates, M. (1980) Complex acetabular fractures: a transtrochanteric lateral surgical approach. *Clinical Orthopaedics and Related Research* **151**, 107–114

Tile, M. (1980) Fractures of the acetabulum. *Orthopedic Clinics of North America* **11**, 481–506

I Injuries of the hip and femur

Dislocations of the hip

Posterior dislocation

Four out of five traumatic hip dislocations are posterior. Usually the bent leg is violently thrust backwards, as when a car hits a tree and the passenger's knee is struck by the dashboard. The impact is liable to fracture the acetabular roof, which displaces with the femoral head; only when the hip is adducted at the moment of impact is dislocation likely to occur without fracture.

Special features

The leg is short and lies adducted, internally rotated and slightly flexed. The femoral head cannot be felt in its socket, but may be palpable in the buttock.

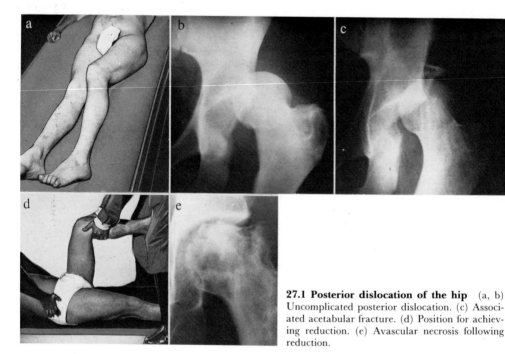

27.1 Posterior dislocation of the hip (a, b) Uncomplicated posterior dislocation. (c) Associated acetabular fracture. (d) Position for achieving reduction. (e) Avascular necrosis following reduction.

X-RAY

In the anteroposterior film the femoral head is seen out of its socket and above the acetabulum. A segment of acetabular roof or femoral head may have been broken off and displaced; oblique films are useful in demonstrating the size of the fragment. If any fracture is seen, other bony fragments (which may need removal) must be suspected.

Treatment

● REDUCE

Deep anaesthesia is essential, preferably with a relaxant. Reduction is more easily effected with the patient lying on a mattress on the floor. An assistant steadies the pelvis; the surgeon flexes the patient's hip and knee to 90 degrees and pulls the thigh vertically upwards. Usually this manoeuvre effects reduction, but sometimes it is necessary also to abduct the flexed hip. X-rays are essential to confirm reduction and to exclude a fracture.

● HOLD

Reduction is stable, but the hip has been severely injured and needs to be rested. The simplest treatment is to apply traction and maintain it for 3 weeks. Alternatively, a plaster spica may be applied with the hip in the neutral position.

● EXERCISE

If the patient is being treated on traction active exercises are permitted, but forced movements are prohibited for fear of myositis ossificans.

At the end of 3 weeks, plaster or traction is removed and the hip x-rayed. In the absence of an associated fracture or myositis ossificans (and provided movements are painless), weight-bearing is permitted.

Complications

EARLY

Fractured acetabulum   A triangular fragment of the acetabulum may have been sheared off during dislocation. If the fragment is small and falls into place when the hip is reduced, traction for 6 weeks and avoiding weight-bearing for a further 6 weeks is probably adequate. But if it is large or imperfectly reduced, it should be fixed in place by screws. If there is more than one fragment it must be assumed that some pieces have entered the joint; operative removal of such débris is important.

Fractured femoral shaft   When this occurs at the same time as hip dislocation, the dislocation is commonly missed. It should be a rule that with every femoral shaft fracture the buttock and trochanter are palpated, and the hip clearly seen on x-ray. Even if this precaution has been omitted, a dislocation should be suspected whenever the proximal fragment of a transverse shaft fracture is seen to be adducted (Helal and Skevis, 1967).

Fractured femoral head   The dislocation may have sheared off a segment of the femoral head. Reduction of the dislocation may automatically reduce the fracture, and this can be confirmed by computerized tomography. Weight-bearing must be deferred for at least 12 weeks. If the head fragment has not been correctly reduced its replacement or excision provides the only hope of regaining reasonable movement at the hip.

Nerve lesions   The sciatic nerve is sometimes damaged but usually recovers. If, after reducing the dislocation, a sciatic nerve lesion and an unreduced acetabular fracture are diagnosed, the nerve should be explored and the fragment correctly replaced.

LATE

Avascular necrosis   The blood supply of the femoral head is seriously impaired in at least 20 per cent of traumatic hip dislocations; if reduction is delayed by more than a few hours, the figure rises to 50 per cent. Avascular necrosis shows on x-ray as increased density of the femoral head; but this change is not seen for at least 6 weeks, and sometimes very much longer.

The avascular head crushes if weight is taken through it; degenerative arthritis follows. If avascular necrosis is diagnosed before the head has begun to collapse, and the patient is relatively young, reduced weight-bearing for a period of up to 2 years might allow the head to revascularize without undue deformation. However, if avascular necrosis quickly leads to degenerative arthritis, an attempt can be made to arthrodese the hip, or the head may be excised and replaced by a metal prosthesis; in older patients a total replacement is better.

Myositis ossificans   It is essential after any injury to prohibit forced movements. Even if they are not the sole cause of myositis ossificans they

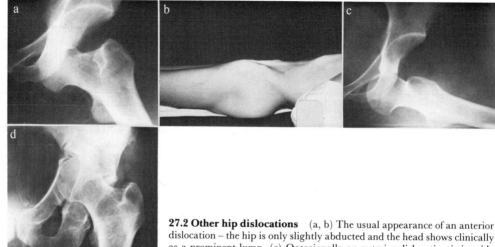

27.2 Other hip dislocations   (a, b) The usual appearance of an anterior dislocation – the hip is only slightly abducted and the head shows clinically as a prominent lump. (c) Occasionally an anterior dislocation is in wide abduction. (d) Central dislocation.

probably increase its severity. At the first suggestion of calcification around the hip, the joint should be rested in a hip spica. The final range will inevitably be restricted.

Unreduced dislocation   After a few weeks an untreated dislocation cannot be reduced by closed manipulation. Open reduction offers the best hope. If joint stiffness or avascular necrosis supervenes, the femoral head or the hip joint can later be replaced.

Anterior dislocation

Anterior dislocation is rare compared with posterior. The usual cause is a road accident or air crash. Dislocation of one or even both hips may occur when a weight falls onto the back of a miner or building labourer who is working with his legs wide apart, knees straight and back bent forwards.

Special features

The leg lies externally rotated, abducted and slightly flexed. It is not short, because the attachment of rectus femoris prevents the head from displacing upwards. Seen from the side, the anterior bulge of the dislocated head is unmistakable. Occasionally the leg is abducted almost to a right angle. The prominent head is easy to feel. Hip movements are impossible.

X-RAY   In the anteroposterior view the dislocation is usually obvious, but occasionally the head is almost directly in front of its normal position; any doubt is resolved by a lateral film.

Treatment and complications

The manoeuvres employed are almost identical with those used to reduce a posterior dislocation, except that while the flexed thigh is being pulled upwards, it should be adducted. The subsequent treatment is similar to that employed for posterior dislocation. Avascular necrosis is the only complication.

Central dislocation
(see also page 432)

A fall on the side, or a car smash, may fracture the acetabular floor and thrust the femoral head into the pelvis. The force is probably transmitted through the greater trochanter.

Special features

The thigh is grazed or bruised, but the leg lies in normal position. The trochanter and hip region are tender. Little movement is possible.

X-RAY   The femoral head is displaced medially, and the acetabular floor fractured.

Treatment

● REDUCE
The surgeon pulls strongly on the thigh and then tries to lever the head outwards by adducting the thigh, using his foot as a fulcrum. In the middle-aged or elderly patient it is wise to be content with

even imperfect reduction. In a young patient, if closed reduction fails, the displacement can sometimes be reduced openly and a large fragment fixed with screws. Lateral traction with a pin or screw through the greater trochanter rarely succeeds.

● HOLD
Whether or not the fracture has been reduced, skeletal traction is applied and a 7-kg pull maintained for 4 weeks.

● EXERCISE
Active use is encouraged from the start. When traction is removed the patient is allowed up with crutches. Weight-bearing is permitted after 8 weeks. The functional result is better than the x-ray appearance would suggest; but unless displacement was only trivial, all movements except flexion and extension remain considerably limited, and degenerative arthritis ultimately develops.

Complications

EARLY
As with other pelvic fractures, visceral injury may be present and shock severe (see page 433).

LATE
Joint stiffness, with or without osteoarthritis, is not uncommon. If total hip replacement is contemplated, it is essential to ensure that the acetabular fracture has united, otherwise the cup will inevitably work loose.

Fractures of the femoral neck

The injury occurs mainly among elderly women (fractures in the young are discussed on page 442). The patient may fall, but often merely catches her foot while walking; the foot twists and the femoral neck is broken by the rotation force. Osteoporosis and trabecular fatigue fractures may have weakened the bone, or it may be the site of a secondary deposit. Only rarely does a fracture occur in an osteoarthritic hip.

Femoral neck fractures have a poor capacity for healing because: (1) by tearing the capsular vessels the injury deprives the head of its main blood supply; (2) intra-articular bone has no contact with soft tissues which could promote osteogenesis; and (3) synovial fluid prevents clotting of the fracture haematoma. Accurate apposition and impaction of bone fragments are therefore of more importance than usual.

Special features

The leg is short and externally rotated. The greater trochanter is too high and too far posterior. Attempts at movement cause intense pain.

X-RAY
The fracture may be high (subcapital), transcervical or basal. The angle of the fracture line is difficult to determine, but the more vertical it is the less favourable is the prognosis. Garden (1971) has described four stages of displacement, which can be correlated with the prognosis (Fig. 27.3). Stages I and II give a good result after internal fixation; stages III and IV have a high rate of non-union and avascular necrosis.

Treatment

Operative treatment is almost mandatory because old people must be got up and active without delay if pulmonary complications and bed sores are to be avoided. Even incomplete fractures (when the patient may be able to walk) are too precarious to be left; they are liable to become complete and to displace. What if operation is considered dangerous? Lying in bed on traction may be even more dangerous, and leaving the fracture untreated too painful.* The principles of treatment are: accurate reduction, secure fixation and early activity.

● REDUCE
With the patient on an orthopaedic table, the hip and knee are flexed and the fractured thigh pulled upwards, then internally rotated, then extended and abducted; the foot is now tied to a footpiece. X-ray control (preferably with an image intensifier) is used to confirm reduction in anteroposterior and lateral views. Accurate reduction of stage

---

*The patient least fit for operation may need it most.

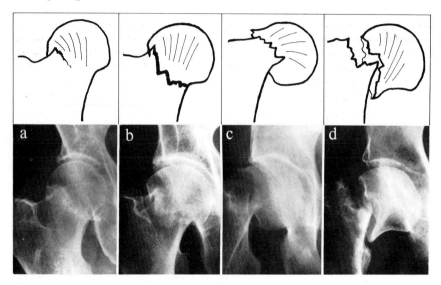

27.3 Garden's classification of femoral neck fractures   (a) Stage I: incomplete (so-called abducted or impacted). (b) Stage II: complete without displacement. (c) Stage III: complete with partial displacement – fragments still connected by posterior retinacular attachment; the femoral trabeculae are malaligned. (d) Stage IV: complete with full displacement – the proximal fragment is free and lies correctly in the acetabulum so that the trabeculae appear normally aligned.

III and IV fractures is important; to fix an unreduced fracture is to invite failure. If a stage III or IV fracture cannot be reduced closed, and the patient is under 60, open reduction through an anterolateral approach is advisable. However, in older patients (and certainly in those over 70) this is seldom justified; if two careful attempts at

closed reduction fail, prosthetic replacement is preferable.

● HOLD
The fracture may be held by: (1). a trifin nail, the least effective method but adequate for fractures which have never been displaced (Garden I and

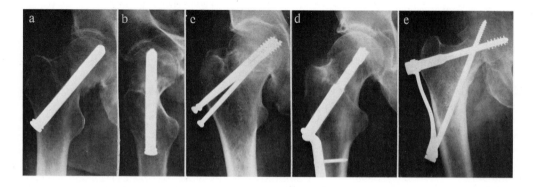

27.4 Fractures of the femoral neck – examples of treatment   (a, b) Trifin nail; (c) multiple screws; (d) sliding nail-plate; (e) Smyth's triangular fixation.

II); (2) threaded pins or, better, lag screws – four or five are required; (3) a sliding device which permits compression or impaction – a stout screw or nail fits inside a sleeve and is attached to a plate screwed to the femoral shaft; (4) triangular fixation (Smyth) or angled blade-plate fixation.

In all cases a lateral incision is used to expose the upper femur. Guide wires (which must be radiologically checked in anteroposterior and lateral views) are used to ensure correct placement of the fixing device; measuring the protruding portion enables the desired length of implant to be calculated. When a single nail or screw is used, it should lie below the middle of the neck and extend into the posterior part of the head.

● EXERCISE
From the first day the patient should sit up in bed or in a chair. She is taught breathing exercises, encouraged to help herself and to begin walking (with crutches or a walker) as soon as possible. To delay weight-bearing may be theoretically ideal but is rarely practicable.

Prosthetic replacement

Some argue that the prognosis for stage III and IV fractures is so unpredictable that prosthetic replacement is always preferable. This underestimates the morbidity associated with replacement. Our policy is, therefore, to attempt reduction and fixation in all cases and to reserve replacement for very frail patients in whom it fails. The least traumatic procedure is an uncemented femoral head prosthesis through a posterior approach. If treatment has been delayed for some weeks and acetabular damage is suspected, total hip replacement is wise.

Complications

General complications such as follow any injury or operation in the elderly are liable to occur, especially calf vein thrombosis, pulmonary embolism, pneumonia and bedsores. In some centres anticoagulants are used routinely. Most of these patients have serious medical disorders and over 30 per cent of them die within 2 years after fracture.

Avascular necrosis The femoral head is mainly supplied with blood by (1) lateral epiphyseal and inferior metaphyseal branches of the medial femoral circumflex artery; and (2) medial epiphyseal arteries in the ligamentum teres. This second group is small or absent in 20 per cent of adults; if in them the first group is damaged (and this is especially liable to occur with displaced fractures), then the head becomes avascular. However, if perfect reduction is securely held, subsequent bone collapse is less severe because the head is well contained in the acetabulum and stress is widely distributed; moreover, fracture union may promote bone regeneration.

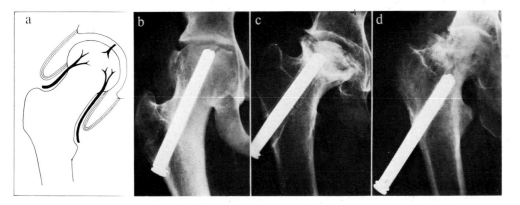

27.5 Avascular necrosis after fracture   (a) Apart from the small amount of blood reaching the head through the nutrient artery and the artery in the ligamentum teres, the main supply is from vessels that run under the retinacular fibres before entering the bone; in this situation they are readily damaged. (b) Segmental necrosis. (c) Massive necrosis. (d) The fracture has united despite avascular necrosis, but the bone has crumbled and the joint is degenerating.

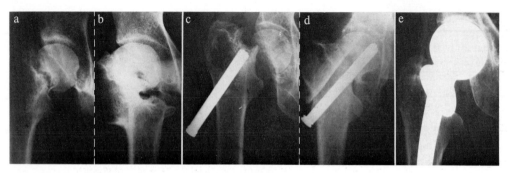

27.6 Fractures of the femoral neck – non-union   (a, b) In this relatively young patient non-union has been treated successfully by osteotomy. (c, d) Another patient, treated by nailing and grafting. (e) In the elderly, replacement by a prosthesis is the usual treatment.

The increased x-ray density due to reactive new bone formation may not become apparent for months or even years. The first indication of necrosis is usually the nail extruding from the head or breaking out of it; the fracture then redisplaces and, if the condition is untreated, non-union occurs. Sometimes the nail is extruded after apparent union of the fracture; a line of separation then develops between living and dead bone, with subsequent refracture. Even if union is secure, the femoral head may eventually collapse and cause degenerative arthritis. The treatment of avascular necrosis with progressive collapse is total joint replacement.

Non-union   Non-union is likely if the fracture line is unduly vertical, if the operation is unskilfully performed (inaccurate reduction or bad nailing) or if the blood supply to the femoral head is diminished. The method of treatment depends upon the cause of the non-union and the age of the patient.

In the relatively young, three procedures are available. (1) If the fracture is unduly vertical but the head is alive, sub-trochanteric osteotomy with nail-plate fixation changes the fracture line to a more horizontal angle. (2) If the reduction or nailing was faulty and there are no signs of necrosis, it is reasonable to remove the nail, reduce the fracture, insert a fresh nail correctly and also to insert a fibular graft across the fracture. (3) If the head is avascular it may be replaced by a metal prosthesis; if arthritis is already present total replacement is necessary.

In elderly patients only two procedures should be considered. (1) If the pain is not severe, a raised heel and a stout stick or elbow crutch are often sufficient. (2) If the pain is considerable, then, no matter whether the head is avascular or not, it is best removed; if the patient is reasonably fit, total joint replacement is performed.

Femoral neck fractures in the young

Ordinary fractures

In young people the femoral neck breaks only if subjected to considerable force. The child's fracture, if undisplaced, may be treated by closed reduction and plaster, but with displacement internal fixation is usually preferred. In young adults all femoral neck fractures are treated by internal fixation. There is a high incidence of avascular necrosis; consequently the patient should not take weight through the leg for 6 months, and then only if the x-ray appearance of the femoral head is normal.

Pathological fractures

In children the neck of the femur may fracture through a cyst. In adolescents the upper femoral epiphysis may slip (page 262), a condition comparable to a fractured neck of femur. Stress fractures are an important cause of unexplained hip pain in army recruits, athletes and ballet dancers.

Avulsions

In adolescents, the lesser trochanter apophysis may be avulsed by the pull of the psoas muscle; the injury nearly always occurs during hurdling. Less commonly the greater trochanter is avulsed by the abductor muscles. With either injury the patient needs rest in bed for only 2–3 days and may then get up using crutches. As soon as he can balance on the affected leg crutches may be discarded, but he is unlikely to resume athletic activities until the following season.

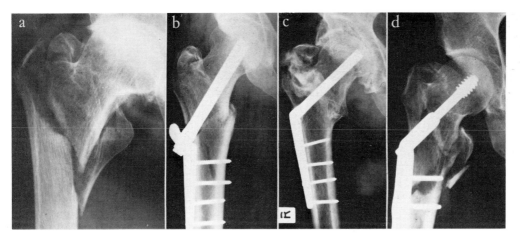

27.7 Intertrochanteric fractures   (a) The medial femoral cortex just below the lesser trochanter is important for stability; (b) fixation with a McLaughlin pin and plate; (c) with a fixed-angle blade-plate; (d) with a sliding screw and plate.

Intertrochanteric fractures

In sharp contrast to intracapsular femoral neck fractures, extracapsular fractures always unite, whether internal fixation is used or not. The patient is usually old and often unfit. Following a fall she is unable to stand. The leg is shorter and more externally rotated than with a cervical fracture (because the fracture is extracapsular) and the patient cannot lift her leg. X-ray often shows considerable displacement. If the lesser trochanter is separated and the medial cortex fragmented, internal fixation may not be stable and weight-bearing should be delayed.

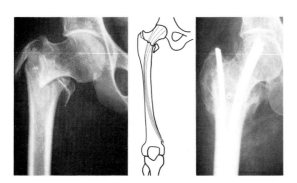

27.8 Intertrochanteric fractures – Ender's nails   The condylocephalic nails are inserted from below and, under x-ray fluoroscopy, guided across the fracture.

Early internal fixation is important and several techniques are available, including blade-plate fixation, a sliding nail or screw fixed to a plate, and Ender's condylocephalic nails (inserted through a small incision just above the medial side of the knee). The essential is to get the patient up and walking (with crutches or a walking aid) as soon as possible; hence the need to restore stability by secure fixation. Avascular necrosis and non-union are almost unknown; but malunion may result in shortening, which is best treated by a raised shoe.

NOTE   The potential complications of operation may be unacceptable in younger patients in whom traction is sometimes preferred, despite the economic and social drawbacks.

Subtrochanteric fractures

Subtrochanteric fracture may occur at any age if the injury is severe enough; but most occur with relatively trivial injury, in elderly patients with osteoporosis, osteomalacia or a secondary deposit. Blood loss is greater than with femoral neck or trochanteric fractures. The head and neck are abducted by the gluteal muscles, and flexed by the psoas.

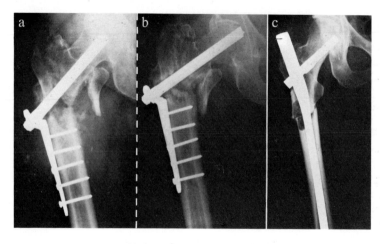

27.9 Subtrochanteric fractures   Fixation with a pin and plate (a) often fails (b). Zickel nail fixation (c) is better.

Special features

The leg lies externally rotated, is short, and the thigh is markedly swollen. Movement is excruciatingly painful.

X-RAY

The fracture is through or below the lesser trochanter. It may be transverse, oblique or spiral, and is frequently comminuted. The upper fragment is flexed and appears deceptively short; the shaft is adducted and is displaced proximally.

Treatment

● REDUCE   The fracture is reduced by strong traction in abduction and flexion.

● HOLD   Reduction can be held only if the flexed abducted position is maintained. This can be achieved in two ways.

Continuous traction   The lower fragment is in line if the patient is nursed in the sitting position. Traction needs to be maintained for 3 months, so the method is not suited to the elderly.

Internal fixation   This is essential for the elderly, and can be used at any age. If the medial cortex is intact, the fracture can be held with a trifin nail high in the femoral neck and head, attached to a long plate screwed to the shaft above and below the fracture line. Low fractures can be fixed with an intramedullary nail. But with neither technique is weight-bearing safe for at least 3 months, and even then coxa vara and shortening are likely to occur. To achieve early weight-bearing (so important for the elderly) without developing coxa vara, the Zickel apparatus or Ender's nails are used.

● EXERCISE   During treatment by traction, the muscles are repeatedly exercised; movement is regained when traction is discontinued.

Following internal fixation the patient is allowed up without delay. If Zickel's technique has been used, full weight-bearing is safe from the start.

Femoral shaft fractures

A spiral fracture is usually caused by a fall in which the foot is anchored while a twisting force is transmitted to the femur. An angulation force or a direct injury may cause a transverse fracture, which is particularly common in motorcycle accidents. A transverse fracture occurring after middle life should be viewed with suspicion; it may be pathological.*

Special features

The patient is usually a young adult. Shock is severe, and with closed fractures fat embolism is common. The leg is rotated externally and may be short and deformed. The thigh is swollen and bruised.

X-RAY

The fracture may be situated in any part of the shaft, but the middle third is the most common site. It may be spiral or transverse, or there may be a separate triangular ('butterfly') fragment on one side. Displacement may occur in any direction. Occasionally there are two transverse fractures, so that a segment of the femur is isolated.

The pelvis should always be x-rayed to avoid missing an associated hip injury or pelvic fracture.

*Old bones break at their ends; if they fracture in the middle, think of metastasis.

Emergency treatment

At the site of the accident, shock should be treated and the fracture splinted before the patient is moved. The injured limb may be tied to the other leg or to any convenient splint. For transport a Thomas' splint is ideal: the leg is pulled straight and threaded through the ring of the splint; the shod foot is tied to the cross-piece so as to maintain traction, and the limb and splint are firmly bandaged together.

Once in hospital and fit for operation the patient is anaesthetized, the splint removed (wound toilet is performed if the fracture was open) and definitive treatment instituted.

Definitive treatment – choice of method

With open fractures internal fixation should be avoided, unless associated injuries dictate otherwise. With closed fractures there is a choice: closed treatment is safe but irksome; open treatment is quick and convenient but not without risk.

The chief drawback of closed treatment is the length of time spent in bed. With functional bracing this can be considerably reduced; indeed, for fractures in the lower half of the femur this is the method of choice, providing the best of all worlds – safety, reliability and a relatively short period of hospitalization (Thomas and Meggitt, 1981). However, the method is not reliable for fractures in the upper half of the femur – the very group in which internal fixation is comparatively easy and dependable. Therefore, provided the necessary expertise and facilities are available, internal fixation may (some would say 'should') be used for transverse fractures in the proximal half of the bone, especially if (1) closed reduction is difficult to maintain, (2) treatment is awkward because the tibia on the same side also is fractured or because the patient is old and frail, or (3) the fracture is through a metastatic tumour.

Closed treatment is preferred if conditions are less than ideal or if the fracture is in the lower half of the bone. Reduction (usually by manipulation under anaesthesia) is maintained by continuous traction. But – and here comes the second controversy – is a splint also necessary? In children clearly no splint is needed. In adults a splint usually is employed; either the traditional Thomas' splint with fixed traction, or (since prolonged knee stiffness is the common sequel) with some modification of the splint which allows knee flexion. Perkins, however, has shown that even in adults no splint is needed; skeletal traction with the leg on a pillow is comfortable, exercises ensure knee mobility, and the fractures join at least as quickly as with a splint. Used intelligently (e.g. traction must not be excessive) this method is very satisfactory; but, since convention dies hard, the techniques of splintage also will be described.

Treatment by fixed traction

● REDUCE

The patient is anaesthetized and manual traction applied by an assistant. The skin is shaved and extension strapping applied. A Thomas' splint of the correct size is threaded over the limb until the ring abuts against the root of the limb. Flannel slings are passed under the limb and secured to the side-bars with safety pins. An attempt is now made to reduce the fracture by manipulation and traction. The traction tapes are pulled tight and tied to the cross-piece of the Thomas' splint. Pads are arranged in front of the flannel slings to maintain the normal forward bow of the femur.

● HOLD

The fixed traction is maintained and tightened as necessary. The slings and pads may need adjustment. X-ray films are taken to ensure that reduction is maintained; lateral angulation of more than 10 degrees is unacceptable.

To avoid undue pressure by the ring of the splint against the ischial tuberosity, the splint is slung from an overhead beam or tied to the foot of the bed which is raised on blocks.

In adults, union may be expected to take 8 weeks for a spiral fracture and 16 weeks for a transverse fracture; consolidation takes twice as long. Once union is fairly well advanced the patient may be allowed up using crutches; but he must take no weight through the leg until consolidation is clinically and radiologically complete.*

● EXERCISE

The patient is taught to lift himself by a 'monkey pole' and to exercise all joints not immobilized. He is also taught quadriceps exercises which he must practise assiduously. When the splint is removed, knee-bending exercises also are started, but it will be many months before a good range of knee flexion is restored.

NOTE Continuous fixed traction is seldom used nowadays: (1) because it is uncomfortable and (2) because the knee often stiffens.

---

*Before consolidation is complete, a fracture – even one that has 'united' – can still 'bend'.

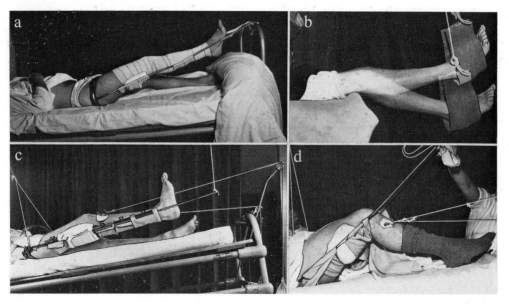

27.10 Fractured shaft of femur (1)   (a) Fixed traction on a Thomas' splint: the splint is tied to the foot of the bed which is elevated. This method should be used only rarely because the knee may stiffen; (b) this was the range in such a case when the fracture had united. One way to minimize stiffness is to use skeletal balanced traction (c); the lower slings can be removed to permit knee flexion (d) while traction is still maintained.

Treatment by balanced traction on a splint

As with fixed traction, a Thomas' splint with slings and pads is used; this is suspended from an overhead beam. The traction, however, is skeletal, through a Steinmann or Denham pin behind the tibial tubercle. Weights (8–10 kg for an adult) are attached, but are not fixed to the cross-piece of the splint; they hang over pulleys at the foot of the bed. Counter-traction is provided by elevating the foot of the bed. The position of the limb is carefully watched and x-ray films are taken to check alignment. From time to time the pads, slings or pulleys need adjustment. With transverse fractures it is especially important to avoid overpulling, which inevitably delays union.

As soon as the patient can lift the straight leg from the splint, knee-flexion exercises are begun, for alignment is maintained by the weights. Once union is well advanced the patient may be allowed up non-weight-bearing with crutches. For fractures in the upper half of the femur added safety is provided by a plaster spica, which is applied at about 8 weeks and kept on for 8 weeks. For fractures in the lower half of the femur

cast-bracing is suitable; in such a brace the patient can usually be allowed up at 4–6 weeks from injury.

Treatment by balanced traction with no splint

In adults the patient is anaesthetized, the fracture reduced by manipulation, and a Denham pin inserted behind the tibial tubercle. A freely swivelling hook is fixed to each end of the pin and a cord attached to each hook. The two cords pass over pulleys at the foot of the bed and a 5-kg weight is attached to each. The leg is cradled on pillows which also prevent backward sag. Exercises are begun without delay; not only quadriceps exercises but also knee bending, which is facilitated by a split mattress (Fig. 27.12).

With fractures in the distal half, the pin can be removed at 4–6 weeks, but only if functional bracing is then used; this technique is demanding and some shortening may result. If this method is not used, and with more proximal fractures, skeletal traction is retained until union is well advanced. The patient then gets up with crutches,

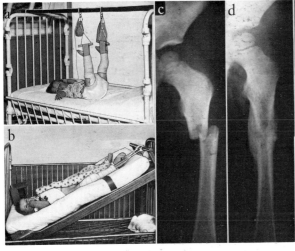

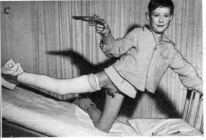

27.11 Fractured shaft of femur (2) (a–d) Traction without a splint is certainly adequate in children, and skin traction is sufficient. (e) Clearly this fracture has united.

but must not take weight through the leg until the fracture is consolidated.

In children skin traction is usually enough. As soon as the leg feels in one piece, and a little callus is visible on x-ray, a hip spica may be applied and worn until consolidation is complete. Knee movement returns rapidly in children.

Treatment by internal fixation

● REDUCE

The patient lies on the uninjured side. Through a lateral approach the fracture is exposed and the bone ends are cleaned.

● HOLD

Much the most efficient method of holding the

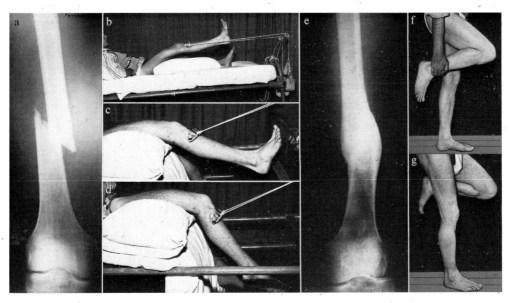

27.12 Fractured shaft of femur (3) Even in the adult, traction without a splint can be satisfactory, but skeletal traction is essential. The patient with this rather unstable fracture (a) can lift his leg and exercise his knee (b, c, d). At no time was the leg splinted, but clearly the fracture has consolidated (e), and the knee range (f) is only slightly less than that of the uninjured left leg (g).

reduction is by an intramedullary (Küntscher) nail which is introduced as follows.

(1) Long drills are driven upwards and downwards from the fracture to expose the medulla, which is then widened with reamers of increasing diameter until it is large enough to take a thick (if possible, 12–14 mm) intramedullary nail.
(2) A long guide is pushed up the proximal fragment until, with the hip flexed and adducted, it emerges in the buttock.
(3) A nail of appropriate length (measured on the other leg before operation) is threaded over the guide and hammered down until it emerges at the fracture.
(4) The guide is withdrawn; the fracture is reduced and rotational alignment is carefully checked. The nail is then hammered home into the distal segment. If the bone is osteoporotic, or the fracture is through a secondary deposit, it is useful to pack acrylic cement into exposed cavities.
(5) An alternative (and easier) method is retrograde insertion, driving the nail directly up the proximal fragment from the site of fracture. When the end is flush, the fracture is reduced under direct vision and the nail punched into the distal fragment.

NOTE   Closed nailing under image intensification is used. It avoids exposing the fracture, but is technically difficult and malrotation is not uncommon.

● EXERCISE

Immediately after operation, exercises to all the leg joints are begun. Within a fortnight the patient should have good muscle control of the limb and good movement of the hip and knee joints. He is then allowed up, weight-bearing if the reduction is stable and the nail fits snugly; otherwise crutches are used and weight-bearing is postponed until the fixation afforded by the nail is reinforced by callus visible on x-ray.

Complications

EARLY

Skin damage   The fracture may be open and the wound then requires excision. Internal fixation should not be used for an open fracture unless the wound is small and other fractures in the same limb justify its use.

Fat embolism   This is so common in young people with fractures of the femur that its presence must be assumed in every case even though clinical manifestations are uncommon; during the first 72 hours the patient must be checked frequently for

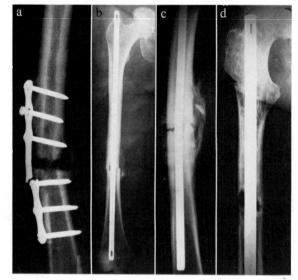

27.13 Fractured shaft of femur (4)   (a) Plating a fractured femur is rarely satisfactory (although Hicks' very strong plates may be adequate). Intramedullary nailing (b) is usually preferred: this young man also had a fractured tibia in the same leg. (c) A delay of 2 weeks before nailing may explain the exuberant callus in this case.
(d) Fracture through a secondary deposit is nearly always treated by nailing.

clinical signs, and the blood gases should be measured soon after admission.

LATE

Delayed union Delayed union occurs with open fractures and also if excessive traction has been used with a transverse fracture. It is essential to ensure that traction is never excessive and to exercise the longitudinal muscles around the fracture repeatedly.

Non-union There is a danger that with delayed union splintage may be discarded too soon. The fracture then angulates and may proceed to non-union. Once non-union is established, the fracture needs operation: the bone ends are freshened, a Küntscher nail is inserted and cancellous bone grafts are packed round the fracture.

Malunion With closed methods there is a risk of angulation, especially if weight-bearing is allowed too soon; with intramedullary fixation malrotation is not uncommon and occasionally is severe enough to warrant operative realignment. There is often shortening, but usually the only treatment necessary is a raised shoe.

Joint stiffness Stiffness of the knee is the commonest complication of a fractured femoral shaft. If the muscles have been exercised, knee movement is likely to return with use even after prolonged splintage. When balanced traction is used, there is no problem in regaining knee movement. After an infected fracture, considerable knee stiffness is almost inevitable, and if it is disabling quadriceps-plasty is useful.

II   Injuries of the knee and leg

Supracondylar fracture of the femur

Supracondylar fractures resemble subtrochanteric fractures (page 443) in two respects: (1) while they may occur in adults of any age who sustain a sufficiently severe injury, they often occur through osteoporotic bone in the elderly; (2) continuous traction is suitable for the young, but for the elderly, early mobilization is so important that internal fixation is preferred.

Direct violence is the usual cause. The fracture line is just above the condyles, but may extend between them. When the lower fragment is intact the pull of gastrocnemius may flex it, endangering the popliteal artery.

Special features

The knee is swollen and deformed; movement is too painful to be attempted. The tibial pulses should always be palpated.

X-RAY

The fracture is just above the femoral condyles and is transverse or comminuted. The distal fragment is often tilted backwards.

NOTE   The entire femur must be x-rayed so as not to miss a proximal fracture or dislocated hip.

Closed treatment

● REDUCE

With displacement reduction is important, and with popliteal artery obstruction it is urgent. A Steinmann or Denham pin is inserted behind the tibial tubercle or through the distal femur (a

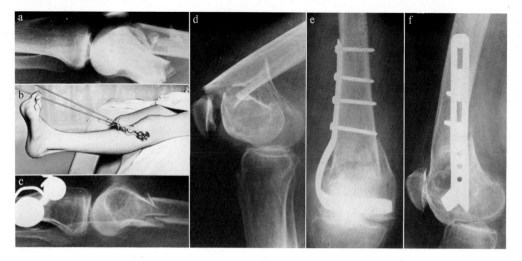

27.14 Supracondylar fractures   (a, b, c) Treatment by traction; (d, e, f) treatment by internal fixation. In both cases note the posterior displacement which may endanger the circulation.

femoral pin should be below the adductor tubercle so as not to interfere with quadriceps exercises). Strong traction is applied by an assistant while the surgeon firmly pushes the fragment into place.

- HOLD
The patient is returned to bed and 9-kg traction is maintained with the knee almost straight. The limb is cradled on pillows or on a Thomas' splint. The fracture takes about 12 weeks to unite and traction must be maintained during that time. The patient is then fitted with a caliper and allowed to take weight. After a further 12 weeks consolidation is usually complete and the caliper may be discarded.

An alternative method is to replace the traction with a cast-brace after 4–6 weeks and allow the patient up and partially weight-bearing with crutches; full weight-bearing is permitted after 12 weeks but the cast-brace is retained until consolidation is complete.

- EXERCISE
Quadriceps muscle exercises are encouraged, but knee movements are not permitted until the fracture has united. Then the caliper is removed and active knee movements are practised.

Operative treatment

If closed reduction fails, or the circulation is not restored, urgent open reduction is essential. In elderly patients open

reduction with internal fixation, though not essential, reduces the time in bed and the danger of knee stiffness.

Through a lateral incision the fracture is exposed, reduced, and held with a specially designed blade plate; with fragile osteoporotic bone it is useful first to pack the interior with acrylic cement. Skin or skeletal traction from below the knee may still be necessary for a few weeks if stability is in doubt but no splint is used and exercises are begun immediately. Unprotected weight-bearing is not permitted until the fracture has consolidated.

Complications

EARLY
Skin damage   is common and wound toilet is then necessary.

Arterial damage   occasionally occurs, and there is danger of gangrene.

LATE
Knee stiffness   is almost inevitable. A long period of exercises is necessary but full movement is rarely regained.

Non-union   may be associated with knee stiffness and indeed may be due to forcing knee movement too soon. The fracture is difficult to treat and, unless great care is exercised, the ultimate range of movement at the knee may be less than that at the fracture.

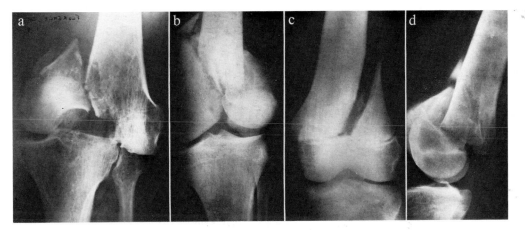

27.15 Other fractures of the lower femur　Manipulative reduction followed by traction is usually the best treatment for condylar fractures (a) and intercondylar fractures (b). Fracture-separation of the lower femoral epiphysis (c, d) may, after reduction, be held in plaster.

Femoral condyle fractures

A direct injury or a fall from a height may drive the tibia upwards into the intercondylar fossa. One femoral condyle may be fractured and driven upwards or both condyles split apart.

Special features

The knee is swollen and may be deformed. There is a tender, 'doughy' feel characteristic of haemarthrosis. The knee is too painful to move, but the foot should be examined to exclude nerve damage.

X-RAY
One femoral condyle may be fractured obliquely and shifted upwards, or both condyles may be split apart so that the fracture line is T-shaped or Y-shaped.

Treatment

Under anaesthetic the haemarthrosis is aspirated.

● REDUCE　A skeletal pin is inserted behind the tibial tubercle. With strong traction and manual compression the fracture can usually be reduced. If closed reduction has failed, operation is advisable; the fracture is then held with a transverse bolt or with lag screws.

　With T-shaped fractures, once the condyles have been bolted or screwed together, the transverse supracondylar fracture can be fixed with an angled blade-plate or treated by traction.

● HOLD　The leg is cradled on pillows and 6-kg traction maintained for 6 weeks; by this time the fracture has usually

united. The patient is then allowed up using crutches, but must not take weight until consolidation is complete, which usually takes 3 months.

● EXERCISE　Quadriceps muscle exercises are vigorously practised from the start. Knee flexion is also encouraged and is facilitated by using a divided mattress; the distal half of the mattress is removed at intervals and active knee movements are practised repeatedly without removing the traction. Movement often improves a previously imperfect reduction because the comminuted femoral condyles are 'moulded' by the intact tibia.

Fracture-separation of lower femoral epiphysis

In an adolescent the lower femoral epiphysis may be displaced (1) laterally by forced abduction of the straight knee or (2) forwards by a hyperextension injury.

Special features

The knee is swollen and perhaps deformed. The pulses in the foot should be palpated because, with forward displacement of the epiphysis, the popliteal artery may be obstructed by the lower femur.

X-RAY
The abduction injury shifts and tilts the epiphysis laterally; the hyperextension injury shifts and tilts it forwards. In either case, a triangular fragment of the shaft is displaced with the epiphysis.

Treatment

- REDUCE   Lateral displacement is corrected by pulling on the straight leg and forcing the knee into adduction. Forward displacement is corrected by pulling with the knee bent and thumbing the fragment into position.

- HOLD   Plaster is applied from the upper thigh to the malleoli, with the knee straight if there was lateral displacement, and 60 degrees flexed if there was forward displacement. The plaster is worn for 6 weeks. The injury may be unstable for much longer than fracture-separation elsewhere; loss of reduction may occur, even in plaster, as late as the third week.

- EXERCISE   Weight-bearing is permitted as soon as the patient can lift his leg. Movement quickly returns when the plaster is removed.

Complications

There is danger of gangrene unless the hyperextension injury is reduced without delay. Interference with growth from damage to the growth disc sometimes occurs.

Tibial plateau fractures

A fall from a height or a direct blow may fracture one tibial condyle or both. The commonest injury is a fractured lateral condyle, for which the term 'bumper fracture' was coined; but the injury is rarely caused by the impact of a car bumper, it is usually a valgus crush. The patient, nearly always aged 50–60, falls with the knee extended and slightly valgus. The lateral tibial condyle is driven upwards and smashed by the lateral femoral condyle, which remains intact.

Special features

The knee is swollen and may be valgus. Bruising is usually extensive and the tissues feel 'doughy' because of haemarthrosis.

X-RAY

Any of the following may be seen: (1) a vertical split of the lateral tibial condyle without displacement; (2) a comminuted crush of the lateral condyle with depression of the fragments; (3) an oblique fracture running downwards and outwards from the tibial plateau; the tibial condyle may be tilted and the upper fibula fractured; or (4) the medial condyle is fractured, and sometimes a transverse line extends across the upper tibia. Because the x-ray shadows overlap, a depressed plateau may be difficult to see on plain films; however, tomography will show the defect.

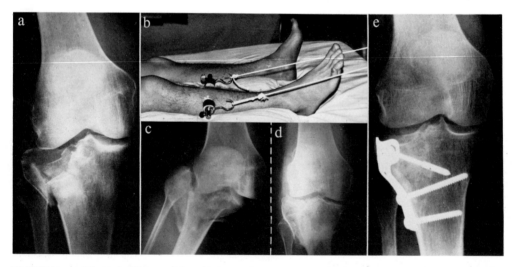

27.16 Fractured lateral tibial condyle   (a) Typical 'bumper' fracture of the lateral tibial condyle. Skeletal traction applied well below the knee (b) is often effective in reducing such a fracture, and in holding it reduced (c, d); it permits early movement, which is important. Open reduction followed by internal fixation (e) is sometimes indicated.

NOTE A crushed lateral condyle usually means that the medial collateral ligament is intact; however, a crushed medial condyle is not infrequently associated with a tear of the lateral ligament. If there is bruising and tenderness on the opposite side of the knee, the joint must be examined with an image intensifier under an anaesthetic to exclude ligament injuries.

Treatment by traction

Treatment by traction is simple and usually produces good results (Apley, 1979). Its sole disadvantage is that the patient must remain in hospital.

● REDUCE
If there is much haemarthrosis the joint is aspirated. A threaded (Denham) pin is inserted through the tibia 7 cm below the fracture. Traction is applied and the condyle manually pushed back into place.

● HOLD
The leg is cradled on pillows and 5-kg traction maintained until the fracture is united, at about 6 weeks. The pin is then removed and the patient is allowed up using crutches. Full weight-bearing should be deferred for a further 6 weeks.

● EXERCISE
Quadriceps muscle exercises are vigorously practised from the very beginning. As soon as the patient can lift his leg, knee flexion is permitted while the traction is maintained. There should be fully controlled extension with flexion to 90 degrees within 4 weeks. Movements often improve a previously imperfect reduction, and articular defects fill in with fibrocartilage.

Treatment in plaster

Treatment in plaster also may give good results, though knee movement takes longer to return; it has the advantage that the patient need not remain in hospital for long.

● REDUCE The fracture is reduced by strong traction and lateral compression.

● HOLD Plaster is applied from the upper thigh to the malleoli with the knee straight. It is removed after 6–12 weeks according to the severity of the injury, and weight-bearing is then permitted.

● EXERCISE Quadriceps muscle exercises are practised within the plaster, and knee movement is regained when the plaster is removed.

Operative treatment

If closed reduction fails, and especially if the condyle is much displaced without comminution, open reduction and levering the condyle back into place is advisable; the condyle may be fixed with a buttress plate and screws; a partially detached meniscus should not be removed if it can be securely sewn back in position. Operative treatment produces admirable x-rays but long-term function is probably no better than with traction and early movement.

Complications

Valgus deformity This is compatible with good function but carries the risk of lateral compartment degeneration in later life.

Joint stiffness Failure to regain full knee bend is an important cause of disability, and is avoided by early movements.

Fractured tibial spine

A hyperextension injury may tear the anterior cruciate ligament (see page 456); sometimes, especially in a child or young adult, the ligament remains intact but the tibial spine is avulsed.

Special features

The knee is held flexed and is swollen. Because of haemarthrosis the joint feels tense, tender and 'doughy'; movement is too painful to be attempted.

X-RAY A lateral film shows the anterior tibial spine elevated from the tibia.

Treatment

● REDUCE Under anaesthesia the joint is aspirated; forcing the knee straight reduces the fracture.
　Sometimes the true nature of the injury is not immediately realized and after a few weeks it may be impossible to straighten the knee even under anaesthesia. Operative reduction is then essential; the tibial spine is anchored by sutures into a cavity gouged out of the upper tibia.

- HOLD   A plaster tube is applied from the upper thigh to the malleoli with the knee straight; it is worn for 6 weeks.

- EXERCISE   Weight-bearing is permitted and the quadriceps muscle vigorously exercised. When the plaster is removed, knee flexion is regained by active use.

Injuries of the upper tibial epiphysis

In a child, resisted extension of the knee usually strains the insertion of the extensor mechanism into the tibial tubercle (Osgood–Schlatter's disease: see page 293). Occasionally a more dramatic avulsion, with displacement, occurs.

Special features

The knee is swollen and the front of the upper tibia is tender. The joint cannot be actively extended.

X-RAY   The entire upper tibial epiphysis may be tilted forwards. Sometimes, when the ligament is attached to a small apophysis separate from the main epiphysis, this apophysis is avulsed and shifted upwards.

Treatment

- REDUCE   Under anaesthesia closed manipulative reduction can usually be achieved. If the small separate apophysis remains displaced it is operatively reduced and sutured in position. Occasionally, when the entire tibial epiphysis cannot be accurately reduced by closed manipulation, it is replaced at operation and held by a screw.

- HOLD   Following reduction, whether closed or open, a plaster tube is applied from the upper thigh to the malleoli with the knee straight. It is worn for 6 weeks.

- EXERCISE   Weight-bearing is permitted at once. Knee flexion quickly returns when the plaster is removed.

Fractured patella

Direct (stellate) fracture

A fall or a direct blow may smash the patella against the femur. The expansions on each side of the patella usually remain intact.

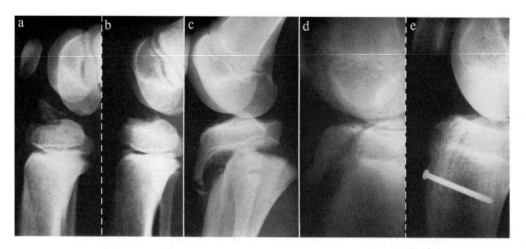

27.17 Other fractures of the upper tibia   A fractured tibial spine (a) usually reduces if the knee is straightened fully (b); only when the fracture is missed (which not uncommonly happens) is open reduction sometimes needed. Fracture-separation of the entire upper tibial epiphysis (c) needs urgent reduction because the popliteal artery may be compressed. (d) Avulsion of the patellar ligament insertion (as distinct from Schlatter's disease) is rare; in this case reduction was held with a screw (e).

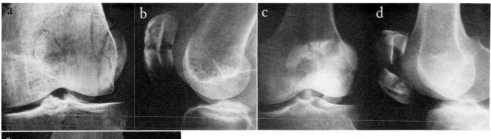

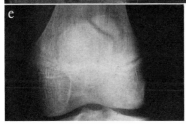

27.18 Fractured patella – stellate   Provided the posterior surface is smooth a stellate fracture of the patella (a, b) can be treated by activity. With gross displacement (c, d) the possibilities are wiring or excision.

(e) A bipartite patella should not be mistaken for a fracture: the line is superolateral (and the condition often bilateral).

Special features

The knee is swollen and held flexed. There is tenderness, and blood in the joint. Because the extensor expansions are intact, the patient can sometimes lift the straight leg.

X-RAY
The films may show (1) one or more fine fracture lines without displacement (the appearance is not to be confused with a bipartite patella in which a smooth line extends obliquely across the supero-lateral angle of the bone); or (2) multiple fracture lines with irregular displacement.

Treatment

ACTIVITY   If there is no displacement, the fracture need not be reduced or held. A tense effusion should be aspirated. A plaster back slab holding the knee straight is worn until quadriceps muscle control is regained. The slab is removed several times a day for active exercises.

OPERATION   If the fragments are displaced the usual treatment is patellectomy. Alternatively, it is worth putting a 'purse-string' wire suture round the patella, tightening it, then hoping to mould the fragments by movement; patellectomy is then reserved for severe comminution or if the patient develops patellofemoral pain.

Indirect (transverse) fracture

Resisted extension of the knee may rupture the extensor mechanism. Typically the patient catches his foot and, to avoid falling, contracts the

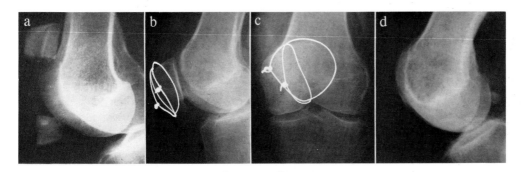

27.19 Fractured patella – transverse   (a) Gap fracture held together by two wires (b, c); it is important that one wire is placed anteriorly. This method is preferred to (d) patellectomy.

quadriceps muscle; but the stair or other obstacle prevents straightening of the knee. In middle life this injury usually fractures the patella transversely and tears the lateral extensor expansions.

Special features

The knee is swollen and extremely tender. Soon after injury a gap is palpable, but later it fills with blood. The patient is unable to lift the straight leg.

X-RAY
The patella is fractured transversely; there is a gap between the two halves and the upper fragment is shifted proximally.

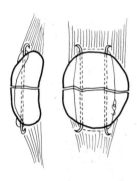

27.20 Transverse patellar fracture – tension band wiring The fragments are transfixed by Kirschner wires; malleable wire is then looped round the protruding ends of the K-wires, passed over the front of the patella and tightened.

Treatment

Operation is essential. Unless the extensor mechanism is repaired, the last 10 or 20 degrees of active extension will be lost and the knee will be unstable.

TECHNIQUE   Through a transverse incision the fracture is exposed and the lateral expansions are repaired with strong catgut sutures. The patella is reconstituted by the tension-band principle. The fragments are reduced and transfixed with two stiff Kirschner wires; flexible wire is then looped tightly around the protruding K wires and over the front of the patella. Any irregularity of the articular surface may be smoothed away by active use; if patellofemoral signs develop later, the patella can then be excised and the knee recovers

more quickly than it does after immediate post-traumatic patellectomy. A plaster back slab is worn until active extension of the knee is regained; the back slab may be removed every day to permit active knee-flexion exercises.

Knee ligament injuries

Acute tears

The fully extended knee is stable, partly because the femoral condyles fit onto the tibial condyles (deepened by the menisci), but chiefly because the capsule and ligaments are taut; in this position sideways tilt, anteroposterior glide and rotation cannot occur. The straight knee may sustain ligamentous injury as a result of hyperextension or of a force applied from either side, but such injuries are rare.

Most ligament injuries occur while the knee is bent, relaxing the capsule and ligaments, and permitting rotation. The damaging force may be a straight thrust (e.g. a dashboard injury forcing the tibia backwards) or, more commonly, a combined rotation and impact injury to the bent weight-bearing knee as in a football tackle. A wide variety of complex injuries may result (O'Donoghue, 1973; Hughston, 1976).

Clinical features

The history is misleading and the signs are deceptive. Partial tears are easy to diagnose, but complete tears are often missed – for three reasons. (1) The story (of a sports injury, fall or road accident) is always imprecise, unless an onlooker can describe it. More important, it seems perverse: thus, with a complete tear (in which nerve fibres also are torn) the patient has little or no pain, and can usually walk or even run in comfort (though he cannot pivot); with a partial tear the knee is painful and the patient lame. (2) Swelling also is worse with partial tears, because haemorrhage remains confined within the joint; with complete tears the ruptured capsule permits leakage and diffusion. (In either case it comes on within an hour or two – much sooner than the effusion of a torn meniscus.) (3) With a

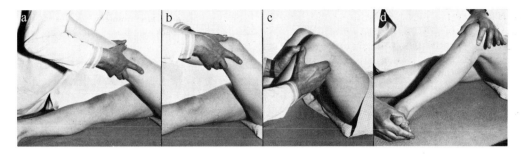

27.21 Knee ligaments   Grips used in examination for abnormal movements. (a) Sideways tilting with the knee straight, and (b) with the knee flexed; (c) anteroposterior glide (this should also be tested flexed only 20 degrees); (d) rotation of the flexed knee.

partial tear attempted movement is painful; the abnormal movement of a complete tear is often painless or prevented by spasm.

The signs in the acute stage are as follows.

● LOOK   Abrasions suggest the site of impact, but bruising is more important and indicates the site of damage.

● FEEL   The doughy feel of a haemarthrosis distinguishes ligament injuries from the fluctuant feel of the synovial effusion of a meniscus injury. Tenderness localizes the lesion, but the sharply defined tender spot of a partial tear (usually medial and 2.5 cm above the joint line) contrasts with the diffuse tenderness of a complete one.

● MOVE   Partial tears permit no abnormal movement, but the attempt causes pain. Complete tears permit abnormal movement which sometimes is painless. To distinguish between the two is critical because their treatment is totally different; *so if there is doubt, examination under anaesthesia is mandatory.*

The important movements are: (1) sideways tilting, examined first with the knee straight, then at 30 degrees of flexion; (2) anteroposterior glide, tested with the knee flexed and the leg neutral, then laterally rotated, then medially; and (3) rotation of the flexed knee in both directions. Undoubted increase of any of these movements (as compared with the normal knee) is an indication for operation.

● X-RAY   Plain films may show that the ligament has avulsed a small piece of bone, the medial ligament usually from the femur, the lateral ligament from the fibula, the cruciate ligament from the tibial spine. Stress films (if neccessary under anaesthesia) demonstrate if the joint hinges open on one side.

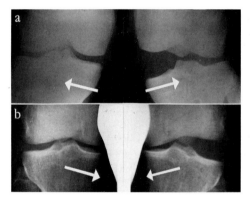

27.22 Ligament injuries   Strain films show (a) complete tear of medial ligament, left knee; (b) complete tear of lateral ligament, left knee. In both, the anterior cruciate also was torn.

Treatment

PARTIAL TEARS

The intact fibres splint the torn ones and spontaneous healing will occur. The hazard is adhesions, so active exercise is prescribed from the start, facilitated by aspirating a tense effusion and injecting local anaesthetic into the tender area. Weight-bearing is permitted but the knee is protected from rotation or angulation strain by a heavily padded bandage or a posterior splint. A complete plaster cast is unnecessary and dis-advantageous; it inhibits movement and prevents weekly reassessment – an important precaution if the occasional error is to be avoided.

COMPLETE TEARS

In theory, healing can occur provided the torn ends are closely apposed and held still in plaster. But the outcome is uncertain. Operation is wiser and affords the best chance of avoiding future instability. The guiding principles are: (1) oper-ate early (the earlier the better and certainly within 14 days); (2) use a generous incision (if posterior structures also are torn and access is inadequate, a second, posterior, incision helps); (3) repair every torn structure tightly and, if possible, by reattachment to bone (staples, or sutures through drill holes, are necessary); (4) protect the repair for 6 weeks in an above-knee plaster with the knee 40 degrees flexed (the leg should be medially rotated if medial structures mainly are involved, laterally rotated with lateral damage).

Complications

Adhesions   If the knee with a partial ligament tear is not actively exercised, torn fibres stick to intact fibres and to bone. The knee 'gives way' with catches of pain; localized tenderness is present and pain on medial or lateral rotation. The obvious confusion with a torn meniscus can be resolved by the grinding test (page 290), or by manipulation and injection under anaesthesia, which is usually curative. If there is still doubt about the possibility of a torn meniscus, arthro-scopy is indicated. Occasionally an abduction injury is followed by calcification near the upper attachment of the medial ligament (Pellegrini –Stieda's disease).

Instability   As the sequel to an injury the knee may continue to give way. The instability tends to get worse and eventually degeneration may fol-low. This important subject is discussed under a separate heading, below.

Chronic ligamentous instability

Instability ('giving way') of the knee may be obvious soon after the acute injury has healed, or it may only become apparent much later. It is usually progressive (a meniscectomy is likely to make it worse) but, except in people engaged in strenuous sport or dancing, the disability is often tolerated without complaint until eventually osteoarthritis supervenes.

Clinical features

The knee collapses with certain strenuous move-ments and this is sometimes accompanied by pain.

The only sign is abnormal movement; this is best considered as a subluxation of the tibia on the femur. It is important to know in which direction (or directions) the tibial condyle sublu-xates; it then immediately becomes clear what movements operation is designed to prevent. Naming the torn structures is less important, but the following guide to the interpretation of the physical signs may be useful.

Tilting into varus   implies a complete tear of the lateral liga-ment; if the posterior cruciate also is torn, tilting can occur with the knee at 0 degrees, otherwise it occurs only with the knee flexed.

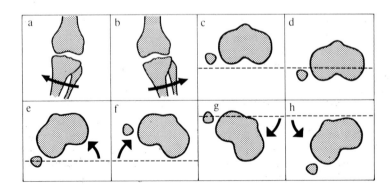

27.23 Knee ligaments – instability Straight subluxations: (a) tilting into varus, (b) into valgus; (c) forward shift, (d) backward.

Rotatory subluxations of tibia: (e) medial condyle forward; (f) lateral condyle for-ward; (g) medial condyle backward; (h) lateral condyle backward.

Tilting into valgus implies a complete tear of the medial ligament; if one or both cruciates also are torn, tilting can occur with the knee at 0 degrees, otherwise it occurs only with the knee flexed.

Forward shift (without rotation) – i.e. a positive anterior drawer sign – means that both the medial ligament and the anterior cruciate are torn. A tear of the medial ligament alone permits forward subluxation of only the medial condyle of the tibia; a tear of the anterior cruciate permits the lateral condyle to subluxate forwards. The various jerk tests also are positive with anterior cruciate injuries.

Backward shift (a positive posterior drawer sign) means that the posterior cruciate ligament is torn. Soon after injury, however, this sign is difficult to elicit unless the arcuate and oblique ligaments also are torn: if only one of these also is torn, only one tibial condyle can be subluxated backwards. Complete tears of all the posterior structures also allow the knee to hyperextend.

Treatment

Stabilization is desirable but late operation often does not succeed and may not last; so conservative treatment is important. Vigorous quadriceps exercises are essential; they are an indispensable preliminary to operation and may allow the patient to lead a normal life even without operation. With the addition of an external brace, games may be possible.

If symptoms are unacceptable or a higher athletic standard is demanded then stabilization must be considered. Stabilization (or reconstruction) involves one or more of the three Rs – *reattachment, reinforcement* and *replacement*. Reattachment implies tightening loose ligaments or capsule by reattaching one or both ends. Reinforcement diverts healthy muscles or tendons to strengthen weak structures. Replacement may involve rerouting living structures, or inserting synthetic materal (such as carbon fibre) to take the place of the ligament and to act as a scaffold along which new fibrous tissue may grow. The more common stabilizing procedures are as follows.

For tilting into valgus The lax medial structures can be tightened by reattaching the upper end more proximally or the lower end more distally. The repair can be reinforced by rerouting the semitendinosus tendon over the medial femoral condyle, or by advancing semimembranosus and sartorius forwards.

For tilting into varus The lateral structures can be tightened and the lateral edge of the arcuate ligament advanced to the posterior edge of the lateral collateral ligament. Reinforcement is possible with the lateral head of the gastrocnemius or a strip of the iliotibial band. If, however, the unstable knee also has a varus deformity, then osteotomy to correct it into slight valgus may be the best treatment.

For forward subluxation of the medial tibial condyle This rotatory instability is often associated with lateral hinge. The same structures are therefore tightened, but the lower end is also moved forwards, or the upper end backwards. A pes anserinus transplant provides additional and dynamic control; the lower two-thirds of the tendon group is detached, reflected upwards and sutured to the patellar ligament.

For forward subluxation of the lateral tibial condyle With this rotatory instability tightening lax structures by reattachment may be possible. A so-called pivot shift operation provides additional control; a strip of fascia lata is detached proximally, looped under the lateral ligament, then threaded through and sutured to the lateral intermuscular septum while the knee is held flexed and externally rotated.

For backward subluxation of the medial tibial condyle The semitendinosus and gracilis can be detached, passed through a hole drilled in the medial femoral condyle to the back of the joint, then through a hole in the tibia and fixed to the front of that bone.

For backward subluxation of the lateral tibial condyle The upper end of the lateral ligament, together with a block of bone and the popliteus tendon, can be advanced upwards and forwards.

In all cases an above-knee plaster with the knee 60 degrees flexed and the tibia rotated so as to relieve tension is worn for 8 weeks. An arduous period of rehabilitation follows; during the early weeks a brace is a wise precaution.

Dislocation of the knee

The knee can only be dislocated by considerable violence, as in a road accident. The cruciate ligaments and one or both lateral ligaments are torn.

Special features

There is severe bruising, swelling and gross deformity. The circulation in the foot must be examined because the popliteal artery may be torn or obstructed. Distal sensation and movement should be tested to exclude lateral popliteal nerve injury.

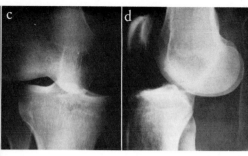

27.24 Dislocations of the knee   (a, b) Postero-lateral dislocation; (c, d) anteromedial dislocation.

(e, f) Traumatic dislocation of the patella.

In addition to the dislocation, the films occasionally show a fracture of the tibial spine (cruciate ligament avulsion) or of the tip of the fibula (lateral ligament avulsion). If there is any doubt about the circulation, an arteriogram should be obtained.

Treatment

● REDUCE

Reduction under general anaesthesia is urgent; this is usually achieved by pulling directly in the line of the leg, but hyperextension must be avoided because of the danger to the popliteal vessels. If reduction is achieved, the limb is rested on

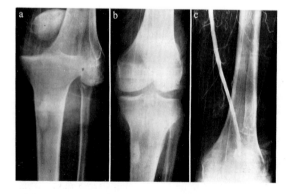

27.25 Knee dislocation and vascular trauma   (a) This patient was admitted with a dislocated knee. After reduction the x-ray (b) looked satisfactory, but the arteriogram (c) showed vascular cut-off at the level of the patella.

a back splint with the knee in 15 degrees of flexion and the circulation is checked repeatedly during the next week. Because of swelling, a plaster cylinder is dangerous.

Occasionally closed reduction fails because the torn medial ligament lies between the femur and the tibial condyles; open reduction must then be performed, the ligament is sutured back into place and the capsule is repaired. Similarly, if there is an open wound, or vascular damage which needs operation, then the opportunity is taken to repair the ligaments and capsule. Otherwise, these structures are left undisturbed.

● HOLD

When swelling has subsided, a plaster is applied and is worn for 12 weeks.

● EXERCISE

Quadriceps muscle exercises are practised from the start. Weight-bearing in the plaster is permitted as soon as the patient can lift his leg. Knee movements are regained when the plaster is removed.

Complications

EARLY

Arterial damage   Popliteal artery damage is common, and early repair is important.

Nerve injury   Nerve injury, especially to the lateral popliteal nerve, may occur but usually recovers.

LATE

Joint instability   Joint instability (increased anteroposterior glide or lateral wobble) usually remains but, provided the quadriceps muscle is sufficiently powerful, the disability is usually not severe.

Dislocation of the patella

While the knee is flexed and the quadriceps muscle relaxed, the patella may be forced laterally by direct violence. It may perch temporarily on the ridge of the lateral femoral condyle and then either slip back into position or be displaced to the outer side, where it lies with its anterior surface facing laterally.

Special features

The knee usually collapses and the patient may fall to the ground. There is obvious (if somewhat misleading) deformity: the displaced patella is not easily noticed but the uncovered medial femoral condyle is unduly prominent and may be mistaken for the displaced patella. The patella can be felt on the outer side of the knee. Neither active nor passive movement is possible.

X-RAY
The patella is seen to be laterally displaced and rotated. In 5 per cent of cases there is an associated osteochondral fracture.

Treatment

- REDUCE   The patella is easily pushed back into place, and anaesthesia is not always necessary. If there is much bruising medially the quadriceps expansion is torn, and immediate operative repair may prevent later recurrent dislocation.

- HOLD   With the knee straight, a plaster back slab is applied. It is worn for 3 weeks.

- EXERCISE   Quadriceps muscle exercises are begun at once and practised assiduously. As soon as the patient can elevate his leg, walking is allowed. When the back slab has been removed, flexion is easily regained.

Complications

The dislocation may recur, either because the quadriceps muscle has not been redeveloped, or because the torn medial capsule has not healed securely (see page 294).

Fractured tibia and fibula

A twisting force applied to the foot may cause a spiral fracture of both bones. The tibia may puncture the skin.

A direct injury crushes the skin and fractures both bones at the same level. An angulation force also breaks both bones at the same level, usually the mid-shaft, and the tibia often pierces the skin. Motorcycle accidents are the commonest cause.

Special features

The skin may be undamaged or obviously divided; sometimes it is intact but has been crushed, and there is danger that it may slough within a few days. The foot is usually rolled outwards and deformity is obvious. The pulses are palpated to assess the circulation, and the toes felt for sensation. Movement at the fracture should not be attempted, but the patient is asked to move his toes.

X-RAY
A spiral fracture is usually in the lower third of the tibial shaft; the fibular fracture also is spiral and usually at a higher level; often there is lateral shift, overlap and outward twist below the fracture.

With a transverse fracture both bones are broken at the same level and there may be shift, tilt or twist in any direction; sometimes there is a separate triangular 'butterfly' fragment.

Closed treatment

With closed fractures the treatment of choice is closed reduction and plaster; if satisfactory reduction is unobtainable, then open reduction followed by internal fixation becomes a reasonable option. With open fractures, internal fixation is best avoided.

A preliminary period of 14 days' traction is useful and, if internal fixation is contemplated, highly desirable. The advantages are: (1) reduction may become sufficiently good to dispense with the need for operation; (2) latent skin damage may become manifest, revealing the hazard of operation; (3) exercises while on traction abolish oedema, restore joint movement and minimize subsequent stiffness; and (4) union occurs more

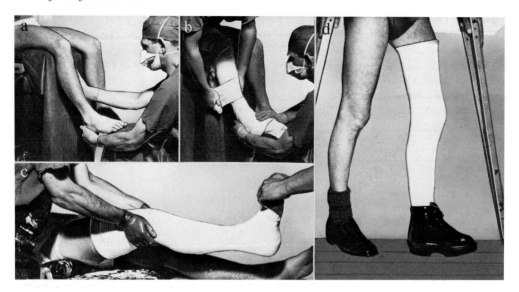

27.26 Fractured tibia and fibula – closed treatment   Reduction is facilitated by bending the knee over the end of the table, with the normal leg alongside for comparison (a). The surgeon holds the position while an assistant applies plaster from the knee downwards (b). When the plaster has set the leg is lifted and the above-knee plaster completed (c); note that the foot is plantigrade, the knee slightly bent, and the plaster moulded round the patella. A rockered boot is fitted for walking (d).

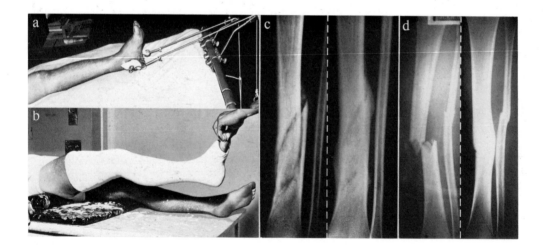

27.27 Fractured tibia and fibula – closed treatment (continued)   Skeletal traction is useful to reduce overlap, and also as provisional treatment when skin viability is doubtful (a). Plaster is applied 10–14 days later (b) using the technique shown in the previous illustration, except that the skeletal pin is retained until the plaster has set. (c, d) Examples of spiral and transverse fractures treated in this way.

rapidly (Smith, 1974). The technique (termed 'provisional treatment' by Perkins) is to apply a 5-kg pull via a Steinmann pin through the calcaneum; the leg is cradled on a pillow or metal frame and the foot of the bed elevated.

Provisional treatment is of course not essential. Many surgeons apply plaster without delay. The technique for such fresh fractures is described below. It is slightly more difficult than that following provisional traction, but the principles and after-care are similar in both cases.

● REDUCE
Reduction is effected by traction and manipulation, preferably with a skeletal pin through the calcaneum or the lower tibia. The bone ends are first accurately apposed, then the alignment corrected; care must be taken to avoid torsional deformity. Skeletal traction is not essential; manual traction on the foot may be effective in achieving reduction, especially if the knee is bent over the end of the table.

● HOLD
The surgeon maintains traction while an assistant applies plaster extending from the upper thigh to the toes with the knee slightly flexed and the foot plantigrade. With fresh fractures the front of the plaster is split.

X-ray films are taken and, if necessary, the plaster is wedged. The pin is removed and the patient returned to bed with the leg elevated. When swelling has subsided the plaster is completed.

Spiral fractures take at least 12 weeks to consolidate, transverse or comminuted fractures a few weeks longer, and open fractures may take 24 weeks. Weight-bearing should be graduated, the amount being guided by comfort, not the calendar. The full above-knee plaster is retained until the fracture is clinically and radiologically consolidated, unless functional bracing techniques are used.

NOTE A severely comminuted fracture is best held by external fixation.

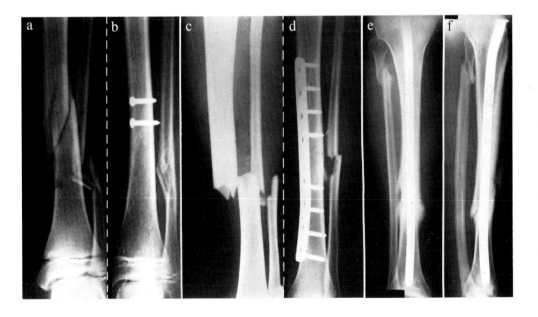

27.28 Fractured tibia and fibula – open treatment   (a, b) Spiral fracture stablized with two screws, facilitating early weight-bearing in plaster. (c, d) Transverse fracture fixed with a plate and screws; movement at the ankle was regained before applying plaster and allowing the patient up. (e, f) A curved intramedullary nail, introduced from above, is sometimes used and facilitates early movement.

● EXERCISE

Right from the start, the patient is taught to exercise the muscles of the foot, ankle and knee. When he gets up, an overboot with a rockered sole is fitted, and he is taught to walk correctly; even if weight is not being taken, he must go through the proper motions of walking. When the plaster is removed, a crêpe bandage is applied and the patient is told that he may either elevate and exercise the limb or walk correctly on it, but he must not let it dangle idly.

FUNCTIONAL BRACING

The full-length above-knee plaster is worn for only a few days, then changed to a functional plaster cast which liberates the knee and takes some pressure on the patellar tendon; weight-bearing in this is permitted after 48 hours. At 3–4 weeks the ankle also is liberated; a splint of plaster or Orthoplast holds the leg and is fixed to a special footpiece by links of malleable polypropylene. The surgeon using this method must master an exacting technique and be prepared to accept some shortening.

Operative treatment

Apart from wound toilet for an open fracture, operative treatment is never essential. However, given ideal surgical facilities, internal fixation has advantages. It is useful when union is likely to be delayed – i.e. when the fracture is unstable or comminuted, when there is a double tibial fracture, and in the elderly.

After provisional treatment by traction for 14 days the tibia is exposed, the fracture ends are meticulously cleaned and then accurately fitted together. Screws alone may suffice for a spiral fracture; but for most cases it is better to use a long and strong plate (preferably a dynamic compression plate) fixed to the bone by screws which penetrate the opposite cortex. An alternative is an intramedullary nail inserted from above, under x-ray control.

'Delayed splintage' is now used. Unless fixation was insecure, the leg is left free in the early postoperative period. Several times daily the physiotherapist encourages knee, ankle and foot movements. When the wound has healed, an above-knee plaster is applied and worn until the fracture has consolidated. Partial weight-bearing is encouraged. Movements, having once been regained, should return rapidly when the plaster is removed. With mid-shaft fractures, if the fixation is good enough to prevent rotation and overlap, a plaster gaiter may be used instead of the full plaster; this prevents angulation and the patient walks normally.

Complications

EARLY

Skin damage   Skin damage is common; even a perforation 'from within' is a compound injury

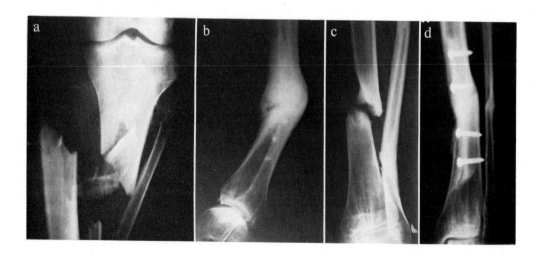

27.29 Fractured tibia and fibula – complications   (a) With this type of fracture skin damage is inevitable and arterial damage not unlikely. (b) Malunion: if the fracture is even slightly angulated in plaster, deformity is liable to increase when weight-bearing begins. (c) Non-union, and (d) a similar case treated with a sliding bone graft.

and should be treated by extending the laceration to permit wound toilet. The wound is left open until it is certain that there is no infection or tissue death; it is then closed by suturing without tension or by skin grafting.

Arterial damage   When skin loss is combined with arterial damage, external fixation is useful (page 346). Volkmann's ischaemia also occurs (especially with proximal tibial fractures) but, because

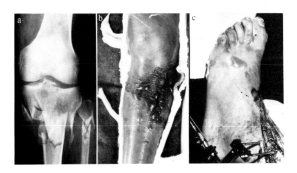

27.30 Fractured tibia and fibula – complications (continued) (a) Although not as severely displaced as the first x-ray in the previous illustration, a fracture at this level is always dangerous. This man was treated in plaster. Pain became intense and when the plaster was split (which should have been done immediately after its application), the leg was swollen and blistered (b). A tibial compartment decompression was performed – but too late; 2 days later (c) the foot became gangrenous.

it is less common in the leg than in the forearm, it is less likely to be diagnosed; minor degrees of ischaemia probably account for the clawing of the toes which sometimes develops.

LATE

Malunion   Slight shortening is usually of little consequence, but rotation and angulation deformity, apart from being ugly, are disabling, because the knee and ankle no longer move in the same plane. Severe deformity can be corrected by osteotomy. Backward angulation (caused by allowing the fracture to sag while plaster is being applied) is common and, if accompanied by a stiff equinus ankle, is dangerous, for when the patient tries to force the foot up in walking the tibia is liable to refracture. This may occur insidiously and lead to non-union.

Delayed union   Union is slow when the fracture is open (especially with infection), if the initial displacement was considerable, if the tibia is fractured in two places, or if the fracture is comminuted. Union may be hastened by weight-bearing (especially with functional bracing) but if delay seems unduly prolonged, bone grafting and internal fixation are indicated.

If the fibular fracture has joined and is splinting the tibia apart, then 2.5 cm of fibula may be excised and a sliding bone graft screwed across the tibial fracture.

Non-union   Non-union may follow bone loss or deep infection; but a common cause is faulty treatment. Either delayed union has not been recognized and splintage discontinued too soon, or the patient with a recently united fracture has walked with a stiff equinus ankle.

Once non-union is established the patient must either wear a permanent splint or the fracture must be operated upon. Compression plating, with its great rigidity, may be adequate, but often grafting is preferred. The bone ends are freshened, fixed with a cortical bone graft and packed with cancellous bone chips; 2.5 cm of fibula is excised and the fracture is then treated in plaster.

Joint stiffness   Joint stiffness is often due to neglect in treatment of the soft tissues; but with the prolonged splintage necessary, and especially in the presence of sepsis, some stiffness may be unavoidable. Limitation of movement at the ankle and foot may persist for 6–12 months after removal of the plaster, in spite of active exercises.

Fracture of one bone only

Fibula

Most spiral fibular fractures are associated with injuries of the ankle or knee; especially with a high fracture the ankle also should be examined and x-rayed.

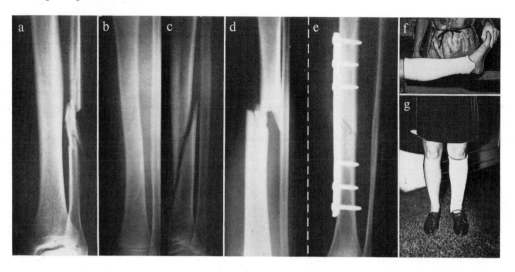

27.31 Fracture of one bone only   (a) Fracture of the fibula alone. (b, c) In this child's leg the spiral fracture of the tibia shows only in one view. (d) Transverse fracture of the tibia alone in the adult: it has been plated (e) and is now so stable that a plaster gaiter (f, g) is the only protection needed.

An isolated fracture of the fibula (usually transverse) may be due to stress or to a direct blow. There is local tenderness, but the patient is able to stand and to move the knee and ankle. Analgesics will control pain, and no other treatment is necessary.

Tibia

In children a twisting injury may cause a spiral fracture of the tibia without fracture of the fibula; this is rare in adults. At any age a direct injury, such as a kick, may cause a transverse or slightly oblique fracture of the tibia alone at the site of impact.

Local bruising and swelling are usually evident, but knee and ankle movements are possible. The child with a spiral fracture may be able to stand on the leg, and, as the fracture may be almost invisible in an anteroposterior film, unless two views are taken the injury can be missed; a few days later an angry mother brings the child with a lump which proves to be callus. Transverse and slightly oblique fractures are easily seen on x-ray but displacement is slight.

Treatment

With displacement, reduction should be attempted. An above-knee plaster is applied as with a fracture of both bones; first a split plaster and then, when swelling has subsided, a complete one. A fracture of the tibia alone takes just as long to unite as if the fibula also were broken; so at least 12 weeks is needed for consolidation and sometimes 24. The child with a spiral fracture, however, can be safely released after 6 weeks; and with a mid-shaft transverse fracture the surgeon may (if he is a skilled plasterer and reduction is perfect) replace the above-knee plaster by a short plaster gaiter.

Complications

An open fracture will, of course, need wound excision; with infection, union will be slow. When closed, isolated tibial fractures, especially in the lower third, may be slow to join, and the temptation is to discard splintage too soon. Even slight displacement may delay union so that open reduction with internal fixation is often preferred. In managing delay, union can usually be hastened by excising 2.5 cm of the fibula, which allows the tibial fragments to impact.

III *Injuries of the ankle and foot*

Ankle ligament injuries

The patient falls or stumbles and the foot inverts under him. As a rule, there is only a partial tear of the lateral ligament and the injury is an ankle sprain. Sometimes, however, the ligament is completely torn and the joint subluxates; the talus momentarily tilts into inversion, then snaps back into position.

Special features

Bruising may be severe (suggesting a complete tear) or may be faint and only appear a day or two after the injury (more likely with a sprain). The ankle is always swollen. Tenderness is usually maximal on the lateral aspect of the joint. Passive inversion is painful, but only with a complete tear of the ligament is the movement excessive. Pain may prevent excessive movement from being demonstrated and, if the injury is severe, inversion must be tested again under local or general anaesthesia.

X-RAY

The x-ray appearance of the resting ankle is normal whether the joint has been sprained or subluxed, for a subluxation reduces itself. X-ray films are taken with both ankles inverted (if necessary, using local or general anaesthesia); these, known as 'stress films', show whether the talus tilts unduly on the affected side ('undue' tilting means 10 degrees more than on the normal side).

Treatment

PARTIAL TEAR

An ankle sprain should be treated by activity. A crêpe bandage is applied and active exercises are begun immediately and persevered with until full

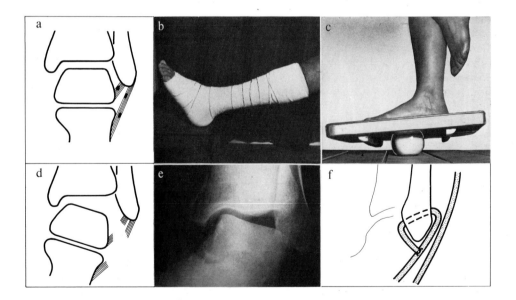

27.32 Ankle sprains   The commonest is a partial tear of the lateral ligament (a). In treatment a crêpe bandage (b) is more efficient than adhesive strapping. The balancing board (c) is a useful method of strengthening the muscles.
A complete tear of the lateral ligament (d) causes recurrent giving way; a strain film reveals talar tilt (e). The operation shown in (f) is simple and effective.

movement is regained. The patient is not allowed to dangle the leg and the bandage is worn until swelling has disappeared. Weight may be taken as soon as the patient will walk, but he must be taught to walk correctly with the normal heel–toe gait. A common cause of prolonged pain is repeated stress due to unstable footwear or weak muscles.

COMPLETE TEAR

Operative repair of acutely ruptured ligaments may be advisable in athletes and dancers. In most patients, however, subluxation can be treated in plaster, which is applied from just below the knee to the toes, with the foot plantigrade. If there is swelling, the plaster is split and replaced when the swelling has subsided. Plaster is worn until the ligament may be expected to have repaired, which takes about 10 weeks. The patient is encouraged to walk normally with the aid of an overboot with a rockered sole. When plaster is removed, a crêpe bandage is worn and movements are regained by active use.

Complications

Adhesions   Following an ankle sprain, adhesions are liable to form unless the foot is actively and correctly used. The patient complains that the ankle 'gives way' and lets him down. Following such an incident, there is tenderness on the outer side and pain on inversion, but no excessive inversion. If active exercises fail to restore full painless movement, the joint should be manipulated under anaesthesia and full range maintained by activity.

Recurrent subluxation   If a complete tear of the lateral ligament was undiagnosed, and consequently unsplinted, the ligament fails to repair and subluxation becomes recurrent. The history is similar to that of adhesions following a sprain; the patient, after an injury, complains that the ankle gives way at intervals. The talus, however, can be inverted further than that of the normal ankle. If the diagnosis is in doubt, the patient should be anaesthetized and both ankles x-rayed in full inversion. If the talus tilts, the injury is a subluxation; if not, the adhesions should be broken down forthwith by manipulation.

Treatment of recurrent subluxation   Raising the outer side of the heel and extending its lower surface laterally ('floated-out heel') may relieve symptoms; but operation is more reliable.

A simple and effective procedure is to detach the peroneus brevis tendon from the muscle, thread it through a hole drilled in the fibula and then sew it back to itself, to the peroneus longus and to the ligamentous structures at the tip of the fibula. Plaster must afterwards be worn for 8 weeks.

Recurrent dislocation of peroneal tendons

The condition is unmistakable, for the patient can demonstrate that the peroneal tendons dislocate forwards over the fibula during dorsiflexion and eversion. Treatment is operative: the superficial cortex of the lower 5 cm of the fibula is hinged backwards and stitched over the peroneal tendons to hold them in their correct position.

Fractures around the ankle

Usually the foot is anchored to the ground while the momentum of the body continues forwards; the patient may stumble over an unexpected obstacle or stair, or into a small depression in the ground, or he may have fallen from a height. The momentum of the body may impose any one of a variety of forces upon the ankle, the most important being external rotation, abduction and adduction. To these an upward thrust is added if the patient has fallen from a height.

Special features

The ankle is swollen, and deformity may be obvious. The site of tenderness is important; if both sides are tender, an injury (bony or ligamentous) must be suspected on both sides.

X-RAY

From a study of the fracture pattern, the type of injury can be deduced, and treatment depends upon its correct identification.

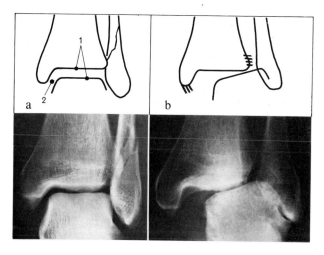

27.33 Ankle fractures – the talus   The position of the talus is all-important. (a) Fracture without subluxation: 1, the surfaces of the tibia and talus are precisely parallel; 2, the distance of the talus from the medial malleolus is normal.
(b) Subluxation – the talus is tilted and unduly separated from the medial malleolus; there is also diastasis (displacement was permitted by a high fracture of the fibula – the Maisonneuve injury).

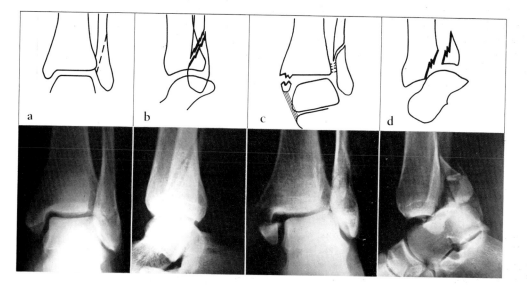

27.34 Ankle fractures – external rotation   (a, b) With an undisplaced external rotation fracture the talus fits the mortise accurately; the fibular fracture may show only in the lateral film. (c) If the fibular fracture is above the tibiofibular ligament there must be a diastasis; here the talus is tilted laterally and the medial malleolus is avulsed; (d) if the posterior margin of the tibia is fractured the talus may be displaced upwards.

Talus   The most important single feature is how accurately the talus fits the mortise. If the mortise is widened or the talus shifted or tilted, subluxation* is present. Usually there is an accompanying mortise fracture and the injury is called a fracture-subluxation. Injuries are classified according to the direction of the damaging force and its consequences.

The mortise   An external rotation force causes a spiral fracture of the fibula. With continuing force, the medial malleolus may be avulsed and fractured transversely. Further rotation may lead to avulsion of a posterior fragment of the tibia, to which the tibiofibular ligament is attached.

*The term 'dislocation' is often used, but 'subluxation' is more accurate.

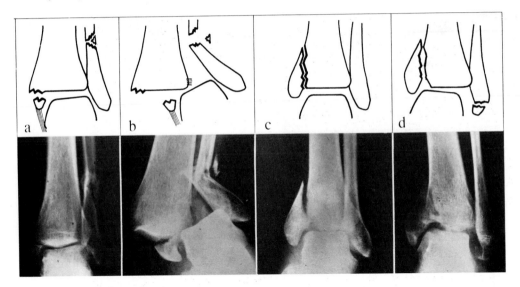

27.35 Ankle fractures – abduction and adduction   (a) Abduction fracture with moderate displacement, (b) with severe displacement and diastasis – note that the fibular fracture is well above the joint. (c) Adduction fracture with slight displacement, (d) with moderate displacement – note that the tibial fracture line is almost vertical.

An abduction force fractures the fibula transversely 5 cm above the joint and may avulse the medial malleolus.

Diastasis may occur in either of the above. The tibiofibular ligament tears, with or without avulsion of its tibial attachment; the ligament tear allows the tibia and fibula to separate and the talus to be driven up between them.

An adduction force causes a near-vertical fracture of the medial malleolus extending upwards from the medial angle of the mortise; the tip of the fibula may also be avulsed.

An upward thrust may split the tibia vertically and this vertical fracture often joins a transverse fracture 5–6 cm above the joint. Sometimes a vertical force shears off the anterior or posterior corner of the lower tibia.

In adolescents, similar injuries occur and may cause fracture-separation of the lower tibial epiphysis.

The fibula   If the fibular fracture is above the tibiofibular joint there must be a diastasis as well. An apparently isolated transverse (avulsion) fracture of the medial malleolus, or a tear of the medial ligament, strongly suggests an associated high fibular fracture (the 'Maisonneuve fracture').

Treatment

Union in perfect position is mandatory at the ankle. Unless closed reduction is perfect and the fracture will unquestionably remain undisplaced (both uncommon), open methods are needed.

Closed methods

Fractures with no trace of displacement clearly require no reduction and are sometimes treated without plaster, the patient being allowed to walk with the ankle in a crêpe bandage. The method is safe only when it is certain that there has not been spontaneous reduction of a displacement. Fractures with displacement are treated as follows.

● REDUCE
First manual traction is applied; then a force is added, the reverse of that which caused the injury. Unless the causal force has been correctly deduced and reversed by manipulation, accurate replacement of the talus is unlikely.

● HOLD
A padded plaster is applied from just below the knee to the toes, with the foot plantigrade; that is, with the foot at an angle of 90 degrees to the leg and neither in varus nor valgus. (The tendency to apply the plaster with the foot inverted must be resisted.) The plaster may need to be split and, if so, it must be completed or replaced when swelling has subsided. An x-ray to confirm reduction must be taken after the plaster has been applied

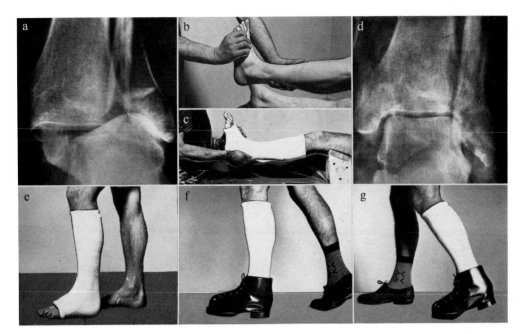

27.36 Ankle fractures – closed treatment An external rotation fracture (a) is reduced by traction followed by internal rotation (b); a below-knee plaster is applied, moulded and held till it has set (c). The check x-ray is usually satisfactory (d). The plaster must be plantigrade (e); a rockered boot permits an almost normal gait (f, g).

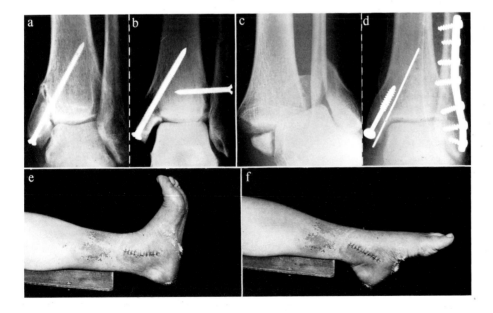

27.37 Ankle fractures – open treatment (a) A large medial fragment needs a malleolar screw; (b) if diastasis is present, a tibiofibular screw may be added; (c, d) if the fibula is displaced its length must be restored and held by internal fixation; (e and f) show this patient exercising his ankle a few days after operation, and before the walking plaster was applied.

and another after it has been changed. With an external rotation injury in which the fibular fracture is below the tibiofibular joint, 6 weeks in plaster is sufficient; all other fractures should be kept in plaster for 12 weeks.

● EXERCISE

An overboot is fitted and the patient is taught to walk correctly as soon as possible. Ankle and foot movements are regained by active exercises when the plaster is removed. As with any lower-limb fracture, the leg must not be allowed to dangle idly. It must be exercised or elevated. After removal of the plaster a temporary crêpe bandage is necessary.

Operative treatment

Operative treatment may be advisable (1) to ensure perfect reduction; (2) to maintain reduction; or (3) to facilitate early movement. The fibula must be restored to full length and this is best achieved with a plate and screws; a large medial malleolar fragment must be fixed in anatomical position with either a screw or semi-rigid pins and tension-band wiring; diastasis requires transverse tibiofibular fixation. Operation is best performed within a few hours of the injury (before swelling is severe) or else after 2 weeks (when severe swelling has subsided). After operation, movements should be regained and then a below-knee plaster worn until the fracture has consolidated.

Complications

Malunion Incomplete reduction is common and, unless the talus fits the mortise accurately, degenerative changes may occur. Sometimes degeneration can be halted or prevented by a corrective osteotomy. If osteoarthritis becomes severe, arthrodesis may prove necessary.

Secondary malunion from epiphyseal arrest in an adolescent is rare.

Non-union Non-union of the medial malleolus occasionally occurs if a flap of periosteum is interposed between it and the tibia. It should be prevented by operative reduction and screw fixation.

Joint stiffness Joint stiffness and swelling of the ankle are usually the result of neglect in treatment of the soft tissues. The patient must walk correctly

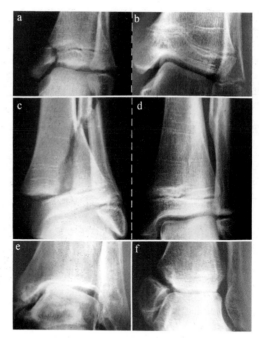

27.38 Ankle fractures – complications (a) Fracture through the epiphysis has disturbed growth, and (b) 3 years later the ankle is no longer horizontal. This contrasts with the two x-rays below in which fracture-separation of the entire tibial epiphysis (c) has, after reduction, grown normally (d). (e) Malunion following failure of reduction in the adult. (f) Non-union of the medial malleolus.

in plaster and, when the plaster is removed, he must, until circulatory control is regained, wear a crêpe bandage and elevate the leg whenever he is not using it actively. Occasionally, several months after the fracture, manipulation under anaesthesia may be needed to restore full movement.

Injuries of the talus

Talar injuries are rare and due to considerable violence, usually a car accident or falling from a height. The injuries include fractures (of the head, neck, body or lateral process of the talus), dislocations (midtarsal, subtalar or total dislocation of the talus) and fracture-dislocations (talar fractures combined with dislocation). Midtarsal injuries are often missed; they have been classified according to the deforming force: longitudinal

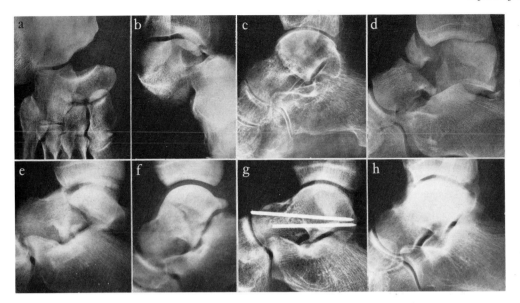

27.39 Talar fractures and dislocations   (a, b) Two views of subtalar dislocation. (c) Talar fracture without displacement, and (d) with considerable displacement. (e, f) Talar fracture before and after reduction by forced plantarflexion. (g) Another method of treatment, by open reduction and internal fixation. (h) Avascular necrosis of the posterior half of the talus following fracture.

compression, plantar and crush varieties are described, as well as medial or lateral displacements, sometimes of a 'swivel' type (Main and Jowett, 1975).

Special features

The foot is obviously deformed and swollen. The skin may have been split or may rapidly necrose. The dorsalis pedis artery should be palpated.

X-RAY

Anteroposterior, lateral and oblique views are needed. The talus is first identified (not always easy); then inspected to see if it is fractured (and if so how the fragments are displaced); next its relationship to the tibia, calcaneum and other tarsal bones is studied (to identify dislocation); finally the midtarsal joint is carefully inspected – the bones must fit precisely and comparison with the normal foot is useful.

Treatment

UNDISPLACED FRACTURES

When displacement is no more than trivial, reduction is not needed. A split plaster is applied and, when the swelling has subsided, is replaced by a complete plaster in the plantigrade position. With fractures of the head, weight-bearing is allowed; with body or neck fractures it is avoided. At 6–8 weeks the plaster is removed and function regained by normal use.

DISPLACED FRACTURES AND FRACTURE-DISLOCATIONS

Reduction is urgent (because the stretched skin soon necroses), but may be difficult. Closed manipulation is tried first, and forced plantarflexion is often the key manoeuvre. If this proves ineffective, a Steinmann pin through the calcaneum can be used to exert powerful traction while a second Steinmann pin transfixes the displaced bone and is used to reduce it. Should this also fail there must be no hesitation in performing open reduction; access can be obtained by osteotomizing the medial malleolus.

It is often expedient to stabilize a reduced fracture with one or two pieces of Kirschner wire, but plaster also is needed. Most of these injuries are stable only with the foot plantarflexed; this unpleasant position is maintained in a split plaster for 2–3 weeks. Then, without anaesthesia, the plaster is removed, and the patient is persuaded to dorsiflex his foot gently; a complete below-knee plaster is then applied with the foot plantigrade and this is worn for a further 6 weeks. When the plaster is removed, the patient is encouraged to exercise the leg and foot, but he should avoid weight-bearing until x-rays show that the talus has not undergone avascular necrosis.

NOTE   An innocuous-seeming flake beneath the lateral malleolus may, on a 20-degree oblique view, prove to be a substantial fragment – the lateral process of the talus. It must be recognized and either fixed back or removed; otherwise considerable loss of function is inevitable.

Complications

Skin damage   Skin damage is common either because the skin has been split or because it is tightly stretched and necroses. Even when a totally detached talus is lying in the wound the bone should not be excised but replaced.

Avascular necrosis   Avascular necrosis of part (usually the posterior half) or all of the talus may occur. The bone becomes dense on x-ray, but it should be remembered that in the lateral view the overlying malleoli normally cause a dense appearance. An avascular talus crushes with weight-bearing; degenerative changes are then inevitable and the ankle may need to be arthrodesed.

Fractures of the calcaneum

The patient usually falls from a height, often from a ladder, onto one or both heels. The calcaneum is driven up against the talus and is split or crushed. The same accident may also have damaged the spine, pelvis or hip, which must always be examined in calcaneal injuries.*

Special features

The heel is broad and a D-shaped bruise appears in the sole. The tissues are thick and tender, and the normal concavity below the lateral malleolus is lacking. The subtalar joint cannot be moved but ankle movement is possible.

X-RAY

Unless every patient with a painful heel after a fall is x-rayed, fractures of the calcaneum will be missed. Lateral and axial films are required. (An axial film is one taken with the x-rays passing obliquely through the sagittal plane of the bone.)

Calcaneal fractures can be classified as chip, split, or crush fractures.

Chip fractures   These comprise (1) vertical fracture of the medial tuberosity; (2) horizontal fracture of the postero-superior corner, sometimes with upward tilt; and (3) fracture of the anterosuperior corner obliquely into the calcaneocuboid joint. All these are rare.

Split fractures   The calcaneum is split into two segments by a vertical fracture which extends from the medial aspect near the back of the bone to the lateral aspect in front. The larger lateral segment is usually shifted laterally and the smaller medial segment displaced upwards. The fracture usually extends into the subtalar joint but the joint may not be severely damaged.

Crush fractures   The fracture line or lines resemble those of split fractures but the portion of the calcaneum which articulates with the talus is driven downwards into the body of the bone. In the lateral x-ray the normal angle between the anterior and posterior parts of the bone (Böhler's angle) is flattened. The subtalar joint is damaged.

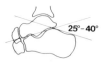

27.40   Calcaneal fractures (1) Böhler's angle (the tuber–joint angle) is normally between 25 and 40 degrees. With crush fractures it is markedly reduced.

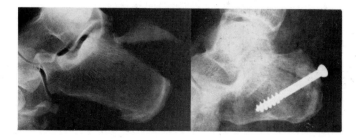

27.41 Calcaneal fractures (2)   Chip fracture of posterosuperior corner fixed by screw.

*'Broken heels – broken back?'

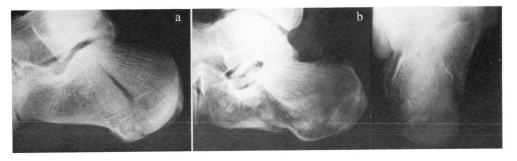

27.42 Calcaneal fractures (3)   (a) Split fracture with little displacement and no joint involvement; (b) lateral and axial views of severe split fracture with considerable joint involvement.

Treatment of chip fractures

If there is no displacement, neither reduction nor splintage is necessary. An elastic bandage is applied and the patient encouraged to walk.

If there is displacement, it is reduced by manipulation under anaesthesia. A below-knee plaster is applied with the foot plantigrade (except when a horizontal fracture can be held reduced only with the foot plantarflexed). An overboot is fitted and the patient is taught to walk. After 6 weeks the plaster is removed, a crêpe bandage is applied and full active use encouraged. If a large fragment of the back of the bone has been avulsed by the tendo Achillis, it should be screwed or wired back into position.

Treatment of split and crush fractures

Three methods are available: (1) closed reduction and plaster; (2) open reduction and bone grafting; (3) functional treatment.

CLOSED REDUCTION AND PLASTER   Lateral spreading of the calcaneum is reduced (if possible) by compressing the bone between the thenar eminences. Upward displacement of the back of the heel is difficult to correct by manipulation; a spike thrust into the bone from behind and used as a lever may help and can be incorporated in the plaster. Following reduction a split plaster is applied and replaced by a complete one when swelling has subsided. It is removed at 6 weeks and exercises are begun, but weight-bearing is not resumed for a further 6 weeks.

OPEN REDUCTION AND GRAFTING   This is often indicated if the thalamic portion of the bone has been crushed. The fracture is exposed from the lateral side and, from within the bone, all articular surfaces are carefully repositioned and the bone restored to as near its original shape as possible. The position can be held by transfixing Kirschner wires, but it is probably better to build up the interior of the bone with cancellous grafts or a bone block. Plaster is used for 6–12 weeks.

FUNCTIONAL TREATMENT   Under general anaesthesia closed reduction can be attempted, as already described. More often this stage is omitted, but in either case the patient is put to bed

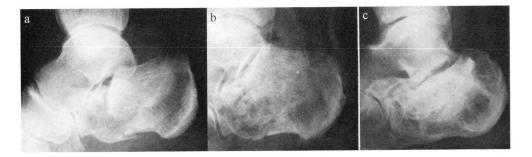

27.43 Calcaneal fractures (4)   (a) Severe crush fracture treated by (b) open reduction and bone grafting (by courtesy of Mr G. R. Fisk who performed the operation); the subtalar joint has been accurately restored and function was good. (c) Another severe crush which was treated by early activity and also regained reasonably good function.

with the leg elevated, and swelling kept to a minimum with elastic bandaging or with a pneumatic compressing stocking. A physiotherapist coaxes the patient to exercise the ankle and foot joints regularly, repeatedly and assiduously. Within 3 or 4 days he is encouraged to put his foot to the ground and take a little weight. He begins walking, using crutches at first, but graduating to full weight-bearing as comfort permits. What he must not do is walk with a stiff foot, or allow the foot to swell; exercise is punctuated by elevation.

CHOICE OF METHOD

This depends on the prognosis and complications. The prognosis is not good; few patients can walk or work comfortably in less than 3 months, many take much longer and some have to change jobs permanently. Stiffness, especially of the subtalar joint, is the bugbear; worse still, the restricted movement may be painful. Consequently the choice of method depends on the prospects of regaining a useful range of comfortable movement.

Closed reduction is never perfect, so plaster merely perpetuates malposition and encourages stiffness. Open reduction can be accurate, it is radiologically rewarding, and it ensures a heel which fits a normal shoe; but to maintain reduction plaster is needed, and full movement is rarely regained. Functional treatment, by insisting on early and repeated activity, moulds the fragments in such a way that a modestly useful range of movement is usually regained; for most patients and most surgeons it is probably the method of choice.

Persistent pain following split or crush fractures may occur, often just below the lateral malleolus. If local anaesthetic injection or manipulation fails to provide relief, a small piece of the medial side of the lower fibula may be excised. Pain when walking on rough ground is usually due to restriction of subtalar movement and may justify arthrodesis. Immediate arthrodesis of all severe calcaneal fractures (or even total excision of the calcaneum!) has been advocated; such pessimism seems unwarranted.

Other tarsal injuries

A crushing force may fracture the scaphoid or cuboid bone or both, and may also cause mid-tarsal dislocation.

Dislocation or displacement is reduced under anaesthesia, and the foot held in plaster for 6 weeks. The patient walks with an overboot. In the absence of displacement, neither reduction nor plaster is required.

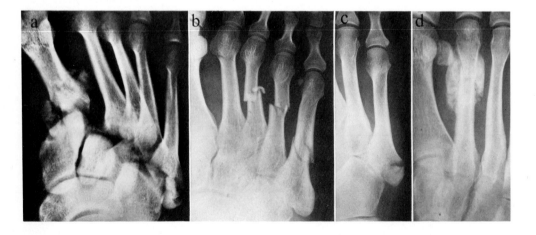

27.44 Metatarsal injuries   (a) Tarsometatarsal dislocation is a serious injury which may endanger the circulation of the foot. (b) Transverse fractures of several metatarsal shafts. (c) Avulsion fracture of the base of the fifth metatarsal. (d) Florid callus in a stress fracture.

Injuries of the metatarsal bones

Rotation injury

If the forefoot is violently twisted, abducted or plantarflexed, tarsometatarsal dislocation may occur. The first metatarsal is either dislocated or fractured near its base; the other metatarsal bones are fractured more distally. The injury is serious and may endanger the circulation of the foot.

Reduction is urgent and is maintained by a padded split plaster. The leg is kept elevated until it is certain that the circulation is satisfactory. After 3 weeks plaster is discarded, active exercises are started, and weight-bearing is resumed at 6 weeks.

Crush injury

Any or all of the metatarsal bones may be fractured by crush injuries. Usually the metatarsal necks fracture and often the overlying skin is damaged. The orthodox treatment is to reduce the fractures by manipulation and to hold them in plaster for a few weeks.

The functional method is as follows. Unless displacement is gross, which is rare, it may be ignored. The leg is elevated and active movements are started immediately. As soon as swelling has subsided, and the patient is comfortable, he is encouraged to walk normally. Malunion rarely results in disability when mobility has been regained.

Traction injury

Forced inversion of the foot may cause avulsion of the base of the fifth metatarsal. Pain may be severe but displacement is slight and the fracture should be disregarded. If early activity is encouraged, and the patient walks as normally as possible in an ordinary shoe, full painless function is rapidly regained.

Stress injury (march fracture)

In a young adult (often a recruit or a nurse) the foot may become painful after overuse. A tender lump is palpable just distal to the mid-shaft of a metatarsal bone. Usually the second metatarsal is affected, especially if it is much longer than an 'atavistic' first metatarsal. The x-ray appearance may at first be normal, although a hair-line crack is sometimes visible; later a large mass of callus is seen.

Unaccountable pain in elderly osteoporotic people may be due to the same lesion; x-ray diagnosis is more difficult because callus is minimal and there may be no more than a pencil-thin periosteal reaction along the metatarsal.

No displacement occurs and neither reduction nor splintage is necessary. The forefoot may be supported with Elastoplast and normal walking is encouraged.

Fractured toes

A heavy object falling on the toes may fracture phalanges. If the skin is broken it must be covered with a sterile dressing. The fracture is disregarded and the patient encouraged to walk in a suitably mutilated boot.

Further reading

Apley, A. Graham (1979) Fractures of the tibial plateau. *Orthopedic Clinics of North America* **10**, 61–74

Barnes, R., Brown, J. T., Garden, R. S. and Nicoll, E. A. (1976) Subcapital fractures of the femur. *Journal of Bone and Joint Surgery* **58B**, 2–24

Collado, F., Vila, J. and Beltrán, J. E. (1973) Condylocephalic nail fixation for trochanteric fractures of the femur. *Journal of Bone and Joint Surgery* **55B**, 774–779

Colton, C. L. (1976) Injuries of the ankle. In *Watson-Jones' Fractures and Joint Injuries*, 5th edn. Ed. by J. N. Wilson. Edinburgh: Churchill Livingstone

Connolly, J. F. and King, P.; Connolly, J. F., Dehne, E. and Lafollette, B. (1973) Closed reduction and early cast-brace ambulation in the treatment of femoral fractures. *Journal of Bone and Joint Surgery* **55A**, 1559–1580; 1581–1599

Epstein, H. C. (1974) Posterior fracture-dislocations of the hip. *Journal of Bone and Joint Surgery* **56A,** 1103–1127

Garden, R. S. (1961) Low-angle fixation in fractures of the femoral neck. *Journal of Bone and Joint Surgery* **43B,** 647–663

Garden, R. S. (1971) Malreduction and avascular necrosis in subcapital fractures of the femur. *Journal of Bone and Joint Surgery*, **53B,** 183–197

Helal, B. and Skevis, X. (1967) Unrecognised dislocation of the hip in fractures of the femoral shaft. *Journal of Bone and Joint Surgery* **49B,** 293–300

Hughston, J. C., Andrews, J. R., Cross, M. J. and Moschi, A. (1976) Classification of knee ligament instabilities. *Journal of Bone and Joint Surgery* **58A,** 159–172; 173–179

Kyle, R. F., Grustilo, R. B. and Premer, R. F. (1979) Analysis of 622 intertrochanteric hip fractures. *Journal of Bone and Joint Surgery* **61A,** 216–221

Lam, S. F. (1971) Fractures of the neck of the femur in children. *Journal of Bone and Joint Surgery* **53A,** 1165–1179

Main, B. J. and Jowett, R. L. (1975) Injuries of the midtarsal joint. *Journal of Bone and Joint Surgery* **57B,** 89–97

Muckle, D. S. (Ed.) (1977) *Femoral Neck Fractures and Hip Joint Injuries.* London: Chapman and Hall

Nicholas, J. A. (1973) The five-one reconstruction for anteromedial instability of the knee. *Journal of Bone and Joint Surgery* **55A,** 899–922

Nicoll, E. A. (1964) Fractures of the tibial shaft. *Journal of Bone and Joint Surgery* **46B,** 373–387

O'Donoghue, D. H. (1973) Reconstruction for medial instability of the knee. *Journal of Bone and Joint Surgery* **55A,** 941–955

Rothwell, A. G. and Fitzpatrick, C. B. (1978) Closed Küntscher nailing of femoral shaft fractures. *Journal of Bone and Joint Surgery* **60B,** 504–509

Sarmiento, A. (1967) A functional below-the-knee cast for tibial fractures. *Journal of Bone and Joint Surgery* **49A,** 855–875

Slocum, D. B. and Larson, R. L. (1968) Pes anserinus transplantation. *Journal of Bone and Joint Surgery* **50A,** 226–242

Smith, J. E. M. (1974) Results of early and delayed internal fixation for tibial shaft fractures. *Journal of Bone and Joint Surgery* **56B,** 469–477

Soeur, R. and Remy, R. (1975) Fractures of the calcaneus with displacement of the thalamic portion. *Journal of Bone and Joint Surgery* **57B,** 413–421

Thomas, T. L. and Meggitt, B. F. (1981) A comparative study of methods for treating fractures of the distal half of the femur. *Journal of Bone and Joint Surgery* **63B,** 3–6

Tile, M. (1980) Fractures of the acetabulum. *Orthopedic Clinics of North America* **11,** 481–506

Overuse Injuries

Overuse syndromes

Whereas most injuries are obvious and direct, those due to overuse are elusive and insidious. They are seen mainly in athletes (hence the unfortunate term 'sporting injuries') and in dancers, but may occur in anyone after overactivity without adequate training.*

Pathology

There are three main causes of overuse trauma: *friction*, *stress* and *ischaemia*.

(1) FRICTION A tendon or bursa may, during joint movement, be subjected to excessive friction within a fibrous sheath or over a bony prominence. An inflammatory reaction starts up ('peritendinitis' or bursitis); swelling occurs and gliding movement is further restricted.

(2) STRESS Repeated or unguarded stress may result in tears of muscle or tendon fibres, incomplete fractures of bone, or impact lesions of articular cartilage (usually of the patella). Occasionally a sudden, excessive force causes a complete rupture of tendon or muscle.

(3) ISCHAEMIA This usually occurs in muscles which are firmly enclosed in fascial compartments (e.g. in the forearm or leg). Ischaemia may be relative, arising only when excessive activity makes demands on the blood supply which cannot be met; or absolute, when intramuscular oedema causes swelling in a tight compartment.

Clinical syndromes

TROCHANTERIC 'BURSITIS'
A ballet dancer or runner complains of pain around the greater trochanter of the femur. There is local tenderness and crepitus in the bursa. Sometimes the tender spot is behind the trochanter, and an x-ray may show calcification in this region; the diagnosis in these cases is probably tendinitis of the gluteus medius.

ILIOTIBIAL BAND FRICTION
This usually occurs in long-distance runners who increase their distance too quickly; it is thought to be due to rubbing of the posterior part of the iliotibial band against the lateral femoral condyle. Pain is felt when the knee reaches about 20 degrees of flexion; the patient walks with a stiff-knee gait and tenderness is localized to a point just behind the lateral condyle. Tensing the iliotibial band by pressing it against the femur and then flexing the knee produces sharp pain at the point of irritation.

PATELLAR TENDINITIS ('JUMPER'S KNEE')
The word 'tendinitis' is customary but inaccurate, since it is the patellar ligament which is affected. The condition is common in both dancers and athletes (especially long-jumpers and high-jumpers). Repeated sudden contraction of the quadriceps at take-off may cause tiny ruptures of fibres at or near the attachment of the ligament to the lower pole of the patella; there is an associated vascular reaction. Pain and tenderness are maximal at the site of the lesion.

*Too much, too soon, too fast.

CHONDROMALACIA PATELLAE ('RUNNER'S KNEE')

The symptoms and signs are those of chondromalacia, though, unlike the usual case which involves adolescent girls, the 'overuse' injury occurs in fit, hard-driving runners. It has been attributed to weakness of the vastus medialis, or to postural abnormalities such as pes valgus and internal rotation of the tibia; whether due to the quadriceps weakness or to mild malalignment of the knee, the patella tends to subluxate laterally during active knee extension, damaging the articular cartilage.

PAINFUL TENDO ACHILLIS

Three syndromes are recognized, though it is doubtful whether they are completely distinct entities.

Peritendinitis (or paratendinitis) is an inflammation around the tendon, which gives rise to pain, diffuse swelling over the tendon, crepitus on moving the foot, and tenderness which remains in one spot regardless of the position of the foot.

Achillis tendinitis causes similar features, except that the tenderness is more clearly in the tendon and shifts as the tendon moves with dorsi- and plantarflexion. It is attributed to small ruptures of tendon fibres.

Calcaneal bursitis presents as a painful heel; tenderness is anterior to the tendo Achillis and more directly on the underlying bone.

All three disorders tend to occur in young athletes who increase their activity, or in older individuals (those over 40) who overstress the tendon by using unaccustomed force in sprinting, climbing or uphill running.

Occasionally, after a period of pain and moderate swelling, the tendon may rupture. This is especially likely after injudicious injection of local anaesthetic or corticosteroids into the substance of the tendon.

MUSCLE TEARS

The clinical picture is similar, whether the area involved is the calf, the quadriceps or the hamstrings. During muscular exertion the patient feels a sharp pain, and sometimes a 'snapping' or 'tearing' sensation. Later, bruising appears and the affected area is tender. Complete muscle tears have been reported, but are very rare.

'SHIN SPLINTS'

This is a term used for pain and tenderness along the posteromedial border of the lower half of the tibia; the symptoms characteristically increase with activity and subside with rest. They may be due to tendinitis, but more serious conditions such as a mild posterior compartment syndrome or a stress fracture of the tibia must be excluded.

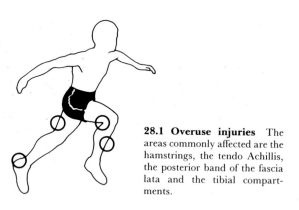

28.1 Overuse injuries The areas commonly affected are the hamstrings, the tendo Achillis, the posterior band of the fascia lata and the tibial compartments.

Treatment

Prevention is better than cure and most overuse injuries can be avoided by adhering to a few simple rules: increases in activity must be graded; training before races must be adequate; changes in activity must be gradual; and warning signals of mild pain at the characteristic sites must be heeded.

Treatment is usually non-specific and consists of reducing activity (rather than complete rest), relieving stress (e.g. on the tendo Achillis, by elevating the heel), and counteracting inflammation (usually by giving anti-inflammatory drugs, occasionally by injecting local anaesthetic and corticosteroids around – but not into – the affected tendon).

Operation may be necessary in resistant cases – to incise the iliotibial band, to release a constricted tendon, or to decompress a tight fascial compartment.

In all cases physiotherapy is important, and is aimed at graded muscle stretching, combined with strengthening exercises.

Index